Diagnostic Testing in Emergency Medicine

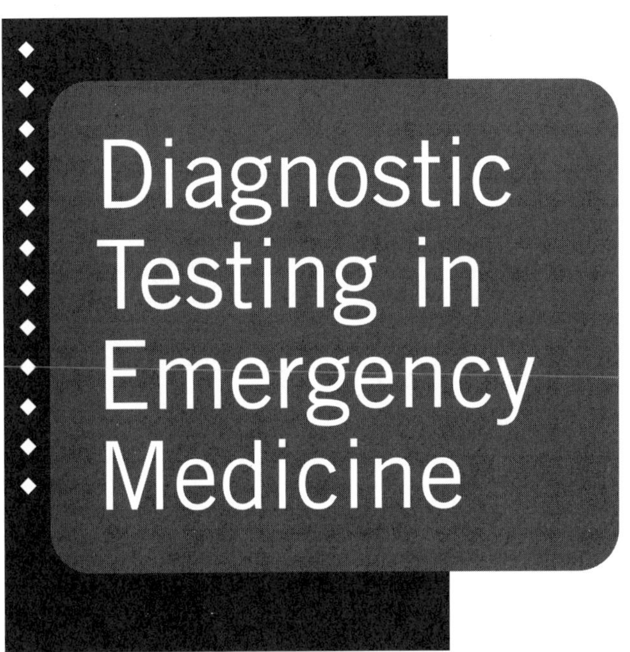

Allan B. Wolfson, M.D., F.A.C.E.P., F.A.C.P.
Associate Professor of Emergency Medicine and Medicine
University of Pittsburgh
Program Director
University of Pittsburgh Affiliated
Residency in Emergency Medicine
Pittsburgh, Pennsylvania

Paul M. Paris, M.D., F.A.C.E.P.
Professor and Chair
Department of Emergency Medicine
University of Pittsburgh
Medical Director
Center for Emergency Medicine
Pittsburgh, Pennsylvania

W.B. SAUNDERS COMPANY
A Division of Harcourt Brace & Company
Philadelphia London Toronto Montreal Sydney Tokyo

W.B. SAUNDERS COMPANY
A Division of Harcourt Brace & Company

The Curtis Center
Independence Square West
Philadelphia, Pennsylvania 19106

Library of Congress Cataloging-in-Publication Data

Diagnostic testing in emergency medicine / [edited by] Allan B. Wolfson, Paul M. Paris. — 1st ed.

p. cm.

ISBN 0–7216–4539–9

1. Emergency medicine—Diagnosis. I. Wolfson, Allan B. II. Paris, Paul M. [DNLM: 1. Emergency Medicine—methods. 2. Diagnostic Tests, Routine. 3. Emergencies. WB 200 D5365 1996]

RC86.7.D54 1996 616.02′5—dc20

DNLM/DLC 95-33470

DIAGNOSTIC TESTING IN
EMERGENCY MEDICINE ISBN 0–7216–4539–9

Printed in the United States of America.

Last digit is the print number: 9 8 7 6 5 4 3 2 1

CONTRIBUTORS

James G. Adams, MD
Instructor of Medicine (Emergency Medicine), Harvard Medical School; Director of Clinical Operations, Department of Emergency Medicine, Brigham and Women's Hospital, Boston, Massachusetts
Prothrombin Time and Partial Thromboplastin Time

Linda G. Allison, MD
Director and Associate Professor, Health Sciences Department, Chatham College, Pittsburgh, Pennsylvania
Spine Radiography for Low Back Pain

William Angelos, MD
Assistant Professor of Emergency Medicine, University of Pittsburgh School of Medicine; Medical Director, Emergency Department, University of Pittsburgh Medical Center, Pittsburgh, Pennsylvania
Urinalysis—Dipstick and Microscopic Examination

Michael Baumann, MD
Instructor of Emergency Medicine, Department of Emergency Medicine, University of Pittsburgh School of Medicine, Pittsburgh, Pennsylvania
The Pregnant Patient

Michael P. Bellino, MD, FACEP
Attending Physician, Director, Coordinator of Information, Emergency Department, Michael Reese Hospital, Chicago, Illinois
Extremity Radiography

John G. Benitez, MD, MPH, FACEP
Assistant Professor, Department of Emergency Medicine, University of Pittsburgh School of Medicine; Medical Director, Pittsburgh Poison Center, Children's Hospital of Pittsburgh, Pittsburgh, Pennsylvania
Spine Radiography for Low Back Pain

Clifton W. Callaway, MD, PhD
Instructor of Emergency Medicine, University of Pittsburgh School of Medicine, Attending Physician, Department of Emergency Medicine, Pittsburgh, Pennsylvania
Serum Electrolyte Determination

Linda Carpenter, MD
Attending Physician, Western Pennsylvania Hospital, Pittsburgh, Pennsylvania
Arterial Blood Gas Analysis

Jeff Coben, MD
Director, Center for Injury Research and Control, Assistant Professor of Emergency Medicine and Assistant Professor of Health Services Administration, University of Pittsburgh Medical School, Pittsburgh, Pennsylvania
Diarrhea

Eric Davis, MD, FACEP
Associate Professor, Department of Emergency Medicine, University of Rochester School of Medicine and Dentistry; Regional Medical Director, Monroe-Livingston Counties, Rochester, New York
Gonorrheal Culture

Theodore R. Delbridge, MD, MPH
Assistant Professor of Emergency Medicine, University of Pittsburgh School of Medicine, Pittsburgh, Pennsylvania
Complete Blood Count

Allan Doctor, MD
Fellow in Critical Care, Harvard Medical School and Children's Hospital, Boston, Massachusetts
Traumatic Aortic Disruption and Aortic Dissection

David Ellis, MD
Assistant Professor, Department of Emergency Medicine, State University of New York at Buffalo; Associate Director, Emergency Department, Erie County Medical Center, Buffalo, New York
Trauma

George L. Ellis, MD, FACEP
Clinical Assistant Professor, State University of New York, Health Science Center at Syracuse, College of Medicine, Syracuse, New York; Chairman, Department of Emergency Medicine, Guthrie Clinic, Robert Packer Hospital, Sayre, Pennsylvania
Superficial Foreign Bodies

John G. Fata, MD
Assistant Professor, Section of Emergency Medicine, Michigan State University College of Human Medicine, East Lansing; Attending Physician, Department of Emergency Medicine, Michigan Capital Medical Center, Lansing, Michigan
Cholescintigraphy

Michael J. Fine, MD, MSc
Associate Professor of Medicine, University of Pittsburgh School of Medicine, Pittsburgh, Pennsylvania
Sputum Gram Stain

Lynda L. Flom, MD
Chief of Pediatric Radiology, The Western Pennsylvania Hospital, Pittsburgh, Pennsylvania
Superficial Foreign Bodies

Phil B. Fontanarosa, MD
Adjunct Associate Professor of Medicine, Division of Emergency Medicine, Northwestern University Medical School, Chicago, Illinois
Chlamydial Culture and Immunoassay and *Cranial Computed Tomography for Nontraumatic Conditions*

Christopher Forsmark, MD
Associate Professor of Medicine, University of Florida College of Medicine, Gainesville, Florida
Liver Function Tests

Jeffrey Garland, MD
Assistant Professor of Medicine, East Carolina University School of Medicine; Staff Physician, Pitt County Memorial Hospital, Greenville, North Carolina
Preoperative and Routine Preadmission Chest Radiography and Electrocardiography

Michael A. Gibbs, MD
Clinical Instructor, Department of Emergency Medicine, University of North Carolina at Chapel Hill School of Medicine, Chapel Hill; Attending Physician, Department of Emergency Medicine, and Medical Director, Air-Medical Services, Carolinas Medical Center, Charlotte, North Carolina
Urologic Trauma

Raquel L. Gibly, MD, FACEP
Clinical Instructor, Department of Emergency Medicine, University of Pittsburgh School of Medicine; Academic Coordinator and Staff Physician, Western Pennsylvania Hospital, Pittsburgh, Pennsylvania
Urinary Tract Infection

Jay M. Goldman, MD
Senior Physician, Department of Emergency Medicine, Kaiser Foundation Hospital, Hayward, California
Cervical Spine Radiography

Michael B. Heller, MD
Clinical Professor of Medicine, Temple University School of Medicine, Philadelphia; Program Director, Emergency Medicine Residence of the Lehigh Valley, Bethlehem, Pennsylvania
Ultrasonography

Alan K. Hodgdon, MD
Clinical Assistant Professor of Emergency Medicine, University of Pittsburgh School of Medicine; Medical Director, Department of Emergency Medicine, Mercy Providence Hospital, Pittsburgh, Pennsylvania
Deep Venous Thrombosis and *Amylase and Lipase*

Kaveh Ilkhanipour, MD, FACEP
Clinical Assistant Professor, Department of Emergency Medicine, University of Pittsburgh School of Medicine; Physician Quality Manager, Department of Emergency Medicine, Mercy Hospital of Pittsburgh, Pittsburgh, Pennsylvania
Serum Magnesium Determination and *Imaging of the Sinuses*

William A. Jenkins, MD
Clinical Instructor of Emergency Medicine, Department of Emergency Medicine, University of Pittsburgh School of Medicine, Pittsburgh; Emergency Medical Services Medical Director and Attending Physician, Westmoreland Regional Hospital, Greensburg, Pennsylvania
Guaiac and Gastroccult

David A. Jerrard, MD, FACEP
Associate Professor, Surgery/Medicine, and Associate Residency Director, Emergency Medicine Residency, University of Maryland School of Medicine, Baltimore, Maryland
Blunt Abdominal Trauma

Dean Johnson, MD
Instructor, Division of Emergency Medical Services, Department of Surgery, University of Maryland School of Medicine; Attending Physician, Emergency Services, Veterans Affairs Medical Center, Baltimore, Maryland
Ascitic Fluid

Scott Jolley, MD
Resident, Affiliated Residency in Emergency Medicine, University of Pittsburgh School of Medicine, Pittsburgh, Pennsylvania
Uric Acid Level

Thomas Russell Jones, MD
Associate Professor, Texas A & M University Health Science Center; Staff Physician, Scott and White Clinic and Hospital, Temple, Texas
Rib Radiographs

Elaine B. Josephson, MD, FACEP
Senior Staff Physician, Department of Emergency Medicine, Henry Ford Medical Center, West Bloomfield, Michigan
Vaginal Wet and KOH Preparations

Raymond B. Karasic, MD
Associate Professor of Pediatrics, University of Pittsburgh School of Medicine; Attending Physician, Emergency Department, Children's Hospital of Pittsburgh, Pittsburgh, Pennsylvania
Fever in Neonates

Laurence Katz, MD
Assistant Professor of Medicine, Director of Emergency Medicine Research, University of Miami School of Medicine, Miami, Florida
Prothrombin Time and Partial Thromboplastin Time and *Type, Screen, and Crossmatch*

Tom Kearns, MD
Attending Physician, Uniontown Hospital, Uniontown, Pennsylvania
Dyspnea

James Kelley, MD
Clinical Instructor, University of Pittsburgh School of Medicine; Attending Physician, Department of Emergency Medicine, Mercy Hospital of Pittsburgh, Pittsburgh, Pennsylvania
Serum Calcium and *Type, Screen, and Crossmatch*

R. Todd Kiskaddon, MD
Assistant Professor, Department of Surgery, Section of Emergency Medicine, Yale University School of Medicine; Attending Physician, Yale-New Haven Hospital, New Haven, Connecticut
Headache

Joanne Gould Kuntz, MD
Clinical Instructor, University of Pittsburgh School of Medicine, Department of Emergency Medicine, University of Pittsburgh School of Medicine; Attending Physician, Department of Emergency Medicine, Mercy Hospital of Pittsburgh, Pittsburgh, Pennsylvania
Thoracentesis and Analysis of Pleural Effusions

Louis Lambiase, MD
Assistant Professor of Medicine, Tulane University School of Medicine, New Orleans, Louisiana
Liver Function Tests

Robert W. Lasek, MD
Associate Professor in Emergency Medicine, Faculty of Emergency Medicine Residency, Geisinger Medical Center, Danville, Pennsylvania
Rib Radiographs

John M. Lorei, MD
Assistant Clinical Professor of Medicine, Department of Emergency Medicine, University of Missouri–Kansas City School of Medicine; Chairman, Emergency Services, St. Luke's Northland Hospital–Barry Road Campus, Kansas City, Missouri
Synovial Fluid Analysis

Bruce A. MacLeod, MD
Clinical Assistant Professor, Department of Emergency Medicine, University of Pittsburgh School of Medicine; Chair, Department of Emergency Medicine, Mercy Hospital of Pittsburgh, Pittsburgh, Pennsylvania
Erythrocyte Sedimentation Rate

Robert J. Maha, Jr., MD
Attending Physician, Mercy Hospital of Pittsburgh, Pittsburgh, Pennsylvania
Suspected Pregnancy

Thomas G. Martin, MD
Assistant Professor of Emergency Medicine, University of Pittsburgh School of Medicine, Department of Emergency Medicine, Medical Director, Toxicology Treatment Program, Pittsburgh, Pennsylvania
Toxicology Laboratory Testing

Thomas P. Martin, MD
Clinical Instructor, University of Pittsburgh School of Medicine; Attending Physician, Department of Emergency Medicine, Western Pennsylvania Hospital, Pittsburgh, Pennsylvania
Modifying Physician Test-Ordering Behavior

Alison J. McDonald, MD, FACEP
Assistant Professor of Surgery/Emergency Medicine, Jefferson Medical College of Thomas Jefferson University; Director, Undergraduate Medical Education for the Emergency Department, Thomas Jefferson University Hospital, Philadelphia, Pennsylvania
Extremity Radiography

Edward A. Michelson, MD, FACEP
Associate Professor of Medicine and Emergency Medicine Residency Program Director, Northwestern University Medical School, Chicago, Illinois
Nausea and Vomiting

Joyce Mitchell-Savinsky, MD
Clinical Instructor, Department of Medicine, Case Western Reserve University, School of Medicine; Associate Residency Coordinator, Department of Emergency Medical Services, Mount Sinai Medical Center, Cleveland, Ohio
Ischemic Chest Pain

W. Scott Morse, MD
Clinical Instructor, Emergency Medicine, University of Pittsburgh School of Medicine; Attending Radiologist, St. Francis Hospital, Forbes Metropolitan Hospital, and Ohio Valley Hospital, Pittsburgh, Pennsylvania
Chest Radiography

Vince Mosesso, MD
Assistant Professor of Emergency Medicine, University of Pittsburgh School of Medicine; Attending Physician, Emergency Department, University of Pittsburgh Medical Center, Pittsburgh, Pennsylvania
Deep Venous Thrombosis

Robert W. Neumar, MD
Assistant Professor of Emergency Medicine, Wayne State University School of Medicine, Detroit, Michigan
Sputum Gram Stain

Kevin O'Toole, MD
Assistant Professor of Emergency Medicine, University of Pittsburgh School of Medicine; Attending Physician, Emergency Department, and Director, Hyperbaric Medicine Program, University of Pittsburgh Medical Center, Pittsburgh, Pennsylvania
Intravenous Pyelography

Thomas S. Pannke, MD
Assistant Clinical Instructor, Department of Surgery, University of Illinois College of Medicine; Staff Physician, Rockford Memorial Hospital, Rockford, Illinois
The 12-Lead Electrocardiogram in Acute Chest Pain

Andrew Peitzman, MD
Professor of Surgery, University of Pittsburgh School of Medicine; Director, Trauma Services, Presbyterian University Hospital, Pittsburgh, Pennsylvania
Urologic Trauma

Louis Profeta, MD
Clinical Associate Professor of Medicine, Indiana University School of Medicine; Department of Emergency Medicine, St. Vincent Hospital and Health Care Center, Indianapolis, Indiana
Cerebrospinal Fluid

Raymond J. Roberge, MD
Clinical Associate Professor of Emergency Medicine, University of Pittsburgh School of Medicine; Vice Chairman, Department of Emergency Medicine, Western Pennsylvania Hospital, Pittsburgh, Pennsylvania
The Acute Scrotum

Loren Rood, MD
Attending Physician, Emergency Department, Winona Memorial Hospital, Indianapolis, Indiana
Soft Tissue Infection

Bruce W. Rosenthal, MD, FAAP, FACEP
Clinical Assistant Professor of Pediatrics, University of Pittsburgh School of Medicine; Chief, Division of Pediatric Emergency Medicine, Mercy Hospital of Pittsburgh, Pittsburgh, Pennsylvania
The Pediatric Patient

Sandra Schneider, MD, FACEP
Professor and Chair, Department of Emergency Medicine, University of Rochester School of Medicine and Dentistry; Chief, Emergency Services, The Strong Memorial Hospital, Rochester, New York
Altered Mental Status

David C. Seaberg, MD
Associate Professor and Residency Director, Division of Emergency Medicine, University of Florida Health Service Center–Jacksonville, Jacksonville, Florida
Amylase and Lipase

Gerhard C. Senula, MD
Medical Director, Emergency Department, Jeannette District Memorial Hospital, Jeannette, Pennsylvania
Muscle Enzymes and Myoglobin

Bern Shen, MD, MPhil
Assistant Professor, Emergency Medicine, University of California, San Francisco, School of Medicine, San Francisco; Research Scientist, Hewlett-Packard Co., Palo Alto, California
Cost Analysis

Linda A. Smith, MD
Clinical Instructor of Emergency Medicine, Department of Emergency Medicine, University of Pittsburgh School of Medicine, Attending Physician, Westmoreland Regional Hospital, Greensburg, Pennsylvania
The Elderly Patient

J. Stephan Stapczynski, MD
Associate Professor and Chair, Department of Emergency Medicine, University of Kentucky College of Medicine; Medical Director, Emergency Department, University Hospital, Lexington, Kentucky
The Febrile Adult and *Blood Cultures*

Andrew Sucov, MD
Assistant Professor of Emergency Medicine, University of Rochester School of Medicine and Dentistry, Rochester, New York
Abdominal Plain Films

Owen T. Traynor, MD
EMS Fellow, Instructor of Emergency Medicine, University of Pittsburgh School of Medicine, Pittsburgh, Pennsylvania
Blood Urea Nitrogen and Creatinine

Michael A. Turturro, MD, FACEP
Clinical Assistant Professor of Medicine, University of Pittsburgh School of Medicine; Vice Chairman and Director of Academic Affairs, Department of Emergency Medicine, Mercy Hospital of Pittsburgh, Pittsburgh, Pennsylvania
Acute Abdominal Pain

Vincent P. Verdile, MD
Associate Professor of Emergency Medicine, Albany Medical College; Vice Chairman, Department of Emergency Medicine, Albany Medical Center Hospital, Albany, New York
Arterial Blood Gas Analysis and *Ultrasonography*

Edward J. Vogel, MD
Attending Physician, Vassar Brothers Hospital, Poughkeepsie, New York
Suspected Pregnancy

Kevin R. Ward, MD
Senior Research Staff, Department of Emergency Medicine, Henry Ford Hospital, Detroit, Michigan
Pulse Oximetry

Steven J. White, MD, FACEP
Assistant Professor, Department of Emergency Medicine, Vanderbilt University School of Medicine, Nashville, Tennessee
Glucose Testing and *Ventilation/Perfusion Nuclear Lung Scan*

Charles Whiteman, MD
Assistant Professor, Department of Emergency Medicine, West Virginia University School of Medicine, Morgantown, West Virginia
Seizure

Robert W. Wolford, MD
Assistant Professor, Michigan State University College of Human Medicine, Lansing; Director, Department of Emergency Medicine, Saginaw Cooperative Hospitals, Inc., Saginaw, Michigan
Evaluation of the Sore Throat and *The 12-Lead Electrocardiogram in Acute Chest Pain*

Donald M. Yealy, MD
Vice Chair and Associate Professor, Department of Emergency Medicine, University of Pittsburgh School of Medicine, Pittsburgh, Pennsylvania
Imaging After Head Trauma

PREFACE

Emergency physicians are increasingly concerned with the efficient use of diagnostic testing, and rightly so. Surprisingly, although diagnostic tests are ordered frequently as an integral part of the evaluation of emergency department patients, explicit guidelines for their appropriate use and their interpretation are still, for the most part, derived from isolated research studies or simply from individual practice experiences.

This book is an attempt to collect under one cover much of the information about emergency department diagnostic testing that has already been established by careful investigation. It also provides a background of factual information and serves as a bedside reference that the emergency physician will find of value in a variety of clinical situations.

The book is organized into three sections. The first addresses such general issues as emergency decision-making, cost-benefit analysis, and ways of modifying the physician's test-ordering behavior. The second section deals with common emergency department patient presentations and complaints and discusses the appropriate use of diagnostic testing for each one. The third and most extensive section addresses the individual tests themselves, summarizing what is known about their indications, their limitations, and their overall utility in the emergency department setting. Whenever possible, limited guidelines are proposed for the appropriate use of each test.

We hope this volume will prove itself useful in stimulating further rigorous investigation into this vitally important area of emergency medicine.

CONTENTS

SECTION I
OVERVIEW

SECTION II
Clinical Syndromes

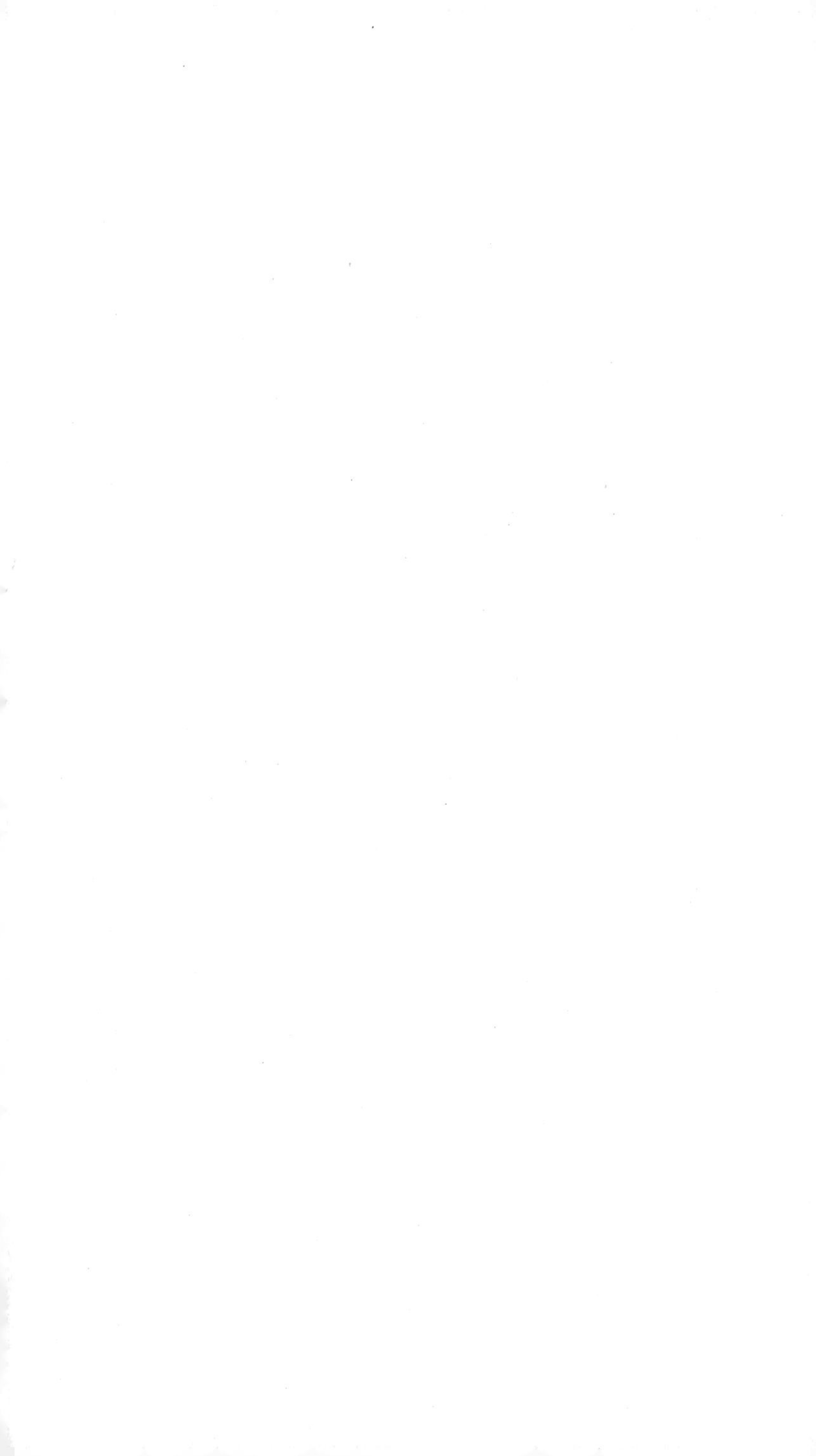

SECTION I
OVERVIEW

Chapter

Diagnostic Testing in the Emergency Department: An Introduction

Allan B. Wolfson

HOW ARE DIAGNOSTIC DECISIONS MADE?

The doctor's mission is to preserve life, limb, and function and to relieve suffering. In the emergency department, these goals must be pursued in the context of the time constraints, limited information, and uncertainty that characterize emergency practice. There is a certain subset of emergency patients who require a stereotyped, cookbook approach to their presenting problem—for example, those suffering from cardiac arrest, altered mental status, or multiple trauma. Most, however, require the physician to gather information rapidly from the history, physical examination, and selected diagnostic tests so as to arrive quickly at a management plan that assures the patient's immediate well-being and provides for access to more definitive care as needed.

How physicians make important decisions such as these has been the subject of much discussion and inquiry. Medical students have long been taught first to elicit data about the patient and the chief complaint, then to generate a differential diagnosis, which is sometimes quite extensive, and finally to "rule in" or "rule out" as many of these potential disorders as possible to arrive ultimately at the diagnosis. According to this paradigm, it is only after the diagnosis has been reached that effective treatment can begin.

Studies of experienced clinicians, however, demonstrate that real-world diagnoses are arrived at in a somewhat different fashion. The experienced clinician appears to function initially by using a combination of pattern recognition and general rules. A diagnostic *hypothesis* is generated, and further information is then elicited with the object of supporting or weakening the initial hypothesis, which is revised and refined in successive steps.

Whether the diagnostic process is that of the medical student or the experienced clinician, one arrives eventually at the same question: When is enough information enough? When has a sufficient degree of diagnostic certainty been reached so that the clinician can confidently proceed with treatment? When is there no further means of increasing the clinician's certainty without a disproportionate or unacceptable increase in "cost"?

More information is good only if it is useful. Making a diagnosis can be defined as knowing that more information would not change a decision to act as if the patient had the disease. Conversely, ruling out a disease has been defined as knowing that more information would not change the decision to act as if the patient did *not* have the disease. In some cases, the initial clinical picture is so clear that no testing is necessary at all. When we are not certain *enough* of the pattern, however, we embark on hypothesis testing.

When it is decided that there is enough information to proceed with management, a diagnosis in the *absolute* sense may still not have been reached. However, the notion of "diagnostic certainty" is often an illusion—it may not actually be impossible to be absolutely certain of a diagnosis, but beyond a certain point more information becomes irrelevant even if the cost of gaining it is not prohibitive.[1]

Emergency medicine is complaint based rather than diagnosis based, and emergency physicians function under severe constraints of time and information. They generally do not have the luxury of being able to perform a definitive diagnostic test or therapeutic trial, even if it were possible or useful. Rather, they try to gather information as efficiently as they can, stay alert for "red flags," and try to guard against common biases and errors.

In the emergency department, it is particularly important to avoid delaying intervention until a diagnosis has been reached with certainty. It is equally important to avoid being led on an often-fruitless search for the cause of every abnormal "objective" result. In either case, the clinician risks allowing a mere number to come between the doctor and the patient.

WHY DO WE ORDER DIAGNOSTIC TESTS?

A tongue-in-cheek list of ten classic reasons for ordering tests was published some years ago[2] and, although modified here, remains essentially true today:

1. "To be complete."
2. "The senior (or attending) said to."
3. "I'll get in trouble if I don't."
4. "If you don't order everything at once, . . ."
5. "As long as he is in the hospital, . . ."
6. "This is an academic institution."
7. "If I don't, I might get sued."
8. "A consultant won't come down unless . . ."
9. "If it were *my* father or mother, . . ."
10. "How do you know he doesn't have it?"

The underlying assumptions here are that testing is harmless (or at least that the benefit is always greater than the cost); that tests don't lie; and that diagnostic certainty, as well as the immediate detection of occult disease, is always both mandatory and beneficial. None of these statements is true, however.[3]

A test is clearly justified when its cost (broadly defined) is less than the benefit it produces—for example, when a quick and inexpensive test can detect a treatable and potentially lethal disease. Testing is clearly *not* justified when an expensive or dangerous test is utilized to diagnose a trivial or untreatable disease. However, a test that can increase diagnostic certainty may be absolutely necessary to justify embarking on a costly or potentially risky treatment.

There are thus some good reasons to order diagnostic tests. Some tests provide objective information that is more reliable than a simple history and physical examination. Others can be useful in guiding treatment. Tests can also help to generate prevalence data that can guide future management strategies.

Clinicians' test-ordering practices are commonly established early in their careers. Medical training has traditionally and often wrongheadedly insisted that it is "good medicine" to test; the ability to spout the results of a plethora of diagnostic tests has long been considered an important component of the honorable sport of roundsmanship. Tests are also ordered for reassurance (ie, to back up a clinical decision with "objective" data) or to comply with patients' expectations or society's medicolegal demands.

Beyond these, many clinicians feel obliged to avoid the discomfort associated with uncertainty. An irrational belief in screening, often accompanied by personal memories of specific cases that were missed, undoubtedly plays a role as well. Busy practice conditions, institutional rules, and peer pressure make it more difficult for the conscientious clinician to ''fight the system.'' Finally, financial incentives, either direct or indirect, may unfortunately operate in some cases as well.

PROPERTIES OF DIAGNOSTIC TESTS

It is easy to forget that diagnostic tests are not absolute measures that perfectly reflect an unchanging reality. Although it is tempting to practice medicine as if there were a strict correspondence between the diagnostic test value and the presence or absence of disease, diagnostic tests *are not* absolutes.

First, there are issues of accuracy and precision. *Accuracy* refers to how closely a test value approaches the ''real'' value of the object being measured. A tympanic membrane thermometer, for example, may yield a reading that only approximates an individual's true temperature as assessed by some ''gold standard'' measurement (eg, the core temperature measured by thermocouple). *Precision* refers to the reproducibility of the value obtained on repeated measurements. A succession of tympanic membrane temperature measurements on the same individual, for example, might yield a series of slightly differing results. Significant limitations of accuracy and precision are characteristic of many commonly used diagnostic tests and clearly limit the degree of credence one may give to certain test results. These imperfections in diagnostic tests stem from causes ranging from improper radiographic technique or blood sample handling to inherent limitations in chemical measurements.

Second is the very real issue of appropriateness. On the one hand, we may be able to tell very accurately and reproducibly exactly what the serum lactate dehydrogenase level or the serum C-reactive protein level is, for example, but that knowledge may not be very helpful in guiding us toward the correct diagnosis and treatment. On the other hand, a semiquantitative urine pregnancy test is often very helpful precisely because the presence of human chorionic gonadotropin very nearly *always* indicates pregnancy and hardly ever anything else.

Even if every measurement or determination were perfectly accurate, 100% reproducible, and appropriate to answer the clinical question at hand, essentially all test values normally vary to one degree or another from individual to individual. That is, rather than there being one absolute ''correct'' value, there is a range of possible values even in normal individuals. What the value of a particular diagnostic test ''should be'' is based on a statistical sampling of a population. Whether a particular test result in a particular individual is normal or abnormal is thus a matter of probabilities rather than certainties.

In a group of individuals who are not ''normal,'' but have the disease being sought by diagnostic testing, test measurements likewise take on a *range* of values, typically with a distribution different from that seen in normal individuals. On the one hand, a test that discriminated perfectly between these two populations, those with disease and those without disease, would yield respective values that did not overlap at all (Fig. 1–1*A*). On the other hand, a test with essentially complete overlap of values (Fig. 1–1*B*) would provide no discrimination whatsoever between diseased and nondiseased individuals and therefore little useful clinical information. Essentially all real-world tests fall somewhere between these two extremes, with some degree of overlap of test values but reasonable discrimination between diseased and healthy individuals (Fig. 1–1*C*).

Test values are generally reported in terms of a range of normal, defined as the range within which 95% of the population will be found. This implies that for any given test 5% of a normal population can be expected to have an "abnormal" value. When a number of independent tests are performed on a normal individual, the probability that at least one will be abnormal increases with the number of tests performed. Thus, when 12 tests are performed (eg, a standard Chem-12 panel), the likelihood that at least one of the results will be outside the normal range approaches 50%. When 20 tests are performed (eg, a standard Chem-20 panel), the odds that at least one result will be abnormal are approximately 2:1 (Table 1–1). If the clinician fails to realize this mathematical fact and, moreover, insists on investigating every abnormal test result through further testing, the stage is set for the "cascade effect," whereby one abnormal test result causes the performance of more tests, each with a certain likelihood of providing a spuriously abnormal result. Test values tend to differ not only between individuals but also within the same individual at different times.

TABLE 1–1. PROBABILITY THAT A HEALTHY PERSON WILL HAVE ABNORMAL RESULTS IN A BIOCHEMICAL PROFILE

No. of Tests	Probability That at Least One Test Will Be Abnormal[a]
1	5
6	26
12	46
20	64
100	99.4

Adapted from Cebul RD, Beck JR: Biochemical profiles: applications in ambulatory screening and preadmission testing of adults. *Ann Intern Med.* 1987;106:403–413.

[a]Assuming that each test in the battery is independent of the others.

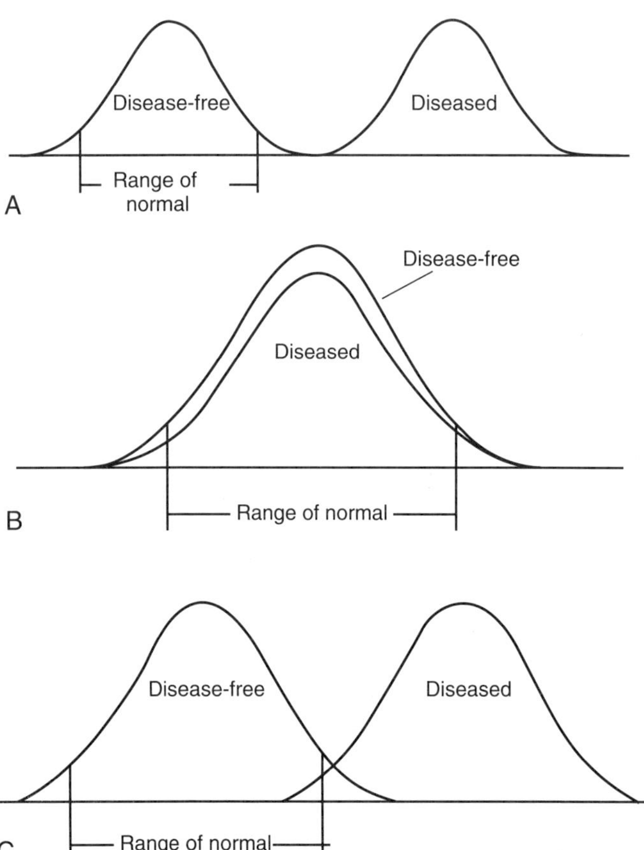

FIGURE 1–1. *A*. A test with complete separation of populations results in perfect diagnostic discrimination. *B*. A test with no separation of the populations results in no diagnostic discrimination. *C*. A test with partial separation of the populations results in partial diagnostic discrimination. From Riegelman RK, Hirsh RP: *Studying a Study and Testing a Test*. Boston: Little, Brown and Company, 1989:142. Published by Little, Brown and Company.

A corollary of these observations is that *all tests yield some false-positives and false-negatives*. A false-positive is a test result that is abnormal even though the individual being tested is disease free. A false-negative is a test result that falls within the normal range even though the individual being tested does indeed have disease. The false-positive and false-negative rates are characteristics of each individual diagnostic test and can be determined empirically, assuming that there is some gold standard available to define the presence or absence of disease.

The utility of performing a test depends on its false-positive and false-negative rates and on the consequences of acting on the basis of a positive or negative test result. If there are too many false-positives, a significant number of individuals without disease are incorrectly labeled as having disease, with the attendant additional costs and risks. If the false-negative rate is too high, a significant number of patients with disease are falsely labeled as disease free, with the corresponding potentially negative consequences.

One must take into account not only the monetary costs of testing, which may be considerable, but also the potential side effects entailed (eg, radiation exposure, arterial puncture). False-positive and false-negative test results may actually lead the clinician *away* from the correct diagnosis and appropriate management. There are also the potential costs of the cascade effect that may be induced. One must add to this the difficult-to-quantitate but real costs of making resources unavailable for other patients, creating potential delays in diagnosis, and causing inconvenience and anxiety in the patient.

A simple principle to follow is that *a test should be ordered only if the result will affect the patient's management*. Although larger issues of screening, routine testing, and public health cannot ultimately be ignored and are considered to be within the purview of emergency practice in some settings, they do not apply to the emergency practitioner's primary task at hand.

SENSITIVITY AND SPECIFICITY

Diagnostic tests are characterized by properties termed sensitivity and specificity. These are independent of the *prevalence* of the disease in the population of interest.

Sensitivity is determined by looking at patients with disease. It is defined as the proportion of individuals with a disease who are labeled positive by the test or, in shorthand, "positivity in disease" (Table 1–2). A highly sensitive test is nearly always positive in the presence of disease. It is therefore useful in *ruling out* disease when it is *negative* and is thus desirable for use in screening. A highly sensitive test is also desirable when the disease being tested for is both severe and treatable enough that we would not want to miss the opportunity to diagnose it. The V/Q scan is an example of a highly sensitive test that can be used to rule out a potentially severe and readily treatable disorder, thus

Sensitivity = positivity in disease

Specificity is defined as the proportion of individuals without disease who are labeled negative by the test or, in shorthand, "negativity in health" (see Table 1–2). A highly specific test is nearly always negative in healthy people; it is therefore very useful in *ruling in* disease when it is *positive*. A highly specific test is desirable when we want to be sure the patient has the disease in question before embarking on a relatively costly or dangerous course of treatment. The EKG is an example of a reasonably specific test that can be used in the emergency department to diagnose acute myocardial infarction amenable to thrombolytic therapy, thus

Specificity = negativity in health

Setting up a simple outcome grid provides a useful way of visualizing these concepts. If we take a group of patients, some of whom have a disease (as determined by some gold standard) and some of whom do not, and perform the diagnostic test of interest on all of them, we end up with four groups of patients, as shown below:

		Disease +	**Disease** −
Test	+	TP	FP
	−	FN	TN

A certain number of individuals have the disease and test positive ("true-positive," TP). A number of others do *not* have the disease and test negative ("true-negative," TN). Because diagnostic tests are by nature imperfect, however, there will be a certain number of normal individuals who test positive ("false-positive," FP), as well as a certain number of diseased individuals who test negative ("false-negative," FN) (see Table 1–2).

As a practical illustration, assume that for a particular diagnostic test and a particular population the number of individuals in each of these four categories is found to be as follows:

		Disease +	**Disease** −
Test	+	800	100
	−	200	900

patients' ultimate diagnosis in order to be calculated. In deciding whether to order a test on a patient in whom the diagnosis is suspected, the clinician may find it useful to know the test's sensitivity and specificity in the appropriate patient population.

It is more often the case, however, that one needs to know the significance of a positive or negative test *result*. The proportion of patients with a positive test who actually have the disease in question is known as the *predictive value of the positive* (disease in positivity, see Table 1–2). This proportion can be calculated by looking again at the outcome grid from page 8, reproduced here. This time, read across from left to right rather than up and down. The top row represents all patients who have a positive test, numbering 900. Of these, 800 have the disease. Therefore, the predictive value of a positive test is 800/900 or 89%.

		Disease	
		+	−
Test	+	800	100
	−	200	900

The clinician likewise would like to know the significance of a negative test result. What proportion of patients with a negative test result are actually free of disease? This proportion, called the *predictive value of the negative* (health in negativity, see Table 1–2), is calculated by reading across the second row of the outcome grid, which shows all patients who have a negative test result. There are 1100 of these individuals, and of these 900 are seen to be free of disease, yielding a predictive value of the negative of 900/1100 or 82%.

Predictive values enable the clinician to estimate the likelihood that a positive test result is in fact a false-positive or that a negative test result is in fact a false-negative. The critical feature of the predictive value of the positive and predictive value of the negative is that, for any given test sensitivity and specificity, they are critically dependent on the prevalence of disease in the population being tested.

The example in Table 1–3 demonstrates the dramatic difference in the positive predictive value of a test when it is applied to two different populations, one with a disease prevalence of 10% and the other with a disease prevalence of only 0.1%. In the former, any positive test result is as likely to be a false-positive as a true-positive; hence, the predictive value of the positive is 50%. In the latter group, where there is a low disease prevalence, a positive test result is more than 100 times as likely to be a false-positive as a true-positive because the disease itself is so rare in this population. Note that in the example *the test's sensitivity and specificity are the same in both groups.*

TABLE 1–3. POSITIVE PREDICTIVE VALUE (PPV) AND PREVALENCE

	Disease Prevalence = 10%		Disease Prevalence = 0.1%	
Test	***Disease Present***	***Disease Absent***	***Disease Present***	***Disease Absent***
Positive	900	900	9	999
Negative	100	8100	1	8991
Total	1000	9000	10	9990
	PPV = 900/1800 = 50%		PPV = 9/1008 = 0.9%	

From Woolf SH, Kamerow DB: Testing for uncommon conditions: The heroic search for positive test results. *Arch Intern Med.* 1990;150:2452.

Testing conditions: size of population, 10,000; sensitivity of test, 90%; and specificity of test, 90%.

This example demonstrates the very limited utility of even an extremely specific test when the underlying likelihood of disease is low. A positive test is of very questionable significance, and a negative test simply confirms what one already suspected. In fact, before the test was even ordered, one would know that a positive result would probably be more prudently ignored than acted upon. An example of this phenomenon occurs when HIV testing is carried out in populations with a low prevalence of infection.

Similarly, if a disease is extremely prevalent in a population or if it is thought to be extremely likely in the patient being evaluated, even a very sensitive diagnostic test is likely to be of limited value. In this case, it is because a negative test is far more likely to represent a false-negative than a true-negative. A negative test result may perhaps best be ignored, and a positive one will simply confirm the initial clinical impression.

The critical dependency of predictive values on disease prevalence and the algebraic demonstration of this fact are usually referred to as Bayes' theorem. The analysis of the utility of diagnostic tests as they depend on disease prevalence is referred to as Bayesian analysis.

These concepts are demonstrated graphically in Figure 1–3, which depicts post-test probabilities (analogous to the predictive value of the positive and predictive value of the negative) as functions of the pretest probability (analogous to the prevalence of disease in the population being tested). In Figure 1–3, the diagnostic test has a quite impressive sensitivity of 90% and specificity of 90%. Note that, for a low pretest probability, even a positive test result still implies a rather low likelihood of disease, whereas a negative test result simply makes the presence of

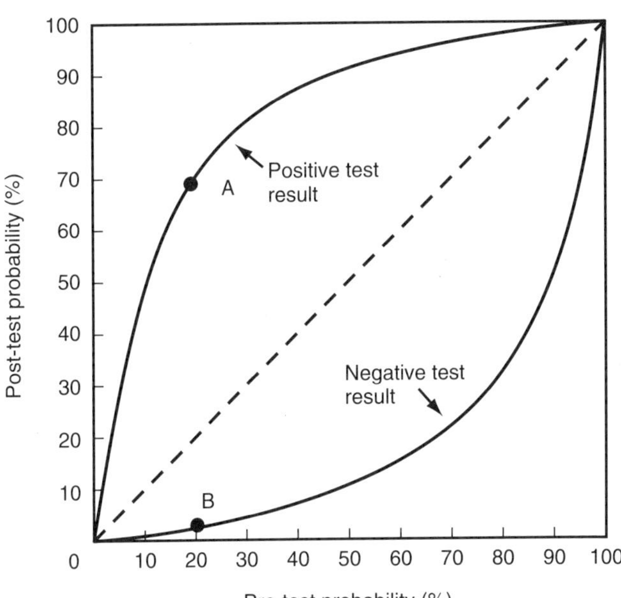

FIGURE 1–3. Relationship between pre- and post-test probability. Sensitivity = 90% and specificity = 90%. From Komaroff AL, Berwick DM: Decision theory and medical practice, in Isselbacher K, et al (eds): *Update IV/Harrison's Principles of Internal Medicine*, New York: McGraw-Hill; 1983. Reproduced with permission of McGraw-Hill, Inc.

disease even less likely. For example, a *positive* EKG stress test in a young nonsmoking female with atypical chest pain may still be associated with a far lower likelihood of significant coronary artery disease than a *negative* test in an elderly male smoker.

Similarly, when the pretest probability is high, a negative test result still implies a rather high likelihood of disease, whereas a positive test result simply makes it even more likely that disease is present.

THE REAL WORLD OF THE EMERGENCY DEPARTMENT

Where does all this information leave the emergency practitioner? One conclusion that can be drawn from the aforementioned observations is that a diagnostic test provides the greatest yield of information when it is applied to the patient in whom the pretest probability of disease is within the middle range of values. To derive the most benefit from a *positive* diagnostic test, the key is to increase the prior probability ("prevalence") of disease before testing. For a *negative* test to add information, one wants to minimize the prior probability of disease prevalence. The diagnostic test is thus used to modify one's estimate of the probability of disease and to move that estimated probability either upward beyond the threshold at which one will decide to treat or downward beyond the threshold at which one will decide not to treat. In fact, the entire diagnostic process can be represented as a series of diagnostic tests (the first and most critical of which is the history and physical examination) that is pursued until the probability that the patient has the disease is either high enough to justify instituting treatment or low enough to justify a decision not to treat.

In practical terms, the sensitivity and specificity of each diagnostic test have not generally been available to the clinician at the bedside. It is not always possible to estimate disease prevalence or even, given a suitable history and physical examination, the pretest probability of disease. Nevertheless, the preceding provides a framework within which the role of diagnostic testing in patient care can be understood. Using this framework enables us to analyze how we go about making clinical decisions at the bedside and to begin to improve the way we employ diagnostic testing in caring for our patients.

The remainder of this book addresses the particulars of this process as they are pursued every day in the emergency department.

REFERENCES

1. Kassirer JP: Our stubborn quest for diagnostic certainty: A cause of excessive testing. *N Engl J Med.* 1989; 320:1489.
2. Hardison JE: To be complete. *N Engl J Med.* 1979; 300:193.
3. Woolf SH, Kamerow DB: Testing for uncommon conditions: The heroic search for positive test results. *Arch Intern Med.* 1990; 150:2451.
4. Riegelman RK, Hirsch RP: *Studying a Study and Testing a Test.* Boston: Little, Brown and Company, 1989.
5. Komaroff AL, Berwick DM: Decision theory and medical practice, in Isselbacher K, et al (eds): *Update IV. Harrison's Principles of Internal Medicine.* New York: McGraw-Hill; 1983:243.

Chapter

Cost Analysis

Bern Shen

This chapter outlines issues of cost analysis as they apply to diagnostic testing in emergency medicine. There are different types of cost analysis and different definitions of costs, benefits, and effectiveness. Yet, all are intended ultimately to guide the physician's clinical decision making at the bedside.

The assessment of practice and technology in medicine differs from that in most businesses in several important ways. First, cost analysis in medicine is necessarily colored by the differences in underlying motivations between medicine and business. The traditional role of the physician as the individual patient's advocate often directly conflicts with societal fiscal imperatives. The underlying purpose behind medical cost analysis is not to cut costs and increase profits but to reestablish the connection between cost and value.[1]

Second, measures of outcome are technically complex. Much of the thrust of cost analysis can be seen as a progression toward improved definitions of optimal care. Not only must a diagnostic test or therapeutic maneuver be "efficacious" (under ideal conditions) but it must be shown to be "effective" (under nonideal conditions) as well.[2, 3] Furthermore, care must also be "appropriate"—although defibrillation often terminates ventricular tachycardia, chemical conversion may be preferred in the stable patient.[4]

The structure of the health care market, however, discourages such assessments. Moreover, providers of health care also become major determinants of health care demand on behalf of patients, a potential conflict labeled the "agency relationship" by economists.[5] With third-party coverage, the "connection between value and cost has been cut."[1] Patients and health professionals alike do not directly bear the full cost of the health care they consume or prescribe[6] and tend to demand more services than they otherwise might.[5] Confusion sometimes results from the use of various terms involving the word "cost."[7] Perhaps the most straightforward type of cost analysis is purely *identification and quantification of costs,* without consideration of the benefits thereby derived. The unit of measurement is simply number of dollars. Using this framework, if one diagnostic test or therapeutic option is less expensive than another of equal sensitivity and specificity, it is superior. Cost identification has two serious limitations. First, it looks only at cost and ignores the health benefits that motivated the expenditure. Second, it entails considerable complexity.

Cost-effectiveness analysis addresses these criticisms by measuring health outcomes as well as the cost of diagnostic or therapeutic maneuvers. To do this, health benefits need to be converted to a common unit of measurement, such as number of lives saved, hospital admissions averted, or millimeters of mercury blood pressure reduced. The unit of measurement is thus dollars per life saved, dollars per hospital admission averted, and mm Hg lowered.

This figure is not particularly useful by itself; rather, it derives much of its meaning from comparing one alternative test or treatment with another. A dollar spent on test A is a dollar not spent on test B. Expressed in economic terms, the advantage of one alternative over the next best alternative is the "marginal return."[8]

A weakness of cost-effectiveness analysis is its limited ability to compare two alternatives in which outcomes cannot easily be measured in the same unit (eg, a defibrillator that costs $A per episode of return of spontaneous circulation vs a rapid CK-MB test that costs $B per hospital admission averted). *Cost-benefit analysis* attempts to broaden our ability to compare disparate options by converting the benefits into a common dollar unit. Assuming this comparison can be made, it then becomes possible to directly match one diagnostic or therapeutic maneuver against an apparently unrelated one.[9, 10]

Difficulties of Cost Analysis

Cost analysis can be tricky, particularly when applied to compare different health care programs and populations.[11, 12] How does one account for the many dimensions of health (social functioning, mental state, physical functioning)? How does one assign relative values to less than "perfectly healthy" life, particularly for different individuals? How much reliance can be placed upon measurements involving proxy variables (eg, process variables rather than outcome variables) when these may be the only ones that can practically be assessed?[13] A number of complex, multidimensional clinical conundrums may actually represent "tossups," in which it really does not matter which option is chosen.[14]

Unfortunately, even when an intervention is identified as cost effective, there may be additional factors that prevent its implementation. Preventative health advice, a simple and an effective health intervention well within the purview of emergency medicine, is sadly underutilized for a number of nonmedical reasons including motivation, training, and financial constraints.[15] Such discrepancies suggest that cost-benefit calculations are likely to be unrealistic and of limited applicability if all options for interventions are not included in the analysis.

Definition of Costs and Benefits

"Cost" means different things to different people. It is usually but not always expressed in dollars, which makes it a convenient proxy term for the actual disparate resources being consumed; in turn, cost must be distinguished from "charges" to the consumer.

Decisions are not made in a vacuum; opting for one test or treatment means foregoing others because of limited time, money, staff, or other resources. Thus, the real cost of choosing one action is not simply the expenditure involved but also includes the *opportunity cost,* the benefit lost by not using the same resources in the most highly valued alternative way.[5]

Technology Assessment, Practice Guidelines, and Future Trends

The W. K. Kellogg Foundation and the National Fund for Medical Education have proposed five recommendations for improving health cost effectiveness:[16]

- Develop and validate indices of cost and effectiveness
- Explore the ethical issues involved in conflicts between therapeutic and fiscal imperatives
- Research ways to improve the physician-patient relationship to foster a more participative patient role in health promotion
- Develop a database and improve teaching techniques for structured clinical problem solving
- Educate physicians to become agents of change in fostering cost-effective health care

Although "big-ticket," highly technical items including intensive care are attractive targets for cost cutters, they actually constitute only about 1% of total annual Medicare costs.[17] Perhaps counterintuitively, high-volume chronic and recurrent needs of frail (not necessarily old) patients, rather than heroic intensive interventions, account for the majority of health care costs.[18, 19] If, as has been suggested, up to 60% of "little-ticket" diagnostic tests in teaching hospitals are ordered inappropriately or unnecessarily, even a 10% reduction of such testing nationwide would save about $12.5 billion a year.[20]

Interventions targeting patients could include cost sharing[19, 21] and patient education.[17, 22] A great deal of waste results from an academic imperative for diagnostic completeness.[23, 24] In particular, the cost of "wanting to know" may no longer be justified.[25, 26]

REFERENCES

1. Eddy D: The challenge. *JAMA.* 1990;263:287–290.
2. Roper W, Winkenwerder W, Hackbarth G, et al: Effectiveness in health care: An initiative to evaluate and improve medical practice. *N Engl J Med.* 1988;319:1197–1202.
3. Rose M, Leibenluft R: Antitrust implications of medical technology assessment. *N Engl J Med.* 1986;314:1490–1493.
4. Murphy D, Matchar D: Life-sustaining therapy; a model for appropriate use. *JAMA.* 1990;264:2103–2108.
5. Drummond M, Stoddart G, Labelle R, et al: Health economics: An introduction for clinicians. *Ann Intern Med.* 1987;107(1):88–92.
6. Davis C: Reforming the US health care financing system, in Virgo J (ed): *Health Care: An International Perspective.* Edwardsville, IL: International Health Economics and Management Institute; 1984:49.
7. Doubilet P, Weinstein M, McNeil B: Use and misuse of the term ''cost effective'' in medicine. *N Engl J Med.* 1986;314(4):253–256.
8. Eddy D: *Assessing Health Practices and Designing Practice Policies: The Explicit Approach.* Philadelphia: American College of Physicians; 1992.
9. Anderson J, Bush J, Chen M, et al: Policy space areas and properties of benefit-cost/utility analysis. *JAMA.* 1986;255(6):794–795.
10. Steinbach J, Hardison W: Comparing health care options using the cost-benefit utility ratio. *JAMA.* 1986;255:747.
11. Emery D, Schneiderman L: Cost-effectiveness analysis in health care. *Hastings Ctr Rep.* 1989; July/Aug:8–13.
12. Hillman A, Eisenberg J, Pauly M, et al: Avoiding bias in the conduct and reporting of cost-effectiveness research sponsored by pharmaceutical companies. *N Engl J Med.* 1991;324(19):1362–1365.
13. McNutt R: How effective is cost effectiveness? *J Gen Intern Med.* 1988;3:203–204.
14. Kassirer J, Pauker S: The toss-up. *N Engl J Med.* 1981;305:1467–1469.
15. Becker M: Practicing health promotion: the doctor's dilemna. *Ann Intern Med.* 1990;113:419–422.
16. Cunningham R, Friedman CP, Weever B, Lake KE: Conference recommendations, in Cunningham R, Friedman CP, Weever B, Lake KE (eds): *Medical Education: Making the Grade in Cost Containment.* Battle Creek, MI: WK Kellogg Foundation; 1986:24–30.
17. Webster J, Berdes C: Ethics and economic realities—goals and strategies for care toward the end of life. *Arch Intern Med.* 1990;150:1795–1797.
18. Avorn J: Benefit and cost analysis in geriatric care; turning age discrimination into health policy. *N Engl J Med.* 1984;310:1294–1301.
19. Shapiro M, Ware J, Sherbourne C: Effects of cost sharing on seeking care for serious and minor symptoms. *Ann Intern Med.* 1986;104(2):246–251.
20. Taylor R: Ethical aspects of medical economics. *Neurol Clin.* 1989;7:883–900.
21. O'Grady K, Manning W, Newhouse J, et al: The impact of cost sharing on emergency department use. *N Engl J Med.* 1985;313(8):484–490.
22. Safran C, Phillips P: Interventions to prevent readmission; the constraints of cost and efficacy. *Med Care.* 1989;27(2):204–211.

23. Dans P: The great zebra hunt—a view of internal medicine from the walk-in clinic. *Pharos.* 1978; July:2–6.
24. Hardison J: To be complete. *N Engl J Med.* 1979;300:193–194.
25. Bryant M, Tepas J, Talbert J, et al: Impact of emergency room laboratory studies on the ultimate triage and disposition of the injured child. *Am Surg.* 1988;54(4):209–211.
26. Reuben D: Learning diagnostic restraint. *N Engl J Med.* 1988;310:591–593.

Chapter

Modifying Physician Test-Ordering Behavior

Thomas P. Martin

Escalating health care costs and ongoing efforts to implement health care reform have led to a wide-ranging reassessment of how health care resources are allocated in this country. A focus of this examination has been physician practice patterns. Given physicians' central role in selecting diagnostic and therapeutic strategies, how and why physicians order diagnostic tests have become the subject of a significant body of research over the past 20 years.

Numerous studies have examined specific interventions aimed at modifying physician practice patterns. Most of these studies, however, have shown mixed results, have had transient effects, or have suffered from methodologic shortcomings that have interfered with interpretation of the results.

Investigators now realize that a multitude of factors affects physicians' clinical decisions. Efforts to encourage physicians to be more cost-effective utilizers of limited health care resources may require fundamental changes in every phase of physicians' professional lives, from medical education to the medicolegal practice environment. The penetrance of managed care into the health care industry is yet another variable that will profoundly affect physician practice patterns, including diagnostic test selection.

Several factors have led to a focus on the physician as the target of efforts to control health care costs. First, physicians are the primary figures directing patient care. As such, they determine diagnostic test use and select therapeutic options. Second, there is an exceptionally wide range of diagnostic test utilization among physicians.[1, 9, 14] Schroeder and colleagues documented an almost 17-fold difference in laboratory test utilization among faculty members at a university-affiliated outpatient clinic.[10] Third, there is mounting evidence that physicians use tests inappropriately.[48] A growing body of literature suggests that coagulation studies,[46] electrocardiograms,[15] and chest roentgenograms[24] are often utilized inappropriately or obtained unnecessarily. Within the emergency department setting, skull films,[5, 42, 43] cervical spine films,[19] electrolyte tests,[6] and leukocyte count and differential[12, 40] have been examined and frequently found to be overutilized. Finally, several studies have found no correlation between increased testing and better patient outcome in selected settings.[7, 35, 47]

Recognition of the monetary and nonmonetary costs of unnecessary, low-yield studies fueled much of the interest in early, interventional studies.

INTERVENTIONAL STUDIES

The past 25 years have seen numerous interventional studies directed at improving physician use of diagnostic testing. In general, these studies have been based at academic institutions and have been directed at resident physicians. Techniques employed fall into five categories: (1) education, (2) feedback, (3) administrative changes, (4) incentives, and (5) physician participation.[26]

Predicated on the concept that, given appropriate information, physicians will become more discriminating and, therefore, efficient utilizers of health care resources, many studies have investigated *educational* interventions. These include grand rounds and attending rounds presentations and education manuals.[16, 30, 37] Whereas some studies have documented significant reductions in selected test use, many have failed to document any reduction in testing.[11, 16] Critics of these studies have cited short follow-up times and have noted a return to baseline test usage when the intervention was removed. Schroeder and colleagues found that the cost of materials and faculty time, in their study, exceeded the cost savings produced by the reduction in laboratory testing.[16]

Interventions involving *feedback* have, similarly, taken many forms, with both the content and means of delivery serving as study variables. Information provided to the physician has included costs of required studies,[2, 38] variance from practice patterns of colleagues,[34] and results of prior tests.[28] The delivery source of this information has varied from respected superiors to interactive computer screens.[28] Results of these studies, however, have again been mixed. The generalizability of these studies as well as other interventional studies centered on academic institutions have also been challenged.

Administrative interventions have included (1) modification of test-ordering forms to require a reason for selection of a test,[39] (2) groups of tests to answer a particular clinical question (eg, a "hypothyroid panel"),[13] and (3) absolute limitations on the number of tests that could be ordered.[20] In some cases, proponents of these studies have been criticized for looking at patient charges rather than at hospital costs as an endpoint and for failing to monitor overall testing as opposed to reduction in the use of selected tests.

Incentives have been both positive and negative in nature. Studies have used financial rewards such as contributions to educational book funds for physicians who achieved target reductions in test use.[37] Negative incentives are best characterized by the peer review system.[18]

The final category of intervention is *physician participation.* This intervention involves recruitment or enrollment of physicians into study groups and focus groups, formed to develop and implement appropriate guidelines for test use. This strategy is based on management theory principles suggesting that individuals are more willing to accept change when they are integrated into the decision-making process.[21] Results with this type of intervention have been encouraging as business management principles have been increasingly embraced by the health care industry.

These five types of interventions, employed alone or in combination, have produced mixed and, occasionally, contradictory results. As noted, their results have been challenged because of methodologic and design flaws. The findings of these interventional studies indicate that outside influences appear to neutralize or dampen the potential positive effects of education, feedback, administrative changes, incentives, and physician participation. These unrecognized influences have been the focus of a second area of investigation and scholarly opinion on physician use of diagnostic testing.

GLOBAL ASSESSMENT OF THE PHYSICIAN DECISION-MAKING PROCESS

Williams and Eisenberg,[11] authors of one of the best-designed and well-controlled interventional studies that failed to produce a reduction in unnecessary testing, attempted to identify the external factors and influences that prevented their interventions from having maximal effect. These investigators believed that strategies to change physician practice patterns might be developed to address these issues and thereby, potentially, be more effective.[17]

Williams and Eisenberg used a three-stage sequential Delphi technique to survey 280 physicians, including residents, academic internists, and community internists. Participants were asked to offer reasons for excessive testing in their own practices. The initial solicitation was in the form of an open questionnaire. In the second and third mailing, participants were asked to rank the most commonly cited explanations from the first questionnaire.

The study found that reasons provided by physicians for excessive testing varied widely among the physicians groups. Whereas both medical residents and faculty internists (commenting on the practice of residents) identified inexperience, habitual ordering of groups of tests, and pressure from superiors as explanations for excessive testing, community physicians cited fear of malpractice and routine screening among their top three answers. The investigators concluded that individual physicians or groups of physicians may have very different rationales for their selection of diagnostic studies. The study also illustrated the multitude of factors that affect the physician decision-making process. The second phase of their questionnaire listed 47 different reasons that physicians had provided to explain overutilization of diagnostic studies.

Williams and Eisenberg[17] suggested that efforts to modify physician practice patterns must begin with an acknowledgment of factors that physicians identify as important influences on their selection of diagnostic studies. These efforts must also be individualized to the target physician group. Interventions directed at community physicians, for example, would need to address concerns about malpractice and provide guidelines on the appropriate use of diagnostic testing in screening for disease.

FACTORS INFLUENCING PHYSICIAN DECISION MAKING

Whereas an exhaustive review of every factor bearing on the physician decision-making process would be an impossible task, several topics deserve mention in the context of influencing diagnostic test selection.

Undoubtedly, diagnostic testing is fueled by something more than the physician's intellectual curiosity and satisfaction. Physicians confront a patient population that is accustomed to ready availability of the most sophisticated medical diagnostic and therapeutic technology. Further, patients are buffered from having to consider costs by third-party payer and managed care programs. Physicians frequently feel compelled to pursue every diagnostic avenue for fear of being found negligent by omission. Diagnostic testing has become a factor to determine the adequacy of an evaluation.[36] Notably, fear of litigation was the third most commonly cited reason for excessive or unnecessary testing by community physicians in the Williams and Eisenberg survey.[17]

Physicians have little support for using diagnostic studies judiciously. Standards of care or practice guidelines are not uniformly accepted as the ideals against which treatment decisions are judged. Further, many existing guidelines fail to meet the necessary standards of validity, reliability, clinical applicability and flexibility, multidisciplinary development, and provision of a means to ensure periodic review.[3] For example, one study found that the standard of care, to which we hold physicians regarding the prompt administration of antibiotics to children suspected of having bacterial meningitis, bears little resemblance to the actual practice of qualified physicians in a university pediatric emergency department.[44]

Deficiencies in our system of medical education have also been cited as contributing to excessive testing. Criticisms have included inadequate training in medical economics and the cost of diagnostic testing[31, 45, 50]; failure to teach analytic approaches to medical diagnosis[16, 22]; focus of medical education within tertiary care centers, without adequate exposure to primary care settings; and inappropriate emphasis on diagnostic testing during the clinical years of medical school.[4] Although many medical schools have implemented curriculum changes to address these problems, it is unclear what impact these modifications in medical education will have on the next generation of practicing physicians.

The means by which new technologies are introduced to the medical community have also been considered as causes of excessive testing. Dixon described a four-step process of development, diffusion, domination, and disillusionment that he believed characterized the course that new technologies or clinical policies follow, as they proceed from introduction to widespread use and, on occasion, to eventual disfavor and replacement by a new practice or innovation.[8]

In his review, Dixon outlines the dangers of our current methods of technology or policy innovation. He points out that the medical literature frequently lags behind innovations and fails to provide timely guidance on appropriate use. Early literature is often limited to reports of potential applications of the new technology and uncontrolled studies, frequently using surrogate endpoints, to support the innovation's merit. Supported on physicians' willingness to accept some degree of empiricism and early literature, the policy or technology enters widespread use and general acceptance. It then frequently becomes difficult to perform the necessary controlled studies to determine the true value of the innovation because of the imperative that has developed to make the technology available to every patient. Where there is little perceived risk to the patient (eg, MRI scanning), the necessary studies may never be undertaken.

Other issues having an impact on physician use of diagnostic testing, which have been examined in the medical literature, include physician risk preference,[25, 27] the role of consultants,[49] the prevalence of subspecialists, and the fee-for-service health care delivery systems.[32]

MANAGED HEALTH CARE

The emergence and increasing penetrance of managed health care in the United States will undoubtedly have an impact on physician test ordering. Whereas many of the interventional studies performed in the 1970s and 1980s reported only transient effects and return to baseline test usage when the intervention was removed, HMOs now represent a major change in the practice environment. The development of a consistent relationship between the health maintenance organization administration and the physician will now allow interventions, such as incentives, feedback, and administrative changes, to be implemented on a permanent basis and may produce more substantial and long-lasting changes in physician practices, including diagnostic testing.

The impact of managed health care on physician practice is now being examined. Health maintenance organizations have previously demonstrated success in reducing physician use of diagnostic testing.[33] Variations in the rates of usage of cesarean sections[23] and rates of hospital admissions for patients with acute chest pain[29] have been studied. An unexpected finding of Pearson's study of patients with chest pain was that HMO membership was associated with higher rates of hospital admission for patients at low and medium risk for myocardial infarction, suggesting that organizational factors beyond financial incentives may have an important role in the admission decision.[29]

How managed health care will affect emergency physician practice and to what degree remains unanswered. Buffered from capitation and the administrative and financial incentives of HMOs, it is unlikely that emergency physicians in departments that see patients from both HMOs and other insurance groups will substantially change their practice. The impact of HMOs on emergency physician practice must be studied in settings were the emergency physician is vested in the administrative and financial workings of the organization. Such information is not yet available.

SUMMARY

In controlling the major portion of diagnostic testing, physicians are an appropriate target of efforts to modify physician practices and thereby reduce health care expenditures. The selection of diagnostic studies is a complex process involving numerous factors that include medical education, patient-physician relationship, and medical and medicolegal practice environments. Effective strategies to influence physician practices must acknowledge and address these factors to produce and maintain significant reductions in diagnostic testing and other focus areas. Managed health care will undoubtedly change the practice of medicine, including diagnostic test selection, but the magnitude of this influence in both the emergency department and other settings remains unknown.

REFERENCES

1. Noren J, Frazier T, Altman I, et al: Ambulatory medical care: A comparison of internists and family-general care practitioners. *N Engl J Med.* 1980;302:11–16.
2. Cummings KM, Frisof KB, Long MJ, et al: The effect of price information of physicians' test ordering behavior: ordering of diagnostic tests. *Med Care.* 1982;20:293–301.
3. Garnick DW, Hendricks AM, Brennan TA, et al: Can practice guidelines reduce the number and cost of malpractice claims? *JAMA.* 1991;266:2856–2860.
4. Eichna LW: Medical school education, 1975–1979: a student's perspective. *N Engl J Med.* 1980;303:727–734.
5. Masters SJ, McClean PM, Arcares JS, et al: Skull x-ray examination after head trauma: Recommendations by a multidisciplinary panel and validation study. *N Engl J Med.* 1987;316:84–91.
6. Lowe RA, Wood AB, Burney RE, et al: Rational ordering of serum electrolytes: Development of clinical criteria. *Ann Emerg Med.* 1987;16:260–269.
7. Martin SP, Donaldson MC, London CD, et al: Inputs into coronary care during 30 years: A cost effective study. *Ann Intern Med.* 1974;81:289–293.
8. Dixon AS: The evolution of clinical policies. *Med Care.* 1990;28:201–220.
9. Griner PF, Medical Housestaff, Strong Memorial Hospital: Use of laboratory tests in a teaching hospital: long term trends. *Ann Intern Med.* 1979;90:243–248.
10. Schroeder SA, Kenders K, Cooper JK, et al: Use of laboratory tests and pharmaceuticals. *JAMA.* 1973;225:969–973.
11. Williams SV, Eisenberg JM: A controlled trial to decrease the use of diagnostic tests. *J Gen Intern Med.* 1986;1:8–13.
12. Callaham M: Inaccuracy and the expense of the leukocyte count in making urgent clinical decisions. *Ann Emerg Med.* 1986;15:774–781.
13. Wong ET, Lincoln TL: Ready! Fire! . . . Aim! An inquiry into laboratory test ordering. *JAMA.* 1983;250:2510–2513.
14. Bertakis KD, Robbins JA: Utilization of hospital services:A comparison of internal medicine and family practice. *J Fam Pract.* 1989;28:91–96.
15. Goldberger AL, O'Konski M: Utility of the routine electrocardiogram before surgery and on routine hospital admission. *Ann Intern Med.* 1986;105:552–557.

16. Schroeder SA, Myers LP, McPhee SJ, et al: The failure of physician education as a cost containment strategy: The report of a prospective controlled trial at a university hospital. *JAMA.* 1984;252:225–230.
17. Williams SV, Eisenberg JM, Pascale LA, Kitz DS: Physicians' perception about unnecessary diagnostic tests. *Inquiry.* 1982;19:363–370.
18. Peterson SE, Rodin AE: Prudent laboratory usage, cost containment and high quality medical care: Are they compatible? *Hum Pathol.* 1987;18:105–108.
19. Fischer RP: Cervical radiographic evaluation of alert patients following blunt trauma. *Ann Emerg Med.* 1984;13:905–907.
20. Griner PF: Training house staff in effective laboratory use, in Connelly DP (ed): *Clinical Decisions and Laboratory Use.* Minneapolis: University of Minnesota Press; 1982:131–139.
21. Wachtel TJ, O'Sullivan P: Practice guidelines to reduce testing in the hospital. *J Gen Med.* 1990;5:335–341.
22. Politser PE: Medical education for a changing future: New concepts for revising texts. *Med Educ.* 1987;21:320–333.
23. Tussing AD, Wojtowycz MA: Health maintenance organizations, independent practice associations and cesarean section rates. *Health Services Res.* 1994;29(1):75–93.
24. Tape TG, Mushlin AI: The utility of routine chest radiographs. *Ann Intern Med.* 1986;104:663–670.
25. Ornstein SM, Market GP, Johnson AH, et al: The effect of physician personality on laboratory test ordering for hypertensive patients. *Med Care.* 1988;26:536–543.
26. Eisenberg JM: Modifying physician pattern of laboratory use, in Connelly DP (ed): *Clinical Decisions and Laboratory Use.* Minneapolis: University of Minnesota Press; 1982:145–157.
27. Nightingale SD: Risk preference and laboratory use. *Med Decision Making.* 1987;7:168–172.
28. Tierney WM, McDonald CJ, Martin DK, et al: Computerized display of past test results. *Ann Intern Med.* 1987;107:569–574.
29. Pearson SD, Lee TH, Lindsey E, et al: The impact of membership in a health maintenance organization on hospital admissions rates for acute chest pain. *Health Services Res.* 1994;29(1):60–73.
30. Marton KI, Tul V, Sox HC: Modifying test-ordering behavior in the outpatient medical clinic: a controlled trial of two educational interventions. *Arch Intern Med.* 1985;145:816–821.
31. Lawrence RS: The role of physician education in cost containment. *J Med Educ.* 1979;54:841–847.
32. Franks P, Clancy CM, Nutting PA: Gatekeeping revisited—protecting patients from overtreatment. *N Engl J Med.* 1992;327:424–429.
33. Berwick DM: Feedback reduces test use in a health maintenance organization. *JAMA.* 1986;255:1450–1454.
34. Gortmaker SL, Bickford AF, Mathewson HO, et al: A successful experiment to reduce unnecessary laboratory use in a community hospital. *Med Care.* 1988;26:631–642.
35. Griner PF, Liptzin B: Use of the laboratory in a teaching hospital. Implications for patient care, education and hospital costs. *Ann Intern Med.* 1971;75:157–163.

36. Kassirer JP: Our stubborn quest for diagnostic certainty: a cause of excessive testing. *N Engl J Med.* 1989;320:1489–1491.
37. Martin AR, Wolf MA, Thibodeau LA, et al: A trial of two strategies to modify the test ordering behavior of medical residents. *N Engl J Med.* 1980;303:1330–1336.
38. Tierney WM, Miller ME, McDonald CJ: The effect on test ordering of informing physicians of the charges for outpatient diagnostic tests. *N Engl J Med.* 1990;322:1499–1504.
39. Kroenke K, Hanley JF, Copley JB, et al: Improving housestaff ordering of three common laboratory tests. *Med Care.* 1987;25:928–935.
40. Badgett RG, Hansen CJ, Rogers CS: Clinical usage of the leukocyte count in emergency room decision making. *J Gen Intern Med.* 1990;5:198–202.
41. Feinstein AR: The 'chagrin factor' and qualitative decision analysis. *Arch Intern Med.* 1985;145:1257–1259.
42. Bessen HA, Rothstein RJ: Futility of skull radiography for nontraumatic conditions. *Ann Emerg Med.* 1982;11:605–609.
43. Bell RS, Loop JW: The utility and futility of radiographic skull examination for trauma. *N Engl J Med.* 1971;284:236–239.
44. Meadow WL, Lantos J, Tanz RR, et al: Ought ''standard care'' be the ''standard of care?'' *Am J Dis Child.* 1993;147:40–44.
45. Greene HL, Goldberg RJ, Beattie H, et al: Physician attitude toward cost containment: the missing piece of the puzzle. *Arch Intern Med.* 1989;149:1966–1968.
46. Erban SB, Kinman JL, Schwartz S: Routine use of prothrombin and partial thromboplastin times. *JAMA.* 1989;262:2428–2432.
47. Griner PF: Treatment of acute pulmonary edema: conventional or intensive care. *Ann Intern Med.* 1972;77:501–506.
48. Eisenberg JM, Williams SV, Garner L, et al: Computer based audit to detect and correct overutilization of laboratory tests. *Med Care.* 1977;15:915–921.
49. Braham RL, Ron A, Ruchlin HS, et al: Diagnostic test restraint and the specialty consultation. *J Gen Intern Med.* 1990;5:95–103.
50. Hudson JI, Braslow JB: Cost containment education efforts in United States medical schools. *J Med Educ.* 1979;54:835–840.

Chapter

The Pediatric Patient

Bruce W. Rosenthal

This chapter describes normative laboratory data for selected biologic variables pertinent to the emergency department setting, and the age- and sex-related differences that are observed in the developing child. The reader is reminded that "normal values" often differ among laboratory settings, owing to varying methods of sample collection and analysis. Accordingly, for valid test result interpretation, the normal reference ranges for a specific laboratory processing site must be reviewed.

BLOOD SAMPLE COLLECTION

Among other factors, RBC hemolysis occurring during blood sample collection contributes to inaccurate test results. The influence of hemolysis on the measurement of selected analytes is listed in Table 4–1.

Measures can be taken to limit RBC hemolysis and other sources of sample artifact. For capillary samples obtained by the "skin puncture technique," alcohol applied to the skin should be allowed to dry completely before puncture and blood droplets are collected. Excessive squeezing of the extremity or scraping of the collection tube across the surface of the skin should be avoided.[2] Adverse osmotic and mechanical effects on the RBC membrane are thus avoided.

For samples collected by venipuncture, hemolysis induced by turbulent blood flow can be minimized by utilizing a small-bore needle connected to a controlled, low-pressure vacuum source (eg, a commercially available vacuum container system). Measurement artifact can also be introduced by maneuvers that increase venous stasis or accumulation of by-products of local tissue metabolism.[3] Accordingly, prolonged tourniquet application and fist pumping should be avoided.

HEMATOLOGY

Normal values for the most commonly ordered hematology studies are given in Table 4–2. Hemoglobin and hematocrit values are highest at birth, presumably in compensation for the relative hypoxia of the

TABLE 4–1. THE EFFECT OF HEMOLYSIS ON SOME COMMONLY MEASURED ANALYTES

Analyte	Result	Analyte	Result
Acid phosphatase	↑	Creatine kinase	↑
Aldolase	↑	Iron	↑
Amino acids	↑	Lactate dehydrogenase	↑
Ammonia	↑	Magnesium	↑
Aspartate aminotransferase	↑	Phosphorus	↑
Alanine aminotransferase	↑	Potassium	↑
Bilirubin	↓	Total protein	↑

↑, increased; ↓, decreased.

From Hicks JM, Boeckx RL (eds): *Pediatric Clinical Chemistry*. Philadelphia: WB Saunders; 1984. With permission.[1]

intrauterine environment. This early RBC bounty is followed closely by a "physiologic anemia," in which hemoglobin values fall as low as 7 g/dL at 3 to 6 weeks of age in premature infants and 9.5 g/dL at 6 to 8 weeks of age in term infants.[4] However, similar values should be considered "abnormal" and indicative of a "symptomatic anemia" in patients with tachycardia, tachypnea, irritability, poor feeding, or even apnea. Thereafter, red cell mass gradually increases, reaching adult levels during adolescence. Racial differences exist also, with hemoglobin levels in black children averaging 0.5 g/dL lower than in white children of similar age and socioeconomic status.[4] Blood specimens obtained by the capillary or skin puncture technique often yield hemoglobin values 1 to 2 g/dL higher than those by peripheral or central venous samples.[4]

Age-related differences exist also with regard to total white blood cell (WBC) counts and to the proportion of the various circulating forms. Although wide range variation occurs in all age groups, the total WBC count is highest at birth and diminishes gradually throughout childhood. As a general guideline, total WBC counts exceeding 20,000 in the neonatal period and 15,000 thereafter should be considered abnormal. Except at birth, lymphocytes are the predominant cell population until the normal adult granulocyte predominance pattern is reached at about 7 years of age.

With regard to the red cell indices, mean corpuscular hemoglobin concentration remains relatively stable throughout childhood, whereas mean corpuscular volume (MCV) demonstrates considerable maturational change. Owing to the large RBC size of the newborn, the MCV is highest at birth, reaching a nadir at about 6 months of age and rising thereafter. Beyond infancy, the lower limits of normal for MCV can be approximated by the formula 70 + age in years.

TABLE 4–2. HEMATOLOGIC VALUES DURING INFANCY AND CHILDHOOD

	Hemoglobin (g/dL)		Hematocrit (%)		Reticu-locytes	Leukocytes (WBC/mm³)[a]		Neutrophils (%)		Differential Counts				
										Lymphocytes (%)	*Eosinophils (%)*	*Monocytes (%)*		
Age	*Mean*	*Range*	*Mean*	*Range*	(%) Mean	*Mean*	*Range*	*Mean*	*Range*	*Mean*	*Mean*	*Mean*	MCV[b]	MCHC[c]
2 wk	16.5	12.0–20.0	50	42–66	1.0	12,000	(5000–21,000)	40	(40–80)	48	3	9	105	31
3 mo	12.0	9.5–14.5	36	31–41	1.0	12,000	(6000–18,00)	30		63	2	5	95	—
6 mo–6 y	12.0	10.5–14.0	37	33–42	1.0	10,000	(6000–15,000)	45		48	2	5	76–81	32–35
7–12 y	13.0	11.0–16.0	38	34–40	1.0	8000	(4500–13,500)	55		38	2	5	86	34
Adult														
Female	14.0	12.0–16.0	42	37–47	1.6	7500	(5000–10,000)	55	(35–70)	35	3	7	90	34
Male	16.0	14.0–18.0	47	42–52									88	34

[a]WBC = white blood cell.

[b]MCV = mean corpuscular volume.

[c]MCHC = mean corpuscular hemoglobin concentration.

From Behrman RE, Kliegman RM (eds): *Nelson Textbook of Pediatrics.* 14th ed. Philadelphia: WB Saunders; 1992. With permission.[4]

TABLE 4–3. NORMAL VALUES FOR SCREENING COAGULATION TESTS

Assay	Normal Adult	Term Neonate	Age at Which Adult Values Are Reached
aPTT (sec)	44	55 ± 10	2–9 mo
PT (sec)	13 (12–14)	16 (13–20)	1 wk

Other hematologic laboratory determinations pertinent to the pediatric patient in the emergency department include coagulation tests (Table 4–3) and sedimentation rates (Table 4–4).

CEREBROSPINAL FLUID

The cytology and chemistry of the cerebrospinal fluid (CSF) in the neonate are quite different from those in the older infant and child (Table 4–5). At birth, the CSF of a term infant may have up to 500 RBCs and 22 WBCs with a slight preponderance of polymorphonuclear leukocytes (PMNs). After the 1st month of life, normal CSF should contain no RBCs, at most 7 WBCs, and no more than a single PMN. Total protein concentration is highest at birth, but values decline to stable levels by 1 and 3 months of age in term and preterm infants, respectively. Cerebrospinal fluid glucose values are lower in neonates and infants, corresponding to the lower blood glucose values observed in these age groups.[5, 7, 8]

TABLE 4–4. ERYTHROCYTE SEDIMENTATION DATA

	Age		
		Adults	
Method	***Childhood (mm/hr)***	MALE (mm/hr)	FEMALE (mm/hr)
Westergreen	0–10	0–10	0–15
Wintrobe	0–20	0–9	0–20
Micro-ESR	1–8		

Data from Oski FA, DeAngelis CD, Feigan RD, et al (eds): *Principles and Practice of Pediatrics*. 2nd ed. Philadelphia: JB Lippincott; 1994; Prakash O, Mohan M: *Indian Pediatr.* 1990;27:1133–1138.[5, 6]

TABLE 4–5. CEREBROSPINAL FLUID COMPOSITION

	Age		
Test	*Preterm Neonate*	*Term Neonate*	*Child*
WBC (× 10^6 cells/L)	0–25	0–22	0–7
Polymorphonuclear count (%)	57	61	0
Glucose (mg/dL)	24–63	34–119	40–80
Protein (mg/dL)	65–150	20–170	5–40
Pressure (mm/H_2O) (decubitus position)			10–28

Data from Oski FA, et al, 1994[5]; Sarff LD, et al, 1976[7]; and Ellis R, 1994.[8]

Cerebrospinal fluid opening pressure values for relaxed patients in a flexed lateral decubitus position range between 10 and 28 cm H_2O.[9]

CHEMISTRIES

The reference intervals for selected clinical chemistry analytes are given in Table 4–6. Most age-related differences can be explained on the basis of maturing physiologic process or changing body mass. For example, total alkaline phosphatase and lactic dehydrogenase values reflect isoenzyme activity associated with skeletal growth and periods of rapid metabolic turnover. Thus, postpubertal levels of these variables are lower than at any other period during childhood.[1]

BLOOD GAS VALUES

Although reference data are limited, it appears likely that adult values for arterial blood gas measurements in children are reached just beyond the newborn period (Table 4–7). In selected clinical circumstances, arterialized capillary samples may provide valuable information about acid-base status and ventilatory exchange. Arterialized blood gas results from well-perfused neonates are shown in Table 4–8. Good correlation has been shown between capillary and arterial values for both pH and P_{CO_2}, but P_{O_2} results thus obtained should be viewed as minimum values at best.[13]

Measurements of central venous pH and P_{CO_2}[14] in critically ill patients and peripheral venous pH and P_{CO_2}[15] in healthy adults appear to correlate relatively well with arterial blood gas results. It is well established that arterial and venous measurements of oxygen tension correlate very poorly. Unfortunately, the validity of these measurements has never been established for the pediatric population.

URINALYSIS

Concentration and Dilution

Beyond infancy, the kidney is capable of achieving specific gravities as low as 1.001 during water diuresis or as high as 1.035 during states of volume depletion. Specific gravities of random urine specimens in healthy, nonstressed patients vary between 1.015 and 1.025, whereas ranges between 1.024 and 1.030 are typical following overnight fluid restriction.[1]

Blood and Protein

Some of the commonly used commercial dipstick methods for identifying heme-containing compounds in the urine are extremely sensitive, detecting as little as 0.02 to 0.03 mg/dL of free hemoglobin or about 15 to 20 erythrocytes per microliter. Thus, given the normal variability of urinary RBC excretion, trace reactions may be seen occasionally.[16]

Urinary protein excretion is highest in the neonatal period, declining in early childhood toward adult values. Accordingly, trace reactions to urinary protein (15 to 30 mg/dL) are common, and 1+ reactions (30 to 100 mg/dL) may be seen occasionally in very young children.[17] Stronger reactions are a cause of greater concern, but they may be attributable to a variety of nonpathologic factors including upright body posture, physical exertion, and increased urine concentration.[18]

Cellular Elements

Traditionally, visualization of more than three to five WBCs and one or two RBCs per high-power field, following urine centrifugation, has been considered abnormal. However, this semiquantitative methodology is associated with a significant degree of sampling error and unreliability. More accurate and reliable cell counts can be obtained utilizing unspun urine and a counting (hemocytometer) chamber. Thus measured, more than 10 WBCs[19, 20] and five RBCs per cubic millimeter[20] are considered to be abnormal.

TABLE 4–6. CLINICAL CHEMISTRY VALUES

	1–7 d	1 mo	3 mo	6 mo	1 y	3 y	6–9 y	10 y	Adult
ALT (U/L)	0–53	0–37						3–28	m: 7–46 f: 4–35
AST (U/L)	14–70				13–64	16–46		15–40	m: 8–46 f: 7–34
GGT (U/L)	13–198			m: 5–65 f: 5–35					m: 9–69 f: 3–33
ALK phos (U/L)		80–270				80–390	115–460	60–280	30–115
LDH (U/L)	40–348	150–360					130–300		m: 70–178 f: 42–166
Bilirubin (mg/dL)									
Pre-term (1—7d)	Full term (1—7d)	1 mo and older: Total <1.5							
0–1 d <8	<6	Direct <0.4							
1–2 d <12	<8								
3–5 d <16	<12								

Amylase (U/L)	5–65			35–125			40–125
Total protein (g/dL)	5.0–7.5						6.0–8.0
Albumin (g/L)	3.0–5.0				3.5–5.0		
Calcium, total (mg/dL)		8.0–11.0		8.5–10.5			
Calcium (ionized mmol?L)	1.17–1.41		1.32–1.58				1.17–6.32
Sodium (mEq/L)			135–145				
Potassium (mEq/L)	3.5–6.0				3.5–5.0		
Chloride (mEq/L)			100–110				
Bicarbonate (mEq/L)	18–25					20–28	
Blood urea nitrogen (mg/dL)		5–20					
Creatinine (mg/dL)	0.3–1.0	0.2–0.4		0.3–0.8		m: 0.4–1.5 f: 0.5–1.3	m: 0.6–1.3 f: 0.4–1.1

	Term neonate		
	<3d	3–7d	>7d
Glucose (mg/dL)	>35	>45	750

ALT—alanine aminotransferase.
AST—asparate aminotransferase.
GGT—gamma-glutamyl transferase.
ALK phos—alkaline phosphatase.
LDH—lactate dehydrogenase.
→ —Values obtain through adulthood.
Modified from Oski FA, De Angelis CD, Feigon RD, et al (eds): *Principles and Practice of Pediatrics,* 2nd ed. Philadelphia: JB Lippincott; 1994.[5]
Data from references 1, 10, and 11.

TABLE 4–7. ARTERIAL BLOOD GAS VALUES OF PATIENTS BREATHING ROOM AIR AT SEA LEVEL

	Adult/Child	1–7 Days after Birth
PaO_2 (mmHg)		
Normal	97	72–75
Acceptable	>80	>50
SaO_2		
Normal	98%	>90%
Acceptable	>95%	—
pH	7.35–7.45	7.35–7.40
$PaCO_2$ (mmHg)	35–45	33.35

From Shapiro BA, Peruzzi WT, Templin R (eds): *Clinical Application of Blood Gases.* 5th ed. Philadelphia: Mosby; 1994. With permission.[12]

TABLE 4–8. CAPILLARY BLOOD GAS VALUES IN THE NEONATE

	Arterial Blood Gas	Capillary Blood Gas
pH	7.38 ± 0.01	7.40 ± 0.01
PCO_2 (mmHg)	40.8 ± 1.1	39.5 ± 1.0
PO_2 (mmHg)	76.5 ± 2.3	52.3 ± 1.4

From Courtney SE, Weber KR, Breakie LA, et al: *Am J Dis Child.* 1990;144:168. With permission.[13] Copyright 1990, American Medical Association.

REFERENCES

1. Hicks JM, Boeckx RL (eds): *Pediatric Clinical Chemistry*. Philadelphia: WB Saunders; 1984.
2. National Committee for Clinical Laboratory Standards: *Procedures for the Collection of Diagnostic Blood Specimens by Skin Puncture,* 3rd ed., vol. 11, no. 11. Villanova, PA; 1991.
3. Bermes EW, Young DS: General laboratory techniques and principles, in Burtis CA, Ashwood ER (eds): *Teitz Textbook of Clinical Chemistry*. 3rd ed. Philadelphia: WB Saunders; 1991.
4. Behrman RE, Kliegman RM (eds): *Nelson Textbook of Pediatrics*. 14th ed. Philadelphia: WB Saunders; 1992.
5. Oski FA, DeAngelis CD, Feigan RD, et al (eds): *Principles and Practice of Pediatrics*. 2nd ed. Philadelphia: JB Lippincott; 1994.
6. Prakash O, Mohan M: Erythrocyte sedimentation rate: its use in pediatric practice. *Indian Pediatr*. 1990;27:1133–1138.
7. Sarff LD, Platt LH, McCracken GH: Cerebrospinal fluid evaluation in neonates: comparison of high-risk infants with and without meningitis. *J Pediatr*. 1976;88:273.
8. Klein JO: Neonatal sepsis. *Semin Pediatr Infect Dis*. 1994;5:3.
9. Ellis R: Lumbar cerebrospinal fluid opening pressure measured in a flexed lateral decubitus position in children. *Pediatrics*. 1994;93:622–623.
10. Meites S (ed): *Pediatric Clinical Chemistry*. 3rd ed. Washington, DC: American Association for Clinical Chemistry; 1988.
11. Schwartz GJ, Haycock GB, Spitzer A: Plasma creatinine and urea concentration in children: normal values for age and sex. *J Pediatr*. 1976;88:828–830.
12. Shapiro BA, Peruzzi WT, Templin R (eds): *Clinical Application of Blood Gases*. 5th ed. Philadelphia: Mosby; 1994.
13. Courtney SE, Weber KR, Breakie LA, et al: Capillary blood gases in the neonate. *Am J Dis Child*. 1990;144:168.
14. Phillips B, Peretz DI: A comparison of central venous and arterial blood gas values in the critically ill. *Ann Intern Med*. 1969;4:745.
15. Gambino SR: Normal values for adult human venous plasma pH and CO_2 content. *Tech Bull Med Tech*. 1959;29:132.
16. Norman ME: An office approach to hematuria and proteinuria. *Pediatr Clin North Am*. 1987;34:545.
17. Miltenyi M: Urinary protein excretion in healthy children. *Clin Nephrol*. 1979;12:216.
18. Vehaskari VM, Robson AM: Proteinuria, in Edelman CM (ed): *Pediatric Kidney Disease*. 2nd ed. Boston: Little, Brown; 1992.
19. Hoberman A, Wald ER, Reynolds EA, et al: Pyuria and bacteriuria in urine specimens obtained by catheter from young children with fever. *J Pediatr*. 1994;124:513.
20. Stansfield JM: The measurement and meaning of pyuria. *Arch Dis Child*. 1962;37:257.

Chapter

The Pregnant Patient

Michael Baumann

The human body undergoes remarkable changes during pregnancy. Under the influence of maternal as well as fetal hormones, the nonpregnant physiology is adapted to an environment safe for both mother and the developing fetus. Recognition of the physiologic and anatomic changes of pregnancy and their impact on clinical chemistry and hematology values is essential to the effective emergency treatment of the pregnant female.

COMPLETE BLOOD COUNT

There is a slowly progressive increase in maternal blood volume until approximately the 32nd week of gestation. The average increase is 40 to 50%.[1, 2] The increased blood volume is composed of plasma as well as cellular components and occurs to compensate for the fetal needs, the maternal loss at delivery, the increased skin flow that occurs during pregnancy, and the relative increase in kidney perfusion.

HEMATOCRIT

Many factors affect red blood cell (RBC) production, but the net result is a progressive increase in RBC mass until the third trimester. Because RBC production does not increase as much as blood volume, there is a dilutional anemia, resulting in a fall of the hematocrit of 10 to 15%.[2] Anemia in pregnancy has been defined as a hemoglobin concentration of less than 10 to 12 or a hematocrit less than 32. The hematocrit is quite variable and should be used with caution as the sole marker for anemia.

WHITE BLOOD CELLS

Leukocytosis occurs during normal pregnancy and has been variously reported to be in the 10,000 to 16,000 range. A good guideline is that the white blood cell (WBC) count typically doubles in the last two trimesters. White blood cell counts of 25,000 or greater have been reported at term. The increase in WBC count is due primarily to an increase in neutrophils and demargination rather than to an increase in production. Thus, the WBC count is difficult to use as a marker for infection in the pregnant female. Leukocytosis generally returns to normal within 1 to 2 weeks after delivery.

PLATELETS

The platelet count can remain normal or fall during pregnancy but is rarely less than the lower limit of normal. The mild thrombocytopenia is partially due to the dilutional effects of increased blood volume, whereas the platelet half-life remains stable.

COAGULATION STUDIES

Pregnancy is regarded as a "hypercoagulable state." The erythrocyte sedimentation rate increases on average to 78 mm/h, a change attributed to increased fibrinogen level and alteration in plasma proteins.

Fibrinogen increases to up to twice the nonpregnant value.[2, 3] A normal fibrinogen level in the third trimester should be regarded with suspicion and may be an indication of disseminated intravascular coagulation.

Coagulation factors VII, VIII, IX, and X also increase during pregnancy, while factor XI decreases slightly. Factor XIII is reduced up to 40%.[1, 2] These changes do not appear to have much effect on coagulation or coagulation studies—bleeding times, clotting times, PT, and PTT are all relatively normal during pregnancy.[1]

PLASMA PROTEINS

Total plasma protein concentration is decreased during pregnancy; this is the result of an expansion in the plasma volume and an unchanged rate of synthesis. The normal albumin-to-globulin ratio of 1.4:1 is decreased to about 1:1 in the pregnant state.

GENITOURINARY SYSTEM

An increase in renal plasma flow (RPF) as well as an increase in glomerular filtration rate (GFR) results in a decrease in blood urea nitrogen (BUN), serum creatinine, and uric acid levels. Renal plasma flow increases by as much as 25% in the first two trimesters; glomerular filtration rate increases even more, up to 50% through the third trimester. Typical BUN and creatinine levels in late pregnancy are <10 and 0.5, respectively.[4–6] Normal values for either BUN or creatinine in a pregnant female may actually reflect renal insufficiency.

The increased RPF and GFR often result in glycosuria. Although excess glucose in the urine is common during pregnancy, the finding mandates careful follow-up and a glucose tolerance test to assess for diabetes of pregnancy. Proteinuria in pregnancy is not considered abnormal until it exceeds 500 mg in a 24-hour urine collection.

ARTERIAL BLOOD GASES

Acid-base balance during pregnancy is one of compensated respiratory alkalosis. Progesterone directly stimulates the respiratory center of the medulla, causing an increase in respiratory rate. There is also an increase in tidal volume. The result is a decrease in the P_{CO_2} to the low 30s after the first trimester. The pH remains normal because of a compensatory increase in renal excretion of bicarbonate. The net effect is a decreased serum bicarbonate, a decreased P_{CO_2}, and an increased P_{O_2}.[1, 5, 15] A normal P_{CO_2} in the pregnant female should suggest respiratory acidosis and a potentially serious pulmonary problem.

CALCIUM, MAGNESIUM, PHOSPHORUS

The majority of calcium in the blood is in the bound state. The decrease in serum albumin concentration during pregnancy thus results in a lowered total serum calcium level. Ionized calcium, however, remains within the normal nonpregnant range throughout pregnancy.[8]

Magnesium has been reported to decrease in normal pregnancy but is generally believed to remain close to the lower limit of normal.[13, 14]

Phosphorus levels are unaffected by normal pregnancy.

SODIUM, POTASSIUM, CHLORIDE

Serum sodium levels in the pregnant female decrease by an average of 4 mEq/L as a result of the expanded plasma volume.[12]

Potassium and chloride levels are unchanged in the normal pregnancy.

LIVER AND PANCREATIC ENZYMES

Bilirubin levels during pregnancy have been reported in various studies to be increased, decreased, and unchanged. The unconjugated bilirubin may be decreased owing to the low serum albumin but it is usually within the nonpregnant normal range.

There is no reported change in AST, ALT, GGT, or LDH levels. These enzymes thus remain good markers for liver disease in pregnancy.

The alkaline phosphatase level is markedly elevated after the 20th week because of increased production of the placental component. Before the 20th week it remains within the nonpregnant normal range. Serum amylase levels are reported to be unchanged in pregnancy.[11] An elevated amylase level during the pregnant state should thus provoke consideration of the same diagnoses considered in the nonpregnant state. Different populations have been shown to have varying amylase levels, and the appropriate normal range should be used.

Total creatinine kinase levels show a modest decrease in pregnancy, but remain within the normal non-pregnant range.[11]

REFERENCES

1. Pearlman MD: Blunt abdominal trauma during pregnancy, in Tintinalli J (ed.): *Emergency Medicine: A Comprehensive Study Guide,* 3rd ed. New York: McGraw-Hill Inc; 1992; 60:414–417.
2. Peck T, Arias F: Hematologic changes associated with pregnancy. *Clin Obstet Gynecol.* 1979;22:785.
3. Chesley L: Plasma and red cell volumes during pregnancy. *Am J Obstet Gynecol.* 1972;112:440.
4. Caton W et al: Circulating red cell volume and body hematocrit in normal pregnancy and the puerperium. *Am J Obstet Gynecol.* 1951;61:1207.
5. Kydd D: Hydrogen ion concentration and acid-base equilibrium in normal pregnancy. *J Biol Chem.* 1931;91:63.
6. Mack HC: The plasma proteins. *Clin Obstet Gynecol.* 1960;3:336.
7. Venning E: Endocrine changes in normal pregnancy. *Am J Med.* 1955;19:712.
8. Pitkin R: Calcium metabolism in pregnancy: A review. *Am J Obstet Gynecol.* 1975;121:724.
9. Winston J, Levitt M: Renal function, renal disease and pregnancy, in *Complications of Pregnancy: Medical, Surgical, Gynecologic, Psychosocial and Perinatal.* 4th ed. Baltimore: Williams & Wilkins; 1991.
10. Hytten F, Lind T: *Diagnostic Indices in Pregnancy.* Basel: Ciba-Geigy; 1973.
11. Lind T: Clinical chemistry of pregnancy. *Adv Clin Chem.* 1980;21:1.
12. Gallery E, Brown M: Control of sodium excretion in human pregnancy. *Am J Kidney Dis.* 1987;9:290.

13. Spatling L, Disch G, Classen H: Magnesium in pregnant women and the newborn. *Mag Res.* 1989;2:4.
14. Kurzel R: Serum magnesium levels in pregnancy and preterm labor. *Am J Perinatol.* 1991;8:119.
15. Lim V, Katz A, Lindheimer M: Acid-base metabolism in pregnancy. *Am J Physiol.* 1976;231:1764.

Chapter

The Elderly Patient

Linda A. Smith

One of every five patients seen in the emergency department (ED) is 65 years of age or older,[1] and approximately half of elderly patients presenting to the ED are hospitalized.[2, 3] Appropriate diagnostic testing in the geriatric patient presents a challenge to even the most experienced clinician. Illnesses often appear atypically in the elderly, and the usual indications for testing have not been validated in this population. Moreover, reference intervals for laboratory tests have traditionally been derived from studies of healthy young adults. These established norms (Table 6–1) may or may not, however, apply equally well to the population of elderly patients.

This chapter addresses some of the diagnostic tests that are commonly ordered for geriatric patients in the ED, emphasizing the normal physiologic changes associated with aging; the often atypical presentations of

TABLE 6–1. LABORATORY PARAMETERS THAT REMAIN UNCHANGED WITH AGING

Electrolytes (sodium, potassium, chloride, bicarbonate)
Creatinine
Blood urea nitrogen
Hemoglobin and hematocrit
White blood cell count
Platelet count
Coagulation studies (PT and PTT)
Liver function tests

disease in geriatric patients; and the interpretations of test results as they apply to the geriatric patients.

RESPIRATORY SYSTEM

Predictable age-related changes in pulmonary physiology[1, 4, 5] include a progressive decline in the forced vital capacity (FVC) and forced expiratory volume at 1 second (FEV_1). This results mostly from the loss of elastic recoil of the chest wall and elastic tissues of the lung. There is also a progressive loss of alveolar units, resulting in cystic areas of the aging lung described as "senile emphysema." The progressive loss of surface area also results in changes in the normal ventilation/perfusion ratio, shunting of blood, impaired oxygen uptake, and arterial desaturation. As a result, the normal arterial oxygen tension falls approximately 0.4% per year.[6]

Sorbini and coworkers[6] suggest a formula to predict PaO_2 in the elderly:

$$\text{Predicted } PaO_2 = 109 - (0.43 \times \text{age})$$

A simple guideline is that the expected PaO_2 of a patient 70 years of age is simply 70 mm Hg, with a range of ±10 mm Hg. The PaO_2 at other ages differs from this value in an inverse fashion by about 1 mm Hg per year. Thus, at 65 years of age the expected PaO_2 is 75 mm Hg (± 10 mm Hg).[1]

The alveolar-arterial oxygen gradient (A-a gradient) has been evaluated in a number of studies and has been found to be increased in healthy geriatric subjects.[8–10] The arterial CO_2 tension ($PaCO_2$) does not change with age, but central and peripheral chemoreceptor function does decline with age, resulting in a diminished ventilatory response to hypoxia and acidosis.

The change in normal arterial blood gas (ABG) values with age is crucial in interpreting results in certain patients. Pulmonary embolism (PE) in particular can be a difficult diagnosis to make in the elderly. Bell and coworkers[7] identified undiagnosed PE in as many as 90% of previously hospitalized elderly adults at autopsy.[7] Table 6–2 presents an approach to the evaluation of ABG and A-a gradient values in the elderly.

CARDIOVASCULAR SYSTEM

The effects of aging on the electrocardiogram (ECG) have been reviewed concisely by Simonson[11] and others.[12, 13] The amplitude of the

TABLE 6–2. INTERPRETATION OF ABG AND A-a GRADIENT VALUES IN THE ELDERLY

Predicted PaO_2 = 109 − 0.43 (age)	
or	
expected PaO_2 of 70 (± 10 mm Hg) at age 70	
with variation of 1 mm Hg per year	
Calculated A-a gradient	
$[FIO_2 \times (PB - 47 \text{ mm Hg})] / [(PaCO_2 \times 1.25) - PaO_2)]$	
Predicted A-a gradient	
Nonelderly upper limits of normal	= 8 to 20 mm Hg
Elderly upper limits of normal	= 20 to 28 mm Hg
Skoridin[9]	4 + (age/4)
Mellemgaard[10]	2.5 + 0.21 (age)
Harris[11]	0.264 (age) − 0.43

QRS and T waves decreases with aging, and the axis shifts leftward. Fibrosis of the septum may result in the loss of R wave amplitude in V_1 and V_2. Electrocardiographic intervals remain nearly constant. Of interest is an increase in premature beats.[14]

Atypical presentation of myocardial infection (MI) is the rule rather than the exception in patients over the age of 85. A number of studies have shown that the most frequently reported symptom in patients over 85 with MI is shortness of breath rather than chest pain.[15, 16] In addition, symptoms of confusion, syncope, stroke, and weakness in association with MI increase in frequency with aging.[15]

In addition to atypical presentations, complicating the diagnosis of acute MI in the ED setting are nonspecific T wave inversions and ST segment depressions, which are common in the elderly. The use of serum cardiac enzymes for the diagnosis of acute MI is unchanged in the elderly.

RENAL AND METABOLIC SYSTEMS

The kidneys of older patients are smaller in size and have a lower blood flow and glomerular filtration rate (GFR) than those of younger individuals. Renal blood flow decreases about 10% per decade, so that the 600 mL/min blood flow typical of a 20 year old is only 300/min in the average 80 year old.[17] This decrease is believed to be related both to decreased cardiac output and age-related vascular changes. The GFR falls at a rate of about 8 to 10 mL/min/1.7 m²/decade. The fall in creatinine clearance is not accompanied by a rise in the serum creatinine concentration because lean body mass also decreases with age.[18] The blood urea nitrogen also remains relatively unchanged with aging.[19, 20]

A higher threshold exists for the appearance of glycosuria in the older patient with hyperglycemia. Glycosuria may not occur until serum glucose levels are greater than 300 mg/dL, implying that urine glucose testing may be unreliable as a screen or monitor of diabetic control in elderly patients.[32]

Electrolyte balance and serum electrolyte levels remain constant despite the aging process. Two noteworthy articles address electrolyte abnormalities in the elderly. Lowe and associates,[21] in a study of serum electrolyte determinations in ED patients, found that although more than half of patients had one or more values that fell outside the normal range, only about 15% affected diagnosis or therapy. These clinically significant abnormalities occurred most frequently in patients 81 to 90 years of age and next most frequently in the group 71 to 80 years of age. From these data, Lowe and associates suggested a set of "optimal criteria" with a 98.8% sensitivity for identifying such clinically significant electrolyte abnormalities. A second study, by Singal and coworkers,[21a] attempted to validate Lowe's criteria in a population of elderly patients (defined as age 55 years and older) and had similar results.

The urinary tract is the most common site of infection in the elderly and the most common source of bacteremia in this population.[24–29] Asymptomatic bacteria is reported in up to 60% of all older adult patients, depending on the age, comorbid diseases, and living situation (ie, institutionalized or not).[22–25] Bacteriuria is often associated with fecal incontinence, perineal contamination, poor hygiene, inadequate emptying of bladder, and previous instrumentation. Urine specimens for culture should be collected from a new catheter because indwelling catheters are often colonized with multiple bacterial specimens that may not represent true bladder flora.

ENDOCRINE SYSTEM

Diabetes is easily and commonly tested for in the ED. Random blood glucose levels less than 150 mg/dL are generally accepted as normal in the elderly. Values over 200 mg/dL are taken to indicate definite diabetes, whereas blood values between 150 and 200 mg/dL are considered "borderline" and require further evaluation.[33]

HEMATOLOGIC SYSTEM

The complete blood count (CBC) is one of the most commonly ordered blood tests in the ED. The interpretation of hemoglobin and hematocrit values in the elderly patient is controversial. Some argue that senile anemias occur as a consequence of aging,[34] whereas others argue that anemia in the elderly is more often a consequence of disease and that physicians' lack of concern about anemia in the elderly serves only to delay the diagnosis of disease.[35–37]

The total leukocyte count does not change significantly with aging.[38] Although there may be a slight decrease in the leukocyte count, values fall within accepted norms. The slight decline is usually attributed to a decrease in the total lymphocyte count.[39] The neutrophils of elderly individuals secrete fewer enzymes and are activated more slowly in response to infection. There is a diminished ability to kill phagocytized bacteria.[27, 40]

Platelets circulate in normal numbers despite advancing age, although structural and functional changes have been described. Prothrombin time (PT), partial thromboplastin time (PTT), and bleeding time are not affected by age in healthy individuals.[41]

There is little agreement on the interpretation of the erythrocyte sedimentation rate (ESR) in the elderly. Older studies utilized the Wintrobe sedimentation rate; newer studies have utilized the Westergren ESR. Furthermore, the ESR may be affected by bleeding disorders, malignancy, and serum protein levels, among other factors, all of which must be taken into account when attempting to define the role of age per se. Nevertheless, some investigators accept an ESR of 40 mm/h as "normal" in the aged patient, indicating at least that the ESR tends to increase with age.[42, 43]

GASTROINTESTINAL SYSTEM

Functionally, the liver remains unchanged with aging.[44, 45] The anatomy and function of the gallbladder also change minimally.

Elderly patients free of pancreatic disease have normal pancreatic exocrine function when compared with a healthy control population.[46]

Liver function tests remain essentially stable in the elderly. A study of 43 healthy subjects over the age of 50 who had normal liver biopsy findings showed no correlation between age and values for serum bilirubin, alkaline phosphatase, or SGOT.[4]

In another study, Tietz and colleagues[47] selected 167 presumably healthy individuals over the age of 60 and measured liver enzyme activities over a 2-year period. Among individuals who remained healthy over this period, there were small increases in alkaline phosphatase (men: 4.8%; women: 6.3%), AST (men: 2.7%; women: 1.4%), ALT (men: −1.7%; women: 2.8%), and LDH (men: 1.1%; women: 3.6%).

SUMMARY

Although the indications for diagnostic testing have not been as well established in the elderly as in younger adults, this population should probably be considered a "high-yield" group for unsuspected clinically significant laboratory abnormalities. Medication use and underlying illness occur more frequently in the elderly, and the presentation of many illnesses may be deceptively nonspecific. The clinician must be aware of the alterations in laboratory values that occur with normal aging to distinguish manifestations of illness from the changes of the normal aging process.

REFERENCES

1. Bosker G, Schwartz GR, Jones JS, et al: *Geriatric Emergency Medicine*. St. Louis: Mosby-Yearbook; 1993:20.
2. Eliastram M: Elderly patients in the emergency department. *Ann Emerg Med.* 1989;18:1222–1229.
3. Lowenstein SR, Crescenzi CA, Kern DC, et al: Care of the elderly in the emergency department. *Ann Emerg Med.* 1986;15:528–535.
4. Hazzard WR, Bierman EL, Blass JP, et al: *Principles of Geriatric Medicine and Gerontology.* New York: McGraw-Hill; 1994:555.
5. Turner JM, Mead J, Wohl ME: Elasticity of human lungs in relation to age. *J Appl Physiol.* 1968;25(6):664–671.
6. Sorbini CA, Grassi V, Solinas E, Muiesan G: Arterial oxygen tension in relation to age in healthy subjects. *Respiration.* 1968;25:3–13.
7. Bell WR, Simon TL, DeMets DL: The clinical features of submassive and massive pulmonary emboli. *Am J Med.* 1977;62:355–360.
8. Skorodin MS: Respiratory disease and A-a gradient measurement. *JAMA.* 1984;252(10):1344.
9. Mellemgaard K: The alveolar-arterial oxygen difference: Its size and components in normal man. *Acta Physiol Scand.* 1966;67:10–20.
10. Harris EA, Kenyon AM, Nisbet HD, et al: The normal alveolar-arterial oxygen tension gradient in man. *Clin Sci Mol Med.* 1974;496:89–104.
11. Simonsen E: The effect of age on the electrocardiogram. *Am J Cardiol.* 1972;29:64–73.
12. Bachman S, Sparrow D, Smith LK: Effect of aging on the electrocardiogram. *Am J Cardiol.* 1981;48:513–516.
13. Rodstein M: The ECG in old age: Implications for diagnosis, therapy, and prognosis. *Geriatrics.* 1977;32:76–79.
14. Okajima M, Scholmerich P, Simonson E: Frequency of premature beats. *Minn Med.* 1960;751–753.
15. Bayer AJ, Chadha JS, Faraq RR, et al: Changing presentation of myocardial infarction with increasing old age. *J Am Geriatr Soc.* 1986;34:263–266.
16. Pathy MS: Clinical presentation of myocardial infarction in the elderly. *Br Heart J.* 1967;29:190–199.

17. Sobel JD: Bacterial etiologic agents in the pathogenesis of urinary tract infection. *Med Clin North Am.* 1991;75:253.
18. Rowe JW, Andres R, Tobin JD, et al: The effect of age on creatinine clearance in man: A cross-sectional and longitudinal study. *J Gerontol.* 1976;31(2):155–163.
19. Campbell H, Greene WJ, Keyser JW, et al: Pilot survey of hemoglobin and plasma urea concentrations in a random sample of adults in Wales. 1965–66. *Br J Prev Soc Med.* 1968;22:41–49.
20. Kane RL, Ouslander JG, Abrass IB: *Essentials of Clinical Geriatrics.* New York: McGraw-Hill; 1994:60.
21. Lowe RA, Wood AB, Burney RE, et al: Rational ordering of serum electrolytes: development of clinical criteria. *Ann Emerg Med.* 1987;16(3):260–269.
21a. Singal BM, Hedges JR, Succop PA: Prediction of electrolyte abnormalities in elderly emergency patients. *Ann Em Med.* 1991;20(9):964–968.
22. Abrutyn E, Mossey J, Levison M, et al: Epidemiology of asymptomatic bacteriuria in elderly women. *J Am Geriatr Soc.* 1991;39:388–393.
23. Nicolle LE, Brunka J, McIntyre M, et al: Asymptomatic bacteriuria, urinary antibody, and survival in the institutionalized elderly. *J Am Geriatr Soc.* 1992;40:607–613.
24. Abrutyn E, Mossey J, Berlin JA, et al: Does asymptomatic bacteriuria predict mortality and does antimicrobial treatment reduce mortality in elderly women? *Ann Intern Med.* 1994;120:827–833.
25. Tronetti PS, Gracely EJ, Boscia JA: Lack of association between medication use and the presence or absence of bacteriuria in elderly women. *J Am Geriatr Soc.* 1990;38:1199–1202.
26. Jacobs G: Infectious disease emergencies in the geriatric population. *Clin Geriatr Med.* 1993;9(3):559–575.
27. Whitelaw DA, Rayner BL, Wilcox PA: Community-acquired bacteria in the elderly: a prospective study of 121 cases. *J Am Geriatr Soc.* 1992;40:996–1000.
28. Esposito AL, Gleckman RA, Cram S, et al: Community-acquired bacteremia in the elderly: Analysis of 100 consecutive episodes. *J Am Geriatr Soc.* 1980;28(7):315–319.
29. McCue JD: Gram negative bacillary bacteremia in the elderly: Incidence, ecology, etiology, and mortality. *J Am Geriatr Soc.* 1987;35:213–218.
30. Setra U, Serventi I, Lorenz P: Bacteremia in a long term care facility: Spectrum and mortality. *Arch Intern Med.* 1984;144:1633–1635.
31. Gleckman R, Blagg N, Hibert D, et al: Community acquired bacteremia urosepsis in the elderly patients: A prospective study of 34 consecutive episodes. *J Urol.* 1982;128:79–81.
32. Garner BC: Guide to changing lab values in elders. *Geriatr Nurs.* 1989;10:144–145.
33. Caird FI: Problems of interpretation of laboratory findings in the old. *Br Med J.* 1973;4:348–351.
34. Lipschitz DA, Mitchell CO, Thompson C: The anemia of senescence. *Am J Hematol.* 1981;11:47–54.
35. Htoo MS, Kofkoff RL, Freedman ML: Erythrocyte parameters in the elderly: An argument against new geriatric normal values. *J Am Geriatr Soc.* 1979;27(12):547–551.

36. Smith JS, Whitelaw DM: Hemoglobin values in aged men. *Can Med Assoc.* 1971;105:816–825.
37. Kelly A, Munan L: Haematologic profile of natural populations: Red cell parameters. *Br J Hematol.* 1977;35:153–160.
38. Kelso T: Laboratory values in the elderly. *Emerg Med Clin North Am.* 1990;8(2):241–254.
39. Carrd FI, Andrews GR, Gallie TB: The leukocyte count in old age. *Age Aging.* 1972;1:239–244.
40. McLauglin B et al: Age related differences in granulocyte chemotaxis and degranulation. *Clin Sci.* 1986;70:59.
41. Jeppesen ME: Laboratory values for the elderly, in Carnevali DL, Patrick M (eds): *Nursing Management for the Elderly,* 2nd ed. Philadelphia: JB Lippincott; 1986;102–142.
42. Schapera R: The significance of erythrocyte sedimentation rates in aged persons. *S Afr Med J.* 1982;62(11):394–396.
43. Sparrow D, Rowe JW, Silbert JE: Cross-sectional and longitudinal changes in the erythrocyte sedimentation rate in men. *J Gerontol.* 1981;36(2):180–184.
44. Popper H: Aging and the liver, in Popper H, Schaffner F (eds): *Progress in Liver Diseases.* Vol 8. New York: Grune & Stratton; 1986:659.
45. Tauch H, Sato T: Hepatic cells of the aged, in Kitani K (ed): *Liver and Aging.* Amsterdam: Elsevier-North Holland: 1978;3.
46. Gullo L, Ventrucci M, Naldoni P, et al: Aging and exocrine pancreatic function. *J Am Geriatr Soc.* 1986;34:790–792.
47. Tietz NW, Wekstein DR, Shuey DF, et al: A two-year longitudinal reference range study for selected serum enzymes in a population more than 60 years of age. *J Am Geriatr Soc.* 1984;32:563–571.

SECTION II
CLINICAL SYNDROMES

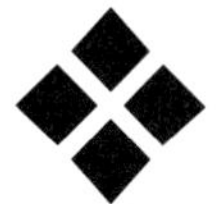

Chapter

Ischemic Chest Pain

Joyce Mitchell-Savinsky

Chest pain is a common presenting complaint in the emergency department (ED), accounting for approximately 2% of patient visits.[1] Although the etiologies of chest pain syndromes are numerous, the serious and life-threatening causes include myocardial ischemia/infarction (MI), pulmonary embolism, and aortic dissection or rupture. Of these, MI is the most common, and missed MI accounts for almost 20% of the total malpractice dollars forfeited in this country.[1] This chapter focuses on diagnostic testing in the evaluation of myocardial pain syndromes.

MISSED DIAGNOSIS

In determining the methods utilized to diagnose MI, it is also important to define the characteristics of that group of patients in whom diagnosis is most frequently missed and to recognize the consequences of missed diagnosis. A conservative approach to patients with suspected MI results in frequent admissions to the hospital and in particular to intensive care units (ICUs). Of these, only approximately 30% "rule in" as having an acute MI (AMI). Despite this, about 4 to 8% of patients presenting to the ED with AMI are incorrectly diagnosed and discharged.[2, 3]

In a multicenter prospective investigation, Lee and associates[2] studied 3077 ED patients with chest pain. Of the 477 patients with AMI, 96% were admitted and 4% were discharged. Acute myocardial infarction was diagnosed by characteristic enzyme changes [creatine kinase (CK)-MB and LDH1 > LDH2], ECGs demonstrating new pathologic Q waves, ^{99m}Tc stannous pyrophosphate scans showing focal uptake in the absence of a history of previous MI, or sudden death within 72 hours in discharged patients. They found that patients with missed AMIs had less typical symptoms, no previous history of angina or MI, and less suspect ECGs, and were significantly younger. ECGs were misread in eight patients (23% of the missed AMIs), and nine (26%) were discharged despite the fact that the physician recognized ischemic symptoms or ECG changes of ischemia. More importantly, patients with missed AMI had significantly higher death rates than those with MI who were admitted to the hospital. The investigators did not study the impact of myocardial salvage techniques on the morbidity of those patients discharged and therefore untreated.

Zarling and colleagues[4] suggested that incorrect diagnoses are caused by atypical presentation, misleading diagnostic tests, and failure to consider the diagnosis. In their retrospective study of autopsy cases, premortem diagnostic accuracy was greatly decreased in those cases with either atypical history or nondiagnostic laboratory studies.

DIAGNOSTIC TESTING

The clinician has relied classically on the patient's history as well as specific diagnostic tests when determining the presence or absence of MI. Of these tests, the ECG has been the standard initial evaluation tool. In addition, cardiac enzymes [CK, lactate dehydrogenase (LDH), and their isoenzymes], serum myoglobin, two-dimensional echocardiography, and nuclear scans have been studied in the initial evaluation of chest pain patients. For emergency physicians, the ECG and measurement of serum CK and its MB isoenzymes provide the most useful tools because of their availability on a 24-hour basis in most hospitals.

ELECTROCARDIOGRAM

Difficulties in the use of the ECG at first presentation in the diagnosis of AMI have been reported.[5] Normal initial ECGs have been reported in 6 to 10% of patients with AMI.[6]

In 1976, McGuinness and coworkers[5] studied 877 patients admitted to the ICU with suspected AMI that was thought to have occurred within the previous 48 hours. Of the 449 patients with diagnosed AMI at the end of the ICU stay, initial ECGs were definitive in 51%, probable in 27%, doubtful in 7%, and negative (''no MI'') in 16%. Serial ECGs helped to diagnose MI in 84%. The investigators concluded that the ECG becomes more helpful with time in the diagnosis of MI and that serial ECGs rather than a single initial examination were vital in the overall assessment.

Rouan and associates[6] specifically looked at the incidence of normal or nonspecific ECGs in patients subsequently diagnosed with AMI. They clearly defined subgroups of ECG findings and excluded from the nonspecific/normal subgroup any patients with ST elevations or Q waves in more than two leads; new ischemia or strain; old infarction, ischemia, or strain; or any other old or new abnormality. In this study they found that 7% of patients with documented AMI presented with an initial ECG finding of nonspecific ST-T wave change or normal. In following these patients they also found that the peak CK levels were significantly lower and that there tended to be a lower death rate. The mortality rate of patients who were mistakenly discharged, however, was higher than that of those who were admitted. From these follow-up data, these investigators suggested that patients admitted with suspected AMI and normal ECGs might be considered for a step-down unit rather than an ICU because the infarcts tended to be smaller and the number of complications was fewer.

Other studies have examined the correlation between the initial ECG and in-hospital life-threatening complications of AMI. Of 167 patients in a study by Brush and associates,[7] 15% had negative ECGs initially and yet proved to have infarction. Electrocardiograms were considered positive if they had evidence of infarction, ischemia, strain, left ventricular hypertrophy (LVH), left bundle branch block (LBBB), or paced rhythm. The life-threatening complications of ventricular fibrillation (VF), sustained ventricular tachycardia (VT), or heart block occurred in 42 of 302 patients with an initially positive ECG and in one of 167 with an initially negative ECG. They concluded that patients suspected of MI who have negative initial ECGs can be admitted to a step-down unit. It is important to note, however, that, of these 167 patients with negative initial ECGs, only 25 proved to have AMI and one developed ventricular tachycardia (VT).

Slater and colleagues[8] found that AMI evolved in 11 of 107 patients (10%) with normal ECGs and six of 73 patients (8%) with only minimal ECG changes. Compared with those patients in their study with initially abnormal ECGs, there were significantly fewer life-threatening complications in the group of MI patients with normal or minimally abnormal initial ECGs. These workers suggested from their study that these patients, therefore, may be appropriate for admission to an intermediate care unit rather than the ICU. Complications in these patients included two episodes of sustained VT, one respiratory arrest, two heart blocks, and one asystole; one would therefore question the safety of admitting these patients to a step-down unit.

Zalenski and coworkers[9] found that patients with initially positive ECGs were older, had a history of MIs and a greater incidence of AMIs, and had more immediate life-threatening complications than patients with initially negative ECGs.

From these and other studies[10] it is clear that initially normal or minimally changed ECGs do not exclude the diagnosis of AMI and that AMI is present in up to 20% of patients. The issue of whether patients with suspected AMI and minimal or no ECGs can be admitted to a step-down unit because of the reduced incidence of life-threatening complications remains in question. The life-threatening aspects of potential complications still require that patients be monitored carefully. The quality and capabilities of each hospital's step-down unit will determine whether these patients with normal or minimally abnormal ECGs can be managed in that setting.

CREATINE KINASE AND ITS ISOENZYMES

The correlation of AMI with an elevation of a serum enzyme level was first noted with serum aspartate aminotransferase in 1954. The association of CK elevation and AMI was discovered in 1960, and the MB isoenzymes were discovered in the early 1970s. The classic use of CK and its MB isoenzyme is among the World Health Organization's criteria for the diagnosis of AMI. Detectable elevations of CK-MB can also be seen in conditions of muscle breakdown, such as marathon running and muscular dystrophy, because modest amounts of this isoenzyme are found in skeletal muscle.[11] Total CK rise as well as an elevation of CK-MB has been reported in aortic dissection.[12, 13]

Emergency department evaluation of acute chest pain patients focuses mainly on CK and its isoenzymes because they are released more rapidly than other myocardial enzymes after acute cellular damage. Creatine kinase and CK-MB begin to rise at 4 to 8 hours after the onset of MI, with peaks at 12 to 24 and 12 to 20 hours, respectively. Lactate dehydrogenase begins to rise at 8 to 12 hours after onset of myocardial damage, with peaks at 72 to 144 hours; aspartate aminotransferase (AST) begins its rise at 8 to 12 hours, with peaks at 18 to 36 hours.[11] Thus, for detection of myocardial damage, the CK/CK-MB measurement provides the earliest changes.

The utilization of CK and CK-MB in the evaluation of chest pain in the ED has been studied and discussed extensively. Multiple investigations have demonstrated that total CK determinations in the ED are of no value in the decision-making process of diagnosing AMI.[14–19] Patients presenting early in the course of the evolution of AMI might not demonstrate CK elevations, and a high total CK might originate in other body tissues, especially skeletal muscle.

Lee and colleagues[17] studied the utility of CK-MB measurements in patients with acute chest pain whose total CKs were elevated. Of 639 patients studied, 105 were subsequently diagnosed with AMI. The sensitivity of an isolated CK-MB measurement in this study was 34%, but it was better than an isolated total CK determination. The sensitivities of both total CK and CK-MB were improved in patients who presented more than 4 hours after the onset of symptoms. The investigators concluded that measurements of these enzymes in a single blood sample were not sufficiently sensitive to be used in the decision to admit or discharge acute chest pain patients.

A study with similar findings was done by Hedges and colleagues,[20] who also evaluated the CK-MB as a screening tool in patients who would otherwise have been discharged from the ED. Three of five AMI patients who were discharged (60%) had elevated CK-MBs. These investigators concluded that, although enzyme determinations were not useful in admission decision making, they might be useful as a final screening evaluation in patients who would otherwise be discharged.

In a pilot study, Gibler and associates[21] utilized a newer immunochemical assay for CK-MB. This assay is reportedly more sensitive than the standard electrophoretic method and, therefore, could be expected to detect smaller rises in CK-MB. In this study of 183 patients, they found that the sensitivity of a single initial CK-MB was only 50 to 62.1% but increased to 83 to 96.4% 3 hours later. This suggested that the test might be useful in preventing some AMI patients from being discharged from the ED, increasing the number of thrombolysis candidates, and helping to decide which patients should be admitted to the CCU.

Several studies have evaluated other complications of enzyme and isoenzyme rises. Shell and coworkers[22] found that the CK-MB rose earlier in patients with nontransmural rather than transmural MIs. They suggested that this reflected reperfusion to ischemic myocardium. Frequently these patients present with nondiagnostic ECGs, and an earlier CK-MB rise may be useful in the ED evaluation of these patients.

Yusuf and associates[23] looked at the significance of an elevated CK-MB level in the presence of normal total CK in patients with AMI. The failure to detect elevated total CK was thought to be due to sampling frequency in patients with small MIs. The study included serial measurements of enzymes and is therefore not freely applicable to ED evaluations. The findings suggested that some small MIs may remain undiagnosed if the MB isoenzyme is not also measured despite a normal total CK.

Quale and colleagues[19] utilized total CK determinations 6 hours apart to decide whether patients believed to have unstable angina were at risk for MI and therefore required ICU admission. Of 96 patients with normal consecutive enzyme levels, only 2% developed AMI. They suggested that this evaluation could reduce the number of ICU admissions in patients with unstable angina.

The conclusion from these studies is that, although utilized in the ultimate diagnosis of AMI, initial CK and CK-MB determinations in the ED cannot be relied upon to rule out a diagnosis of AMI or to enable the clinician to confidently make decisions to discharge a patient or arrange for admission to an immediate care setting.

OTHER TESTING

Myoglobin

Serum myoglobin has been found to rise rapidly after myocardial damage and to peak at 4 hours.[24, 25] Gibler and associates[25] compared myoglobin with CK-MB in the evaluation of 59 chest pain patients presenting to the ED and subsequently admitted. Of 21 patients with documented AMI, myoglobin levels were positive in 13 initial presentations and in 21 patients at 3 hours, whereas CK-MB was elevated in 3 and 19, respectively. Other studies have confirmed this rapid rise in myoglobin, but it has not become a routine tool in the evaluation of chest pain patients. This is due to its lack of specificity because of its presence in striated muscle. In addition, rapid assays for myoglobin are not widely available on a 24-hour basis.

Nuclear Scans

Mace[26] reported on a small group of patients with acute chest pain who were evaluated in the ED by portable thallium scintigraphy. There were six positive scans, three indicating infarction and three ischemia. Normal scans were seen in 14 patients who had undiagnosed chest pain at discharge and one who had angina. The limitations of scintigraphy included expense and low availability, failure to identify lesions <2.5 cm in diameter, and the fact that defects are best detected only within the first 6 hours. Its specificity is also limited,[27] especially in distinguishing old from new defects.[26]

Echocardiography

Studies of the echocardiographic detection of regional wall motion abnormalities (RWMA) support the use of this tool in the evaluation of selected patients who present to the ED with acute chest pain.

Horowitz and colleagues[27] studied 80 patients admitted to ICU with chest pain, excluding those patients who had other reasons for having RWMA (eg, valvular heart disease, previous MI, cardiomyopathy, significant pericardial effusion). Of 33 patients with documented AMI, 31 demonstrated RMWA; the remaining two had uncomplicated non-transmural AMIs. Of 32 patients without AMI, five had RWMA; three of these patients had significant coronary artery disease documented on subsequent angiography. Adequate echocardiograms could not be obtained in 15 patients. These investigators also noted that serious cardiovascular complications were seen only in the patients who demonstrated RWMA (10 of 36). The investigators suggested that echocardiography was useful in identifying a high-risk group of patients who were likely to have AMI and to experience complications requiring ICU admission. They noted, however, that this diagnostic tool was limited by technical difficulties in obtaining high-quality studies. The presence of previous MI may also cause persistent RWMA, thus decreasing specificity.

Arvan and Varat[28] compared echocardiography with ECG in the diagnosis of non-Q wave AMI. Restricting their population to those patients who had no preexisting causes of RWMA, they found accuracy of the two modalities to be comparable.

Sabia and coworkers[29] studied 180 patients presenting to the ED with acute chest pain to determine whether echocardiography was superior to conventional methods in diagnosing AMI and limiting hospital admissions. Technically adequate echocardiograms were obtained in 29 of 30 patients with enzyme-documented AMI. Of these 29, 27 demonstrated RWMA. Nine had initial diagnostic ECG changes, three had normal ECGs, and ten had nonspecific ECG changes. Of 13 patients who developed in-hospital complications, all had demonstrated RWMA but only four had had diagnostic ECGs initially. In those patients without AMI, 60 of 140 with technically adequate studies had RWMA; these included 31 patients with previous MI and 32 patients with already diagnosed significant coronary artery disease. These investigators concluded that the detection of RWMA was superior to conventional diagnostic methods in evaluating acute chest pain patients in diagnosing AMI, predicting in-hospital complications, and reducing hospital admissions. Two patients with AMI were not detected by echocardiography, and, although these patients did not suffer subsequent complications, the effect on morbidity had they been discharged was not addressed.

Echocardiography in the ED holds promise for in-depth evaluation of patients with chest pain, but serious limitations remain. The availability not only of equipment and technicians but also of expert interpretation may be limited.[30] Technically adequate studies are not always possible. Previous conditions, especially past MI, may alter regional wall motion and yield false-positives. False-negatives have been found in all studies thus far.

CONCLUSION

The emergency physician is often the ''gatekeeper'' in deciding which chest pain patients are admitted and which are admitted to either an ICU or a step-down unit. The tools available for the evaluation of these patients in the ED appear to have limited diagnostic accuracy. The initial ECG and CK/CK-MB analyses are readily available but lack the sensitivity to be used as the sole determinants for admission. Echocardiography shows promise in the early diagnosis of AMI but at present is limited in its availability; more important, it too has been demonstrated to be less than 100% accurate. The emergency physician is left, therefore, employing clinical judgment as the foundation of decision making in evaluating chest pain patients for admission.

REFERENCES

1. Hedges JR, Kobernick MS: Detection of myocardial ischemia/infarction in the emergency department patient with chest discomfort. *Emerg Med Clinics North Am.* 1988;6(2):317–340.
2. Lee TH, Rouan GW, Weisberg MC, et al: Clinical characteristics and natural history of patients with acute myocardial infarction sent home from the emergency room. *Am J Cardiol.* 1987;60:219–224.
3. Schor S, Behar S, Modan B, et al: Disposition of presumed coronary patients from an emergency room: A follow-up study. *JAMA.* 1976;236:941–943.
4. Zarling EJ, Sexton H, Milnor P: Failure to diagnose acute myocardial infarction: The clinicopathologic experience at a large community hospital. *JAMA.* 1983;250(9):1177–1181.
5. McGuinness JB, Begg TB, Semple T: First electrocardiogram in recent myocardial infarction. *Br Med J.* 1976;2:449–451.
6. Rouan GW, Lee TH, Cook EF, et al: Clinical characteristics and outcome of acute myocardial infarction in patients with initially normal or nonspecific electrocardiograms (a report from the Multicenter Chest Pain Study). *Am J Cardiol.* 1989;64:1087–1092.
7. Brush JE Jr, Brand DA, Acampora D, et al: Use of the initial electrocardiogram to predict in-hospital complications of acute myocardial infarction. *N Engl J Med.* 1985;312:1137–1141.
8. Slater DK, Hlatky MA, Mark DB, et al: Outcome in suspected acute myocar-

dial infarction with normal or minimally abnormal admission electrocardiographic findings. *Am J Cardiol.* 1987;60:766–770.

9. Zalenski RJ, Sloan EP, Chen EH, et al: The emergency department ECG and immediately life-threatening complications in initially uncomplicated suspected myocardial ischemia. *Ann Emerg Med.* 1988;17:221–226.
10. Stark ME, Vacek JL: The initial electrocardiogram during admission for myocardial infarction: Use as a predictor of clinical course and facility utilization. *Arch Intern Med.* 1987;147:843–846.
11. Lee TH, Goldman L: Serum enzyme assays in the diagnosis of acute myocardial infarction: Recommendations based on a quantitative analysis. *Ann Intern Med.* 1986;105:221–233.
12. Davidson E, Weinberger I, Rotenberg Z, et al: Elevated serum creatine kinase levels: An early diagnostic sign of acute dissection of the aorta. *Arch Intern Med.* 1988;148:2184–2186.
13. Georgiou D, Brundage BH: Chest pain and increased CK-MB enzyme levels. *Chest.* 1990;98:442–447.
14. Seager SB: Cardiac enzymes in the evaluation of chest pain. *Ann Emerg Med.* 1980;9:346–349.
15. Viskin S, Heller K, Gheva D, et al: The importance of creatine kinase determination in identifying acute myocardial infarction among patients complaining of chest pain in an emergency room. *Cardiology.* 1987;74:100–110.
16. Nowakowski JF: Use of cardiac enzymes in the evaluation of acute chest pain. *Ann Emerg Med.* 1986;15:354–360.
17. Lee TH, Weisberg MC, Cook EF, et al: Evaluation of creatine kinase and creatine kinase-MB for diagnosing myocardial infarction: Clinical impact in the emergency room. *Arch Intern Med.* 1987;147:115–121.
18. Lee TH, Cook EF, Weisberg M, et al: Acute chest pain in the emergency room: Identification and examination of low-risk patients. *Arch Intern Med.* 1985;145:65–69.
19. Quale J, Kimmelstiel C, Lipschik G, et al: Use of sequential cardiac enzyme analysis in stratification of risk for myocardial infarction in patients with unstable angina. *Arch Intern Med.* 1988;148:1277–1279.
20. Hedges JR, Rouan GW, Toltzis R, et al: Use of cardiac enzymes identifies patients with acute myocardial infarction otherwise unrecognized in the emergency department. *Ann Emerg Med.* 1987;16:248–252.
21. Gibler WB, Lewis LM, Erb RE, et al: Early detection of acute myocardial infarction in patients presenting with chest pain and nondiagnostic ECGs: Serial CK-MB sampling in the emergency department. *Ann Emerg Med.* 1990;19:1359–1366.
22. Shell WE, DeWood MA, Kligerman M, et al: Early appearance of MB-creatine kinase activity in nontransmural myocardial infarction detected by a sensitive assay for the isoenzyme. *Am J Med.* 1981;71:254–262.
23. Yusuf S, Collins R, Lin L, et al: Significance of elevated MB isoenzyme with normal creatine kinase in acute myocardial infarction. *Am J Cardiol.* 1987;59:245–250.
24. Roxin L-E, Cullhed I, Groth T, et al: The value of serum myoglobin determinations in the early diagnosis of acute myocardial infarction. *Acta Med Scand.* 1984;215:417–425.

25. Gibler WB, Gibler CD, Weinshenker E, et al: Myoglobin as an early indicator of acute myocardial infarction. *Ann Emerg Med.* 1987;16:851–856.
26. Mace SE: Thallium myocardial scanning in the emergency department evaluation of chest pain. *Am J Emerg Med.* 1989;7:321–328.
27. Horowitz RS, Morganroth J, Parrotto C, et al: Immediate diagnosis of acute myocardial infarction by two-dimensional echocardiography. *Circulation.* 1982;65(2):323–329.
28. Arvan S, Varat MA: Two-dimensional echocardiography versus surface electrocardiography for the diagnosis of acute non-Q wave myocardial infarction. *Am Heart J.* 1985;110:44–49.
29. Sabia P, Afrookteh A, Touchstone DA, et al: Value of regional wall motion abnormality in the emergency room diagnosis of acute myocardial infarction: A prospective study using two-dimensional echocardiography. *Circulation.* 1991;84(suppl I):I-85–I-92.
30. Hauser AM: The emerging role of echocardiography in the emergency department. *Ann Emerg Med.* 1989;18:1298–1303.

Chapter

Dyspnea

Tom Kearns

Fundamental to the practice of emergency medicine is a rapid assessment and institution of measures to ensure adequate airway and acceptable oxygenation and ventilation.

The causes of dyspnea are legion, and the diagnostic approach to each patient must be individualized. Fortunately, most cases do not present a diagnostic dilemma. In general, the diagnosis will be apparent after the history and physical examination, with a chest roentgenogram and arterial blood gases or pulse oximetry evaluations providing confirmation and initial estimate of the severity of the disease process. Ancillary studies serve primarily to confirm the clinical impression, quantify the magnitude of the illness, and gauge the response to the therapeutic interventions.

Nevertheless, there are occasions when the cause of a patient's respiratory distress is not readily apparent on initial evaluation, and diagnostic testing becomes vital in patient management. This chapter offers a framework for the integration of diagnostic testing into the initial evaluation of the dyspneic patient. For this purpose, the causes of dyspnea can be divided into four broad categories: lesions of the upper respiratory tract, the lower respiratory tract, and the cardiovascular system, and central nervous system and metabolic derangements.

UPPER RESPIRATORY TRACT

Compromise of the upper airway classically occurs as acute or subacute dyspnea with or without stridor. Causes include foreign bodies, croup, angioedema, epiglottitis/supraglottitis, abscess, hematoma, and traumatic airway disruption. These conditions all have the potential to progress unpredictably to complete airway obstruction and respiratory arrest.

A lateral soft-tissue radiograph of the neck is the initial diagnostic procedure of choice. This study should be undertaken in the emergency department (ED) while the patient is being closely monitored. A portable film is usually adequate but if the patient must leave the department he or she must be accompanied by a physician and resuscitation equipment.

Important findings associated with *epiglottitis* and *supraglottitis* include ‘‘thumblike’’ swelling of the epiglottis and swelling of the aryepiglottic folds. Unfortunately, radiographs are of limited sensitivity in adults with epiglottis; one retrospective study found a true-positive rate of only 43%.[1] In *croup,* a gradual narrowing of the air column, the ‘‘steeple sign,’’ is usually well demonstrated on an anteroposterior (AP) view.[2] An important, though nonspecific, clue to the diagnosis of upper airway compromise, particularly in children, is dilation of the hypopharynx; this is especially pronounced in croup.[3]

Aspirated foreign bodies are an important cause of dyspnea, particularly in children less than 4 years old. Ingested coins impacted in the esophagus may also cause airway compromise by impinging on the child's relatively compressible adjacent trachea. Plain radiographs and direct and indirect visualization have been the mainstays of diagnosis.

Traditionally, one expects esophageal coins to lie in the coronal plane (seen as a disk on an AP radiograph) and tracheal coins in the sagittal plane (seen as a line on an AP film). These findings lack specificity, however, and should not be completely relied upon. An important next step is to obtain a lateral radiograph, which may demonstrate the coin within the tracheal air column. Indirect evidence of foreign bodies includes atelectasis, pneumonia, and asymmetric hyperinflation. Suspected radiolucent esophageal foreign bodies should be evaluated with a barium swallow. Some investigators have suggested having the patient swallow a barium-soaked cotton ball to identify an impaction, but this test also lacks documented sensitivity and specificity and may be dangerous. Fluoroscopy to detect mediastinal abnormalities and asymmetric lung expansion is a useful and often-overlooked modality.[4]

Definitive diagnosis is based on visualization of the upper airway by direct, indirect, or fiberoptic laryngoscopy and possibly bronchoscopy or endoscopy. Because of the risk of precipitating complete airway obstruction, these procedures should be carried out under controlled conditions by a consultant who is prepared to create a surgical airway if necessary.

LOWER RESPIRATORY TRACT

Fortunately, most causes of dyspnea associated with lower respiratory tract pathology are apparent on physical examination and chest roentgenography.

The combination of fever, purulent sputum, and radiographic infiltrate points to pneumonia. Experienced clinicians are familiar with the many variations in the clinical presentation of this common entity. The challenge here lies not so much in making the general diagnosis but rather in identifying specific pathogens. Although lacking in sensitivity and specificity,[5] certain classic radiologic patterns may be helpful. Lobar consolidation with pneumococcal disease, multiple densities progressing to abscess formation from *Staphylococcus aureus*, bulging of the interlobar fissures in *Klebsiella* pneumonia, and the features of the atypical pneumonia syndrome have all been well described.[6]

Presumptive microbiologic diagnosis is usually based on an examination of spontaneously expectorated, induced, or nasotracheally suctioned sputum. Infectious disease texts have long recommended the usefulness of this procedure, and it does have the advantage of being readily available in the ED. Because of the difficulty of obtaining specimens that originate in the lower respiratory tract and the inevitable contamination from passing through the oropharyngeal secretions, this time-honored test must be viewed with some caution. There is in fact a paucity of data supporting the reliability of sputum Gram stains. In previously healthy children and adults with a classic presentation and a sputum Gram stain showing gram-positive diplococci and sheets of polymorphonuclear leukocytes, initial therapy with pencillin for presumed streptococcal pneumonia is warranted.[7] For all other patients, however, basing initial antibiotic therapy solely on the Gram stain is not definite. One is better advised to use an antibiotic with a broad-enough spectrum to cover all likely pathogens, with further modifications of therapy after culture and sensitivity results are available and the clinical response to empiric treatment can be observed.[8]

Other diagnostic modalities may provide additional information. For example, blood cultures are positive in 10 to 30% of patients with pneumonia and may provide a specific microbiologic diagnosis, particularly in immunocompromised and elderly patients.[11]

In selected cases the accuracy of sputum examination may be improved by obtaining specimens via bronchoalveolar lavage or transtracheal aspiration. Although the results are not readily available in the ED, direct fluorescent antibody testing of sputum is the test of choice for diagnosing *Legionella* pneumonia.

Special mention should be made of *Pneumocystis carinii* pneumonia, as 70 to 80% of patients with the acquired immunodeficiency syndrome will eventually be infected. The chest x-ray findings, although nonspecific, typically consist of bilateral perihilar infiltrates extending peripherally. Definitive diagnosis is made by visualizing the organism on a silver stain of material obtained by bronchoscopy and bronchoalveolar lavage.[12] Immunofluorescent staining techniques may improve the accuracy of induced sputum examination but are still investigational.[13] Elevated serum lactate dehydrogenase levels may provide a useful clue in the ED.[14] Gallium scanning may be positive even before the development of radiographic signs, with a sensitivity of 98%; however, specificity, calculated from pooled data, is only 47%.[15, 16]

It is also important for the emergency physician to consider the increasing prevalence of tuberculosis in indigent and immigrant populations, as well as in immunocompromised patients, and to obtain sputum acid-fast bacillus stains and cultures on patients who are at risk. If a pleural effusion is present, diagnostic thoracentesis may be undertaken in the ED. The yield of this test is greatly increased by combining it with a pleural biopsy, a procedure generally performed by a pulmonary or infectious disease consultant.

Another very common cause of dyspnea in emergency patients is exacerbation of both reactive and obstructive airway disease (asthma and chronic obstructive pulmonary disease). Useful diagnostic information may be obtained by bedside spirometry and measurement of peak expiratory flow rates. In particular, peak flows have become popular in the ED because they are inexpensive and easy to perform and often eliminate the need for arterial blood gases.[17] Their utility in predicting the need for admission is controversial.[18, 19]

Chest radiographs rule out pneumonia and pneumothorax as causes of dyspnea in patients with airway disease are part of many evaluations. However, routinely evaluating chest radiographs in both adult and child asthmatics has been questioned. The incidence of clinically significant radiograph findings in adults presenting with uncomplicated asthma has been reported to range from 0 to 2.2%.[20–22] The data from pediatric studies are more difficult to interpret, being largely retrospective and strongly biased toward sicker patients.[23, 24] Nevertheless, the incidence of important findings is quite low. Some patients, over the course of many years, will make multiple ED visits for acute asthma exacerbations. If radiographs are taken every time, the cumulative radiation dose may become significant. Therefore, radiography should be withheld in patients in whom the diagnosis is established and who respond appropriately to bronchodilators.

CARDIOVASCULAR CAUSES

The major cardiovascular causes of dyspnea include congestive heart failure, myocardial ischemia, pericardial tamponade, and pulmonary embolism.

Diagnostic testing of patients with congestive heart failure (CHF) relies primarily on the CXR, ECG, and ABG. Appropriate laboratory studies might include CBC, electrolytes, cardiac enzymes, and, in cases of new-onset CHF, thyroid function studies. Pulse oximetry is a useful continuous monitor of the patient's condition. Although early reports suggested that pulse oximetry is unreliable under conditions of low cardiac output,[25] further data have demonstrated clinical reliability in patients with cardiac indices <2.2 L/min/m^2.[26, 27] In practice, if the oximetry signal is adequate, the saturation measurement will also be reasonably accurate. Invasive monitoring and measurement of pulmonary artery pressures may prove invaluable but are generally reserved for the ICU setting.

Because dyspnea is well described as an anginal equivalent,[28] if the history is suggestive one should obtain an ECG and consider admission to a monitored setting for serial ECGs and cardiac enzyme determinations and appropriate cardiac evaluation.

Cardiac tamponade of any etiology may occur with dyspnea. Emergency department ultrasonography is gaining popularity as a rapid, accurate, and noninvasive means of establishing the presence or absence of pericardial fluid.[29] In appropriate cases, central venous access should be obtained for pressure monitoring and diagnostic or therapeutic pericardiocentesis performed. The aspiration of nonclotting blood may indicate a pericardial source but, as with so many other findings in clinical medicine, this lacks sensitivity and specificity and should not be solely relied upon.

The signs and symptoms of pulmonary embolism (PE) are protean, and noninvasive diagnostic testing often lacks specificity. The difficulty is compounded by the fact that effective therapy is available but is associated with significant morbidity. When one is considering the diagnosis of PE, the initial studies are CXR, ABG, and ECG. The chest x-ray, although often abnormal, generally demonstrates a nonspecific effusion or infiltrate or elevation of a hemidiaphragm. Two radiologic findings suggestive of PE are a wedge-shaped pleural-based density

(Hampton hump) and relative oligemia with a dilated pulmonary artery (Westermark sign), but these are seen quite uncommonly. The most frequent ABG finding is hypoxia, seen in 88% of patients.[31] However, 12% of patients with proven PE have a normal Po_2. Some clinicians have proposed that an increased A-a gradient (normal 10 to 30 mmHg) may be a more sensitive indicator of PE, but others have termed this unreliable.[29] The ECG may show evidence of acute right heart strain with the classic $S_1Q_3T_3$ pattern but is usually unhelpful.

Unfortunately, the common diagnostic modalities are either insensitive or nonspecific for PE, and no single finding or combination of findings has proved adequate for definitive confirmation or exclusion.

The diagnostic standard has long been pulmonary angiography. One should proceed directly to pulmonary angiography in cases of high clinical suspicion, hemodynamic compromise, or relative contraindication to anticoagulation. Regrettably, the test itself has significant morbidity and mortality, with one large series reporting a 3.5% incidence of major complications and a 0.2% mortality rate.[30] Allergy to intravenous contrast material limits its utility in some individuals. In addition, emergency angiography may not be available in small or rural hospitals.

Ventilation/perfusion (V/Q) lung scans are minimally invasive, have a negligible morbidity, are relatively easy to perform, and are widely available. As such they have assumed a role as the primary diagnostic modality in most patients with suspected pulmonary emboli. A normal perfusion scan excludes significant pulmonary emboli with a sensitivity approaching 100%.[34] The presence of multiple perfusion defects that are not matched with ventilation defects (ie, a high-probability scan) has been associated with at least an 88% incidence of angiographically documented pulmonary emboli, with a sensitivity of 41% and a specificity of 97%.[35] In the appropriate clinical setting this is accepted by most clinicians as adequate proof of a pulmonary embolus (PE) and mandates treatment.

Unfortunately, most scans fall into the low- or intermediate-probability categories. These findings are neither sensitive enough to rule out PE nor specific enough to confirm the diagnosis and thus have limited clinical utility.[36] Indeed, in patients with a high clinical suspicion of PE, even a normal perfusion scan may miss 2%.[37] A more detailed discussion of V/Q scanning appears elsewhere in this volume.

Recognizing the limitations of V/Q scanning, some workers have suggested an alternative strategy of evaluating patients for deep venous thrombosis on the theory that the absence of significant thrombi militates against PE. When combined with a low-probability scan and a low clinical suspicion, this is perhaps sufficient evidence to exclude PE with adequate sensitivity.[40] Nevertheless, the data are limited and the current consensus favors pulmonary angiography in questionable cases.[41] The details of both invasive and noninvasive lower-extremity testing are also covered elsewhere in this volume.

CENTRAL NERVOUS SYSTEM AND METABOLIC CAUSES

Hyperventilation in compensation for metabolic acidosis may appear as dyspnea, and characteristic abnormalities of the arterial blood gas values point to the correct diagnosis. This vital information is not provided by pulse oximetry. Although it is rapidly gaining popularity in EDS because of its noninvasive nature, pulse oximetry is still primarily a *monitoring* and not a *diagnostic* tool.

Centrally mediated anxiety-related hyperventilation—panic disorder or the so-called hyperventilation syndrome—commonly appears as dyspnea. Despite the intensity of the symptoms, no specific diagnostic test is available.[42] Classically, one expects the arterial blood gas values to demonstrate a relatively pure respiratory alkalosis, although there are no data to support the sensitivity or specificity of this finding. In young patients in whom the diagnosis can be made on clinical grounds, no diagnostic testing is necessary. Nevertheless, because there are a number of serious conditions that may be confused with hyperventilation, if there is any doubt about the diagnosis an evaluation consisting of ABG, CXR, ECG, electrolytes, and CBC has been recommended.[38]

Any one of a number of disorders causing hypoxia or hypoxemia, especially when they occur acutely, may appear with dyspnea. Once again, the ABG, coupled with a CBC, usually provides a working diagnosis. Of particular importance to the emergency physician are the toxidromes involving limitation of oxygen-carrying capacity and the inhibition of cellular respiration. Carbon monoxide (CO) levels as low as 10% may occur with dyspnea as part of the symptom complex.[44] The diagnosis is made by measuring a carboxyhemoglobin level. One should remember that ABGs measure Po_2, which is normal in CO poisoning, as is the *calculated* oxygen saturation. It is important to obtain an oxygen saturation *measured* with a cooximeter. Pulse oximetry registers carboxyhemoglobin as oxyglobin and yields a falsely elevated saturation reading.[45] Patients with poisoning with cyanide or hydrogen sulfide may present in a similar manner.

REFERENCES

1. Stankiewicz JA, Bowes AK: Croup and epiglottitis: a radiologic study. *Laryngoscope*. 1985;95:1159.

2. Keats TE: *Emergency Radiology*. Chicago: Year Book Medical Publishers; 1984;177.
3. Swischuk LE: *Emergency Radiology of the Acutely Ill or Injured Child.* Baltimore: Williams & Wilkins: 1986:137.
4. Mu L, Sun DQ, He P, et al: Radiological diagnosis of aspirated foreign bodies in children: review of 343 cases. *J Laryngol Otol.* 1990;104(10):778–782.
5. MacFarlane JT, Miller AC, Roderick Smith WH, et al: Comparative radiographic features of community acquired legionnaire's disease, pneumococcal pneumonia, mycoplasma pneumonia and psittacosis. *Thorax.* 1984;39:28.
6. Schillinger D: Pneumonia, in Harwood-Nuss A, Linden C, Luten RC, et al (eds): *The Clinical Practice of Emergency Medicine.* Philadelphia: JB Lippincott; 1991:910.
7. Gleckman R, De Vita J, Hibert D, et al: Sputum gram stain assessment in community-acquired bacteremic pneumonia. *J Clin Microbiol.* 1988;26:846.
8. Brown RB: Management of pneumonia by emergency department physicians. *Curr Ther Res.* 1991;49:651.
9. Perlino CA: Laboratory diagnosis of pneumonia due to *Streptococcus pneumoniae. J Infectious Dis.* 1984;150:139.
10. Guzzetta P, Toews GB, Robertson KJ, et al: Rapid diagnosis of community-acquired bacterial pneumonia. *Am Rev Respir Dis.* 1983;128:461.
11. Bentley DW: Bacterial pneumonia in the elderly: clinical features, diagnosis, etiology, and treatment. *Gerontology.* 1984;30:297.
12. Ognibene FP, Shelhamer J, Gill V, et al: The diagnosis of *pneumocystis carinii* pneumonia in patients with the acquired immunodeficiency syndrome using subsegmental bronchoalveolar lavage. *Am Rev Respir Dis.* 1984;129:929–932.
13. Kovacs JA, Ng VL, Masur H, et al: Diagnosis of *Pneumocystis carinii* pneumonia: improved detection in sputum with use of monoclonal antibodies. *N Engl J Med.* 1988;318:589.
14. Bukata WR: Medical emergencies in AIDS patients. *Emerg Med Acute Care Essays.* 1991;15(6):1.
15. Murray JF, Felton CP, Garay SM, et al: Pulmonary complications of the acquired immunodeficiency syndrome. *N Engl J Med.* 1984;318:1682–1688.
16. Woolfenden JM, Carrasquillo JA, Larson SM, et al: Acquired immunodeficiency syndrome: GA-67 citrate imaging. *Radiology.* 1987;162:383.
17. Martin TG, Elenbaas RM, Pingleton SH: Use of peak expiratory flow rates to eliminate unnecessary arterial blood gases in acute asthma. *Ann Emerg Med.* 1982;11:70.
18. Thomas MG, Elenbaas RM, Pingleton SH: Failure of peak expiratory flow rate to predict hospital admission in acute asthma. *Ann Emerg Med.* 1982;11:466.
19. Nowak RM, Pensler MI, Sarkar DD, et al: Comparison of peak expiratory flow and FEV_1 admission criteria for acute bronchial asthma. *Ann Emerg Med.* 1982;11:25.
20. Zieverink SE, Harper AP, Holden RW, et al: Emergency room radiography of asthma: an efficacy study. *Radiology.* 1982;145:27–29.
21. Findley LJ, Sahn SA: The value of chest roentgenograms in acute asthma in adults. *Chest.* 1981;80:535–536.

22. Aronson S, Gennis P, Kelly D, et al: The value of routine admission chest radiographs in adult asthmatics. *Ann Emerg Med.* 1989;18:1206–1208.
23. Rushton AR: The role of the chest radiograph in the management of childhood asthma. *Clin Pedlatr.* 1982;21:325–328.
24. Zieverink SE, Harper AP, Holden RW, et al: Emergency room radiography of asthma: an efficacy study. *Radiology.* 1982;145:27–29.
25. Tremper KK, Hufstedler SM, Barker SJ, et al: Accuracy of a pulse oximeter in the critically ill adult: effect of temperature and hemodynamics. *Anesthesiology.* 1985;63:A175.
26. Palve H, Vuori A: Pulse oximetry during low cardiac output and hypothermia states immediately after open heart surgery. *Crit Care Med.* 1989;17:66.
27. Palve H, Vuori A: Accuracy of three pulse oximeters at low cardiac index and peripheral temperature. *Crit Care Med.* 1991;19:560.
28. Murphy C: Acute dyspnea, in Callaham (ed): *Current Therapy in Emergency Medicine.* Toronto: B. C. Decker; 1984;177.
29. Whye D, Barish R, Almquist T, et al: Echocardiographic diagnosis of acute pericardial effusion in penetrating chest trauma. *Am J Emerg Med.* 1988;6:21.
30. Allingham JD: A clinically oriented nomogram for the derivation and interpretation of alveolar-arterial oxygen gradients. *Ann Emerg Med.* 1980;9:323.
31. The urokinase pulmonary embolism trial; a national cooperative study. *Circulation.* 1973;47(suppl 2):1–108.
32. Overton DT, Bocka J: The alveolar-arterial gradient in patients with documented pulmonary embolism. *Ann Emerg Med.* 1987;16:501.
33. Mills SR, Jackson DC, Older RA, et al: The incidence, etiologies, and avoidance of complications of pulmonary angiography in a large series. *Radiology.* 1980;136:295.
34. Fedullo PF, Shure D: Pulmonary vascular imaging. *Clin Chest Med.* 1987;8:53.
35. The PIOPED Investigators: Value of the ventilation/perfusion scan in acute pulmonary embolism. *JAMA.* 1990;263:2753.
36. Hull RD, Hirsh J, Carter CJ, et al: Diagnostic value of ventilation-perfusion lung scanning in patients with suspected pulmonary embolism. *Chest.* 1985;88:819.
37. Hull RD, Raskob GE, et al: Low-probability lung scan findings: A need for change. *Ann Intern Med.* 1991;114(2):142.
38. McBride H, La Morte WW, Menzoian JO, et al: Can ventilation-perfusion scans accurately diagnose acute pulmonary embolism? *Arch Surg.* 1986;121:754–757.
39. Sors H, Safran D, Stern M, et al: An analysis of the diagnostic methods for acute pulmonary embolism. *Intens Care Med.* 1984;10:81.
40. Feied CF: Diagnosis and management of pulmonary embolism. *Clin Courier.* 1991;9:1.
41. Quinn RJ, Butler SP, et al: A decision analysis approach to the treatment of patients with suspected pulmonary emboli and an intermediate probability lung scan. *J Nucl Med.* 1991;32:2050.
42. Stoop A, de Boo T, Lemmens W, et al: Hyperventilation syndrome: measurement of objective symptoms and subjective complaints. *Respiration.* 1986;49:37.
43. Sinkinson CA, Rosenbaum JF, Teicher MH: Panic attacks: what most physicians don't know. *Emerg Med Rep.* 1990;11:201.

44. Olson KR: Carbon monoxide poisoning, in Harwood-Nuss A, et al (eds): *The Clinical Practice of Emergency Medicine.* Philadelphia: JB Lippincott; 1991:513.
45. Vegfors M, Lennmarken C: Carboxyhaemoglobinaemia and pulse oximetry. *Br J Anaesth.* 1991;66:625.

Chapter

Acute Abdominal Pain

Michael A. Turturro

Diagnostic studies of patients with acute abdominal pain often do little more than confirm the clinical diagnosis. Because there is often significant overlap in test results between severe and trivial causes, these tests frequently cause diagnostic confusion.

Many studies of patients with acute abdominal pain have been retrospective and have evaluated laboratory and radiographic results in patients with confirmed diagnoses. In addition, the diagnostic tests examined are typically far from 100% sensitive or specific for a given diagnosis. It is therefore difficult to apply published statistics to the individual emergency department (ED) patient who presents with an array of undifferentiated signs and symptoms. In conjunction with careful clinical evaluation, judicious use of diagnostic studies may be helpful to the clinician in making a presumptive or probable diagnosis. Although diagnostic studies are frequently ordered on a routine basis for patients with undifferentiated abdominal pain, few offer specific answers.

CAUSES OF ACUTE ABDOMINAL PAIN

The differential diagnosis the emergency physician must consider in any patient with acute abdominal pain is enormous, and similar clinical and laboratory findings occur with many of these disorders. Consequently, an exact diagnosis may not be attainable in the ED, although life-threatening and operative disease must still be ruled out. Diagnostic studies in acute abdominal pain should generally be employed to answer a specific question (eg, Does the patient have an operative disorder?).

The most common "surgical" cause of acute abdominal pain is

acute appendicitis.[1] As a consequence, many clinical studies evaluating clinical and laboratory findings in patients with acute abdominal pain focus on this diagnosis. As with many other abdominal disorders, "classic" history and physical and laboratory findings are frequently inconsistent or absent in patients with this condition.

Despite technologic advances, physicians are little better than their predecessors in identifying the specific cause of acute abdominal pain in the majority of patients. "Nonspecific abdominal pain" or "abdominal pain of undetermined etiology" remain the most common diagnosis in published series of patients presenting with undifferentiated acute abdominal pain.[1–3]

HISTORY AND PHYSICAL EXAMINATION

Clinical features remain the primary means of making a diagnosis, and the clinician's experience is an important factor.[4] Thus, a meticulous history and physical examination are paramount. History and physical findings may be vague in the very young and very old, adding further to the difficulty of establishing a diagnosis. In the elderly, findings may be subtle or absent, and one needs to have a heightened index of suspicion for significant pathology. Likewise, in certain populations, most notably alcoholic and psychiatric patients, the history may be difficult, and physical findings may be unimpressive despite significant pathology. Historical features may be unobtainable in young children with abdominal disease. An acute onset and peritoneal signs, when present, are the best indicators of a serious disorder. In the aforementioned patient populations, a greater reliance on diagnostic studies is often necessary.

DIAGNOSTIC TESTING

Commonly ordered diagnostic tests in patients with unspecified abdominal pain are listed in Table 9–1. Many of these tests are further discussed in later chapters but are discussed here in their relationship to acute abdominal pain. Although diagnostic tests are generally most useful in confirming a clinical diagnosis, they rarely serve to rule one out. Clinicians should bear in mind the advice, "Treat the patient, not the lab result."

TABLE 9–1. COMMONLY ORDERED DIAGNOSTIC STUDIES IN PATIENTS WITH ACUTE ABDOMINAL PAIN

Test	Cost ($)[a]	Utility
Complete blood count	25	+/−
WBC differential	25	+/−
Electrolytes, BUN, creatinine, glucose	60	+/−
Amylase	20	+[b]
Lipase	50	+ +[b]
Liver function tests (SGOT, SGPT, alkaline phosphatase, GGTP only)	60	+/−
Urinalysis (routine and microscopic)	20	+ +[b]
βHCG (urine or serum qualitative)	25	+ + +
Cervical Gram stain	20	+ +[b]
KOH/wet prep	25	+ +[b]
Radiography (with interpretation)		
Plain	145	+[b]
Intravenous pyelography	325	+ + +[b]
Computed tomography (with contrast)	1100	+ +[b]
Ultrasonography	350–500	+ +[b]
Nuclear hepatobiliary scan	635	+ + +[b]

[a]Approximate patient charge, The Mercy Hospital of Pittsburgh, May 1995.
[b]When specific diagnosis is suspected.

Leukocyte Count

A complete blood cell count with differential is often routinely ordered in patients with acute abdominal pain. Unfortunately, some patients with serious disease have normal leukocyte counts upon presentation, and many patients with insignificant disease have elevated white blood cell counts.[1]

Leukocyte and absolute granulocyte counts cannot reliably distinguish patients with surgical disease from patients with nonsurgical disease. Although the *mean* leukocyte count may be higher among a group of patients with serious abdominal disease, this finding does not help the clinician who is concerned about an individual patient. Patrick et al[1] noted that extreme elevation of the leukocyte count (above 20,000/mm^3) increases the *likelihood* of serious disease. Leukocyte counts in the lower range of normal (between 3000 and 5000/mm^3) are uncommon in patients with significant pathology. Unfortunately, these extremes are found in only a minority of patients who present with acute abdominal pain. An elevated white blood cell count or a left shift, combined with typical historical features and physical findings for a given disorder, may increase the *likelihood* that the disorder is present.[5]

Electrolytes

Significant electrolyte abnormalities in patients with acute abdominal pain are uncommon unless there is a coexisting history of significant volume loss.[6, 7] Abnormalities may also be present in alcoholic patients, diuretic therapy patients, patients with mental status changes, and elderly patients. In the majority, however, routine ordering of electrolyte laboratory tests is not warranted.

Amylase

One must not equate hyperamylasemia with pancreatitis because there are many other causes of elevated serum amylase levels. Several of these are causes of acute abdominal pain. In addition, pancreatitis may exist without hyperamylasemia, most commonly in chronic pancreatitis. Clinical findings are more predictive of pancreatitis than amylase levels.[8]

Typically, acute pancreatitis causes extreme elevation of the serum amylase, and other disorders rarely cause a similar elevation.[9] One can improve the diagnostic yield for acute pancreatitis by adding a serum lipase determination and by considering an amylase elevation of at least three times the upper limit of normal as presumptive evidence of pancreatitis.[9] Use of this cutoff will improve the specificity from 76% (using upper limit of normal) to 98% but will lower the sensitivity from 97 to 84%.[9] Pancreatic isoenzyme assays are not helpful to confirm pancreatitis. Calculation of urinary amylase clearance is not likely to be worthwhile.[11]

Liver Function Tests

Liver function tests are often ordered in suspected hepatitis or cholecystitis. Typically, the alkaline phosphatase and gamma-glutamyltranspepsidase (GGTP) are more significantly affected with biliary obstruction, and aspartate aminotransferase (AST, SGOT) and alanine aminotransferase (ALT, SGPT) are more significantly affected with parenchymal damage.

Hepatic enzyme elevations are frequently absent in acute biliary colic.[12] Therefore, liver function tests cannot be relied upon to help make a diagnosis of biliary colic. One should not be confused by a normal result in a patient with typical clinical findings. Enzyme elevations may be helpful, however, in determining the degree of obstruction or hepatic dysfunction in documented cases of cholecystitis.[12]

Urinalysis

The presence of pyuria and bacteriuria in patients with urinary symptoms such as dysuria, frequency, urgency, or flank pain is sufficient to make a presumptive diagnosis of urinary tract infection. The presence of pyuria without bacteriuria or urinary symptoms should, however, alert the clinician that another condition may be present. Any inflammatory process contiguous to the urinary tract (eg, appendicitis) may cause pyuria.[13] One should also be cautious in ascribing mild (less than 10 WBCs/high power field) pyuria to urinary tract infection, particularly in the absence of urinary symptoms. Similarly, the presence of hematuria with flank pain is indictive of renal colic. Renal colic may occur without hematuria, however. There are other causes of hematuria in patients with acute abdominal pain. In elderly or hypertensive patients with hematuria and back pain, one must be alert to the possibility of a leaking abdominal aortic aneurysm.

Gynecologic Studies

Perhaps no other test is as highly sensitive and specific and as inexpensive and easy to perform as current βHCG assays. Because inaccurate menstrual histories are common[14] and the information gained from a βHCG result often has important clinical implications, this test should be ordered routinely in any woman of childbearing age who presents with acute abdominal pain. Endocervical cultures are also indicated to screen for gonorrhea and chlamydial infection. Endocervical Gram stains and vaginal wet preparation may lead to a presumptive diagnosis of an infectious disorder.

Electrocardiography

An electrocardiogram should be performed on all patients with upper abdominal pain who have known coronary artery disease or are over 40 years old because myocardial ischemia may masquerade as abdominal pain. In addition, patients with gastrointestinal hemorrhage may develop myocardial ischemia as a result of blood loss.

Abdominal Imaging

In the majority of patients with acute abdominal pain, plain abdominal radiography adds little additional information to the history and physical findings and rarely influences patient management.[15–17] Abdominal radiographs should be ordered selectively and not routinely. The highest yield of abnormalities occurs in the elderly and in patients with suspected bowel obstruction, perforation viscus, foreign body ingestion, or mesenteric ischemia.[18, 20, 21] Contrary to popular opinion, plain abdominal radiographs have a low sensitivity and predictive value for ureterolithiasis.[22] Subtle findings are frequently present in operative disease such as appendicitis and cholecystitis, but these are rarely specific for the diagnosis. Although found on less than 10% of plain films in adults with appendicitis, the presence of an appendicolith in a patient with a suspicious clinical picture is a highly specific indicator of this disease.[23–25]

Typically, both a supine and an upright or left lateral decubitus view are obtained. The upright abdominal view adds little information except when free air is visualized. An upright chest radiograph has a higher sensitivity for this finding and requires less radiation.[15, 26]

More sophisticated tests are often utilized to confirm a diagnosis. Computed tomography provides excellent visualization of solid organs and the retroperitoneum and is the best imaging procedure to use to diagnose intraabdominal abscess and disruption of the abdominal aorta. Nuclear imaging studies have a high degree of accuracy for acute biliary obstruction and are useful when ultrasound is equivocal or unavailable.[27]

Sonography is commonly utilized to verify the presence of gallstones and to confirm biliary dilatation suggestive of acute cholecystitis. It also can confirm acute urinary obstruction due to ureteral stones. Transvaginal sonography is extremely useful in the diagnosis of suspected ectopic pregnancy and may reveal other gynecologic causes of lower abdominal pain in women.[28] Several centers have reported using ultrasonography with great success to confirm an impression of appendicitis.[29, 30] A negative study result does not rule out the disease. Indicative findings include demonstration of localized ileus, abscess, intraperitoneal fluid, or appendicolith.[31] Ultrasound in patients with undifferentiated abdominal pain sometimes reveals unsuspected biliary disease but rarely affects acute management.[32, 33]

SUMMARY

Diagnostic studies in acute abdominal pain play a secondary role to clinical signs and symptoms. The judicious, selective use of these modalities and appreciation of the limitations of each test are critical to the skillful practice of emergency medicine. Keeping these facts in mind, one can rationally optimize the use of diagnostic testing in patients with acute abdominal pain.

REFERENCES

1. Patrick GL, Stewart RJ, Isbister WH: Patients with acute abdominal pain: White cell and neutrophil counts as predictors of the surgical acute abdomen. *NZ Med J*. 1985;98:324–326.
2. Brewer RJ, Golden GT, Hitch DC, et al: Abdominal pain: An analysis of 1000 consecutive cases in a university hospital emergency room. *Am J Surg*. 1976;131:219–223.
3. deDombal FT: The OMGE acute abdominal survey: Progress report, 1986. *Scand J Gastroenterol*. 1988;23(suppl144):35–42.
4. Ellis H: The OMGE acute abdominal and laboratory diagnosis. *Contemp Issues Clin Biochem*. 1985;2:33–37.
5. Nauta RJ, Magnant C: Observation versus operation for abdominal pain in the right lower quadrant. *Am J Surg*. 1986;151:746–748.
6. Lowe RA, Wood AB, Burney RB, et al: Rational ordering of serum electrolytes: Development of clinical criteria. *Ann Emerg Med*. 1987;16:260–269.
7. Lowe RA, Arst HF, Ellis BK: Rational ordering of serum electrolytes in the emergency department. *Ann Emerg Med*. 1991;20:16–21.
8. Hoffman JR, Jaber AJ, Schriger DL: Serum amylase determination in the emergency department evaluation of abdominal pain. *J Clin Gastroenterol*. 1991;13:401–406.
9. Lin X, Wang S, Tsai Y, et al: Serum amylase, isoamylase, and lipase in the acute abdomen. *J Clin Gastroenterol*. 1989;11:47–52.
10. Pace BW, Bank S, Wise L, et al: Amylase isoenzymes in the acute abdomen: An adjunct in those patients with elevated total amylase. *Am J Gastroenterol*. 1985;80:898–901.
11. Farrar WH, Calkins WG: Sensitivity of the amylase-creatinine clearance ratio in acute pancreatitis. *Arch Int Med*. 1978;138:958–962.
12. Dunlop MG, King PM, Gunn AA: Acute abdominal pain: The value of liver function tests in suspected cholelithiasis. *J R Coll Surg Edinburgh*. 1989;34:124–127.
13. Hiatt JR: Management of the acute abdomen: A test of judgment. *Postgrad Med*. 1990;87(5):38–51.
14. Ramoska EA, Saccheti AD, Nepp M: Reliability of patient history in determining the possibility of pregnancy. *Ann Emerg Med*. 1989;18:48–50.
15. Paterson-Brown S: Strategies for reducing inappropriate laparotomy rate in the acute abdomen. *Br Med J*. 1991;302:1115–1118.
16. Campbell JPM, Gunn AA: Plain abdominal radiographs and acute abdominal pain. *Br J Surg*. 1988;75:554–556.
17. Field S, Guy PJ, Upsdell SM, et al: The erect abdominal radiograph in the acute abdomen: Should its routine use be abandoned? *Br Med J*. 1985; 290:1934–1936.

18. DeLacey GJ, Wignall BK, Bradbrooke L, et al: Rationalizing abdominal radiography in the accident and emergency department. *Clin Radiol.* 1980;31:453–455.
19. Eisenberg DL, Heinecken P, Hedgecock MW, et al: Evaluation of plain abdominal radiographs in the diagnosis of abdominal pain. *Ann Surg.* 1983;197:464–469.
20. Lee PWR: The plain X-ray in the acute abdomen: A surgeon's evaluation. *Br J Surg.* 1976;63:763–766.
21. McCook TA, Ravin CE, Rice RP: Abdominal radiography in the emergency department: A prospective analysis. *Ann Emerg Med.* 1982;11:7–8.
22. Mutgi A, Williams JW, Nettleman M: Renal colic. Utility of the plain abdominal roentgenogram. *Arch Intern Med.* 1991;151:1589–1592.
23. Hollerman JJ, Bernstein MA, Kottamasu SR, et al: Acute recurrent appendicitis with appendicolith. *Am J Emerg Med.* 1988;6:614–617.
24. Guy PJ, Pailthorpe CA: The radio-opaque appendicolith—its significance in clinical practice. *J R Army Med Corps.* 1983;129:163–166.
25. Shin MS, Ho KJ: Appendicolith. Significance in acute appendicitis and demonstration by computed tomography. *Dig Dis Sci.* 1985;30:184–187.
26. Piper KJ: Reappraisal of the erect abdominal radiograph. *Radiography.* 1987;53:19–21.
27. Grossman SJ, Joyce JM: Hepatobiliary imaging. *Emerg Med Clin North Am* 1991;9:853–874.
28. Kivikowski AI, Martin CM, Smeltzer JS: Transabdominal and transvaginal ultrasonography in the diagnosis of ectopic pregnancy: A comparative study. *Am J Obstet Gynecol.* 1990;163:123–128.
29. Jefferey RB: Sonography in acute appendicitis. *Diagn Radiol.* 1990;41:24.
30. Scwwerk WB et al: Ultrasonography in the diagnosis of acute appendicitis: a prospective study. *Gastroenterology.* 1989;97:630.
31. Forel F, Filiatrault D, Grignon A: Ultrasonic demonstration of appendicolith. *J Can Assoc Radiol.* 1983;34:66–67.
32. Kuuliala IK, Niemi LK: Sonography as an adjunct to the plain film in the evaluation of acute abdominal pain. *Ann Clin Res.* 1987;19:355–358.
33. Walsh PF, Crawford D, Crossling FT, et al: The value of immediate ultrasound in acute abdominal conditions: A critical appraisal. *Clin Radiol.* 1990;42:47–49.

Chapter

Suspected Pregnancy

Robert J. Maha, Jr., and Edward J. Vogel

Diagnosing pregnancy is of great importance in emergency medicine. A positive pregnancy test result can markedly change the diagnostic and therapeutic approach to a patient, whereas a negative test result can narrow the differential diagnosis in the female with abdominal pain or symptoms suggestive of pregnancy.

The history, physical examination, and laboratory findings all play a role in the diagnosis of pregnancy. The patient's history is often unreliable,[1] and a pregnancy test should be performed on all females capable of childbearing if a positive result will alter treatment.

Indications for pregnancy testing in the emergency department include

- Symptoms suggestive of pregnancy such as abnormal or missed menses, morning sickness, breast engorgement, abdominal fullness, and urinary frequency or hesitancy
- Physical signs of pregnancy such as obvious uterine enlargement, Chadwick sign, and hyperpigmentation
- Suspicion of pathologic pregnancy such as ectopic pregnancy, threatened abortion, or molar pregnancy
- Patients receiving potentially teratogenic drugs
- Patients sustaining abdominal trauma
- Comatose or mentally impaired patients
- Patients potentially in need of prenatal counseling (eg, substance abusers) and those diagnosed with HIV or herpes
- Rape victims
- Patients undergoing radiographic studies or invasive procedures. In general, 10 rads of ionizing radiation is considered the upper limit of safe exposure during pregnancy. With a maternal abdomen/pelvic shield, the following fetal radiation dosages occur:[2]

Chest radiograph	8 millirads
KUB radiograph	300 millirads
Pelvis radiograph	350 millirads
Pelvis CT scan	74–2000 millirads (depending upon fetal distance from section scanned)

LABORATORY TESTING

HCG Testing

The laboratory diagnosis of pregnancy is based upon the detection of human chorionic gonadotropin (HCG) in the urine or serum. Human chorionic gonadotropin is a glycoprotein produced by embryonic trophoblastic tissue during pregnancy and is needed to maintain the corpus luteum. The HCG molecule is composed of two subunits, alpha and beta. The beta subunit is specific for HCG, but the alpha subunit is a component of other glycoproteins such as thyroid-stimulating hormone, follicle-simulating hormone, and luteinizing hormone.

The quantitation of HCG is confusing because of the presence of two HCG immunoassay reference standards. The first standard developed is actually referred to as the second international standard (second IS). The more recent standard, known as the international reference preparation (IRP), is preferred for radioimmunoassay use. The conversion between the two standards can be calculated using the equation 1.8 × second IS = IRP. Clinicians must know which reference standard is employed in their hospital to interpret test results accurately.

Human chorionic gonadotropin can be detected in the serum within 24 hours of blastocyst implantation or 9 to 13 days after ovulation.[3] Human chorionic gonadotropin rises exponentially with a doubling time that averages approximately 2 days. This "rule" for doubling is somewhat oversimplified. In actuality, the HCG doubling time depends on gestational age, ranging from 1.5 days very early in pregnancy to 3.5 days at 7-weeks gestation.[4, 5] Of clinical value is the knowledge that pregnancies with a rise in HCG of less than 66% over a 48-hour period usually represent either an abnormal intrauterine pregnancy likely to abort or an ectopic pregnancy.[6] In normal pregnancy, levels peak approximately 60 days after ovulation, followed by a slight decline and a plateau extending until approximately 2 weeks postpartum.[7]

A number of laboratory tests have been developed to measure HCG as an indicator of pregnancy. An ideal emergency department pregnancy test would combine high sensitivity and specificity while being inexpensive, fast, and easily standardized.

Bioassays, developed in the 1920s, were the first laboratory tests used to diagnose pregnancy.[8] Bioassays are based upon eliciting predictable hormonally induced physiologic responses in living organisms injected with urine specimens containing HCG. These tests are labor intensive, expensive, slow, and difficult to standardize.

The first immunoassay test for pregnancy was developed in 1960.[9] In general, immunoassays lack the sensitivity, specificity, and speed needed for emergency department pregnancy testing.[10]

Radioimmunoassays (RIAs) were developed in the 1970s[11] and provided a significant improvement in pregnancy testing. In this test, the patient's serum and a radioisotope-labeled HCG are added to an anti-HCG antibody. The resultant complex of anti-HCG antibody and radioisotope-labeled HCG is analyzed for radioactive activity. Human chorionic gonadotropin in the patient's serum competes with the radiolabeled hormone for binding to antibody. The amount of radioactivity detected is thus inversely proportional to the HCG in the patient's serum. The test allows for both qualitative and quantitative testing.

Radioreceptor assays (RRAs), also developed in the 1970s, are similar to RIAs but use animal tissue with HCG receptor sites instead of antibodies against HCG. They are faster than RIAs but less sensitive. Solid-phase immunoassays have been developed, including enzyme-linked immunosorbent assays (ELISAs), immunoenzymatic assays, and immunoconcentration assays.

The widely used ICON-II HCG immunoconcentration assay (Hybritech Inc., San Diego, CA) uses two different monoclonal antibodies to detect HCG in serum or urine. Each of the monoclonal antibodies binds to a different portion of the HCG molecule. One of them is embedded in a test membrane to which the urine or serum specimen is added. Any HCG present in the specimen forms a complex with the membrane-bound anti-HCG monoclonal antibodies. The second anti-HCG monoclonal antibody, which is linked to the enzyme alkaline phosphatase, is then added and binds to a different site on the HCG molecules that have already been immobilized as described. Thus, the HCG molecule is "sandwiched" between the two anti-HCG monoclonal antibodies and immobilized in a membrane-bound complex.

A washing step is performed to remove any alkaline phosphatase–linked antibody that is not part of a membrane-bound complex. A color developer is added, which reveals a blue color in the presence of alkaline phosphatase. The intensity of this blue color is proportional to the amount of alkaline phosphatase bound in the sandwich, which in turn is proportional to the amount of HCG present in the original serum or urine specimen. Positive and negative reference zones are also used to provide internal controls.

Enzyme-linked immunoconcentration assays have been tested extensively and appear to be the best pregnancy tests available for emergency department use.[12–15] Human chorionic gonadotropin can be reliably detected at levels <25 IU/L in the serum and <50 IU/L in the urine.[16] Because levels of 50 IU/L are reached within 1 week of implantation, early diagnosis of pregnancy is thus possible. This advantage is valuable for the evaluation of potential ectopic pregnancy. It also allows for the early detection of normal pregnancy, permitting the clinician to take this into account when making the decision to order radiographic or pharmacologic interventions.

The sensitivity and specificity of enzyme-linked immunoconcentration assays approach 100%.[12] These assays are rapid, taking approximately 5 minutes to perform, and are easy to perform, making them amenable to bedside use by emergency department staff. The cost is relatively modest, with a wholesale price of approximately $10 per test. For these reasons, enzyme-linked immunoconcentration assays are currently the best qualitative pregnancy tests available for the emergency department.

Quantitative serum HCG measurement is also needed in certain emergency department cases. This is especially true when used in conjunction with ultrasonography to establish a ''discriminatory zone'' for management of a potential ectopic pregnancy. Serial quantitative HCG measurements can also be initiated in the emergency department for the evaluation of a potentially abnormal pregnancy including ectopic pregnancy, blighted ovum, threatened abortion, or hydatidiform mole. Quantitative measurements can detect HCG to a level of 5 IU/L. Quantitative methods are more time consuming and costly than qualitative levels, however, and are often not available on an emergency basis to the emergency department.

Progesterone Testing

The desire to expedite the diagnosis of ectopic pregnancy, and thereby to decrease associated morbidity and mortality, led to investigations of the utility of serum progesterone measurements. Serum progesterone levels can be especially useful in noncompliant patients in whom a single laboratory value allows identification of an abnormal pregnancy that might otherwise remain unknown and untreated.

After the initial rise of the serum progesterone in the luteal phase, a normal intrauterine pregnancy maintains a constant level of serum progesterone for the first 8 weeks of gestation. By contrast, progesterone production is diminished in ectopic pregnancies regardless of gestational age.[17] Thus, a single quantification of serum progesterone allows identification of a normal intrauterine pregnancy regardless of gestational age. In patients undergoing pharmacologic induction of ovulation, progesterone levels may be misleading, however, because of multiple corpora lutea.[18]

A single progesterone level is valuable in managing complicated first-trimester pregnancies with HCG levels below the ''discriminatory zone.'' Two retrospective studies[19, 20] show progesterone levels of <15 ng/mL to be highly predictive of an abnormal pregnancy. Using this cutoff, 100% sensitivity for ectopic pregnancies was noted, and all but one abnormal intrauterine gestation was identified. The prospective study by Stovall et al,[21] which included significantly more patients than in previous retrospective studies, noted that 81% of ectopic pregnancies, 93% of abnormal intrauterine pregnancies, and 11% of normal pregnancies had progesterone levels <15 ng/mL. Fewer than 4% of abnormal intrauterine pregnancies and fewer than 2% of ectopic gestations had serum progesterone >25 ng/mL. Using the 25 ng/mL cutoff, normal pregnancy was identified with a sensitivity of only 61%, but the specificity was 97%. Therefore, a serum progesterone level of >25 ng/mL is strongly correlated with a normal intrauterine gestation. By contrast, a progesterone value <15 ng/mL suggests an abnormal pregnancy, although as many as 11% of normal intrauterine pregnancies fall below this value.

COMBINING ULTRASOUND AND LABORATORY STUDIES IN THE EVALUATION OF POTENTIAL ECTOPIC PREGNANCY

The number of hospitalizations for ectopic gestations in the United States nearly tripled in the 1970s.[22] The timely diagnosis of ectopic pregnancy is important for limiting not only mortality but also morbidity.

Combining pelvic ultrasonography with laboratory testing allows the clinician to differentiate the normal intrauterine pregnancy, the abnormal intrauterine pregnancy, and the ectopic pregnancy. Ultrasonography is well suited to confirming intrauterine pregnancies. In doing so, it essentially rules out the possibility of extrauterine pregnancy, with the exception of the rare heterotopic pregnancy, said to occur in only one of 4000 conceptions.[23] The incidence of heterotopic pregnancies may be increased nearly 10-fold, however, in patients undergoing ovulation induction because of infertility.[24] Less commonly, sonography can identify an ectopic pregnancy by visualizing an extrauterine fetus.

The discriminatory zone of HCG was originally defined as a range of HCG values at which a normal intrauterine pregnancy should be visualized by transabdominal ultrasound. This value has been defined as between 6000 and 6500 mIU/mL (IRP). At this level approximately 94% of intrauterine gestations would be revealed by transabdominal sonography.[25]

The lack of an intrauterine gestational sac when the zone is exceeded is associated with an ectopic gestation in 86% of patients.[26] Approximately 75% of ectopic gestations have HCG concentrations less than the discriminatory zone for abdominal ultrasound at the time of first evaluation.[27]

Patients with multiple gestations demonstrate higher levels of HCG for any given gestational age. Therefore, ultrasound findings consistent with intrauterine gestation may be lacking within the discriminatory zone for multiple gestation pregnancies.

Owing to its higher resolution, transvaginal ultrasound affords earlier diagnosis than does transabdominal ultrasound. This increased resolution results from the lack of intervening soft tissues, the absence of a distended bladder (which compresses small gestational sacs), and the direct proximity of the transducer to the area of interest. By allowing a lower discriminatory zone, transvaginal ultrasound allows for more timely diagnosis, earlier medical or surgical intervention, decreased morbidity, increased future fertility, and most likely lower maternal mortality.

Various discriminatory zones for the identification of intrauterine gestations by transvaginal ultrasound have been reported in the literature. A cutoff as low as 1000 mIU/ml (IRP) has been reported by some clinicians who define a gestational sac as either an eccentrically located intrauterine fluid collection or a fluid collection surrounded by a thickened border representing a chronic reaction.[28] The gestational sacs defined in this manner have included intrauterine fluid collections as small as 1 mm,[29] but it is probably more reasonable to expect visualization of an intrauterine sac at levels of approximately 1500 mIU/mL. This finding corresponds to a gestational age of 35 days from the last menstrual period's 1st day.[30] Discriminatory values of up to 3000 mIU/mL (IRP) may be more reasonable in some hospitals, depending to a great part upon the level of experience of the sonographer and the resolution of different imaging systems. Until a "gestational sac," which contains a fetal pole or yolk sac, has been identified, an ectopic pregnancy cannot be ruled out.

Transvaginal imaging can also be useful in identifying abnormal complex adnexal masses sometimes seen with ectopic pregnancy. Identification of these adnexal masses has a sensitivity of 93%, specificity of 99%, and positive predictive value of 98% for the diagnosis of ectopic pregnancy.[28] When the threshold of 1000 mIU/mL was combined with ultrasonographic visualization of an adnexal mass, a sensitivity of 97% was attained, with specificity and positive predictive value remaining the same. Transvaginal ultrasonography is also useful in detection of cul-de-sac fluid, which may help in selection of cases for diagnostic culdocentesis or laparoscopy.

REFERENCES

1. Ramoska EA, Saccetti AD, Nepp M: Reliability of patient history in determining the possibility of pregnancy. *Ann Emerg Med.* 1989;18:48–50.
2. Wyte CD: Diagnostic modalities in the pregnant patient. *Emerg Med Clin North Am.* 1994;12(1):35–36.
3. Catt KJ, Dufau ML, Valukaitis JL: Appearance of HCG in pregnancy plasma following the initiation of implantation of the blastocyst. *J Clin Endocrinol Metab.* 1975;40:537–540.

4. Pittaway DE: BHCG dynamics in ectopic pregnancy. *Clin Obst Gynecol.* 1987;30(1):129–134.
5. Fritz MA, Guo S: Doubling time of HCG in early normal pregnancy: Relationship to HCG concentration and gestational age. *Fert Steril.* 1987;47(4):584–589.
6. Kadar N, Caldwell BV, Romero R: A method of screening for ectopic pregnancy and its indications. *Obstet Gynecol.* 1981;58(2):162–166.
7. Seifer DB, Flynn SD: Clinical application of human chorionic gonadotropin, in Henry JB (ed): *Clinical Diagnosis and Management by Laboratory Methods.* Philadelphia: WB Saunders; 1991:474–481.
8. Aschein S, Zondek B: Das Hormon des Hypophysencorderloppe: Test Objeckt Zum Nachaueis das Hormons. *Klin Wochenschr.* 1927;6:248.
9. Wide L, Gemzell CA: An immunologic pregnancy test. *Acta Endocrinol.* 1960;35:261.
10. Honingman B: Selected serology: Pregnancy testing, hepatitis A and B, and infectious mononucleosis. *Emerg Med Clin North Am.* 1986;4(2):299–314.
11. Vaitukaitis JL, Braunstein GD, Ross GT: A radioimmunoassay which specifically measures HCG in the presence of human luteinizing hormone. *Am J Obstet Gynecol.* 1972;113(6):751–758.
12. Gennis P, Hain L, Anderson HF, et al: Utility of a sensitive bedside serum pregnancy test. *Ann Emerg Med.* 1987;16(6):659–660.
13. Stovall TG, Kellerman AL, Ling FW, et al: Emergency department diagnosis of ectopic pregnancy. *Ann Emerg Med.* 1990;19(10):1098–1103.
14. Tsokos N, Masters AM, Boyne P: Emergency serum and urine HCG analysis with the ‘‘Tandem ICON’’ procedure. *Aust NZ J Obstet Gynaecol.* 1986;26:284–286.
15. Cartwright PS, Victor DF, Moore RA, et al: Performance of a new enzyme-linked immunoassay urine pregnancy test for the detection of ectopic gestation. *Ann Emerg Med.* 1986;15(10):1198–1199.
16. Valkirs GE, Barton R: ImmunoCentration—a new format for solid-phase immunoassays. *Clin Chem.* 1985;31(9):1427–1431.
17. Hubinot CJ, Thomas C, Schwers JF: Luteal function in ectopic pregnancy. *Am J Obstet Gynecol.* 1987;156(3):669–674.
18. Gelder MS, Boots CR, Younger JB: Use of a single random serum progesterone value as a diagnostic aid for ectopic pregnancy. Abstract P-100, American Fertility Society Program and Abstracts. Birmingham, AL: AFS, 1989:S101–S102.
19. Matthews CP, Coulson PB, Wild RA: Serum progesterone levels as an aid in the diagnosis of ectopic pregnancy. *Obstet Gynecol.* 1986;68:390–394.
20. Yeko TR, Gurill MJ, Hughes LH, et al: Timely diagnosis of early ectopic pregnancy using a single blood progesterone measurement. *Fertil Steril.* 1987;48(6):1048–1050.
21. Stovall TG, Ling FW, Cope BJ, et al: Preventing ruptured ectopic pregnancy with a single serum progesterone. *Am J Obstet Gynecol.* 1989;160:1425–1431.
22. Dorfaran SF: Ectopic pregnancy mortality, United States, 1979 to 1980: Clinical aspects. *Obstet Gynecol.* 1984;64:386–390.
23. Bello GV, Schonholz D, Moshiipur J, et al: Combined pregnancy: The Mount Sinai experience. *Obstet Gynecol Surv.* 1986;41:603.

24. Leach RE, Ory SJ: Modern management of ectopic pregnancy. *J Reprod Med.* 1989;34(5):324–328.
25. Kadar N, Devore G, Romero R: Discriminatory HCG zone: Its use in the sonographic evaluation for ectopic pregnancy. *Obstet Gynecol.* 1981; 58(2):156–161.
26. Romero R, Kadar N, Jeanty P, et al: Diagnosis of ectopic pregnancy: Value of the discriminatory HCG zone. *Obstet Gynecol.* 1985;66(3):357–360.
27. Daus K, Mundy D, Graves W, et al: Ectopic pregnancy. What to do during the 20-day window. *J Reprod Med.* 1989;34(2):162–166.
28. Cacciatore B, Stenman U, Ylostalo P: Diagnosis of ectopic pregnancy by vaginal ultrasound in combination with a discriminatory serum HCG zone of 1000 IU/L (IRP). *Br J Obstet Gynaecol.* 1990;97:904–908.
29. Cacciatore B, Tiitinen A, Stenman U, et al: Early pregnancy: Serum HCG levels and vaginal ultrasound findings. *Br J Obstet Gynaecol.* 1990;97:899–903.
30. Fossum GT, Davajan V, Kletzky OA: Early detection of pregnancy with transvaginal ultrasound. *Fertil Steril.* 1988;49(5):788–791.

Chapter

Headache

R. Todd Kiskaddon

Headache is the primary reason for presentation in 2.5% of all emergency department visits.[1] By its nature, headache is a subjective complaint and seldom associated with objective physical findings and thus is often particularly troublesome to evaluate. In a busy emergency department the perceived importance of the complaint may be influenced by the physician's perception that the patient may only have a low pain tolerance or may be a drug seeker.

Whereas a majority of headaches are so-called muscle tension headaches, 20 to 24% of patients' seeking treatment suffer from vascular- or migraine-type cephalgia, and 1% have some other underlying organic process (Table 11–1).[1, 2] Although most headaches are benign, any suspicion of serious findings, such as meningitis, tumor, abscess, or intracranial hemorrhage, mandates investigation with more advanced diagnostic modalities. The challenge for the emergency physician is to ascertain the cause of the patient's complaint while maximizing diagnostic sensitivity and minimizing cost and invasiveness.

Obtaining a detailed history and performing a physical examination,

TABLE 11–1. COMMON CAUSES OF HEADACHE

Muscular	Organic
Strain	Stroke
Tension/depressive	Embolic
Cervical arthritis	Thrombotic
Myositis	Hemorrhagic
	Bleed
Vascular	Subdural/epidural
Migraine	Subarachnoid/aneurysm
Classic	Post-traumatic
Atypical	Infection
Cluster	Meningitis/encephalitis
Episodic	Sinusitis
Chronic	Abscess
Variant	HIV related
Hypertensive	Inflammatory
Toxic	Arteritis/vasculitis
Arteritis/vasculitis	Cervical arthritis
	TMJ dysfunction
	Neuralgia
	Neoplastic
	Primary
	Metastatic

Adapted from Freitag FG, Diamond M: Emergency treatment of headache. *Med Clin North Am.* 1991;75(3):749–761.

including comprehensive neurologic and eye examinations, are the fundamental means of diagnosing the cause of headache. Patients who present to the emergency department with well-established complaints of chronic head pain should be fully evaluated if there is any new component to the headache or any change in its character. For instance, patients who suffer from vascular or migraine headaches require no further testing if the headache is consistent with the usual pattern and adequate evaluation has been performed in the past. Additional testing is indicated only if the diagnosis remains in doubt after the initial history and physical examination.

BLOOD TESTING

Blood tests are of little value in the primary diagnosis of headache. "Baseline" testing or screening adds little to the evaluation, while increasing cost and prolonging the patient's stay in the emergency department. Although electrolyte derangements, such as hyponatremia and hypercalcemia, may be associated with headache, routine electrolyte screening, for example, will yield abnormalities in fewer than 1% of patients.

Directed testing, such as carbon monoxide levels and toxicology screens, is indicated when the history is suggestive but should not be considered routine. Thus, a patient with persistent anorexia or vomiting related to the complaint may benefit from electrolyte determination.

Pregnancy should be identified prior to nonemergent radiologic studies and institution of drug therapies. Other tests, such as white blood cell count and blood cultures, may be part of the overall workup for the patient with a headache who may appear septic, but these will not by themselves be helpful in identifying the cause of head pain in the emergency department setting.

Perhaps the only exception to the rule that in most cases blood studies have little role in the emergency department evaluation of headache is the utility of the erythrocyte sedimentation rate (ESR) in older patients with headaches. Headache is reported in 70 to 90% of patients with giant cell arteritis (GCA, also termed temporal arteritis),[2] and an ESR greater than 40 mm/h is reported to be 70 to 90% sensitive for detecting GCA.[2, 3] This is an important diagnosis because early steroid therapy may prevent the sequelae of optic nerve infarction or major arterial occlusion that occurs in about 50% of untreated patients.[1] Although GCA is rare in individuals under the age of 50, it should be considered in younger patients who have symptoms such as visual loss, temporal tenderness or ''beading,'' jaw claudication, malaise, or polymyalgia rheumatica. Temporal artery biopsy has been considered the standard for the diagnosis of GCA, but a positive biopsy specimen may be obtained in as few as 10 to 30% of GCA patients.[2–4] The diagnosis in biopsy-negative cases is made on the basis of responses to steroid therapy or characteristic angiographic findings.

LUMBAR PUNCTURE

The role of lumbar puncture (LP) in the evaluation of headache, as well as its proper place in the diagnostic sequence, is the topic of some debate. The LP has long been the standard for diagnosis in cases of meningitis and subarachnoid hemorrhage (SAH), but its use has been limited by the possibility of its precipitating cerebral herniation in patients with either obvious or occult elevated intracranial pressure (ICP).

In patients with suspected bacterial meningitis, examination of the cerebrospinal fluid (CSF) leads to rapid diagnosis and allows for directed rather than empiric antibiotic therapy. Although it is possible to predict in most cases the most likely bacterial pathogens, LP is crucial to the management of the immunocompromised hosts. In these patients, CSF analysis should include a search for diverse opportunistic pathogens in addition to the standard studies.

In children, bacterial meningitis causes a compensated increase in ICP secondary to cerebral edema and acute hydrocephalus. Nevertheless, only about 5% of patients manifest signs of brain herniation.[5] Although some studies purport to show a temporal association between LP and cerebral herniation in as many as 30% of meningitis-associated herniation deaths in children, a cause-and-effect relationship has not been unequivocally established.[3, 5, 6] Thus, one retrospective study of 445 children with meningitis suggested a 4.3% rate of herniation as assessed by clinical criteria.[7] Autopsy results confirmed herniation in only five cases (1.1%), and, of the eight cases noted to have the closest temporal relationship between LP and herniation, six (and possibly seven) were already exhibiting signs of herniation at the time of LP.[7, 8]

Although it is not clear that LP will cause cerebral herniation, the removal of significant amounts of CSF or the precipitation of a CSF leak in the presence of signs of impending herniation would appear to risk accelerating herniation. Profound, persistent, or progressive obtundation, posturing or loss of tone, lateralizing neurologic findings, third nerve palsy, and papilledema are all considered contraindications to LP as a primary diagnostic modality. Cranial computed tomography (CT) screening should be performed prior to LP in these cases; however, its sensitivity is only 64 to 82% in detecting impending herniation. Thus, a normal scan cannot rule out a risk of herniation even when ICP is dangerously high.[7]

Lumbar puncture should be delayed (but broad-spectrum antibiotics should be administered at once) in cases of headache due to suspected meningitis when signs of high ICP are present. Blood cultures, urine antigen screening, and delayed CSF examination may provide acceptable alternatives to immediate LP in these cases.[5, 7, 9]

Lumbar puncture is also useful in the diagnosis of SAH. Because of the variability in bleeding sites, the clinical presentation of SAH is variable. The most common feature is sudden severe headache noted in as many as 65 to 85% of patients.[2, 10, 11] Despite an incidence of <1% in the general population, one study reports that improper diagnosis and treatment of SAH is responsible for 5% of medical malpractice litigation.[12]

Patients who present with either sudden unexplained head pain or altered mental status should undergo head CT scanning in the emergency department. Computed tomography reliably detects SAH in most cases and can often localize the source of bleeding, but it may miss 5 to 25% of subarachnoid bleeds.[1, 9, 13] In the face of a clinical suspicion of SAH, a negative CT should be followed by LP, which is considered the standard. The finding of persistently nonclotting blood in serial tube samples suggests strongly that headache or meningismus is secondary to SAH rather than infection.

The LP may rarely yield a false-negative result in the presence of a true SAH. Patients with a typical presentation but negative initial CT and LP who are shown subsequently to have had a bleed may have had prodromal head pain secondary to a small, contained aneurysmal leak or "aneurysmal stretch."[2] Patients with minor bleeds who have normal spinal taps within the first few hours after the onset of symptoms appear to belong to a small group in whom the subarachnoid blood has not had time to reach the lumbar region of the spinal canal.[9] A repeat LP is indicated if suspicion for SAH remains high. A positive LP should be followed by angiography to identify the aneurysm or other source of bleeding. There is a 20% incidence of multiple aneurysms in patients with SAH.

IMAGING PROCEDURES

Plain Films

Plain skull radiographs have essentially no role in the evaluation of nontraumatic head pain. Sinus films, long considered a screening standard for clinically diagnosed sinusitis, have been all but replaced by CT, which is comparable in expense and superior in detail, while exposing the patient to less radiation.[15]

Computed Tomography and Magnetic Resonance Imaging

Although the CT scan may be overused for screening, it has become an irreplaceable diagnostic tool for the evaluation of acute head pain and neurologic impairment in the emergency department (Table 11–2). Acute bleeding from epidural, subdural, subarachnoid, or intraparenchymal hemorrhage is usually easily seen on regular noncontrast head CT. Computed tomography is superior to magnetic resonance imaging (MRI) in the detection of acute bleeding. In SAH, a positive CT scan makes an LP unnecessary, thereby avoiding additional complications and allowing the patient to directly undergo angiography.

Major structural alterations in the brain are also apparent on CT. These include mass effect, atrophy, hydrocephalus, vascular malformations, and edema. Immunocompromised patients, including those with AIDS, who present with headache should have a screening CT prior to

TABLE 11–2. CRITERIA FOR ORDERING HEAD COMPUTED AXIAL TOMOGRAPHY SCAN

Clinical suspicion of hemorrhage or infarction
Evidence of acute increase in intracranial pressure
Acute onset of localizable neurologic findings
Suspected head injury with altered mental status
Open or depressed skull fracture
Screening scan prior to lumbar puncture in patients with signs of increased intracranial pressure

Adapted from Freitag FG, Diamond M: Emergency treatment of headache. *Med Clin North Am.* 1991;75(3):749–761.

LP. They are more likely to have characteristic diagnostic findings (eg, ring-enhancing lesions due to brain abscess or toxoplasmosis). Other pathology associated with head pain, such as sinusitis and bone disease, is also detectable on CT.

Despite the broad utility of CT, several caveats apply to the interpretation of a normal CT in the presence of an abnormal clinical examination. Whereas acute bleeding is readily apparent on CT (except in cases of severe anemia), subacute hemorrhage may appear isodense. Thus, a subdural hematoma that is several weeks old may be missed on unenhanced CT. Deposits of hemosiderin, ferritin, and methemoglobin in old bleeding sites are easily detected by MRI, making it a more sensitive diagnostic tool in this situation. Similarly, traumatic shear injury, often found after head trauma, is detectable on MRI but rarely on CT.[14] Computed axial tomography is also inferior to MRI in evaluating the posterior fossa; thus, even with a normal CT, any symptoms suggestive of a posterior fossa lesion require further evaluation of the patient.

Although still not as widely available as CT, MRI is becoming the standard of care for the definitive diagnosis of many types of intracranial pathology. Magnetic resonance imaging can more clearly characterize neoplastic disease and localize pathologic lesions. Vascular disorders, temporomandibular joint pathology, and inflammatory neuropathy may also be detected on MRI. Gadolinium can be used to enhance the meninges in inflammatory states such as encephalitis and meningitis.[14]

Despite MRI's superior resolution capabilities, the associated expense and the necessity to provide dedicated staffing for both imaging and interpretation will probably continue to limit its use in the emergency setting. Other important limiting factors include distance from the emergency department; contraindication for patients with ferromagnetic foreign bodies (including some aneurysm clips) and pacemakers; relatively long scanning time; and relatively inaccessible patients with critical needs during scanning.

Angiography

Angiography is seldom used in the emergency department for the evaluation of headache. Its major role is in definitive diagnosis and intervention in cases of SAH, cerebral aneurysm, and arterial dissection. For less emergent indications (eg, temporal arteritis), angiography may be postponed pending the results of other diagnostic studies.

CONCLUSION

Headache in emergency department patients may be due to a variety of causes. The seriousness of a headache can easily be underestimated, resulting in serious morbidity or death. The challenge to the emergency practitioner is to develop an organized and a consistent approach to the evaluation of the patient with this complaint, minimizing interventional expense and morbidity while maintaining the highest sensitivity for detecting significant disease. Despite the existence of highly accurate and readily available diagnostic modalities, a careful medical history and physical examination continue to be the clinician's most valuable tools.

REFERENCES

1. Freitag FG, Diamond M: Emergency treatment of headache. *Med Clin North Am.* 1991;75(3):749–761.
2. Couch JR: Headache to worry about. *Med Clin North Am.* 1993;77(1):141–167.
3. Hunder GG: Giant cell (temporal) arteritis. *Rheum Dis Clin North Am.* 1990;16(2):399–409.
4. Ellis ME, Ralston S: The ESR in the diagnosis and management of the polymyalgia rheumatica/giant cell arteritis syndrome. *Ann Rheum Dis.* 1983;42:168–170.
5. Haslam RHA: Role of computed tomography in the early management of bacterial meningitis. *J Pediatr.* 1991;119(1):157–159.
6. Addy DP: When not to do a lumbar puncture. *Arch Dis Child.* 1987;62:873–875.
7. Rennick G, Shann F, de Campo J: Cerebral herniation during bacterial meningitis in children. *Br Med J.* 1993;306:953–955.
8. Obaro SK: Avoiding coning in childhood meningitis. *Br Med J.* 1993;306:1691–1692.
9. Kooiker JC: Spinal puncture and cerebrospinal fluid examination, in Roberts JR, Hedges JR (eds): *Clinical Procedures in Emergency Medicine.* 2nd ed. Philadelphia: WB Saunders; 1991:969–984.

10. Calvert JM: Premonitory symptoms and signs of subarachnoid hemorrhage. *Med J Aust*. 1966;1(16):65–67.
11. Okawara SH: Warning signs prior to rupture of an intracranial aneurysm. *J Neurosurg*. 1973;38:575–580.
12. Karcz A, Holbrook J, Burke MC, et al: Massachusetts emergency medicine closed malpractice claims: 1988–1990. *Ann Emerg Med*. 1993;22:553–559.
13. Grossman RI, Heller MB, Raskin RH: Severe headache: Initial measures. *Patient Care*. 1993;27(9):124–143.
14. Prager JM, Mikulis DJ: The radiology of headache. *Med Clin North Am*. 1991;75(3):525–544.
15. Levine HL: Otorhinolaryngologic causes of headache. *Med Clin North Am*. 1991;75(3):677–692.

Chapter

Altered Mental Status

Sandra Schneider

The patient who presents to the emergency department (ED) with an acute alteration in mental status poses both a diagnostic and a therapeutic challenge. An altered level of consciousness is an important symptom in any patient, but especially in the elderly, in whom it may be a more frequent and more prominent indication of physical illness than other signs such as fever or pain.[1] The assessment in many patients is complicated by an abnormal baseline mental status.

This chapter addresses the utility of diagnostic tests in establishing a diagnosis and therapy for patients with an *acute* alteration in mental status. Unfortunately, few good studies are available on this subject, and among them few deal with the initial evaluation.

DIFFERENTIAL DIAGNOSIS

An altered mental status is generally caused by a focal effect on the reticular activating system (RAS) or a widespread effect on both the hemispheres. Focal effects on one hemisphere rarely affect the level of consciousness. The hemispheres are more sensitive than the RAS to the effects of electrolyte imbalance, acid-base disturbances, loss of glucose or oxygen substrates, and toxins (exogenous or endogenous).

TABLE 12–1. CAUSES OF ALTERED MENTAL STATUS

Primary CNS Disease	
Cerebrovascular	Subarachnoid hemorrhage Intracerebral hemorrhage (hypertensive) Thrombotic or embolic stroke Vasculitis
Trauma	Subdural hematoma Epidural hematoma Contusion Concussion
Infection	Encephalitis (eg, viral, herpes) Meningitis (eg, viral, bacterial)
Neoplastic	Tumor (with or without mass effect) Carcinomatous meningitis
Seizure	Epilepsy Secondary to mass/drug
Psychiatric	Catatonia Depression Locked-in syndrome
Systemic Disease Affecting the Nervous System	
Pulmonary	Hypoxemia Hypercapnea
Metabolic	Thyroid disorder Adrenal crisis Acid/base imbalance Glucose abnormality Temperature abnormality Dehydration
Cardiovascular	Embolus (particularly to CNS) Hypotension Hypertension
Infectious	Sepsis Pneumonia (particularly in the elderly)
Gastrointestinal	Hepatic failure
Gastrourologic	Renal failure Toxemia of pregnancy
Musculoskeletal	Myasthenia gravis

TABLE 12–1. CAUSES OF ALTERED MENTAL STATUS *Continued*

Exogenous Toxic Substances	
Drugs	Aliphatic alcohol (eg, ethanol, methanol, isopropanol) Anxiolytic (eg, sedative-hypnotic, benzodiazepine) Anticholinergic Anticonvulsant Antidepressant Antihistamine Barbiturate Bromide Opiate Tranquilizer Mood elevator/hallucinogen (eg, LSD, PCP, cocaine, amphetamines, nutmeg, jimsonweed) Salicylate
Toxic gases	Carbon monoxide Cyanide
Industrial compounds	Lead, mercury, organic solvents, cyanide
Withdrawal from Substances	
Narcotics Muscle relaxer (particularly baclofen) Barbiturate Benzodiazepine Alcohol Sedative-hypnotic	

There are many approaches to the patient with altered mental status in the ED. It is important to have a systematic differential diagnosis such as that in Table 12–1 as a reference in determining the cause of the impairment of consciousness in the specific patient.

INCIDENCE

There are few studies that examine the actual incidence of altered mental status and basically none that examine *all* patients as they would present to an ED. Most large epidemiologic studies exclude patients who recover in the ED (hypoglycemia, narcotic overdose) and trauma victims. Although altered mental status is a common prehospital complaint, its actual incidence is not published. In one study of naloxone, the University of California Los Angeles Emergency Medicine Service (UCLA-EMS) attended to 730 patients for acute mental status change in 1 year, but these were only the cases in which naloxone was used.[2] In one hospital in Peoria, Illinois, 0.6% of patients were brought in by medics for altered mental status.[3]

Altered mental status in children is less common than in adults, accounting for 0.03% of pediatric patients seen in one emergency care unit per year.[4]

Levey[5] studied 500 patients over the age of 12 who were admitted to the hospital and remained comatose for at least 6 hours. Patients whose coma was caused by trauma or drugs were excluded. Over 40% of these patients had coma as a result of hypoxic/ischemic insult (only 5% of this group ultimately made a good recovery). The next largest groups were "other cerebral disease" (29%), hepatic encephalopathy (10%), and subarachnoid hemorrhage (8%). A large "miscellaneous" group (12%) was due to unspecified metabolic causes.

Purdie[6] et al retrospectively reviewed charts of patients with the diagnosis of "acute organic brain syndrome" (including acute confusion, acute organic psychosis, and acute metabolic encephalopathy) who required admission to the hospital (including drug-induced problems but excluding obvious trauma, correctable causes, and cases in which the diagnosis was made in the ED, eg, subarachnoid hemorrhage). The leading cause of altered mental status was drug related, with a large number (44%) due to street drugs. Use of anticholinergics (including tricyclic antidepressants) was also common. In this study, 44% of the patients had an underlying chronic organic brain syndrome, and within this group the acute exacerbation was most commonly due to environmental change ("sundowning"), dehydration, infection, or seizures.

Age is an important determinant of the differential diagnosis. Younger patients tend to be involved with illicit and toxic substances or trauma. Patients aged 20 to 49 are most likely to have an altered mental status secondary to drugs or poisoning (more than 60%).[7] In the elderly, medications, particularly anticholinergics and over-the-counter medications, are a common cause of altered mental status change, particularly in patients with Alzheimer disease. Elderly patients are more likely to suffer from systemic disease and many have two or more causes for their altered mental status.[1] Disorders that would cause only minimal or no discernible effect in a younger patient may produce coma in an elderly patient.

DIAGNOSTIC URGENCY

To establish the best sequence of investigations for a particular patient, one must consider not only the likelihood of the disease occurring in the patient but also the diagnostic urgency. For example, hypoglycemia is devastating to cerebral tissue and rapidly correctable; its diagnostic urgency is high.

Few immediately reversible causes of altered mental status are found in the ED, most commonly hypoglycemia and opiate overdose. The "coma packet" consisting of naloxone (up to 10 mg, given in 1 to 2 mg doses) and 50% dextrose (25 mL), with or without thiamine (100 mg), should be considered for every patient with a worsened level of consciousness. A rapid bedside check of glucose concentration is preferable to dextrose administration when available.

With the exception of the few immediately correctable situations, nearly all patients with acute mental status changes require admission to the hospital. Therefore, the primary task of the ED is not to decide disposition or definitive diagnosis but to initiate workup and treatment in those instances when time is related to morbidity and mortality. Table 12–2 lists those disorders in which there is diagnostic urgency. These disorders should be the focus of our diagnostic endeavors.

THE EVALUATION OF THE PATIENT WITH ALTERED MENTAL STATUS

History and Physical

A detailed history should be obtained from family members, witnesses, paramedics, and the patient when possible. Differentiation should be made between sudden and subacute onset of the mental status change. A sudden onset suggests an alteration of cerebral perfusion (arrhythmia) or an intracerebral disorder (cerebral hemorrhage, trauma, seizure). A subacute onset suggests a metabolic disorder (hypoxia, hypoglycemia) or drug overdose. Some intracranial hemorrhages (subdural hematoma) may have either acute or subacute onset.

Respirations

Tachypnea due to respiratory failure or acidosis or a decrease in respiration due to sedative or hypnotics overdose mandates an arterial blood gas evaluation, regardless of pulse oximetry reading.

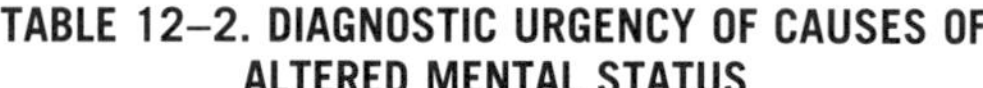

TABLE 12–2. DIAGNOSTIC URGENCY OF CAUSES OF ALTERED MENTAL STATUS

Diagnostic Urgency	Treatment
Immediately Reversible	
Narcotic overdose	Naloxone
Hypoglycemia	D-50 (and thiamine)
Benzodiazepine overdose	Flumazenil (if available)
Critical	
Hypotension	Fluids, pressors
Hypertension	Vasodilators (dependent on cause)
Hypoxia	Oxygen, airway
Hypercapnea	Bicarbonate, increase ventilation
Acid base imbalance	Bicarbonate, adjust ventilation
Urgent	
Sepsis	Fever reduction, fluids, antibiotics
Hyperthermia	Temperature reduction
Hypothermia	Rewarming
Diabetic ketoacidosis and hyperosmolar coma	Fluids, insulin
Renal failure	Dialysis
Hyponatremia	Saline (0.9–3%)
Hypernatremia	Saline (0.45–0.9%)
Hypocalcemia	Calcium chloride or gluconate
Hypercalcemia	Diuretics, saline
Seizures	Prophylaxis
Toxic ingestion	Gastric lavage, charcoal
Toxic exposure	Decontamination, specific antibodies
CNS catastrophe	Normalization of vital signs, hypocapnia (P_{CO_2}, possibly diuretics, mannitol, steroids)

BEDSIDE DIAGNOSTIC TESTS

Bedside diagnostic tests are rapid, inexpensive, and helpful in focusing treatment if not in establishing the diagnosis.

Glucose Estimation

Hypoglycemia is a common cause of altered mental status. In one study, it accounted for 45% of altered mental status patients seen by paramedics.[3] In addition to diabetics, patients with fulminant liver failure, sepsis, malnutrition, chronic alcoholism, or insulinoma may become acutely hypoglycemic. Patients may receive exogenous insulin either through intentional overdose or therapeutic error. Therefore, bedside estimation of glucose or empiric administration of dextrose is *mandatory* in all patients with altered mental status.

In one study of 51 patients with altered mental status, nearly 20% had serum levels of glucose <80 mg/dL; 80% of these were <60 mg/dL. After 50 mL of 50% dextrose, the serum glucose rose an average of 166 mg/dL.[10] Although glucose levels <80 mg/dL may cause an altered mental status, levels <60 mg/dL may be noted in patients without mental status change.

Blood Alcohol Level

Bedside alcohol estimators (eg, saliva sticks and breath analyzers) are useful not only diagnostically but also for following intoxicated patients. Alterations in cognitive function (particularly attention, motor coordination, and reaction time) are seen at ethanol levels >100 mg/dL in social drinkers.[11] These same effects may occur at higher levels in chronic alcoholics.[11] It is unlikely for alcohol to cause coma below a blood concentration of 200 mg/dL.[12] Fatalities from respiratory depression may occur at dose levels exceeding 500 mg/dL.[13]

Patients with high alcohol concentrations should be expected to improve within 8 hours of initial assessment. Failure to improve, or presence of coma out of proportion to alcohol level, should prompt a thorough search for another cause. Head injury is common in these patients, and an early computed tomography scan is indicated for patients with trauma, sudden collapse, focal neurologic signs, low alcohol concentration, or protracted recovery.

Pulse Oximetry

Pulse oximetry should be used to screen all patients with altered mental status for occult hypoxemia. Minor alterations in oxygen saturation (95% or less) should lead to the use of supplemental oxygen and arterial blood gas values. An oxygen saturation of 90% correlates with a Po_2 as low as 60. Oximetry readings of 90% and below suggest severe hypoxemia requiring immediate oxygenation, with or without intubation. Pulse oximetry may give spurious readings or fail to register in cases of vasoconstriction or hypothermia.

Noninvasive CO_2 Measuring Devices

Quantitative end tidal CO_2 levels correspond to venous Pco_2 levels. Devices have not been adapted for use in nonintubated patients, however. Transcutaneous P_{CO_2} devices do not correlate well with actual measurements but can indicate trends.

Arterial Blood Gas

Although pulse oximetry measures oxygen saturation, it does not measure P_{CO_2} or pH abnormalities. Therefore, arterial blood gases should be measured on all patients with unexplained altered mental status.

Arterial blood gas values may be spuriously altered by either hypothermia or hyperthermia. The P_{O_2} measurement is spontaneously increased by 7.2% and P_{CO_2} by 4.4% for each degree below 37°C.[17] Although correction of these values during the treatment of hypothermia is controversial, correction is necessary before reaching conclusions about the cause of coma or altered mental status. Opposite changes are seen with hyperthermia but are less likely to be severe. Air bubbles in the syringe may decrease the P_{CO_2} and increase the P_{O_2}. Excessive heparin causes a falsely acidotic reading.[18]

Severe metabolic acidosis (pH <7.20) leads to a variety of metabolic and cellular changes. Simple metabolic acidosis rarely causes acute mental status change.[19] Patients with metabolic acidosis due to hyperosmolar coma, ketoacidosis, or ingestion (salicylate, methanol, ethylene glycol) have other variables contributing to coma.

Acute severe metabolic alkalosis (bicarbonate >50 mmol/L) may be associated with agitation and clouding of consciousness but rarely with stupor or coma.[20] The frequent association with abnormalities in potassium, calcium, and P_{CO_2} may contribute to central nervous system symptoms.

The presence of hypoxemia is an important finding. In one study of 310 non–drug/trauma coma patients, hypoxia/ischemia was the most common cause (nearly 40%).[21] The P_{O_2} reflects only the amount of oxygen dissolved in the plasma, however, and does not represent *oxygen-carrying capacity*. A more important reflection of the adequacy of *pulmonary gas exchange* is the $A\text{-}aO_2$ gradient, which is less than 15 in young normal patients but increases in older patients. Elevation over 30 at any age is abnormal.

Chemicals that displace oxygen from hemoglobin (eg, carbon monoxide), cyanide, anemia, and high-affinity hemoglobin do not affect the P_{O_2} measurement despite tissue hypoxia. Metabolic acidosis with respiratory distress should suggest these possibilities. Pulse oximetry gives normal readings in these related clinical situations.

Patients with normal baseline neurologic function and normal oxygen-carrying capacity generally tolerate hypoxemia to a P_{O_2} of 60. Below

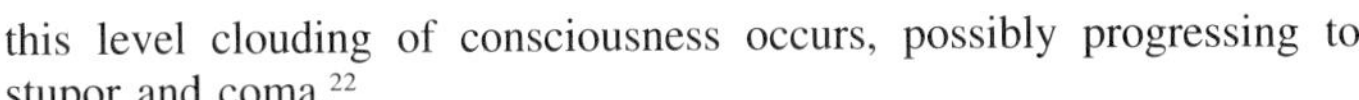

this level clouding of consciousness occurs, possibly progressing to stupor and coma.[22]

Unlike metabolic acidosis, respiratory acidosis is a common cause of altered mental status. Elevation of P_{CO_2} and acidosis suggests acute ventilatory failure. A normal mental status may be present even with a P_{CO_2} as high as 60 to 80. In one study, coma correlated with $P_{CO_2} > 80$ and presence of acidosis.[23]

Hemoglobin/Hematocrit

Severe anemia should not by itself cause altered mental status. Acute loss of red blood cells (and oxygen-carrying capacity) from sudden hemorrhage is reflected in hypotension and tachycardia. Chronic severe red blood cell losses (<7.5 g/dL) are compensated for by increased cardiac output and decreased hemoglobin affinity for oxygen, allowing increased tissue oxygenation. Because P_{O_2} measures the dissolved oxygen in the plasma, it remains normal despite a major loss of hemoglobin.

Electrolytes

Electrolyte abnormalities are responsible for only a few nontraumatic coma cases[5] but may *contribute* to the mental status change in many more.

Sodium

Hyponatremia more often causes seizures than coma or lethargy. In one report, 77% of hyponatremic patients who experienced seizures developed an altered mental status that lasted several hours to days.[20] Patients who developed symptoms did so at sodium levels <115 mmol/L and had a rapid fall in serum sodium levels, usually over less than 48 hours.[20] Hyponatremia due to acute water intoxication (ie, developing over less than 24 hours) is associated with serious manifestations and poor outcome. In contrast, chronic hyponatremia (ie, developing over days to weeks) causes less severe symptoms despite similar sodium levels.[24]

Hypernatremia causes stupor and coma in infants. Among adults, hypernatremia most often occurs in association with severe dehydration and hyperosmolar coma. In the latter, the level of consciousness is correlated with serum osmolality. The sodium concentration is lowered by the presence of large quantities of osmolar substances, mainly glucose. In this situation, to provide an indication of free water balance, the measured sodium value should be corrected by increasing the sodium concentration by 1.3 to 1.6 mmol/L for every 5.56 mmol/L (100 mg/dL) increase in glucose over 100 mg/dL.[25]

Calcium

Hypocalcemia rarely occurs in health but may occur in severe sepsis, pancreatitis, burns, or acute renal failure or after thyroidectomy/parathyroidectomy. The finding of tetany with diffuse muscle spasm or positive Chvostek or Trousseau sign should lead one to suspect hypocalcemia. Seizures are more common than coma.[20]

Falsely low calcium levels occur in the presence of hypoalbuminemia. Ionized calcium levels remain normal. The calcium must be corrected by the following formula: for every decrease in albumin of 1.0 mg% there should be a decrease in the total calcium of 0.8 mg%. Alkalosis increases calcium binding to protein, lowering free calcium.

Hypercalcemia causes mental status changes ranging from mild personality alterations to psychosis. Rapid increases of calcium to levels greater than 14 mg/dL (3.5 mmol/L) commonly result in stupor or coma, although there is considerable individual variation.[20] The most common cause of hypercalcemia in the adult is malignant disease.

Magnesium/Phosphate

Hypomagnesemia causes agitation and hallucinations but rarely stupor or coma. Hypermagnesemia occurs most commonly in renal failure patients because of their inability to excrete magnesium generally taken as antacids. There is some suggestion that the hypotension and respiratory depression with high levels of magnesium may be more responsible for the mental status changes than direct ionic effect.[29]

Severe hypophosphatemia (<1 mg/dL) may cause altered mental status, seizures, or coma.[30, 31] Although severe hypophosphatemia may be observed with prolonged hyperventilation and respiratory alkalosis, these do not cause true phosphate depletion, and patients are not symptomatic.[32] Symptoms occur more frequently in patients with hypophosphatemia secondary to chronic alcoholism, poor dietary intake, and ingestion of phosphate-binding antacids.[32] The exact cause of CNS effects is unknown.[30]

Hyperglycemia

The two major disorders of hyperglycemia are diabetic ketoacidosis and hyperosmolar coma. Stress, pain, and elevated catecholamines elevate the glucose level transiently. Although these findings share some common pathways (dehydration, insulin resistance), they may occur in completely different ways. Diabetic ketoacidosis often appears with signs of acidosis (tachypnea, abdominal pain), whereas hyperosmolar coma appears (usually in the elderly) with profound dehydration and hypoperfusion. Patients who develop hyperosmolar coma are generally debilitated, often without previous diagnosis of glucose intolerance. Alteration in mental status can be directly correlated with osmolality (Table 12–3).

Blood Urea Nitrogen/Creatinine

A sudden rise in blood urea nitrogen (BUN) and creatinine, such as with acute renal failure, causes altered mental status both in level of consciousness and cognitive function, but the degree of azotemia does not correlate well with mental status changes. Patients may have stupor with a BUN of 50 mg/dL or be symptom free with levels of 200 mg/dL.[26]

Blood Osmolality

Osmolality >350 mOsm/kg is associated with a decreased level of consciousness.[27] Osmolality levels >400 represent a clear emergency.

Some exogenous materials (eg, ethanol, methanol, ethylene glycol) contribute to serum osmolality. Because these substances are not measured, a "gap" may be seen between the calculated and measured osmolality.

An osmolar gap of >6 should suggest the presence of one of the substances listed in Table 12–4. The concentration of the substance involved can be calculated; however, it is important to confirm these levels with standard toxicology screen evaluations.

SPECIALIZED TESTS

Computed Tomography Scans

Computed tomography (CT) of the head has revolutionized our approach to neurologic emergencies. The CT scan is superb at disclosing intracerebral bleeding as well as extracerebral bleeding in the form of epidural, subdural, and subarachnoid hemorrhages. A patient with a head injury and an altered level of consciousness has a one in 32 chance of having a significant intracranial process.[33] This number is even higher

TABLE 12–3. GLASGOW-LIEGE SCALE

Eye Opening	Score	Verbal Response	Score	Motor Response	Score	Brain Stem Reflexes	Score
Spontaneously	4	Oriented	5	Obeys	6	Frontoorbicular	5
To speech	3	Confused	4	Localizes	5	Vertical oculovestibular	4
To pain	2	Inappropriate	3	Withdraws	4	Pupillary light	3
No response	1	Incomprehensive	2	Abnormal flexion	3	Horizontal oculovestibular	2
		No response	1	Extension	2	Oculocardiac	1
				No response	1	No response	0

Frontoorbicular reflex—percussion of glabella contracts orbicularis oculi muscle. Vertical oculovestibular reflex—ice water simultaneously in both ears causes vertical deviation of at least one eye. Pupillary light reflex—present in at least one eye. Horizontal oculovestibular reflex—ice water in one ear leads to lateral deviation of at least one eye. Oculocardiac reflex—increasing pressure on the eyeball causes heart to slow.

TABLE 12–4. EFFECT OF SUBSTANCES ON SERUM OSMOLALITY

An Increase in Serum Osmolality of 1 mOsm/Kg H_2O Caused by	Corresponds to a Concentration of (mg/dL)
Methanol	2.6
Ethanol	4.3
Ethylene glycol	5.0
Acetone	5.5
Isopropyl alcohol	5.9

From Kulig K, Duff JR, Linden CH, et al: Toxic effects of methanol, ethylene glycol, and isopropyl alcohol. *Top Emerg Med.* 1984;6:16. ©1984 Aspen Publishers, Inc.

(one in four) in the presence of a skull fracture.[33] The diagnostic accuracy of CT approaches 100% for acute bleeding, excluding subarachnoid hemorrhage. One exception is the isodense subacute subdural hematoma, which may be difficult to differentiate from normal brain tissue.[34, 35]

Subarachnoid hemorrhages account for 8% of nontraumatic comas. Sensitivity of the CT scan is estimated to be 55 to 91%.[36, 37] Therefore, when subarachnoid hemorrhage is considered, a normal CT scan warrants lumbar puncture. Combined, the two have a sensitivity approaching 100%.

Lumbar Puncture

There are two indications for lumbar puncture (LP) in the ED workup of altered mental status—suspected subarachnoid hemorrhage and suspected CNS infection. Lumbar puncture should be routinely performed on patients suspected of having subarachnoid bleeds with normal CT scans. A false-positive LP finding may occur because of bleeding during the procedure (eg, nicking, transecting a vessel). Differential red blood cell count (between the first tube of CSF and the last tube) has been used to distinguish between a bloody tap and true blood in the CSF. However, a patient may have both a bloody tap and a subarachnoid hemorrhage. Therefore, unless the fluid is completely clear on the last tube, one cannot state with total assurance that a subarachnoid hemorrhage has not occurred.

Children, particularly those aged 6 to 12 months, are at greatest risk for meningitis.[38] Nearly 70% of all cases of meningitis occur before the age of 5 years.[39] The signs of meningitis differ among age groups. The neonate <8 weeks old may present with mild fever, vomiting, irritability, or failure to feed. Older infants and toddlers present with fever, often with febrile seizures, and focal neurologic signs (sixth nerve palsy). The progression of their disease may be extremely rapid. Adults present with less prominent headache, stiff neck, and fever. Meningitis due to gram-negative and other unusual organisms may occur in immunosuppressed hosts, after head trauma or neurosurgery, or in patients with ventricular shunts.

Lumbar puncture is the procedure of choice to establish the diagnosis of meningitis and is performed when acute mental status changes occur with signs of toxicity (fever, chills, headache). Fulminant meningitis, however, may lead to significant cerebral edema, especially in children, making an LP potentially dangerous.[40] Computed tomography scan prior to LP when feasible may be warranted.[40]

Encephalitis due to viruses and bacteria may cause coma. Patients present with fever, headache, and altered mental status. Cerebrospinal fluid opening pressure is high (180 to 400 mm), and classically there is leukocytosis (polymorphonuclear cells)[26] with elevated CSF protein but normal glucose levels.[26] CT or MRI may be helpful in establishing the diagnosis of herpes simplex encephalitis.[41]

OTHER TESTS

Toxicology Screen

Poisoning, either accidental or intentional, is the most common cause of altered mental status, particularly in those aged 20 to 49. Very often the diagnosis is obvious (suicide notes, empty pill bottles) but at times is more subtle (therapeutic misadventures, over-the-counter medications) or completely unsuspected (cyanide, carbon monoxide). One study examined all causes of unknown coma, eliminating all cases of *known* poisoning and trauma.[7] Poisoning was the most common cause of coma (52%), including two patients who poisoned themselves while hospitalized for other reasons. More than half of the patients ingested more than one responsible agent.

Urine screens are qualitative tests used to identify drugs that have a rapid elimination time, such as barbiturates, cyclic antidepressants, and sedative-hypnotics. Blood samples, however, are quantitative. Acid or neutral drugs are better detected in blood screens, whereas drugs with large volumes of distribution are better detected in urine screens.[41]

Standard drug screens may or may not include the substance taken by an individual patient. For example, because fentanyl is not on standard screens, patients may respond to naloxone but have a negative toxicology screen evaluation. Analysis of gastric contents may also lead to false-negative toxicology results, because many screens are designed

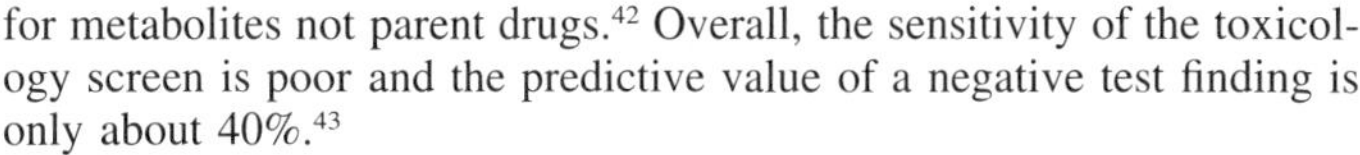

for metabolites not parent drugs.[42] Overall, the sensitivity of the toxicology screen is poor and the predictive value of a negative test finding is only about 40%.[43]

Blood Cultures

Blood cultures should be obtained from patients with altered mental status and signs of sepsis, fever, or neutropenia. In some patients (such as those at risk for endocarditis), multiple blood cultures may be necessary to detect infection.[44] Although it is prudent to draw the first set of blood cultures in the ED before initiating antibiotics, bacteremia can be detected even after antibiotics are initiated.

Other Tests

Reye syndrome occurs with abnormal behavior, nausea, and vomiting, followed by signs of increased intracranial pressure. The CT scan is normal, but there are elevations of the serum ammonia and hepatic

TABLE 12–5. THE WORKUP OF A PATIENT WITH ALTERED MENTAL STATUS

1. Stabilize vital signs
2. Correct reversible causes: hypoglycemia, opiate overdose, and benzodiazepine overdose
3. Assess oxygenation through pulse oximetry; if O_2 Sat is <95%, obtain arterial blood gases
4. History and physical: look for obvious head trauma, signs of poisoning/ingestion, and hypotension
5. If cause undetermined, obtain
   a. Electrolytes, BUN, creatinine, CBC and differential, glucose
   b. ECG
6. If cause still is undetermined, obtain
   a. CT scan
   b. Toxicology screen
7. If special situations, order
   a. SGOT—in young children
   b. LP—normal CT, signs of meningitis, fever, immunosuppression, HIV+
   c. Calcium, phosphate, magnesium—in debilitated, malnourished patients
   d. Serum osmolality—intoxication, suicide behavior
   e. Blood cultures—elderly, febrile, immunosuppressed patients
   f. Thyroid functions—hypothermia, hyperthermia
   g. Liver function tests

enzyme levels. Elevated SGOT levels are very helpful in identifying this syndrome in the ED.[47]

Patients with hypothyroidism often present with decreased consciousness and hypothermia. Unexplained hypothermia should suggest hypothyroidism and prompt ordering of thyroid function tests.

SUMMARY

The workup of a patient with altered mental status (Table 12–5) begins with a detailed history and physical examination. Lateralizing signs suggest structural abnormalities and the need for rapid CT evaluation. Absence of lateralizing signs does not eliminate a structural diagnosis. In some patients, when there are no clues to the diagnosis, the only option is a "shotgun" approach in which initial laboratory tests, toxicology screens, and CT scans are obtained simultaneously.

REFERENCES

1. Lipowski ZJ: Delirium in the elderly patient. *N Engl J Med.* 1989;320:578–582.
2. Hoffman JR, Schriger DL, Luo JS: The empiric use of naloxone in patients with altered mental status: A reappraisal. *Ann Emerg Med.* 1991;20:246–252.
3. Thompson RH, Wolford RW: Development and evaluation of criteria allowing paramedics to treat and release patients presenting with hypoglycemia: A retrospective study. *Prehosp Disaster Med.* 1991;6:309–313. (Including personal communication.)
4. Maragos GD: The unconscious child. *Paediatrician.* 1978;7:142–151.
5. Levy DE, Bates D, Caronna JJ, et al: Prognosis in nontraumatic coma. *Ann Intern Med.* 1981;94:293–301.
6. Purdie FR, Honegman B, Rosen P: Acute organic brain syndrome: A review of 100 cases. *Ann Emerg Med.* 1981;10:455–461.
7. Helliwell M, Hampel G, Sinclair E, et al: Value of emergency toxicological investigation in differential diagnosis of coma. *Br Med J.* 1979;2:819–821.
8. Flumazenil (Editorial). *Lancet.* 1988;2:828–830.
9. Danzl D: Accidental hypothermia, in Rosen P, Baker FJ, Barkin RM, et al (eds): *Emergency Medicine: Concepts and Clinical Practice.* St Louis: CV Mosby Co.; 1989:667.
10. Adler PM: Serum glucose changes after administration of 50% dextrose solution: Pre- and in-hospital calculations. *Am J Emerg Med.* 1986;4:504–506.
11. Minocha A, Barth T, Roberson DG, et al: Impairment of cognitive and psychomuscular function by ethanol in social drinkers. *Vet Hum Toxicol.* 1985;27:533–536.

12. Quaghebeur G, Richards P: Comatose patients smelling of alcohol. *Br Med J.* 1989;299:410.
13. Ellenhorn MJ, Barceloux DG: *Medical Toxicology.* New York: Elsevier Science Publishing Co.; 1988:787.
14. Sorensen SC, Matteson K: Naloxone as an antagonist in severe alcohol intoxication. *Lancet.* 1978;2:688–689.
15. Lyon LJ, Anthony J: Reversal of alcoholic coma by naloxone. *Ann Intern Med.* 1982;96:464–465.
16. Nuotto E, Palva ES, Lahdenranta U: Naloxone fails to counteract heavy alcohol intoxication. *Lancet.* 1983;2:167.
17. Reuler JB: Hypothermia: Pathophysiology, clinical setting, and management. *Ann Intern Med.* 1978;89:519–527.
18. Hutchison AS, Ralston SH, Dryburgh FJ, et al: Too much heparin: Possible source of error in blood gas analysis. *Br Med J.* 1983;287:1131–1132.
19. Posner JB, Plum F: Spinal-fluid pH and neurologic symptoms in systemic acidosis. *N Engl J Med.* 1967;277:605–613.
20. Dubois GD, Arieff AI: Clinical manifestations of electrolyte disorders, in Arieff AJ, DeFronzo RA (eds): *Fluid Electrolyte and Acid-Base Disorders.* New York: Churchill Livingstone; 1985.
21. Bates D, Caronna JJ, Cartlidge NEF, et al: A prospective study of nontraumatic coma: Methods and results in 310 patients. *Ann Neurol.* 1977;2:211–220.
22. West JB: *Pulmonary Pathophysiology,* 3rd ed. Baltimore: Williams & Wilkins; 1987;160.
23. Kilburn KH: Neurologic manifestations of respiratory failure. *Arch Intern Med.* 1965;116:409–415.
24. Arieff AI, Guisado R: Effects on the central nervous system of hypernatremic and hyponatremic status. *Kidney Int.* 1976;10:104–116.
25. Macaulay D, Watson M: Hypernatremia as a cause of brain damage. *Arch Dis Child.* 1967;42:485–491.
26. Plum F, Posner JB: Diagnosis of stupor and coma. Philadelphia: FA Davis Co., 1966.
27. Daugirdas JT, Kronfol NO, Tzamaloukas AH, Ing TS: Hyperosmolar coma: Cellular dehydration and serum sodium concentration. *Ann Intern Med.* 1989;110:855–857.
28. Knochel JP: Disorders of magnesium metabolism, in Wilson JD, Braunwald E, Isselbacher KJ, et al (eds): *Principles and Practice of Internal Medicine.* New York: McGraw-Hill Inc.; 1991:1938.
29. Dirks JH, Alfrey AC: Normal and abnormal magnesium metabolism, in Schrier RW (ed): *Renal and Electrolyte Disorders,* 3rd ed. Boston: Little, Brown and Company; 1986.
30. Knochel JP: The pathophysiology and clinical characteristics of severe hypophosphatemia. *Arch Intern Med.* 1977;137:203–220.
31. Silvis SE, Paragas PD: Paresthesias, weakness, seizures, and hypophosphatemia in patients recovering from hyperalimentation. *Gastroenterology.* 1972;62:513–520.
32. Knochel JP: Disorders of phosphorus metabolism, in Wilson JD, Braunwald E, Isselbacher KJ, et al (eds): *Principles and Practice of Internal Medicine,* New York: McGraw-Hill Inc.; 1991:1933.

33. Mendelow AD, Teasdale G, Jennet B, et al: Risks of intracranial haematoma in head injured adults. *Br Med J.* 1983;287:1173–1176.
34. Weisberg LA: Analysis of the clinical and computed tomographic findings in isodense subdural hematoma. *Comput Radiol.* 1986;10:245–252.
35. Slowikowski JS, Cooperberg CI, Ruisi JA, Bertino FJ: Superiority of magnetic resonance imaging over computer tomography for diagnosing isodense bilateral subdural hematomas. *Am J Med.* 1989;86:345–346.
36. Leblanc R: The minor leak preceding subarachnoid hemorrhage. *J Neurosurg.* 1987;6:35–39.
37. Hillman J: Should computer tomography scanning replace lumbar puncture in the diagnostic process in suspected subarachnoid hemorrhage? *Surg Neurol.* 1986;26:547–550.
38. Roberts KB: Meningitis, in *Manual of Clinical Problems in Pediatrics.* Boston: Little, Brown and Company; 1979:10.
39. Hartner DH, Petersdorf RC: Bacterial meningitis and brain abscess, in Wilson JD, Isselbacher KH, et al (eds): *Principles and Practice of Internal Medicine.* New York: McGraw-Hill, Inc.; 1991:2023–2031.
40. Pearce JMS: Hazards of lumbar puncture. *Br Med J Clin Res.* 1982; 285:1521–1522.
41. Neils EW, Lukin R, Tomsick TA, Tew JM: Magnetic resonance imaging and computerized tomography scanning of herpes simplex encephalitis—report of two cases. *J Neurosurg.* 1987;67:592–594.
42. Ellenhorn MJ, Barceloux DG: *Medical Toxicology.* New York: Elsevier Science Publishing Co.: 1988;42–52.
43. Hepler BR, Suthermer CA, Sunshine I: The role of the toxicology laboratory in emergency medicine. *J Toxicol Clin Toxicol.* 1982;19:353–365.
44. Aronson MD, Bor DH: Blood cultures. *Ann Intern Med.* 1987;106:246–253.
45. Caveney S: Molecular integrity of aspirin in relation to Reye's syndrome. *W Va Med J.* 1988;84:186–190.
46. Lecky BRF, Winer JB, Kenwright S: Mild Reye's syndrome in an adult. *J Neurol Neurosurg Psych.* 1984;47:885–886.
47. Mertes S, Bubis S: Diagnostic quality of laboratory tests as evaluated by graphic comparison of "first test" data, with Reye's syndrome "work-up" assays as a model. *Clin Chem.* 1987;33:100–102.

Chapter

Seizure

Charles Whiteman

As with any emergency department patient, diagnostic testing in one with seizures should be guided by a thorough history and physical examination. To facilitate the discussion of the emergency department evaluation of the seizure patient, it is important to consider subgroups of these patients separately.

KNOWN SEIZURE DISORDER

The most common cause of a seizure in an individual on anticonvulsant therapy is a subtherapeutic anticonvulsant level,[1] and the most common reason cited for a subtherapeutic anticonvulsant level is noncompliance with therapy.[1, 2] If the patient arrives in the emergency department awake, alert, and at baseline mental status, the laboratory evaluation should consist only of determination of the anticonvulsant level.[2] Eisner et al[2] found routine metabolic screening to be of little help in evaluating patients with epilepsy presenting to an emergency department after seizure. Although minor laboratory abnormalities were noted, treatment or disposition was not changed. The most common electrolyte abnormality was the serum bicarbonate level (15 to 35 mmol/L), attributed primarily to transient lactic acidosis from major motor seizure. No serum sodium abnormality significant enough to cause seizure activity was noted (129 to 150 mmol/L). All serum magnesium levels fell within the range of 1.4 to 3.2 mmol/L. Serum calcium levels ranged from 8.1 to 10.9 mmol/L and were not believed to be the cause of seizure recurrence. Minor abnormalities of the serum potassium and chloride levels were also noted, but these abnormalities have not been implicated as causes of seizures. Serum glucose abnormalities significant enough to cause seizures in patients with epilepsy were not reported by Eisner et al. Retrospective views by Powers[3] and Krumholz et al[1] have demonstrated similar results when routine metabolic screens were obtained on patients with epilepsy who presented to the emergency department following seizures.

Cranial computed tomography (CT) should be promptly obtained in patients with epilepsy if the history or physical examination is suggestive of acute head trauma, intracranial hemorrhage, or intracranial mass.[4, 5] Routine CT scanning, however, is of little value in the evaluation of this group of patients.

NEW-ONSET SEIZURES

Patients presenting to an emergency department after a first episode of seizure activity have traditionally been evaluated with a large battery of laboratory tests.[6] The incidence of metabolic abnormality as the cause of new-onset seizure has been reported to be between 2.4 and 8%.[3, 6, 7] In prospective evaluations of such patients by Turnbull et al[7] and Eisner et al,[2] no significant abnormalities in the serum electrolytes were identified that were not suspected on the basis of the history and physical examination. As in the group of patients with epilepsy, Eisner et al[2] reported minor abnormalities in the serum electrolytes of the new-onset seizure patients, but none required therapeutic intervention.

In contrast, abnormalities of the serum glucose levels, both hypoglycemia and hyperglycemia, are not uncommonly noted in the first-time seizure patient,[6, 7] and these abnormalities may not be clearly suggested by the history and physical examination. Thus, the serum glucose level should be routinely checked on all new-onset seizure patients.

Both therapeutically and self-administered drugs can result in seizure in otherwise normal individuals.[8, 9] Although no data support routine drug screening of all new-onset seizure patients, screening based on historical or physical findings is appropriate.

Urgent head CT scanning is indicated in patients with a new-onset seizure who also have historical or physical examination findings suggestive of acute head trauma, intracranial hemorrhage, or intracranial mass.

FEBRILE SEIZURES

As in other groups of seizure patients, large batteries of laboratory tests have traditionally been obtained in the emergency department assessment of the patient with a febrile seizure.[8] Nevertheless, Rutter and Smales[10] found routine chemistries and complete blood counts to be of little utility in the evaluation, treatment, or disposition of children with a first febrile seizure. Abnormalities in the serum electrolytes results were noted but reflected dehydration or other clinical syndromes indicated by the history or physical examination.

When a patient presents to the emergency department with a fever and a history of seizure, the possibility of intracranial infection must be addressed. In the absence of signs of increased intracranial pressure, a lumbar puncture should be performed unless the episode can clearly be classified as a febrile seizure. The risks of lumbar puncture in patients with normal intracranial pressure are relatively small (<0.5% for serious complications and usually self-limited).[11] Lumbar puncture is generally believed to be contraindicated in patients with evidence of increased intracranial pressure, whether due to acute meningitis or intracranial mass lesion.[12, 13] Cranial CT should be performed prior to lumbar puncture in these patients. If lumbar puncture is considered to be contraindicated, the etiological agent of acute bacterial meningitis can be identified using bacterial antigen assays on body fluids other than cerebrospinal fluid.[14]

SUMMARY

A standard battery of routine diagnostic tests is not indicated for all seizure patients presenting to the emergency department. Selective laboratory screening based on a thorough history and physical examination can help in the diagnosis and treatment of the seizure patient in the emergency department. Cranial CT is indicated when the history or physical examination suggests acute head trauma, intracranial hemorrhage, or intracranial mass.

REFERENCES

1. Krumholz A, Grufferman S, Orr S, et al: Seizures and seizure care in an emergency department. *Epilepsia.* 1989;30:175–181.
2. Eisner RF, Turnbull T, Howes D, et al: Efficacy of a "standard" seizure workup in the emergency department. *Ann Emerg Med.* 1986;15:33–39.
3. Powers RA: Serum chemistry abnormalities in adult patients with seizure. *Ann Emerg Med.* 1985;14:416–420.
4. Gastaut H, Gastaut JL: Computerized transverse axial tomography in epilepsy. *Epilepsia.* 1976;17:325–336.
5. Forbes SG, Sheedy P, Piepgras D, et al: Computed tomography in the evaluation of subdural hematomas. *Radiology.* 1978;126:143–145.
6. Rosenthal RH, Helm M, Waeckerele J, et al: First time major motor seizure in an emergency department. *Ann Emerg Med.* 1980;9:242–245.
7. Turnbull TL, Vanden H, Howes D, et al: Utility of laboratory studies in the emergency department patient with a new-onset seizure. *Ann Emerg Med.* 1990;19:373–377.
8. Tomlanovich MC, Yee AS: Seizures, in Rosen P, et al (eds): *Emergency Medicine: Concepts and Clinical Practice.* Vol 2. St. Louis: CV Mosby; 1992:1787–1805.

9. Jick H, Slone D, Shapiro S, et al: Drug-induced convulsions. *Lancet.* 1972;2:677–679.
10. Rutter N, Smales ORC: Role of routine investigations in children presenting with their first febrile convulsion. *Arch Dis Child.* 1977;52:188–191.
11. Wiesel J, Rose D, Silver A, et al: Lumbar puncture in asymptomatic late syphilis. *Arch Intern Med.* 1985;145:465–468.
12. Sharp CG, Steinhart CM: Lumbar puncture in the presence of increased intracranial pressure: The real danger. *Pediatr Emerg Care.* 1987;3:39–43.
13. Heldrich FJ, Johnson T: Risk of diagnostic lumbar puncture in acute bacterial meningitis. *Pediatr Emerg Care.* 1986;2:180–182.
14. Siegel JD: New developments in meningitis. *Pediatr Infect Dis.* 1982; 1:3(supplement):S45–S51.

Chapter

14 The Febrile Adult

J. Stephan Stapczynski

In contrast to the extensive number of studies and reviews devoted to the problem of the pediatric patient presenting to the emergency department (ED) with a fever, the published literature concerning the evaluation of the adult patient with a fever is sparse. This is surprising because fever is a common condition in the ED.

Because infection is often equated with fever, three facts deserve mention. First, fever does not always indicate infection.[1] Second, infection does not always cause fever, especially in the very young and very old. Third, the severity of fever does not correlate with the severity of the infectious process.

There is no well-established definition for a discrete body temperature that defines a fever.[2] Human body temperature is surprisingly constant when measured in large populations. There are distinct differences among individuals, however, and even within the same individual, when temperature is measured at different times of the day and at different sites.[3] Body temperature has a diurnal variation, typically lowest in the early morning (around 5 am) and rising to a peak level in the early evening (around 8 pm).[4] The differences in the lowest and highest values range between 0.3 and 1.5°C in normal adults. In young adults, rectal temperatures are typically higher than oral temperatures by about 0.5 to 0.6°C, although the range of difference is from −0.6 to 1.1°C.[3]

With advancing age, mean oral temperatures decrease whereas rectal temperatures remain similar to those in younger adults.[4] Thus, in the elderly, the rectal temperature may be as much as 1.0°C higher than the oral temperature. The finding of an oral temperature within a normal range, therefore, does not exclude an increased core temperature as measured rectally in the elderly.[5]

Without delving into issues of clinical thermometry and body temperature measurement, this review considers an oral temperature equal to or above 38°C to be a fever. Although some individuals without any recognizable illnesses may have body temperatures in this range, this low limit will be sensitive enough to detect most of those patients with significant disorders that disturb body thermoregulation.

CLINICAL PROBLEM

Several studies have documented that 2 to 6% of adult patients presenting to EDs have a fever or history of fever.[6–8] These patients can be divided into two broad groups. The first group presents with specific symptoms, usually localizing to a body area, and have a fever. The second group presents primarily because of fever itself and may have secondary symptoms, such as chills, sweats, or malaise.

The likelihood of a potential cause being responsible for fever in the adult varies according to the patient's age and underlying medical condition.[9, 10] For example, a healthy 19 year old presenting with a fever is most likely to have an infection owing to one of the respiratory viruses, whereas an 80-year-old bedridden patient from a nursing home is more likely to have a bacterial infection of the respiratory or urinary tract. The astute physician uses demographic and historical information to ascertain the likelihood of serious bacterial infections in adults: age, season, previous health status, underlying medical conditions, and location where illness developed.

CLINICAL APPROACH

The approach to the febrile patient in the ED involves detecting a treatable infection—which for practical purposes in most situations means bacterial—or excluding a treatable infection to a reasonable degree of clinical certainty. The evidence collected by the emergency physician that enters into the decision-making process is obtained from the history, physical examination, and ancillary tests available within a clinically relevant time frame. For a patient who presents with a clinical syndrome that, from the symptoms and signs, has a high probability of being due to a bacterial infection, ancillary tests provide little information of use in making diagnostic or therapeutic decisions. Conversely, in a patient with a clinical syndrome that has a very low probability of being due to a bacterial infection (eg, the common cold), ancillary tests also have little utility. Between these two extremes, ancillary tests in the ED are useful in the febrile adult

1. To detect or suggest a disease that is not suspected upon clinical grounds. The value of these ancillary tests is best in patients with an intermediate pretest probability of disease.
2. To confirm and document the clinical diagnosis. The results of these tests may not influence immediate clinical decision making but may have implications for disposition or follow-up.

There are four important questions to ask in the evaluation of the febrile adult:

1. Are there symptoms or signs that suggest a localized process?
2. Is this localized process infectious or noninfectious?
3. If infectious, is the cause bacterial or nonbacterial?
4. Does the patient have cause, based on clinical grounds, for emergency hospitalization?

The patient's general condition—how well the illness is being tolerated—often determines the disposition; relatively ''well'' patients are usually discharged, and ''ill'' patients are usually admitted. There are important exceptions, however. Patients with serious comorbid conditions or underlying immunodeficiencies are usually admitted because of the possibility of serious complications developing rapidly owing to delayed diagnosis or treatment.

In 70 to 85% of febrile adults presenting to the ED, a strongly suggested clinical diagnosis can be made based upon the history and physical examination.[7–9] Ancillary tests in these patients are often inappropriate and without clinical justification.

The evaluation of the febrile patient should consider the epidemiologic setting. Malaria is a common cause of acute undifferentiated fever in Southeast Asia, for example, but not in suburban communities in the United States. Likewise, in the rural areas of the mid-Atlantic region, the otherwise relatively rare infection Rocky Mountain spotted fever becomes a serious diagnostic consideration during the spring and summer. Although most acute febrile illnesses in the United States are infectious, usually due to a respiratory virus, the majority of these remain without an etiology because diagnostic techniques are elaborate, costly, and time consuming and do not influence patient management or outcome.

History and Physical Examination

A comprehensive physical examination is always valuable but not always possible in a busy department and not always necessary for many patients. In most cases, important physical findings will be guided by symptoms elicited from the history, and these symptoms point to a localizing source.[7, 11] Some findings, although not localizing, are indicative of generalized sepsis or bacteremia.[12] Signs such as tachycardia, hypotension, tachypnea, or hyperventilation are associated with a 37 to 47% positive blood culture rate.[13]

Physical examination skills are less than 100% sensitive. For example, physical findings of pulmonary consolidation may be absent in 6 to 25% of patients with a radiographic infiltrate.[7, 15]

Clinical Impression

After the history and physical examination, it is useful to classify the patient's illness according to a syndrome, if possible: eg, upper respiratory infection (nasal congestion, rhinitis, sinus congestion, sore throat), acute pharyngitis (sore throat, cervical adenopathy), lower respiratory infection (productive cough), and gastroenteritis (nausea, vomiting, diarrhea). This clinical impression then guides the remainder of the evaluation.

For each of these syndromes, according to the age of the patient and underlying host status, there is a relatively limited number of most likely pathogens. For example, in a young, healthy adult with an upper respiratory infection syndrome, the causes are overwhelmingly viral. A bacterial etiology is not a realistic consideration. For therapeutic and patient disposition decisions, additional ancillary testing is not necessary. For an elderly patient who presents with an lower respiratory infection, however, bacterial pneumonia is likely. A chest radiograph is indicated.

Patients without focal symptoms or signs present a challenge.[7, 8] The possibility of a clinically occult bacterial infection exists and is similar to that in a febrile infant. Mellors et al[7] first developed the multivariate risk index on ED patients that was also studied by Leibovici et al[11] on inpatients. The results were similar (Table 14–1). Additional conclusions of these studies are

1. A significant portion of adults with fever unexplained by history

TABLE 14–1. MULTIVARIATE INDEX FOR CLINICALLY OCCULT BACTERIAL INFECTION (FEBRILE ADULT PATIENTS WITHOUT LOCALIZING SYMPTOMS OR SIGNS)

Score One Point for Each Factor

Age ≥50 years
Diabetes mellitus
WBC ≥15,000
Neutrophil band count ≥1500
ESR ≥30 mm/h

	Emergency Department Patients[a]	
Score	*Bacterial Infection*	*Bacteremia*
0	1/21 (5%)	0/21 (0%)
1	15/45 (33%)	3/45 (7%)
2	15/38 (39%)	6/38 (16%)
≥3	17/31 (55%)	12/31 (39%)
	Hospitalized Patients[b]	
Score	*Bacterial Infection*	*Bacteremia*
0	1/11 (0%)	0/11 (0%)
1	12/44 (27%)	5/44 (11%)
2	13/41 (32%)	7/41 (17%)
≥3	9/17 (53%)	6/17 (35%)

[a]After history and physical examination in ED.
[b]After initial assessment on inpatient unit including ancillary tests.
Data from Mellors JW et al: *Arch Intern Med.* 1987;147:666–671. ©1987 American Medical Association; data from Leibovici L et al: *Arch Intern Med.* 1990;150:1270–1272. ©1990 American Medical Association.

or physical examination had a bacterial infection (about 30%) often with bacteremia (about 15%).

2. These clinically occult infections were most often due to common bacteria in common locations (Table 14–2).

3. The incidence of diagnostically positive abnormalities from the routine use of urinalysis (UA) was 16 and 13% and from chest radiography 4 and 3%, respectively, in the two studies. Routine UA and chest radiography detected approximately half of clinically occult infections (Table 14–3).

4. Increasing age, underlying illness, leukocytosis, or left shift on the white blood cell differential was associated with increased risk of bacterial infection.

5. In the study by Mellors et al,[7] about two thirds of patients with clinically occult infections presented with general findings that led to hospital admissions based upon physician judgment. Of the approximately one third that were sent home, the incidence of bacterial infection was about 20%.

TABLE 14–2. CAUSE OF CLINICALLY OCCULT BACTERIAL INFECTIONS (FEBRILE ADULT PATIENTS WITHOUT LOCALIZING SYMPTOMS OR SIGNS)

	Reference 6	Reference 10
Urinary[a]	22 (6)	15 (5)
Respiratory	8 (1)	3 (1)
Endocarditis	3 (3)	2 (2)
Other		
Osteomyelitis	1 (0)	0
Axillary abscess	1 (0)	0
Retroperitoneal	1 (0)	0
Paracolonic abscess	1 (0)	0
Sigmoid colon	1 (1)	0
Peritonitis	0	2 (1)
Dysentery	0	2 (0)
Ascending cholangitis	0	1 (0)
Meningitis	0	1 (1)
Primary bacteremia	10 (10)	8 (8)
Total	48 (21)	34 (18)
n = total patients	135	113

Data from Mellors JW et al: *Arch Intern Med.* 1987;147:666–671. ©1987 American Medical Association; data from Leibovici L et al: *Arch Intern Med.* 1990;150:1270–1272. ©1990 American Medical Association.

ANCILLARY TESTS

White Blood Cell Count and Differential

Studies of unselected emergency patients have noted that the white blood cell count (WBC) is of low utility in clinical decision making.[16–18]

TABLE 14–3. YIELD OF URINALYSIS AND CHEST RADIOGRAPH IN PATIENTS WITH CLINICALLY OCCULT BACTERIAL INFECTION

	Urinalysis	Chest Radiograph
Reference 6[a]	22/135	6/135
Reference 10[b]	15/113	3/113

[a]After history and physical examination in ED.
[b]After initial assessment on inpatient unit including ancillary tests.
Data from Mellors JW et al: *Arch Intern Med.* 1987;147:666–671. ©1987 American Medical Association; data from Leibovici L et al: *Arch Intern Med.* 1990;150:1270–1272. ©1990 American Medical Association.

Overall, the total WBC and differential is insensitive in detecting bacterial infections and lacks specificity to exclude them as well.

In selected subgroups, the WBC count can be used to increase the confirmation of bacterial infection in (1) adults with fever unexplained by history and physical examination,[7, 11] (2) febrile patients with history that suggests leukopenia,[19] and (3) febrile elderly adults (age >70).[10] In febrile adults without localizing symptoms or signs, a WBC count over 15,000/mm^3 is associated with a 56% incidence of bacterial infection and a 28% incidence of bacteremia, compared with incidences of 32 and 13%, respectively, in patients with a WBC less than 15,000/mm^3.[7] In neutropenic patients with a fever, a neutrophil count below 1000/mm^3 is associated with a 20 to 30% incidence of bacteremia.[7, 19] In the febrile elderly population, a WBC count over 14,000/mm^3 is associated with a 50% incidence of bacterial infection, compared with a 33% rate in those with a WBC count below 14,000/mm^3.[10] Although there is clearly an increased risk of bacterial infection in these three groups when the WBC count is "abnormal," the unanswered question is whether the detection of an abnormal WBC actually affects the decision process. Does it trigger a more intensive evaluation to detect a bacterial infection than otherwise would have been performed? A single conclusion can be drawn, and the answer depends upon the clinical circumstances and the physician's judgment.

It is also worth noting the value of the *white blood cell differential* in detecting bacterial infection in two of these groups: the febrile adult patient without localizing symptoms or signs and the febrile elderly patient (age >70). In the febrile adult without localizing symptoms or signs, an absolute neutrophil band count over 1500/mm^3 was associated with a 50% incidence of bacterial infection and a 20% incidence of bacteremia, compared with rates of 28 and 12%, respectively, in patients with counts below 1500/mm^3.[7] In the febrile elderly, a white blood cell differential with ≥6% neutrophil bands was associated with a 78% incidence of bacterial infection, compared with a 29% incidence with <6% bands.[10]

Abnormal total WBC count and elevated percentage of neutrophilic bands are associated with increased risk of bacterial infection and bacteremia in these groups. The risk is only relative—these infections can be absent with abnormal values or present with normal values. Is it possible to develop low-risk criteria using a combination of WBC and differential counts that would identify some patients who are at such low risk for bacterial infection that further testing is not useful? In the multivariate analysis of Mellors et al that evaluated febrile adults without localizing symptoms or signs (assuming age less than 50, absence of diabetes, ESR less than 30 mm/h), those with a total WBC count less than 15,000/mm^3, and an absolute neutrophil band count less than 1500/mm^3, the incidence of bacterial infection was 3% (2/32), and the incidence of bacteremia was 0% (0/32).[7, 11] Preliminary data from another study of febrile adults, with and without localizing symptoms and signs, indicate that, for those younger than 60, with a total WBC count less than 10,000/mm^3 and an absolute neutrophil band count less than 800/mm^3, the incidence of bacterial infection was 5% and the rate of bacteremia was 0%.[8] Although the numbers of patients studied have been small and the conclusions are tentative, a combination of the total WBC and differential may be useful to exclude bacterial infection in some subgroups of febrile adults and may obviate the need for further ancillary testing.

Erythrocyte Sedimentation Rate

In unselected febrile adults, the ESR does not appear to be a useful test in discriminating between those with serious bacterial infections and those without.[20] Similar to the relative risk with leukocytosis, an increased ESR is associated with an increased incidence of bacterial infection. In their study of the febrile adult without localizing symptoms or signs, Mellors et al found that an ESR above 30 mm/h had a sensitivity of 83% and a specificity of 44% for detecting bacterial infections.[7] For bacteremia, the sensitivity was 85% and the specificity was 39%. The incidence of bacterial infection and bacteremia in patients with an ESR greater than 30 mm/h was 50 and 30%, respectively, with corresponding rates of 20 and 10% in patients with an ESR less than 30 mm/h. By itself, the ESR had only modest utility but remained an independent factor in the multivariate analysis.[7, 11]

Urinalysis

Urinalysis is useful in febrile patients with urinary symptoms: internal dysuria, frequency, urgency, and flank or abdominal pain.[21] In patients with acute pyelonephritis syndrome (fever, chills, flank pain, nausea, vomiting) or patients with subclinical pyelonephritis (dysuria but with "upper tract infection"), the UA is almost always "positive" with pyuria (>5 WBC/high-power field).[21] As such, a positive result is enough to terminate further diagnostic evaluation and begin empiric treatment. A negative result indicates strongly against a urinary tract infection being the cause of the fever in an otherwise healthy adult. In immunosuppressed or neutropenic patients, a urinary tract infection may be present without pyuria, and a "negative" UA does not exclude the need for a urine culture.[11, 31]

As noted previously, the UA is also useful in (1) the febrile adult patient without localizing symptoms or signs[7, 11] and (2) the febrile elderly patient to detect a clinically occult urinary tract infection.[9, 10]

Chest Radiograph

Using a radiographically visible infiltrate as the standard, clinical examination has deficiencies in detecting pneumonia. Of patients with a radiographic infiltrate, 6 to 25% may lack auscultatory findings on clinical examination.[7, 15] Conversely, abnormal auscultatory findings have been reported in 20 to 62% of patients without a radiographic infiltrate.[23–25] Thus, the chest x-ray (CXR) remains the most accurate technique for diagnosing pneumonia in the ED.

The development of decision rules to predict the absence or presence of pneumonia has met with mixed success. Singal et al[23] attempted to develop low-yield criteria, which, if present, would obviate the need for chest radiography. The univariate predictors for a radiographic infiltrate were the presence of fever, cough, and rales.[23] For patients without these findings, the incidence of pneumonia was three of 67 (4.5%). These researchers concluded that they could not devise any clinically useful low-yield criteria that improved upon an experienced clinician's probability estimate of pneumonia. Heckerling et al[25] developed a clinical prediction rule based on five factors: fever, tachycardia (pulse >100/min), rales, decreased breath sounds, and absence of asthma. This prediction rule was derived from one patient set and validated on two other sets. The overall prevalence of pneumonia in each set was 12.4, 30, and 21.5%, respectively. Combining the three sets and assuming a patient had a fever but no other findings, the incidence of pneumonia was 17 of 452 (4%, 95% confidence index (CI) of 2.3 to 5.7). Mellors et al and Leibovici et al found clinically occult pneumonia in 4 and 3% of their febrile adults, respectively,[7, 11] and Jochelson et al found pneumonia in three of 75 (4%) febrile neutropenic patients without pulmonary symptoms.[26] A reasonable conclusion from these studies is that febrile adults have about a 4% incidence of pneumonia (radiographic infiltrate) in the absence of any pulmonary symptoms or signs. The development of low-yield criteria to exclude pneumonia clinically is likely to be limited by this baseline incidence.

The CXR results may not influence therapeutic or disposition decision making. If, for example, the physician plans to treat the patient with antibiotics based upon the clinical presentation of fever and productive cough, the results of a CXR have little influence. Likewise, in patients who have pneumonia but are otherwise healthy and clinically tolerating the infection (not hypoxic, toxic, or in respiratory distress), outpatient management is acceptable and the CXR results will have little influence on that decision.

Blood Cultures

Three studies have found that the routine use of blood cultures (BCs) in febrile adult emergency patients does not improve disposition decision making, has a low yield, increases cost, produces many false-positives, and imposes the added liability of requiring the physician to discharge patients with positive cultures for follow-up evaluation.[27–29] Thus, the unrestricted use of BCs in the ED has little utility.

For the febrile adult without localizing symptoms or signs and a score of zero on the multivariate score of Mellors et al, BCs had a low yield: none of 32 (0%, CI 0 to 10%).[7, 11] Although the numbers of patients are small, the data suggest that BCs have little use in such individuals. Studies of hospitalized patients have also been performed to develop prediction criteria for bacteremia,[30–32] but the prevalence of bacteremia is higher than in either the outpatient or ED setting. The incidence of bacteremia predicted for the lowest risk group is 1 to 2%. This value may be applicable for use in the ED when patients with serious comorbid conditions present with fever. Aronson and Bor concluded that, when the incidence of bacteremia is greater than 1%, BCs appear to be useful.[33]

Emergency department BCs have a role in situations in which the BC is the primary modality of diagnosis, ie, suspected bacterial endocarditis. Two populations that may present to the ED should have BCs drawn: intravenous drug users[34–36] and patients with prosthetic heart valves.[37]

Blood cultures drawn in the ED have also been found to be positive in patients with cellulitis, gastroenteritis, pyelonephritis, and pneumonia. Depending upon the syndromes, host factors, and organisms, the rate of bacteremia in febrile adults is as low as 1% in patients with simple cellulitis and as high as 60% in patients with suppurative thrombophlebitis. In most of these cases, a bacteriologic diagnosis can be made from the primary site, and the disposition decision is based on clinical grounds. There is little justification for routinely performing ED BCs in patients with these clinical syndromes.

SPECIAL PATIENT POPULATIONS

Certain patient subgroups have increased incidences of bacterial infections. With rare exception, however, there is little in the medical literature to validate a diagnostic approach or to evaluate the utility of ancillary tests in the assessment of these patients when they present with fever. In general, their evaluation during an ED presentation must include both a symptom- and sign-directed approach as well as testing to detect clinically occult infections. The extent of such testing necessary to make diagnostic, therapeutic, and disposition decisions in the ED has not been well studied.

HIV

HIV-infected patients are susceptible to a wide range of infectious disorders, a range far too wide to review in this discussion.[38] Whereas HIV patients are commonly considered to be at risk primarily for nonbacterial infections, they are also at increased risk for bacterial pathogens such as *Nocardia, Listeria, Salmonella*, and mycobacteria, as well as for increased disease severity in infections of *Salmonella, Shigella*, pneumococcus, *Haemophilus influenzae*, and *Campylobacter.*[39]

The febrile HIV-positive patient's evaluation is primarily directed by signs, symptoms, and physical findings. The physical examination should include looking carefully for focal infections: oral lesions or ulcerations, thrush, sinus tenderness, retinal lesions, fluctuant lymphadenopathy, focal rales, abdominal tenderness, hepatosplenomegaly, perirectal ulceration or swelling, and alterations in the neurologic findings.

Two serious opportunistic infections in HIV patients may appear with fever alone: cryptococcosis and *Mycobacterium avium* complex infection. Therefore, a broad diagnostic evaluation is recommended, even in patients with fever as the sole symptom: CBC, urinalysis, urine culture, BC, electrolytes, blood urea nitrogen, creatinine, liver function tests, and perhaps serum cryptococcal antigen. Additional blood tests and cultures are guided by symptoms and physical findings. Chest radiographs are recommended because lung infections are frequent and may occur with few symptoms or findings. When the $CD4^+$ lymphocyte count falls below 200/mm^3, the lung is the most common site of infection, often with *Pneumocystis carinii.*

In general, hospitalization is required for the HIV patient with a new fever, especially in the presence of dyspnea, neutropenia, thrombocytopenia, or a toxic appearance. If the ED evaluation is nondiagnostic and the patient is tolerating the fever without other symptoms, discharge is appropriate, but further assessment should be arranged within 2 days.

Intravenous Drug Users

The evaluation of febrile intravenous drug users is complicated because of the possibility of endocarditis and the inability to accurately predict its presence or absence upon ED evaluation.[34–36] Studies from municipal hospitals in New York City, Boston, and Newark found that the most common infection in the febrile intravenous drug user was pneumonia, seen in 33 to 38%. The incidence of bacterial endocarditis was 6 to 13%. Other serious bacterial infections in these febrile patients were pneumonia, cellulitis, abscess, septic arthritis, and pyelonephritis. Importantly, only a minority of patients, 15 to 32%, had "minor" illnesses.

Although some clinical features or ancillary test results were associated with occult bacterial infection or endocarditis, no single feature or combination was accurate enough to guide the evaluation or disposition decisions. In the study by Marantz et al, two of seven (28%) of the patients predicted to have a minor illness upon ED evaluation developed major illness during hospitalization[34]; three of the 28 (11%) of the patients predicted *not to have* endocarditis did indeed *have* endocarditis. In the study by Samet et al, 9% of patients predicted *not to have* bacteremia *had* positive blood cultures (7 of 79), and 4% of patients predicted *not to have* endocarditis did indeed *have* endocarditis (6 of 140).[35]

If the initial evaluation is nondiagnostic, admission is not mandatory but 24- to 48-hour follow-up of BC results is required. If this is not possible because of likely noncompliance, hospitalization during this period is recommended as the safest course of action.[54]

Alcoholics

Alcoholics are at increased risk for infection, the most common being pneumonia.[40] Most infections are clinically apparent, with the exception of spontaneous bacterial peritonitis (SBP) and, possibly, endocarditis. Spontaneous bacterial peritonitis typically occurs with fever and diffuse abdominal pain. Paracentesis is therefore indicated when these symptoms are present in a patient with ascites.

Recommended ancillary tests include CBC, analysis of electrolytes, coagulation studies, UA, BCs, and chest radiograph. Abdominal paracentesis is required when an alcoholic patient with ascites presents with a fever, the clinical evaluation is nondiagnostic, and no infection can be found in the lungs or urinary tract (upon chest radiograph and UA).

Alcoholics with infections tend to do poorly and have an increased incidence of complications; moreover, compliance with outpatient regimens is usually poor. Hospitalization should be the norm.

Neutropenia

The evaluation of the febrile neutropenic patient is based upon the consistent findings that rapid administration of broad-spectrum antibiotics reduces the mortality from bacterial infection, most typically gram-negative sepsis.[41]

Although the physical examination should be directed by localizing symptoms, if present, careful attention must be paid to areas that may harbor focal infection but that may not manifest symptoms in the neutropenic patient: teeth, sinuses, ears, lungs, perineal and perirectal areas, and any skin lesions.[22] Urinalysis, urine culture, and BCs are indicated. Review articles recommend chest radiography, even in the absence of pulmonary symptoms, but the yield of such an approach is unknown. A study of 75 febrile neutropenic patients without symptoms or signs of pneumonia found three (4%) with new radiographic infiltrates.[26] These investigators did note, however, that the detection of the infiltrate before the development of symptoms did not affect treatment or the clinical course. Clearly, any patient with pulmonary symptoms or signs should have chest radiography performed.

Cancer

Fever is a common problem in patients with cancer; the largest single cause of such episodes is infection.[42] The major risk factor for bacterial infection is neutropenia, usually related to chemotherapy.[43] Cancer may also provide the basis for local infection by obstructing the normal flow of air, bowel contents, bile, or urine. Other causes for fever in cancer patients include antineoplastic drugs, blood transfusions, and radiation-induced tumor necroses, in addition to neoplasias themselves.

The ED evaluation is typically broad for the cancer patient, although the yield from such an approach is unknown.

Diabetes Mellitus

It is well known that diabetes predisposes patients to bacterial infections. The three most common sites are the lungs, urinary tract, and skin.[43] The presence of diabetes increases the risk of a clinically occult infection in febrile adult patients without localizing symptoms or signs.[7, 8, 11] This predisposition appears to be present for both insulin- and non–insulin-dependent diabetes.[7, 11] A CBC, UA, and chest radiograph seem appropriate in febrile diabetics unless they have clear-cut localizing symptoms for which the likelihood of a bacterial etiology is very low (eg, URI).

Elderly Adults

A common theme throughout this discussion has been that elderly adults are more prone to bacterial infection. This observation has been borne out in many different studies.[6–11] Unfortunately, most do not distinguish between those elderly patients who can care for themselves and those who have lost the capacity to care for themselves (the "frail elderly").[44, 45] Frail elderly adults are especially susceptible to infections because of impairments (dementia, immobility, pulmonary aspiration, urinary incontinence) and typical place of residence (nursing homes or extended care facilities).[44] It is in these frail elderly patients that the febrile response to infection may be blunted or absent.[6, 9, 10] The practical point is that a fever in an elderly patient, particularly a frail one, should be considered as evidence of a bacterial infection and thus requires a thorough ED evaluation and admission to the hospital.

SUMMARY

Although the potential causes for fever in adults are many, the majority (70 to 80%) can be diagnosed by a thoughtful history and symptom-directed physical examination. Ancillary tests and cultures should be used intelligently to substantiate the clinical impression and to assist in therapeutic and disposition decisions. For those patients without localizing symptoms or signs, approximately half of the clinically occult bacterial infections are detected by chest radiography and UA. The diagnosis of the other half rests primarily on the results of BCs. In suburban America, the overwhelming majority of clinically occult bacterial infections are cases with common bacteria in common locations; "zebras" are rare.

Patients with underlying immunodeficiencies or comorbid conditions are predisposed to bacterial infections and require more thorough evaluations with ancillary tests and cultures.

Disposition decisions are still based predominantly on clinical condition—how well is the patient tolerating the illness? Similar to a febrile 3 month old, in whom the "septic workup" is "negative" and the patient is discharged home with a follow-up examination scheduled in 24 hours, the febrile adult with a nondiagnostic evaluation in the ED should also be seen again or contacted by phone in 24 hours.

The evaluation of the febrile adult requires a thoughtful history, careful physical examination, and judicious use of ancillary tests but, most of all, intelligence and common sense to decide on a course of action.

REFERENCES

1. Bernheim HA, Block LH, Atkins E: Fever: Pathogenesis, pathophysiology, and purpose. *Ann Intern Med.* 1979;91:261–270.

2. Mackowiak PA, Wasserman SS, Levine MM: A critical appraisal of 98.6° F, the upper limit of the normal body temperature and other legacies of Carl Reinhold August Wunderlich. *JAMA.* 1992;268:1578–1580.
3. Horvath SM, Menduke H, Pierson GM: Oral and rectal temperatures of man. *JAMA.* 1950;144:1562–1565.
4. Weizman ED, Moline ML, Czeiler CA, et al: Chronobiology of aging: Temperature, sleep-wake rhythms, and intrainment. *Neurobiol Aging.* 1982;3:299–309.
5. Downton JH, Andrews K, Puxty JAH: Silent pyrexia in the elderly. *Age Ageing.* 1987;16:41–44.
6. Manning LV, Touquet R: The relevance of pyrexia in adults as a presenting symptom in the accident and emergency department. *Arch Emerg Med.* 1988;5:86–90.
7. Mellors JW, Horwitz RI, Harvey MR, et al: A simple index to identify occult bacterial infection in adults with acute unexplained fever. *Arch Intern Med.* 1987;147:666–671.
8. Stapczynski JS: Evaluation of the febrile adult in the emergency department. (abstr.) *Ann Emerg Med.* 1990;19:481.
9. Keating HJ, Klimek JJ, Levine DS, et al: Effect of aging on the clinical significance of fever in ambulatory adult patients. *J Am Geriatr Soc.* 1984;32:282–287.
10. Wasserman M, Levinstein M, Keller E, et al: Utility of fever, white blood cells, and differential count in predicting bacterial infections in the elderly. *J Am Geriatr Soc.* 1989;37:537–543.
11. Leibovici L, Cohen O, Wysenbeek AJ: Occult bacterial infection in adults with unexplained fever. Validation of a diagnostic index. *Arch Intern Med.* 1990;150:1270–1272.
12. Bone RC, Fisher CJ Jr, Clemmer TP, et al: Sepsis syndrome: A valid clinical entity. *Crit Care Med.* 1989;17:389–393.
13. Bone RC: Toward an epidemiology and natural history of SIRS (systemic inflammatory response syndrome). *JAMA.* 1992;268:3452–3455.
14. Schneiderman H: *Bedside Diagnosis. An Annotated Bibliography of Literature on Physical Examination and Interviewing.* 2nd ed. Philadelphia: American College of Physicians; 1992.
15. Osmer JC, Cole BK: The stethoscope and roentgenogram in acute pneumonia. *South Med J.* 1966;59:75–77.
16. Wenz B, Gennis P, Canova C, et al: The clinical utility of the leukocyte differential in emergency medicine. *Am J Clin Pathol.* 1986;86:298–303.
17. Callaham M: Inaccuracy and expense of the leukocyte count in making urgent clinical decisions. *Ann Emerg Med.* 1986;15:774–781.
18. Badgett RG, Hawen CJ, Rogers CS: Clinical usage of the leukocyte count in emergency room decision making. *J Gen Intern Med.* 1990;5:198–202.
19. Meunier F: Infections in patients with acute leukemia and lymphoma, in Mandell GL, Douglas RG, Bennett RE (eds): *Principles and Practice of Infectious Diseases.* 3rd ed. New York: Churchill Livingstone; 1990:2265–2275.
20. Sox HC, Liang MH: The erythrocyte sedimentation rate. Guidelines for rational use, in Sox HC (ed): *Common Diagnostic Tests. Use and Interpretation.* 2nd ed. Philadelphia: American College of Physicians; 1990:204–226.
21. Komaroff AL: Urinalysis and urine culture in women with dysuria, in

Sox HC (ed): *Common Diagnostic Tests. Use and Interpretation.* 2nd ed. Philadelphia: American College of Physicians; 1990:286–301.
22. Sickles EA, Greene WH, Wiernik PH: Clinical presentation of infection in granulocytopenic patients. *Arch Intern Med.* 1975;135:715–719.
23. Singal BM, Hedges JR, Radack KL: Decision rules and clinical prediction of pneumonia: evaluation of low-yield criteria. *Ann Emerg Med.* 1989;18:13–20.
24. Gennis P, Gallagher J, Falvo C, et al: Clinical criteria for the detection of pneumonia in adults: guidelines for ordering chest roentgenogram in the emergency department. *J Emerg Med.* 1989;7:263–268.
25. Heckerling PS, Tape TG, Wigton RS, et al: Clinical prediction rule for pulmonary infiltrates. *Ann Intern Med.* 1990;113:664–670.
26. Jochelson MS, Altschuler J, Stomper PC: The yield of chest radiography in febrile and neutropenic patients. *Ann Intern Med.* 1988;105:708–709.
27. Eisenberg JM, Rose JD, Weinstein AJ: Routine blood cultures from febrile outpatients. Use in detecting bactermia. *JAMA.* 1976;236:2863–2865.
28. No reference.
29. Stair TO, Lenhart M: Outpatient blood cultures: retrospective and prospective audits in one ED. *Ann Emerg Med.* 1984;13:986–987.
30. Bates DW, Cook EF, Goldman L, et al: Predicting bacteremia in hospitalized patients. A prospectively validated model. *Ann Intern Med.* 1990;113:495–500.
31. Leibovici L, Greenshtain S, Cohen O, et al: Bacteremia in febrile patients. A clinical model for diagnosis. *Arch Intern Med.* 1991;151:1801–1806.
32. Bates DW, Lee TH: Rapid classification of positive blood cultures. Prospective validation of a multivariate algorithm. *JAMA.* 1992;267:1962–1966.
33. Aronson MD, Bor DH: Blood cultures. *Ann Intern Med.* 1987;106:246–253.
34. Marantz PR, Linzer M, Feiner CJ, et al: Inability to predict diagnosis in febrile intravenous drug abusers. *Ann Intern Med.* 1987;106:823–828.
35. Samet JH, Shevitz A, Fowle J, et al: Hospitalization decision in febrile intravenous drug users. *Am J Med.* 1990;89:53–57.
36. No reference.
37. Alvarez-Elcoro S, Mateos-Mora M, Mantecon V: Community-acquired febrile illness in patients with prosthetic heart valves. *South Med J.* 1985;78:1431–1434.
38. Douglas RG, Chamberland ME, Curran JW, et al: Acquired immunodeficiency syndrome, in Mandell GL, Douglas RG, Bennett RE (eds): *Principles and Practice of Infectious Diseases.* 3rd ed. New York: Churchill Livingstone; 1990:1029–1121.
39. Rolston KVI, Uribe-Botero G, Mansell PWA: Bacterial infections in adult patients with the acquired immunodeficiency syndrome (AIDS) and AIDS-related complex. *Am J Med.* 1987;83:604–605.
40. Wrenn KD, Larson S: The febrile alcoholic in the emergency department. *Am J Emerg Med.* 1991;9:57–60.
41. Bodey GP: Antibiotics in patients with neutropenia. *Arch Intern Med.* 1984;144:1845–1851.
42. Bodey GP: Infection in cancer patients. A continuing association. *Am J Med.* 1986;81(suppl 1A):11–26.
43. Serody JS, Cohen MS: Infection in the immunocompromised host, in Brillman JC, Quenzer RW (eds): *Infectious Disease in Emergency Medicine.* Boston: Little, Brown and Company; 1992:367–385.
44. Jones SR: Infection in the elderly, in Mackowiak P (ed): *Fever: Basic Mechanisms and Management.* New York: Raven Press; 1991:233–242.

45. Rhyne RL, Roche RJ: Infection in the elderly, in Brillman JC, Quenzer RW (eds): *Infectious Disease in Emergency Medicine.* Boston: Little, Brown and Company; 1992:343–365.

Chapter

Fever In Neonates

Raymond B. Karasic

Fever is one of the most common symptoms of childhood and provides the impetus for one fifth of all pediatric visits to the emergency department. In older children the evaluation of febrile illnesses is generally straightforward, requiring a carefully performed history and physical examination, supplemented by laboratory testing as needed. In contrast, the approach to fever in infants <3 months of age (neonates) is more complicated and controversial.

The heightened concern about fever in young infants is related primarily to two factors: the known susceptibility of neonates to serious bacterial infections and the lack of specificity of the clinical signs of septicemia. Nevertheless, most episodes of fever do not represent life-threatening diseases but rather self-limited viral infections that require only supportive treatment.[1, 2] The challenge lies in distinguishing the febrile infant with a serious bacterial infection from the many who have mild viral illnesses.

For the purposes of this chapter, fever is defined as a temperature of >38.0°C and the term *young infant* refers to patients <3 months old. Serious bacterial infections include the following bacteriologically confirmed diseases: meningitis, bacteremia, pneumonia, bone and joint infections, urinary tract infections, and enteritis.

CLINICAL ISSUES

Before considering laboratory testing, the physician should make maximal use of the clinical information already at his or her disposal. This includes the findings of the physical examination as well as established data about the prevalence of serious bacterial infections among febrile infants, risk factors that increase the likelihood of serious infection, and utility of clinical judgment.

Although the physical examination remains an integral part of the evaluation of fever at any age, the implications of physical findings are often different for young infants compared with older children. For example, clinicians are traditionally more reluctant to attribute fever to minor focal infections in young infants because of the concern about an accompanying systemic infection. Thus, the presence of acute otitis media in a toddler with fever might obviate the need for laboratory studies, whereas the same diagnosis in a febrile young infant would generally prompt a thorough laboratory evaluation.

Estimates of the prevalence of serious bacterial infection in febrile young infants have been relatively consistent in prospective studies, ranging from about 5 to 10%.[3, 4] Factors that are reported to be associated with an increased risk of serious infection include young age (<1 month),[5] high fever,[6] and toxic appearance.[7] Unfortunately, these associations are of limited practical value because serious bacterial infections can occur in the absence of any recognized risk factors.

The sensitivity of clinical judgment (as measured by the physical examination or use of an infant observation scale) in detecting serious infections in febrile infants has been evaluated prospectively by several investigators.[3, 4, 8] Unfortunately, the majority of studies indicate that the clinical examination is relatively insensitive, even when performed by experienced physicians.[8]

ROLE OF LABORATORY TESTING

Laboratory studies used in the evaluation of young infants with fever generally fall into one of two categories: confirmatory (specific) tests and screening (nonspecific) tests. A confirmatory test (eg, chest radiograph) is used to verify a clinical diagnosis and, with certain studies (eg, stool culture), to provide a specific diagnosis. In contrast, a screening test (eg, white blood cell count) is used to detect the presence of a condition (eg, serious bacterial infection). If the test result is positive, it usually indicates the need for further evaluation or treatment. Although—in clinical practice—confirmatory and screening laboratory tests are frequently obtained at the same time (eg, urine culture and urinalysis), these two categories are addressed separately.

CONFIRMATORY TESTS

Confirmatory tests used in the evaluation of young infants with fever usually are performed to establish the presence or absence of a serious bacterial infection. Despite the emphasis on bacterial infections, certain viruses (eg, herpes simplex virus) are also capable of causing life-threatening infection in this age group. When a particular viral agent is suspected, the workup should include specific tests (eg, viral culture, serological studies) designed to identify that agent.

The confirmatory tests used in the evaluation of febrile young infants are routinely performed as a combination of studies known as the "sepsis workup." The usual components of this battery include examination of the cerebrospinal fluid (CSF); cell count, protein values, glucose level, Gram stain, and bacterial cultures of CSF, blood, and urine. Other studies, such as chest radiographs and stool cultures, are performed more selectively, depending upon the patient's symptoms and signs.

CEREBROSPINAL FLUID EXAMINATION AND CULTURE. The diagnosis of meningitis is based upon the presence of CSF pleocytosis (increased number of WBCs), with or without other CSF abnormalities. For practical purposes, the absence of pleocytosis excludes the diagnosis of meningitis, although there are case reports documenting the recovery of pathogenic bacteria and viruses from acellular CSF. In general, bacterial meningitis is defined by the results of the CSF culture. An exception to this rule would be the situation in which there is CSF pleocytosis and a positive blood culture, despite a negative CSF culture. This combination would also satisfy the definition of bacterial meningitis.

BLOOD CULTURE. Bacteremia is defined as the presence of bacteria in the bloodstream. Because of the inherent difficulty in obtaining blood from small children, the diagnosis of bacteremia in infants is generally based on the results of a single blood culture that has been inoculated with a small volume of blood. Although there is evidence that this practice results in underdetection of bacteremia,[9] collection of a single blood culture nonetheless remains the standard method of diagnosing bacteremia in children.

URINE CULTURE. The diagnosis of urinary tract infection is based upon the culture results of properly collected urine. There are two accepted techniques for obtaining urine for culture from young infants: suprapubic aspiration and bladder catheterization. In contrast, there is ample evidence that urine collection bags are unsatisfactory for obtaining urine for culture because of the high rate of contamination by perineal flora, which results in falsely positive culture results. Suprapubic aspiration of the bladder is a well-established procedure that involves skin antisepsis followed by insertion of a needle directly into the bladder through the lower abdominal wall. Generally, the recovery of any number of organisms from the urine by suprapubic aspiration is considered significant (ie, indicative of urinary tract infection). The main problem with this technique is that the likelihood of successfully obtaining urine by suprapubic aspiration is 50% or lower.[10, 11] For this reason, bladder catheterization probably represents the most practical technique for collecting urine from young infants. When urine is collected by catheterization, urinary tract infection can be defined as the recovery of a single pathogen with a colony count of $>10^4$ organisms per milliliter of urine.[12]

CHEST RADIOGRAPH. Unlike the culture techniques mentioned, the chest radiograph does not provide a specific bacteriologic diagnosis, but it remains the standard method of confirming the diagnosis of pneumonia. Because the yield of chest radiography is low in children who lack respiratory symptoms or signs,[7] chest radiographs should be obtained selectively, rather than routinely, in febrile infants.

SCREENING TESTS

Screening tests relevant to the febrile young infant are nonspecific and readily available tests used to identify serious bacterial infection. To be useful, a screening test must have a high sensitivity. In the case of a febrile young infant, in whom missing a case of serious bacterial infection can have dire consequences, the sensitivity should approach 100%.

Although screening tests (eg, WBC count) are typically performed in the laboratory, they may alternatively represent clinical criteria (eg, toxic appearance) that are designed to detect infants with serious infections. Screening tests can be individual studies or combinations of tests. When multiple tests are used, in general the combination is considered positive when any of the individual tests are positive. This strategy has the advantage of improving sensitivity while minimizing the loss of specificity.

WHITE BLOOD CELL COUNT. The WBC and differential counts are frequently performed in the evaluation of febrile children. In young children with fever, the association between bacteremia and a WBC count of 15,000/mm^3 or greater is well established.[7] Despite this association, the sensitivity of this criterion for detecting bacteremia in febrile children younger than 3 years of age is only 65%.[13] Based on a study of 503 febrile young infants, the sensitivity of the WBC count is only 33% when used as a screen for serious bacterial infections.[14] Fortunately, the WBC and differential counts perform better when used in combination with other tests or criteria.

URINARY SCREENING TESTS. The standard urinalysis has long been used as a screening test to identify the presence of urinary tract infection, with a positive test usually defined by the presence of pyuria or bacteriuria. Concerns have been raised about the insensitivity of microscopic analysis of the urine for detecting urinary tract infection. In a study of 442 febrile infants younger than 8 weeks of age who had urine collected by catheterization or suprapubic aspiration as part of an evaluation for sepsis, only half these infants had pyuria (≥5 WBCs/hpf in centrifuged urine) or bacteriuria (any bacteria/hpf in uncentrifuged urine).[15] Hoberman and colleagues[16] described their experience with an "enhanced urinalysis," in which pyuria was defined as ≥10 WBCs/mm^3 measured by hemocytometer, and bacteriuria was defined as any bacteria per 10 oil immersion fields on a Gram-stained smear. They found the enhanced urinalysis to be superior to standard urinalysis in diagnosing urinary tract infection with respect to sensitivity (84.5 vs 65.6%) and positive predictive value (93.1 vs 80.8%); the negative predictive value using the enhanced technique was 99.3%.[16] Newer screening methods, such as reagent strip tests for nitrite or leukocyte esterase, have also been evaluated, but there is no convincing evidence that they offer a significant advantage over urine microscopy for the diagnosis of urinary tract infection in young children.[17]

LOW-RISK CRITERIA. In 1985 Dagan et al prospectively evaluated 233 infants younger than 3 months of age who were hospitalized for presumed sepsis.[18] The principal goal of the investigation was to establish criteria that accurately identified young infants who were at low risk for having a serious bacterial infection. Infants who were previously healthy were considered to be at low risk if they met the following criteria: no identifiable bacterial infection on physical examination; WBC count between 5000 and 15,000/mm^3; band count <1500/mm^3; and normal urinalysis. All infants not meeting these criteria were categorized as "high-risk." Of the 233 infants enrolled, 144 (62%) were classified as "low-risk"; only one such infant had a serious bacterial infection and no infant in this group had bacteremia. In contrast, 22 (25%) of the 89 infants in the high-risk group had serious infections. Thus, the sensitivity of these criteria (ie, the high-risk criteria) for detecting serious bacterial infection was 95.6%, with a negative predictive value of 99.3%. Although other investigators who have applied these criteria to their own study populations have reported lower sensitivities,[14, 19] the use of low-risk criteria nonetheless can help clinicians identify infants who are unlikely to have serious bacterial infections.

Acknowledging the imperfect sensitivity of low-risk criteria for detecting serious infection, Baskin et al prospectively evaluated an outpatient management strategy for selected febrile infants between 28 and 89 days of age.[14] In this study, ceftriaxone (a third-generation cephalosporin with a long half-life) was administered intramuscularly to 503 infants meeting their low-risk criteria, which included the following: not appearing ill; having no source of infection identified by physical examination; having a peripheral WBC count <20,000/mm^3; a CSF

WBC count <10/mm^3; and a normal urinalysis (<10 WBCs/hpf) or a negative dipstick for leukocyte esterase. At 24 hours after discharge from the emergency department, enrollees returned for reevaluation and administration of a second dose of ceftriaxone. Patients were then followed by telephone 2 and 7 days later. Of the 503 infants, 27 (5.4%) were found to have a serious bacterial infection (including nine episodes of bacteremia) at follow-up. These cases represented the episodes of serious infection that were misclassified by the low-risk criteria in the study. Fortunately, all patients with serious bacterial infections recovered fully after treatment with appropriate antibiotics.

Baker et al evaluated criteria for selecting infants between 29 and 56 days of age who could be safely managed (either as outpatients or inpatients) without antibiotic treatment.[4] Infants were considered to be low risk if they had the following: nontoxic appearance (defined as an Infant Observation Score ≤10); no evidence of bacterial disease on physical examination; peripheral WBC count <15,000/mm^3; normal urinalysis (<10 WBCs/hpf; normal CSF (<8 WBCs/mm^3 and negative Gram stain); and normal chest radiograph. Infants in the low-risk group were assigned to either outpatient or inpatient observation without antibiotics. High-risk infants (ie, those not meeting the low-risk criteria) were hospitalized and treated with antibiotics. Patients not receiving antimicrobial therapy were reexamined 24 and 48 hours after their initial evaluation. Among the 747 infants enrolled, there were 65 episodes of serious bacterial infections. Of the 287 patients classified as low risk, only one had a serious infection, whereas 64 of the 460 children categorized as high risk had serious bacterial infections. Thus, 64 of the 65 cases of serious infection were identified by the screening criteria, yielding a sensitivity of 98% and a negative predictive value of 99.7%. The investigators concluded that selected febrile infants between 1 and 2 months of age can be managed as outpatients without antibiotics.

IMPLICATIONS FOR THERAPY

The availability of screening criteria that have a high sensitivity and negative predictive value provides physicians with several reasonable options for the management of febrile infants. Despite the existence of published guidelines about fever in young infants,[7] many questions remain unanswered, and accordingly there is still need for clinical judgment. The following general recommendations are based on information that is currently available.

- All febrile infants should undergo a careful physical examination by a clinician experienced in the evaluation of young infants.

- Cultures of blood, urine, and—in most cases—CSF should be obtained, along with peripheral WBC and differential counts, urinalysis, and CSF examination.
- Chest radiographs should be performed in infants who have respiratory symptoms or signs.
- Sensitive screening criteria, such as those used by Baker et al,[4] should be applied to allow infants to be classified as either high or low risk.
- Because the safety of outpatient treatment for febrile infants <28 days old has not been established, all such infants should be hospitalized and treated parenterally with antibiotics, pending culture results.
- Similarly, hospitalization and presumptive antimicrobial therapy are recommended for all infants categorized as high risk.
- Only those infants who meet low-risk criteria should be considered for outpatient management.
- Before discharging the infant, the clinician may opt to treat with a dose of ceftriaxone, but this is not mandatory.
- The most important aspect of management is to ensure scrupulous follow-up of all febrile infants after discharge; in general this requires a careful reexamination within 24 hours of the visit. If such follow-up cannot be guaranteed, the child is not a candidate for outpatient management and instead should be hospitalized at the initial encounter.

SUMMARY

Because the clinical signs of serious bacterial infections in young infants are often subtle and nonspecific, laboratory studies are an important component of the evaluation of fever in this age group. In addition to their traditional role in confirming the presence of bacterial infection, laboratory tests can be used in conjunction with clinical criteria to screen for the presence or absence of serious infections. Refinements in screening criteria have permitted the identification of febrile young infants who can be safely discharged from the ED and followed closely as outpatients.

REFERENCES

1. Krober MS, Bass JW, Powell JM, et al: Bacterial and viral pathogens causing fever in infants less than 3 months old. *Am J Dis Child.* 1985;139:889–892.
2. Dagan R, Hall CB, Powell KR, et al: Epidemiology and laboratory diagnosis

of infection with viral and bacterial pathogens in infants hospitalized for suspected sepsis. *J Pediatr.* 1989;115:351–356.

3. Crain EF, Shelov SP: Febrile infants: Predictors of bacteremia. *J Pediatr.* 1982;101:686–689.
4. Baker MD, Bell LM, Avner JR: Outpatient management without antibiotics of fever in selected infants. *N Engl J Med.* 1993;329:1437–1441.
5. Klein JO, Schlesinger PC, Karasic RB: Management of the febrile infant three months of age or younger. *Pediatr Infect Dis.* 1984;3:75–79.
6. Bonadio WA, Romine K, Gyuro J: Relationship of fever magnitude to rate of serious bacterial infections in neonates. *J Pediatr.* 1990;116:733–735.
7. Baraff LJ, Bass JW, Fleisher GR, et al: Practice guideline for the management of infants and children 0 to 36 months of age with fever without source. *Pediatrics.* 1993;92:1–12.
8. Baker MD, Avner JR, Bell LM: Failure of infant observation scales in detecting serious illness in febrile, 4- to 8-week old infants. *Pediatrics.* 1990;85:1040–1043.
9. Karasic RB, Isaacman DJ, Kost SI, et al: Collecting two blood cultures and a larger volume of blood improves detection of bacteremia in children. *Acad Emerg Med.* 1994;1:A21–A22.
10. Gochman RF, Karasic RB, Heller MB: Use of portable ultrasound to assist urine collection by suprapubic aspiration. *Ann Emerg Med.* 1991;20:631–635.
11. O'Callaghan C, McDougall PN: Successful suprapubic aspiration of urine. *Arch Dis Child.* 1987;62:1072–1073.
12. Hoberman A, Chao H-P, Keller DM, et al: Prevalence of urinary tract infection in febrile infants. *J Pediatr.* 1993;123:17–23.
13. Jaffe DM, Fleisher GR: Temperature and total white blood cell count as indicators of bacteremia. *Pediatrics.* 1991;87:670–674.
14. Baskin MN, O'Rourke EJ, Fleisher GR: Outpatient treatment of febrile infants 28 to 89 days of age with intramuscular administration of ceftriaxone. *J Pediatr.* 1992;120:22–27.
15. Crain EF, Gershel JC: Prevalence of urinary tract infection in febrile infants younger than 8 weeks of age. *Pediatrics.* 1990;86:363–367.
16. Hoberman A, Wald ER, Penchansky L, et al: Enhanced urinalysis as a screening test for urinary tract infection. *Pediatrics.* 1993;91:1196–1199.
17. Lohr JA, Portilla MG, Geuder TG, et al: Making a presumptive diagnosis of urinary tract infection by using a urinalysis performed in an on-site laboratory. *J Pediatr.* 1993;122:22–25.
18. Dagan R, Powell KR, Hall CB, et al: Identification of infants unlikely to have serious bacterial infection although hospitalized for suspected sepsis. *J Pediatr.* 1985;107:855–860.
19. Anbar RD, Richardson-de Corral V, O'Malley PJ: Difficulties in universal application of criteria identifying infants at low risk for serious bacterial infection. *J Pediatr.* 1986;109:483–485.

Chapter

Diarrhea

Jeff Coben

Diarrhea is a very common complaint in the clinical practice of emergency medicine, accounting for nearly 5% of all emergency department (ED) visits.[1,2] Most often diarrhea is a benign, self-limited disorder that can be treated symptomatically. On occasion, however, diarrhea can result in serious physiologic insult or be a harbinger of more serious underlying disease. The goal of the initial diagnostic evaluation is to determine which cases merit a more in-depth investigation and are caused by invasive pathogens that may benefit from empiric antibiotic therapy.

Diarrhea has been variously defined as increased stool weight, increased number of stools, or increased stool water content. For the emergency medicine practitioner, the most satisfactory definition appears to be the passage of loose, watery stools causing the patient to seek evaluation. Diarrhea can be further subclassified as acute, chronic, or recurrent. Acute diarrhea can be defined as diarrhea of less than 2 weeks' duration.[3]

This review focuses on the initial evaluation of acute diarrhea, but many of the concepts discussed may also be applied to chronic diarrhea with acute exacerbation or chronic diarrhea not previously evaluated. Although diagnostic evaluation of diarrhea often depends on host factors (age, underlying diseases, immunocompetency) and epidemiologic considerations (seasonal, locational, clustering), certain guidelines can be delineated that apply to the general ED population.

The evaluation of diarrhea should begin with a thorough history and physical examination, the results of which will help guide further diagnostic testing. Often a detailed history including documentation of sick contacts, travel, food ingestion, sexual habits, underlying disease states, medication usage, and associated symptoms will provide a presumptive diagnosis. Physical examination should concentrate on signs of dehydration, abdominal tenderness or mass, stool testing for occult blood, and detection of other possibly associated findings (rash, synovitis, hepatomegaly). Above all, a competent history and physical examination should disclose how seriously ill the patient is at the time of evaluation. Based on these findings, the emergency physician can then rationally determine what, if any, further evaluation is necessary. Further diagnostic testing can be conveniently divided into those tests examining the stool itself and those pertaining to other areas (eg, blood tests, x-rays).

STOOL STUDIES

Fecal Leukocytes

Examination of the stool for fecal leukocytes is generally considered the most useful diagnostic study in patients with acute diarrhea. The question arises whether or not all patients with diarrhea should have this relatively simple, noninvasive test performed. The answer appears to be no, with certain qualifications.

The emergency physician estimates the probability of invasive diarrheal disease and the potential for significant adverse sequelae.[4, 5] For patients with a history of acute, nonbloody diarrhea who appear to be improving and have no physiologic compromise or significant physical findings, it is reasonable not to perform any further diagnostic evaluation. These patients have a low pretest probability of invasive disease, and testing all of them for fecal leukocytes is time consuming and of little benefit in patient management. If the physician has knowledge of an outbreak of invasive disease in a given community or is examining an immunocompromised host, it may be reasonable to test the stool for fecal leukocytes even in the absence of significant physical findings. This approach underscores the need for clinical judgment in obtaining diagnostic studies and, beyond this, the need for discharge instructions that are clear, precise, and specific, directing the patient to return for further testing if the illness becomes more severe or prolonged.

Patients who are acutely ill with diarrhea, have a high fever and heme-positive stools, and appear toxic do not need a fecal leukocyte examination. In these patients one assumes an invasive process is present, and there is no need for a confirmatory test. Even under the best circumstances, there appears to be at least a 15% false-negative rate associated with the fecal leukocyte test.[4] Thus the clinician should not obtain the test in these circumstances unless a negative test result would influence further decision making.

If the fecal leukocyte study is indicated, it should be obtained on a fresh specimen. The literature suggests that the stool should be examined using Wright stain, Gram stain,[6] or Loffler methylene blue[7] or even an unstained specimen.[8] There are no data to support the routine use of one method over another, but the Gram stain is widely available, is frequently used by laboratory personnel, and is often diagnostic in the case of *Campylobacter* enteritis. Gram stain may demonstrate gram-negative rods arranged in characteristic gull-wing configuration in nearly half the cases owing to *Campylobacter* (sensitivity of 43 to 65% and specificity of 95 to 99%).[3, 9, 10]

Various investigators, in differing clinical scenarios, have reported the fecal leukocyte study to have a sensitivity ranging from approximately 15 to 80%[11] in detecting the presence of an invasive enteropathogen. A well-done, ED-based, prospective study from San Francisco General Hospital found a sensitivity of 89%, specificity of 68%, positive predictive value of 71%, and negative predictive value of 87% for the fecal leukocyte test alone.[4] When combined with a positive stool test for occult blood, the sensitivity was 81%, specificity 83%, positive predictive value 81%, and negative predictive value 83%. Although this adult study may have excluded some patients with less severe gastroenteritis and the population included 35% male homosexuals, the results seem applicable to most urban adult ED patients because, when analyzed separately, the sensitivity, specificity, and predictive values were similar for male homosexuals and the rest of the study population. Thus the fecal leukocyte examination is both sensitive and specific for the diagnosis of acute invasive diarrhea. There remains, however, at least a 15% false-negative rate associated with this test.

Cultures, Ova and Parasites, *Clostridium difficile* Analysis

If the history, physical examination, or fecal leukocyte examination indicates a strong likelihood of an invasive enteropathogen, the emergency physician must then decide what, if any, further evaluation is warranted. Unfortunately, there is little guidance in the way of well-designed prospective studies. The consensus of opinion in the current literature suggests that *stool culture* for *Salmonella, Shigella,* and *Campylobacter* is justified when there is a strong suspicion of an invasive organism, because the need for treatment and the antibiotic of choice differ among these pathogens.[1, 6, 11] In contrast, the indiscriminate use of stool cultures can yield positive results in only 1.5 to 2.5% of unselected cases with resultant huge costs per positive result.[12]

Routine stool culture for *Yersinia enterocolitica* requires special techniques, is not cost-effective, and should be requested only if there is clinical or epidemiologic support.[6, 13] Similarly, because the majority of patients with *Vibrio parahaemolyticus* require no therapy,[14] routine cultures for this organism are not justified. The identification of enterotoxin-producing strains of *Escherichia coli* also requires special techniques and does not appear justified in ED patients.

The decision to analyze the stool for *ova and parasites* must be made on a case-by-case basis. Although the majority of acute diarrhea cases are caused by viruses, bacteria, or toxins, on occasion the emergency physician takes a history that suggests parasitosis. Under these circumstances, it seems reasonable to initiate the evaluation with microscopic evaluation for ova and parasites: the recovery rate for amoeba on a single specimen is only 83%.[11, 15] Thus a negative result with a strong clinical suspicion should prompt referral for further evaluation and repeat microscopic examination.

If a patient develops diarrhea after the administration of antibiotics or chemotherapeutic agents, *C. difficile*–associated colitis must be suspected. Fecal leukocytes may or may not be present in this disease.[14, 16] Because this illness continues to carry a significant mortality, testing for *C. difficile* toxin seems warranted and should be ordered in the appropriate clinical setting. *C. difficile* may be present in the feces of normal individuals, making identification of the toxin rather than culture of the organism a requirement for proper diagnosis.

Special Clinical Scenarios

Rotavirus is the most common cause of diarrhea in *infants* and *young children.*[17] Although this agent is not typically classified as ''invasive'' and usually does not result in a positive fecal leukocyte test result, many patients with this disease are febrile or dehydrated and may appear quite ill. Testing for rotavirus by enzyme-linked immunosorbent assay (ELISA) is both sensitive and specific.[18] The decision to test for rotavirus must be made on an individual basis, utilizing knowledge of local epidemiologic patterns and pediatric practices. In general, however, this test adds very little to the evaluation and management of the patient from the perspective of the emergency physician.

Diarrhea in the *homosexual or immunocompromised patient* can be caused by a multitude of opportunistic pathogens. In patients with the acquired immunodeficiency syndrome (AIDS), diarrhea is reported to occur in 30 to 50% of cases in the United States and in up to 90% of cases in Africa and Haiti.[19] The diarrhea, with associated weight loss and wasting, can be quite disabling in these cases. Although early studies frequently failed to identify a causative agent, further studies have isolated one or more enteric pathogens in 45 to 85% of patients with AIDS and diarrhea.[19] The most common organisms cited in the literature include *Mycobacterium avium-intracellulare, Cryptosporidium, Isospora belli, Cytomegalovirus, Herpes simplex, Microsporidia, Candida albicans, Giardia lamblia,* and *Entamoeba histolytica.*[20, 21] In addition, these patients often have simultaneous bacterial infections with *Salmonella, Shigella,* or *Campylobacter.* Thus the diagnostic evaluation of diarrhea in these patients is often complex and frustrating. The considerations previously discussed concerning routine stool cultures are equally valid for this patient population, although some investigators suggest more liberal guidelines. More specific testing for opportunistic pathogens is best left to the specialist with expertise in the management of these patients. Observations that 50 to 69% of identifiable enteric pathogens in AIDS patients are treatable with specific antimicrobial therapy[19] underscore the importance of appropriate referral and evaluation.

Stool Electrolytes and Osmolality

Analysis of stool electrolytes and osmolality is frequently cited as a useful method to distinguish secretory diarrheal disorders (eg, laxatives, cholera, other enterotoxins) from osmotic disorders (eg, lactulose, sorbitol, monosaccharidase deficiency). Interestingly, studies have shown that diarrheal stool, regardless of the cause, has an osmolality comparable to that of serum (280 to 330 mOsm).[22] Thus measurement of osmolality alone is not sufficient to distinguish the underlying pathogenesis. The concept of osmotic gap is useful in these circumstances and has been estimated by the following calculation:

$$\text{Osmotic gap} = \text{measured osmolality} - 2 \times (\text{Na} + \text{K})$$

If the diarrhea is secretory in nature, the osmolality is determined primarily by its electrolyte concentration, and there should be a small gap ($<$50 mOsm/kg) between measured and estimated osmolalities. If the diarrhea is induced by a nonabsorbable substance, the osmolality of the solution is maintained by the nonabsorbable substance, and the osmotic gap will be greater in these cases.[23] Unfortunately, there have been no studies evaluating the use of the osmotic gap in the diagnosis of acute diarrhea in the ED setting. Furthermore, in acute infectious diarrhea, one might anticipate a mixed clinical picture owing to various secretagogues and nonabsorbable foodstuffs resulting from loss of intestinal absorptive capacity. Thus stool electrolyte and osmolality determinations are not currently recommended for the evaluation of acute diarrhea.

SERUM STUDIES

Serum Electrolytes

The utility of serum electrolytes in the evaluation of acute adult gastroenteritis was examined retrospectively in more than 200 patients aged 18 to 56 years.[24] This study found that 11% of the patient population had electrolyte abnormalities but that only 1% had abnormalities that were clinically significant. This suggests that there is no justification for the routine ordering of serum electrolyte studies in adults with gastroenteritis. The generalizability of this study, however, is questionable as the population consisted primarily of young, relatively healthy patients (average age of 28 years, only 27% with abnormal orthostatic vital signs). Thus serum electrolyte studies may be indicated in certain "higher-risk" patients, including those on diuretics, those with chronic liver or kidney disease, and those with symptoms lasting beyond 24 hours. In addition, the utility of serum electrolyte studies and blood urea nitrogen studies in pediatric and geriatric emergency patients has not been similarly studied. Clinical experience suggests that significant abnormalities are much more frequent in these patients. Thus, although routine electrolyte analysis can be safely omitted in otherwise healthy patients with diarrhea, the physician must use clinical judgment in determining which patients require this test.

Complete Blood Count, Liver Function Tests, Blood Cultures

Currently, it is impossible to give specific, literature-based guidelines regarding which patients should have CBC, liver function tests (LFT), or blood culture obtained as part of an evaluation. Once again, the emergency physician should rely on clinical judgment in the ordering of these tests. Certainly the patient with acute, nonbloody diarrhea who lacks abdominal tenderness or signs of toxicity does not require these studies. Conversely, patients with marked dehydration, abdominal tenderness, clinical signs of toxicity, and particularly those who are very young, elderly, or immunocompromised, would warrant further investigation, possibly including CBC, LFT, blood culture, amylase value, and urinalysis. Bacteremia has been documented in up to 43% of AIDS patients with diarrhea,[20] and *Shigella* bacteremia, although rare, has been reported in children and adults, both immunocompetent and immunocompromised.[25] *Salmonella* may also occasionally be recovered from the blood and is particularly prevalent in patients with sickle cell anemia and other hemolytic anemias. The patient with diarrhea and localized abdominal pain also merits further investigation to exclude a surgical process. Once again, CBC, amylase value, LFT, or urinalysis may be useful in these circumstances.

ABDOMINAL RADIOGRAPHS

The usefulness of abdominal radiographs in patients with acute diarrhea has not been adequately evaluated. Most often, abdominal films are nonspecific or reveal a pattern consistent with ileus. Clinical judgment must be exercised in obtaining these studies. Elderly patients, immunocompromised patients, or patients with significant abdominal tenderness appear to be those most likely to benefit from radiologic examination to rule out any occult surgical processes.

SIGMOIDOSCOPIC EXAMINATION

The diagnosis of *C. difficile*–associated colitis is often established by the finding of pseudomembranous lesions in the rectosigmoid area. Although emergency physicians are certainly capable of performing sigmoidoscopy, it is not a procedure done with any regularity in the emergency department. Thus if the emergency physician suspects *C. difficile*–associated colitis, it would seem more prudent to discontinue the antibiotic, obtain stool for *C. difficile* toxin testing, and arrange for sigmoidoscopy by a gastroenterologist.

SUMMARY

The diagnostic evaluation of diarrhea should aid the clinician in distinguishing those cases caused by invasive pathogens and other potentially significant illnesses from those caused by more benign, usually viral, etiologies. This evaluation should be guided by the history and physical examination as well as knowledge of local outbreaks and underlying health status of each patient. For patients who require further evaluation, the fecal leukocyte test remains the most important diagnostic aid. Patients who appear toxic or have blood or leukocytes in the stool or other signs of an invasive process should have a stool culture obtained on a fresh specimen. Young, otherwise healthy patients do not require routine serum electrolyte determination. The remainder of the diagnostic evaluation of the patient with diarrhea is based primarily on clinical judgment. Currently there are insufficient data to support more specific recommendations.

REFERENCES

1. Bitterman RA: General disorders of the large intestine, in Rosen P (ed): *Emergency Medicine: Concepts and Practice.* St. Louis: CV Mosby; 1988.
2. Moffett HL: Common infections in ambulatory patients. *Ann Intern Med.* 1978;89:743–745.
3. Radetsky M: Laboratory evaluation of acute diarrhea. *Pediatr Infect Dis.* 1986;5(2):230–238.
4. Siegel D, Cohen PT, Neighbor M, et al: Predictive value of stool examination in acute diarrhea. *Arch Pathol Lab Med.* 1987;111:715–718.
5. Sox HC: Probability theory in the use of diagnostic tests. *Ann Intern Med.* 1987;104:60–66.
6. Bergquist EJ: The office evaluation of infectious diarrhea. *Primary Care.* 1990;17:852–866.

7. Patel P, Komawar V, Jain MK, et al: Fecal leucocytes in acute diarrhea. *Indian Pediatr.* 1984;21:191–194.
8. Heller MB: Diarrhea and proctitis, in Harwood-Nuss A, Linden C, Luten RC, et al (eds): *The Clinical Practice of Emergency Medicine.* Philadelphia: JB Lippincott; 1991.
9. Ho D, Ault M, Mufata G: Campylobacter enteritis: Early diagnosis with Gram's stain. *Arch Intern Med.* 1982;142:1858–1860.
10. Sazie ESM, Titus AE: Rapid diagnosis of campylobacter enteritis. *Ann Intern Med.* 1982;96:62.
11. Adler PM: Stool examination: culture versus gram stain. *Ann Emerg Med.* 1986;15:337–341.
12. Guerrant RL, Wanke CA, Barrett LJ, et al: A cost effective and effective approach to the diagnosis and management of acute infectious diarrhea. *Bull NY Acad Med.* 1987;63:484–499.
13. Kachoris M, Ruoff KL, et al: Routine culture of stool specimens for Yersinia enterocolitica is not a cost-effective procedure. *J Clin Microbiol.* 1988; 26:582.
14. Bitterman RA: Acute gastroenteritis and colon disorder, in Rosen P (ed): *Emergency Medicine: Concepts and Practice.* St. Louis: CV Mosby; 1988.
15. Thompson J, Hassa R: Intestinal parasites: The necessity of examining multiple stool specimens. *Mayo Clin Proc.* 1984;5A:641–642.
16. Tenesco FJ: Antibiotic associated pseudomembranous colitis with negative proctosigmoidoscopy examination. *Gastroenterology.* 1979;77:295.
17. Fontana M, Zuin G, Paccagnini S, et al: Simple clinical score and laboratory-based method to predict bacterial etiology of acute diarrhea in childhood. *Pediatr Infect Dis J.* 1987;6:1088–1091.
18. Pickering LK: Rotaviruses infection. *Pediatr Infect Dis J.* 1985;85:S2–S6.
19. Smith PD, Janoff EN: Infectious diarrhea in human immunodeficiency virus infection. *Gastroenterol Clin North Am.* 1988;17:587–598.
20. Antony MA, Brandt LJ, Klein RS, et al: Infectious diarrhea in patients with AIDS. *Dig Dis Sci.* 1988;33:1141–1146.
21. Rijpstra AC, Canning EU, Van Ketel RJ, et al: Use of light microscopy to diagnose small-intestinal microsporidiosis in patients with AIDS. *J Infect Dis.* 1988;157:827–831.
22. Shiau YF, Feldman GM, Resnick MA, et al: Stool electrolyte and osmolality measurements in the evaluation of diarrheal disorders. *Ann Intern Med.* 1985;102:773–775.
23. Shiau YF: Clinical and laboratory approaches to evaluate diarrheal disorders. *Crit Rev Clin Lab Sci.* 1987;25:43–69.
24. Olshaker JS, Mason JD: The usefulness of serum electrolytes in the evaluation of acute adult gastroenteritis. *Emerg Med.* 1989;18:258–260.
25. Morduchowicz G, Huminer D, Siegman-Igra Y, et al: Shigella bacteremia in adults. A report of five cases and review of the literature. *Arch Intern Med.* 1987;147:2034–2037.

Chapter

Nausea and Vomiting

Edward A. Michelson

Nausea and vomiting are common reasons for patients to present to the emergency department (ED). Ancillary tests may aid both in determining the cause and in managing the consequences of the associated decreased intake and increased loss of fluid and electrolytes. The laboratory workup of the vomiting patient must take into account the varied gastroenterologic as well as non-GI etiologies. The differential diagnosis of nausea and vomiting encompasses a number of mechanical, metabolic, inflammatory, and psychologic etiologies. Pathologic processes both within and remote to the abdomen may be responsible.

The duration of vomiting and resulting fluid and electrolyte losses coupled with the age and prior general condition of the patient are also important factors. A thorough history and physical examination findings aid in reducing the differential diagnosis, thus restricting the number of tests necessary to diagnose and manage the underlying cause.

INTRAABDOMINAL CAUSES

Diseases causing obstruction to outflow from the stomach or occlusion of the small or large bowel will eventually result in nausea and vomiting. A history of multiple prior abdominal operations increases the likelihood of adhesions, which may be a mechanical cause of obstruction. Peptic ulcer disease in the vicinity of the pylorus may produce pyloric stenosis and obstruction. Likewise, gastric tumors may obstruct gastric outflow at the pylorus. Blood in the lumen of the stomach is very irritating and may cause nausea and vomiting. Patients with a clinical presentation consistent with peptic ulcer disease (PUD) or gastritis should have the vomitus and stool examined for gross or occult blood.

History or examination findings of melena or of bloody emesis or stool should prompt an ED determination of blood counts. These patients will subsequently need endoscopic or radiologic contrast studies of the GI tract to identify the site and cause of bleeding. Patients with emesis of large amounts of blood or passage of significant amounts of blood per rectum should also have a specimen sent early on to the blood bank for crossmatch. Likewise, patients with examination findings of volume depletion coupled with any amount of GI bleeding should be crossmatched early.

Obstruction of the small bowel or colon also results in ileus and vomiting. Intussusception and volvulus are two causes that may appropriately be evaluated by contrast radiographic studies of the colon. In fact, ileocolonic intussusception may be reduced by a barium enema. Likewise, large obstructing tumors of the colon may be visualized on colonoscopy or after barium enema. More commonly, in patients with one or more prior laparotomies, adhesions may block bowel function.

Physical examination findings of ileus are expected in patients with bowel obstructions. Flat and erect radiographs of the abdomen are expected to demonstrate scattered air-fluid levels in the small bowel. These radiographs might also provide evidence of a visceral perforation producing free air under the diaphragm. The addition of left and right lateral decubitus abdominal radiographs may increase the number of patients in whom free air will be found.

A patient with gallbladder disease, including symptomatic cholelithiasis and acute cholecystitis, frequently appears with a history of nausea and vomiting along with right upper quadrant abdominal and occasionally referred back and shoulder pain. The presence of fever and elevated white blood cell count (WBC) in a patient with characteristic right upper quadrant pain and tenderness increases the likelihood of acute cholecystitis. Ultrasonography of the gallbladder in the patient who has not recently eaten may demonstrate stones in the gallbladder or dilation of the common bile duct or cystic duct suggestive of obstruction. Liver function tests may be abnormal in the latter case, although they will likely be normal if the stone is obstructing only the cystic duct.

Acute inflammation of pelvic and retroperitoneal organs may also cause vomiting. Pelvic inflammatory disease frequently appears with fever, vomiting, lower abdominal pain, and elevated WBC count. Peritonitis and peritoneal irritation are also associated with nausea and vomiting. Appendicitis and hepatitis may all also feature vomiting along with characteristic associated pain and tenderness. Elevated WBC count is helpful in diagnosing the former, whereas liver function tests and serology are useful in the latter.

Acute pancreatitis is associated with severe epigastric pain and vomiting. Predisposing factors for pancreatitis, including ethanol abuse, hyperlipidemias, or pancreatic duct stones, coupled with this clinical presentation suggest the need for serum amylase and lipase determinations. Patients with recurrent pancreatitis not associated with chronic use of ethanol should have serum lipids evaluated.

EXTRAABDOMINAL CAUSES

Nausea and vomiting may be the principal and in fact the only symptoms of acute myocardial ischemia or infarction.[1] Although frequently thought to be a sign of inferior wall ischemia, one study demonstrated that infarct size rather than location correlated with nausea or vomiting.[2] In this study of 306 consecutive patients admitted to a CCU with chest pain and ECG changes, the sensitivity of nausea or vomiting for detecting MI was 53%, with specificity of 72% and a positive predictive value of 61%. Hence, patients with risk factors for cardiac disease should have an ECG obtained as part of their ED workup of nausea in the absence of another cause.

Recurrent morning episodes of nausea and vomiting in young women of reproductive age may be the first symptoms of pregnancy. Urine or serum pregnancy tests should confirm the diagnosis and would be mandatory prior to obtaining any radiographs or treating with antiemetics. In contrast to patients with the more severe hyperemesis gravidarum, these patients rarely lose significant fluid or electrolytes and should not require serum electrolyte determinations. Severe, persistent vomiting during pregnancy should prompt the physician to check serum electrolyte, blood urea nitrogen (BUN), creatinine levels, and urinary ketones. Likewise, if there are signs of dehydration in late pregnancy, fetal monitoring or non-stress testing may be desirable to assure the well-being of the fetus.

Increased intracranial pressure may occur with the combination of headache and vomiting, with or without other changes in the neurologic examination. This may be the result of tumor with mass effect,[3] hydrocephalus, or extrinsic compression or swelling of the brain. Persistent emesis following any significant head injury is of concern, raising the possibility of a subdural or epidural hemorrhage. Projectile vomiting or vomiting without preceding nausea suggests the possibility of brain tumor.[5] In both instances CT or magnetic resonance imaging of the head may demonstrate structural lesions or alterations in ventricle size or position that will confirm the diagnosis.

Vertigo may be accompanied by nausea and vomiting, particularly in the older adult population as signs of labyrinthitis. Labyrinthitis of short duration should not cause dehydration or electrolyte depletion. Prolonged nausea and vertigo of many weeks' duration should prompt the physician to test for unilateral hearing loss. If present, acoustic neuroma should be ruled out on head CT scan.

Subarachnoid hemorrhage may be heralded by severe headache, nausea, and vomiting. Once considered, this diagnosis must be excluded by head CT scan, sampling of cerebrospinal fluid for blood or xanthochromia, and possible cerebral angiography.

The nausea and vomiting common with migraine headaches do not require further laboratory evaluation unless symptoms are prolonged or the diagnosis is uncertain.[3]

Likewise, the same symptoms associated with motion sickness should not require further laboratory evaluation.

EMOTIONAL CAUSES

Self-induced vomiting is a component of patients with bulimia nervosa and other eating disorders.[4] These patients frequently also abuse laxatives and diuretics and may be severely malnourished. Determination of serum electrolyte levels, including magnesium and calcium, and blood counts for signs of micro- or macrocytic anemia are suggested. Urinalysis might show signs of fasting ketosis, and serum cholesterol, total protein, and albumen concentrations may be depressed.

Pediatric patients with multiple workup for vomiting and all negative results have often been found to be poisoned with emetic drugs by their parents, guardians, or other caregivers. A drug screen is warranted in such patients, particularly after the negative workup, if the clinician's suspicions are thus raised.

Ingestion of toxins and emetic drugs is another cause of emesis. Emetic agents produce their effect in three ways: by stimulating the vomiting center in the brain, by irritating the stomach, and by psychologically associating with prior episodes of pain or illness. There are case reports of intentional, inadvertent, and unknowing emetic drug ingestion resulting in multiple visits for vomiting.

METABOLIC/TOXIC CAUSES

A number of alterations of normal metabolism may produce vomiting, including hepatic coma, renal failure, and diabetic ketoacidosis (DKA). Elevations in hepatic enzymes, ammonia, BUN, and creatinine may aid the diagnosis of the first two. Patients with diabetic ketoacidosis frequently present with these symptoms. Elevations of blood glucose and the presence of ketones may be determined at the bedside by colorimetric strips and by Clinitest tablets in patients with diabetic ketoacidosis (DKA). Chemistry laboratory confirmation of pH, serum ketones, and glucose may also be helpful. Likewise, diabetics with hypoglycemic reactions may be nauseous as part of the hyperadrenergic response to low blood glucose levels. They should also have a rapid determination of serum glucose level or empiric glucose therapy if there is any delay obtaining the laboratory results.

Uremia is associated with nausea and vomiting and may be assessed by serum BUN and creatinine measurements.

Three endocrine disorders—hyperparathyroidism, Addison disease, and hyperthyroidism—may include nausea and vomiting. When hyperparathyroidism is suspected, serum calcium level should be determined. Adrenocortical deficiency is associated with hyponatremia, hypochloremia, and hyperkalemia as well as elevated BUN. Thyrotoxicosis should be evaluated with serum T_4 and T_3 resin uptake tests.

Certain drugs that are not normally emetic will produce nausea and vomiting in the toxic range. Aminophylline, theophylline, and phenytoin cause nausea and vomiting when taken in toxic amounts. Drug levels should be obtained in patients on these drugs who present with vomiting, particularly if there has been a change in dose, or if the patient may be noncompliant. Lithium and iron both have vomiting as a prominent feature when taken in overdose. A lithium level should be promptly obtained in symptomatic patients on this drug.

Heavy metals cause vomiting as a prominent feature when taken in overdose. Iron may cause an erosive gastritis and possible perforation, producing GI bleeding. Iron levels should be checked in the suspected iron overdose. Iron pills are radiodense and hence may be seen on abdominal radiographs.

Lead toxicity may produce nausea and vomiting. A kidney, ureter, bladder (KUB) study may demonstrate lead-containing paint chips ingested by a child, although films may be normal if the exposure was not recent or if the exposure was to lead-containing dust or fumes. A whole blood lead level, obtained in special lead-free tubes, may confirm the diagnosis of lead toxicity. Finding of basophilic stippling on a blood smear is also suggestive of lead toxicity.

Drug-induced gastritis is a common side effect of nonsteroidal antiinflammatory drugs as well as of certain antibiotics. Bedside testing of stool or gastric contents for occult blood, when positive in patients with the appropriate history, supports this diagnosis.

Vomiting is a common side effect of numerous narcotics and may also be seen in acute withdrawal. Illicit use of narcotics may be confirmed by toxicologic testing. Likewise, various chemotherapeutic agents have nausea and emesis as prominent side effects.

A number of plants when ingested may cause vomiting. Poisonous mushrooms often cause early nausea and vomiting. Microscopic examination of the emesis may demonstrate mushroom spores, confirming the ingestion and aiding mushroom identification.

Food contaminated with enterotoxins produced by *Staphylococcus* may result in vomiting.

OTHER CONSIDERATIONS

Inflammatory pathology of the kidney, including pyelonephritis, glomerulonephritis, and nephrolithiasis, may include nausea and emesis in its clinical presentation. Findings of flank pain or the characteristic colicky pain of kidney stones would direct the clinician to include microscopic and dipstick examination of the urine. Plain radiography of the abdomen is of little value in ruling out kidney stones. Intravenous pyelography (IVP) may demonstrate the stone directly or as a result of delayed visualization of a kidney or a dilated ureter proximal to an obstructing calculus. Absence of red blood cells in the urine does not exclude the diagnosis of nephrolithiasis. Urinalysis and WBC count determinations are indicated in the workup of suspected pyelonephritis.

Vomiting of blood calls for special consideration. Blood is irritating to the stomach and may trigger nausea and vomiting. The presence of blood in emesis, not obvious on gross examination, may be confirmed by an occult test for blood. Bloody emesis may result from blood in the naso-oropharynx that has been swallowed; from varices in the esophagus; from Mallory-Weiss tears of the lower esophagus associated with retching; or from tumors, gastritis, or ulceration of the stomach. Confirmation of hemoglobin and hematocrit values is advisable in any patient with a history of vomiting blood.

Some laboratory tests are indicated to assess the consequences of vomiting. Patients with brief episodes of vomiting are unlikely to develop fluid/electrolyte abnormalities as a result. In the presence of protracted vomiting, poor oral intake, or preexistent dehydration or electrolyte imbalance, measurement of serum electrolytes plus BUN/creatinine is warranted. Hypochloremic metabolic alkalosis may result from excess chloride, sodium, and hydrogen ions lost with emesis. Hypokalemia may also ensue owing to compensatory increased potassium loss by the kidneys.

REFERENCES

1. Gnecchi-Ruscone T, Guzzetti S, Lombardi F: Lack of association between prodromes nausea and vomiting, and specific electrocardiographic patterns or acute myocardial infarction. *Int J Cardiol.* 1986;11:17–23.
2. Herlihy T, McIvor ME, Cummings CC, et al: Nausea and vomiting during acute myocardial infarction and its relation to infarct size and location. *Am J Cardiol.* 1987;60:20–22.
3. Kunkel RS: Acephalgic migraine. *Headache.* 1986;26:198–201.
4. Santangelo WC, Richey JE, Rivera L, et al: Surreptitious ipecac administration simulating intestinal pseudo-obstruction. *Ann Intern Med.* 1989;110:1031–1032.
5. Squires RH Jr: Intracranial tumors. Vomiting as a presenting sign. A gastroenterologist's perspective. *Clin Pediatr.* 1989;28:351–354.

Chapter

Deep Venous Thrombosis

Vince Mosesso and Alan Hodgdon

Diagnosing deep venous thrombosis (DVT) in the pelvis and lower extremities presents a frequent but difficult challenge to emergency medicine physicians. Clinical and autopsy studies have demonstrated that untreated deep venous thrombophlebitis above the knee frequently leads to pulmonary embolism.[1, 2] Although the documented incidence of DVT is about 200,000 to 300,000 per year in the United States, many additional undetected cases are believed to account for most of the 600,000 annual episodes of pulmonary embolism.[3]

The natural history of DVT above the calf is embolization (which occurs in approximately 50% of patients), spontaneous recanalization, or collateral vein formation. Patients without demonstrable proximal DVT (including those with superficial saphenous vein thrombosis above the knee and DVT in the calf) have less than a 10% incidence of clinically evident pulmonary embolism.[4] Thus location is a critical factor regarding the risk of embolization. Often, however, significant morbidity occurs even in the absence of embolization because of venous intimal damage and valvular destruction, leading to venous stasis with its concomitant complications, generally referred to as the postphlebitic syndrome.

Deep venous thrombosis is thought to develop as a result of any of three conditions: mechanical vein injury, hypercoagulable state, or venous stasis. The following clinical risk factors have been demonstrated:

1. Prior history of venous thrombosis.
2. Recent trauma or surgery, especially involving the lower extremities or pelvis, such as hip arthroplasty or prostatectomy.
3. Pregnancy or use of exogenous estrogen.
4. Malignancy, especially adenocarcinoma.
5. Obesity.
6. Recent immobilization or bed rest.
7. Congestive heart failure.
8. Recent myocardial infarction.
9. Age > 40 years.

The number of risk factors present correlates with the risk of DVT in patients who present with pain or swelling. A patient with one risk factor was found to have a 24% risk of DVT, whereas those with four or more risk factors were all found to have DVT.[5] One investigator has suggested that patients with no or one risk factor be considered at low risk, whereas those with two or more be considered at high risk and undergo appropriate studies.[3] The simple use of risk factors has been shown to predict DVT better than physical examination alone.

The question of DVT usually arises when a patient presents complaining of pain or swelling in one leg. Physical examination may point strongly to a different diagnosis, such as a generalized edematous state or a local infection. The physical examination is often nonspecific and, unfortunately, accurate only about half the time.[1] Although the classic picture involves edema, elevated temperature, erythema, tenderness, palpable cord, and deep calf tenderness as well as the Homan sign, numerous studies have clearly shown these findings to lack sensitivity and specificity.[2, 3, 6, 7] Some workers have reported that an increased circumference of the calf or the thigh is somewhat more specific. Others have noted that swelling around one ankle is most predictive of DVT.[1] Owing to the significant expense and morbidity involved in the treatment of DVT, it is imperative that the clinician make a definitive diagnosis before committing the patient to a full course of therapy.

Venography is well established as the standard for making the diagnosis of DVT, but this study is difficult to perform, painful, and requires considerable expertise to interpret properly. This difficulty in interpretation, especially in an area where the anatomy is variable and complex, ensures that the test is neither 100% sensitive nor 100% specific. Venography also carries significant risks, such as contrast-induced phlebitis, allergy, and renal failure. In addition, the potential difficulties of cannulating a foot vein are encountered. These problems have led to the emergence of a number of noninvasive diagnostic modalities.

PLETHYSMOGRAPHY

Plethysmography is a simple and objective noninvasive method based on the concept that acute volume changes in the extremities occur almost exclusively because of changes in vascular volume. Owing to the much greater capacitance of the venous system, volume changes largely reflect only changes in venous blood volume. Plethysmography involves the measurement of changes in calf volume occurring because of extrinsically imposed venous outflow obstruction by the investigator and the subsequent speed of venous outflow after such obstruction is released.

Impedance plethysmography (IPG) involves the measurement of the electrical resistance between two electrodes placed at two different sites longitudinally along the extremity. A positive result indicates that there is significant venous occlusion above the knee. Two parameters are measured:

1. The increase in calf volume after inflation of a thigh cuff to obstruct the venous outflow, thereby reflecting venous capacitance.
2. The rate of decrease in calf volume after release of the tourniquet, thereby reflecting the rate of venous outflow.

These volume changes produce a detectable change in electrical resistance or impedance. Thrombi that do not produce functional venous obstruction (eg, those causing subtotal occlusion or those in the hypogastric or profunda femoris veins) are not detected. Likewise, owing to the low venous capacitance distally, calf DVT is not reliably detected.

False-positive results can occur from unrecognized involuntary muscle contraction in the leg, from extrinsic compression by tumor or gravid uterus, and from other conditions that lead to increased intraabdominal pressure and decreased venous outflow from the legs. Congestive heart failure, cardiogenic shock, hypothermia, arterial insufficiency, pharmacologic vasoconstrictors, and other low-flow states can also cause false-positive results. Most of these conditions, however, should be detected by an experienced operator.

Proponents of IPG point to these factors: the test provides objective data and is only mildly dependent on interpretation and operator technique, the results are reproducible, there is essentially no morbidity, and the test may be done at the bedside.[8] A review of ten studies between 1978 and 1982 revealed a fairly consistent sensitivity of about 94% for proximal DVT[6] and a specificity of about 95%. It has been clearly demonstrated, however, that plethysmographic studies are not sufficiently accurate to be clinically useful for isolated calf DVT.

Much of the research on the clinical utility of impedance plethysmography has been done by Hull, Hirsh, and colleagues.[8, 9] Two major studies reported in 1981 and 1985 showed that serial testing done on the day of the initial visit (day 0) and sequentially on day 1, day 3, day 5 or 7, day 10, and day 14 allows for adequate detection of clinically significant venous thrombosis. The initial study compared IPG and fibrinogen uptake to contrast venography results. Of 634 patients randomized to follow-up by either IPG and fibrinogen scan or by IPG alone, only one patient subsequently developed pulmonary embolism and only 2% of patients developed DVT above the calf that was not detected in the original series of tests. These investigators argue that serial testing by IPG alone to detect propagation of clot to more proximal sites is adequate and that patients not identified initially with an abnormal IPG need not undergo anticoagulation because they have such a low risk of significant clinical sequelae.

NUCLEAR MEDICINE STUDIES

A great variety of nuclear medicine studies have been proposed for diagnosing DVT. Many of these, however, have insufficient or unproven accuracy. They are less widely available than IPG or ultrasound and often require up to 24 to 48 hours for definitive results, making them of limited utility to the emergency physician.

Perhaps the best evaluated of the nuclear medicine techniques is ^{125}I-labeled fibrinogen uptake, which is based on the premise that the labeled fibrinogen will be incorporated into the forming clot as fibrin. This test has been found to have a sensitivity of 90% for calf DVT but of only 60 to 80% for clot in the thigh and is even lower for detecting clots in the pelvic veins.[6] Because of this unacceptably high risk of missing the more clinically significant proximal thrombi, this modality cannot be relied on independently. Moreover, definitive diagnostic results may require images 24 to 48 hours after initial injection. In addition, interpretation is confounded by inactive old thrombi as well as by very small thrombi, recent surgical wounds, hematomas, or acute inflammation. The test is contraindicated in pregnant and lactating females and carries the potential risk common to all human blood products.

Radionuclide venography utilizing ^{99m}Tc-labeled macroaggregated human albumen or human albumen microspheres has been reported to have a sensitivity of 75% and a specificity of 99% in the thigh and 100% sensitivity and specificity in the iliac veins.[6] The test is very poor, however, for calf and popliteal fossa thrombi. In a small study using ^{99m}Tc-labeled albumen, Bornhov[10] studied the utility of scintigraphic readings taken 1 hour after injection into an antecubital vein. He developed screening criteria with a sensitivity of 92% and a specificity of 61% and diagnostic criteria with a sensitivity of 64% and a specificity of 98%. These findings, however, have not been duplicated. Leclerc[11] studied ^{99m}Tc-labeled red blood cells vs venography and found only a 68% sensitivity. Contact thermography, ^{99}Tc-labeled plasmin scintigraphy,[10] and ^{111}In-labeled platelet scintigraphy[12] have all produced dismal results to date.

Perhaps most promising among the newer nuclear medicine techniques is the utilization of ^{111}In-labeled monoclonal anti–fibrin antibody Fab fragments. The studies reported to date[10, 13–15] all involve very small numbers of patients and must be considered very preliminary. This modality does, however, show promise of being sensitive and specific for thrombi throughout the entire lower extremity as well as the iliac veins. Its place in clinical practice will depend on the results of future trials.

Thus, except for use in clinical research protocols, the utilization of any of the nuclear medicine techniques cannot be recommended for the emergency department diagnosis of DVT. Nuclear medicine scans may play an adjunctive role in searching for isolated calf DVT because most other methods are not very reliable in this area. Some physicians treat these patients to prevent proximal propagation or the postphlebitic syndrome.

ULTRASONOGRAPHY

Ultrasonic techniques bring a new dimension of versatility, portability, and timeliness to the emergency clinician's armamentarium for diagnosing DVT. Two types of ultrasonic examination are now available: the Doppler method and the technique of B-mode real-time scanning. Both methods are more convenient and provide more rapid results than either plethysmographic or nuclear medicine studies. They are also less expensive and more reliable than nuclear studies and, in certain circumstances, IPG. Indeed, B-mode real-time scanning has come to the forefront of noninvasive testing. Unfortunately, its weakness is that it is dependent on subjective interpretation and therefore on the skill of the examiner.

Doppler

Doppler ultrasonography takes advantage of the fact that, when an ultrasound beam is reflected back to its source by a moving object (such as flowing red blood cells), there occurs a slight shift in the frequency of the ultrasonic wave—a phenomenon known as the Doppler shift, the magnitude of which is proportional to the velocity of blood flow. If venous channels are patent, changes in velocity associated with respiration are detectable. Velocity changes can also be produced by augmentation techniques, such as by release of a tourniquet or by squeezing of the leg distal to the site of examination. Loss of the normal ebbs and flows in venous velocity is another indicator of outflow obstruction. Doppler ultrasonography has been found to be more reliable than impedance plethysmography in patients with elevated central venous pressure or arterial insufficiency.[6] For anatomic reasons, however, this modality cannot evaluate the hypogastric, profunda femoris, anterior tibial, or peroneal veins.

Although earlier studies reported a sensitivity of 71% and a specificity of 90%, Sumner[2] has reported a sensitivity of 94% and a specificity of 90% in detecting thrombi above the popliteal fossa and 91 and 84%, respectively, for clots below the knee, when compared with phlebography. He also notes that the commonly quoted sensitivity of 70 to 75% includes the consideration that calf thrombi are false-negative (missed) findings in many studies.

Any extrinsic compression of venous outflow causes positive findings by Doppler. These other etiologies include ruptured Baker cyst, hematoma, tumor, ascites, recent surgery, and pregnancy. In current clinical practice, Doppler flow studies are usually combined with B-mode real-time ultrasound, and the combination is termed duplex scanning.

Real-Time B-Mode Ultrasonography

Real-time ultrasound, initially utilized for the diagnosis of DVT by Talbot in 1982,[15a] has since gained much popularity in the initial diagnostic workup of DVT. This modality offers many enticing characteristics: direct anatomic visualization and noninvasiveness, and it can be performed very rapidly and at the bedside, making it feasible in unstable patients.

This noninvasive technique has consistently been shown to be sensitive and specific for venous thrombosis in the femoral-popliteal system. Becker and associates[16] rigorously evaluated and compiled data from 15 articles that they deemed to meet basic methodologic standards. Their review found a mean sensitivity of 96% and a specificity of 99% for clot in the femoral and popliteal veins. Overall (ie, both above and below the knee) sensitivity ranged between 78 and 100%, with a similar specificity. It is important, however, to recognize that it has repeatedly been confirmed that this modality should not be considered reliable in detecting thrombosis either in the calf or in the iliac veins.

Ultrasonographic criteria for a positive result have been generally agreed on. The most definitive is visualization of clot inside a vessel. Experienced ultrasonographers usually can determine this easily, but it has been noted to be a questionable finding with novices. The second criterion is compressibility of individual vessels; noncompressibility is usually due to the presence of intraluminal thrombus. A matter of some debate is the utility of pulsed Doppler flow studies to provide adjunctive information. Becker and coworkers[16] noted no increase in sensitivity or specificity in studies that utilized pulsed Doppler flow technique compared with those that did not. Some workers[17, 18] argue strongly that pulsed Doppler data are necessary for detection of clot in the adductor canal (an area hidden from ultrasonographic visualization) and that it may be helpful in detection of clot in the venous system of the calf.

Another important advantage to real-time ultrasound is that its anatomic visualization allows for the diagnosis of other etiologies of the patient's symptoms. Popliteal cysts, pelvic and inguinal lymphadenopathy, popliteal hematoma, and traumatic arterial aneurysms may all be detected using this technique.

Although a fairly large number of studies suggest that real-time ultrasonography is the best noninvasive test for DVT of the popliteal and femoral veins, a number of limitations must be kept in mind. Most importantly, the clinician must not forget that this method is not sensitive for either calf or iliac thrombosis. Second, many of the studies have involved patients in whom there was a high enough risk or a great enough clinical suspicion for them to be referred for contrast venography. These may represent a selection bias, although screening in asymptomatic patients has yielded satisfactory results as well. Third, causes of false-positive results, including congestive heart failure, venous insufficiency, and extrinsic venous compression, should be considered. Finally, ultrasonography is quite dependent on operator skill and experience. Therefore, before emergency physicians wholeheartedly adopt this diagnostic aid, large-scale clinical studies of patients presenting to the emergency department with signs or symptoms consistent with DVT should be undertaken.

OTHER MODALITIES

Both computed tomography with intravenous contrast and magnetic resonance imaging have been recommended as accurate diagnostic tools for DVT.[19–21] These modalities must be considered experimental, however, at this time. Although they potentially offer the advantage of greater anatomic detail and more accurate detection of pelvic thrombosis, formal criteria for positive results have not yet been established.

A CLINICAL APPROACH

Given this information on available modalities and using principles of decision analysis modeling,[4] the following approach to the diagnosis of DVT may be suggested.

Since DVT cannot be reliably diagnosed clinically, some imaging study is necessary. Neither treatment without proper diagnosis nor nontreatment is without significant risk.

The initial imaging study of choice is either duplex scanning (the combination of Doppler flow with B-mode real-time ultrasound) or IPG, depending on local availability and expertise. Both are accurate and reliable for clinically significant DVT, and both are noninvasive. They are also reasonably available and relatively inexpensive. Because these modalities are somewhat operator dependent, however, an awareness of who performs and interprets these procedures and what equipment they use is essential to ensure maximum reliability.

In patients with significant clinical likelihood of DVT, if either test result is positive and there are no contraindications to anticoagulation, the patient is begun on heparin, usually in the emergency department.

If confounding factors are present that could make the test finding falsely positive or if the test finding itself is equivocal, further workup is required. This usually consists of contrast venography or the alternate test that was not performed initially—either IPG or duplex scan. Venography provides a reliable alternative but carries a 3% risk of causing thrombophlebitis in the limbs examined. The incidence of nondiagnostic or unsuccessful venograms is about 9%.

Studies do seem to confirm that two noninvasive tests are better than one. This depends on the incidence of DVT in the population being examined, however. As the incidence of DVT in symptomatic legs in the population falls, the risk of the venogram in terms of morbidity and mortality rises, making two noninvasive studies, such as duplex ultrasound/IPG, more attractive. Clinical acumen, personal experience, and local availability of resources must be used to answer difficult questions until further research or technologic advances provide a definitive solution.

REFERENCES

1. Hobson RW II, Mintz BL, Jamil Z: Diagnosis of acute deep venous thrombosis. *Surg Clin North Am.* 1990;70:143–157.
2. Sumner DS: Noninvasive tests in the diagnosis and management of thromboembolic disease. *Surg Ann.* 1986;18:1–28.
3. Turnbull TL, Linblad R: Deep venous thrombosis and thrombophlebitis, In Harwood-Nuss A, Linden C, et al (eds): *The Clinical Practice of Emergency Medicine.* Philadelphia: JB Lippincott; 1991:887–889.
4. Tintinalli JE, et al: *Emergency Medicine: A Comprehensive Study Guide.* 2nd ed. New York: McGraw-Hill; 1988:245–256.
5. Venta ZA, Venta ER, Mumford LM: Value of diagnostic tests for deep venous thrombosis: A decision analysis model. *Radiology.* 1990;174:433–439.
6. Hirsh J, Hull RD, Raskob GE: Clinical features and diagnosis of venous thrombosis. *J Am Coll Cardiol.* 1986;8:114B–127B.
7. Spritzer CE, Sussman SK, Blinder RA, et al: Deep venous thrombosis evaluation with limited flip angle, gradient re-focused MR imaging. *Radiology.* 1988;166:371–375.
8. Hull RD, Hirsh J, Carter CJ, et al: Diagnostic efficacy of impedance plethysmography for clinically suspected deep-vein thrombosis. *Ann J Intern Med.* 1985;102:21–28.
9. Hull R, Hirsh J, Sackett D, et al: Replacement of venography in suspected venous thrombosis by impedance plethysmography and I-fibrinogen leg scanning: A less invasive approach. *Ann Intern Med.* 1981;94:12–15.
10. Bornhov S, Dahlstrom JA, Nilsson J: Diagnosis of deep vein thrombosis with a new radionuclide method—^{99}Tcm-albumin test. *Acta Med Scand.* 1988;224:571–576.
11. Leclerc JR, Wolfson C, Arzoumanian A, et al: Technetium-99m red blood cell venography in patients with clinically suspected deep vein thrombosis: a prospective study. *J Nucl Med.* 1988;29:1498–1506.
12. Farlow DC, Ezekowitz MD, Rao SR, et al: Early image acquisition after administration of indium-111 platelets in clinically suspected deep venous thrombosis. *Am J Cardiol.* 1989;64:363–368.

13. Alavi A, Gupta N, Palevsky HI, et al: Detection of thrombophlebitis with In-labeled anti-fibrin antibody: Preliminary results. *CA Res.* 1990;50:(suppl)958–961.
14. Alavi A, Palevsky H, Gupta N. Radiolabeled antifibrin antibody in the detection of venous thrombosis: Preliminary results. *Radiology.* 1990; 175:79–85.
15. Lensing AW, Prandoni P, Brandjes D, et al: Detection of deep venous thrombosis by real-time B-mode ultrasonography. *N Engl J Med.* 1989;320:342–345.
15a. Talbot SR: Use of real-time imaging in identifying deep venous obstruction: A preliminary report. *Bruit.* 1982;6:41–46.
16. Becker DM, Philbrick JT, Abbitt PL: Real-time ultrasonography for the diagnosis of lower extremity deep venous thrombosis: The wave of the future? *Arch Intern Med.* 1989;60:283–288.
17. Cavaye D, Kelly AT, Graham JC, et al: Duplex ultrasound diagnosis of lower limb deep venous thrombosis. *Aust NZ J Surg.* 1990;60:283–288.
18. O'Leary DH, Kane RA, Chase BM: A prospective study of the efficacy of B-scan sonography in the detection of deep venous thrombosis in the lower extremities. *J Clin Ultrasound.* 1988;16:1–8.
19. Bauer AR, Flynn RR: Computed tomography diagnosis of venous thrombosis of the lower extremities and pelvis with contrast material. *Surg Gynecol.* 1988;167:12–15.
20. Erdman WA, Jayson HT, et al: Deep venous thrombosis of extremities: Role of MR imaging in the diagnosis. *Radiology.* 1990;174:425–431.
21. Rollins DL, Semrov CM, Friedell ML, et al: Progress in the diagnosis of deep venous thrombosis: The efficacy of real-time B-mode ultrasonic imaging. *J Vasc Surg.* 1988;7:638–641.

Chapter

Evaluation of the Sore Throat

Robert W. Wolford

Sore throat, either alone or as part of a symptom complex, is a frequent complaint of children and adults seeking care in the emergency department. This chapter reviews the important causes of sore throat, describes laboratory tests to aid in its diagnosis, and suggests an approach to assist in emergency department decision making.

ETIOLOGIES

The diagnosis and treatment of sore throat have traditionally focused on infections caused by group A beta-hemolytic (GABH) streptococci. It has been shown that early treatment reduces the frequency of nonsuppurative complications of GABH streptococcal pharyngitis (ie, rheumatic fever).[1] Early treatment also hastens the resolution of symptoms,[2, 3] speeds the clearance of organisms from the pharynx,[4] and may reduce the frequency of suppurative complications.

Group A beta-hemolytic streptococcal pharyngitis most often occurs in patients during their early school years (5 to 7 years old) and early teens (12 to 13 years old) and then decreases in frequency with increasing age.[5] Although it is usually considered uncommon in children less than 3 years of age, Schwartz and coworkers[6] found positive GABH streptococcal cultures in 35% of sore throat patients between 22 and 35 months of age, 19% of patients between 13 and 24 months, and 17% of patients less than 12 months of age.

Beta-hemolytic streptococci, other than group A, may also cause pharyngitis.[7, 8] The clinical presentations of infections caused by these organisms are identical to those of GABH streptococcal pharyngitis.

The ability of clinicians to correctly identify patients with GABH pharyngitis has been found to be poor. To improve the accuracy of clinical diagnosis and to reduce unnecessary throat cultures, a number of clinical scoring systems have been developed.

Centor and colleagues[9] developed a decision rule using four clinical variables, based on 286 emergency department patients >15 years of age, to determine the likelihood of GABH pharyngitis (ie, positive throat culture; Table 19–1). The same decision rule was evaluated in 555 adult outpatients at the University of Nebraska.[10] Culture results were found to closely approximate those predicted by the decision rule.

TABLE 19–1. CENTOR DECISION RULE

Clinical Variables
Anterior Cervical Adenopathy
Tonsillar Exudate
Absence of Cough
History of Fever

Prediction of Positive Culture

No. of Variables Present	*Probability of Positive Culture (%)*
0	~2.5
1	~6.5
2	~15
3	~32
4	~56

From Funamura JL, Berkowitz CD: Applicability of a scoring system in the diagnosis of streptococcal pharyngitis. *Clin Pediatr.* 1983;22:622–626.

Breese[11] developed a nine-factor "score card" for use in children (Table 19–2). Funamura and Berkowitz[12] evaluated the Breese score card in 892 clinic patients. They found a score of >28 points to have a positive predictive value of 40 to 59% and a score <28 points to have a negative predictive value of 57 to 80%.

Sore throat may also be caused by *Neisseria gonorrhoeae.* Although this is an uncommon etiology of pharyngitis in the general population, patients of sexually transmitted disease clinics may have gonococci cultured from the oropharynx 8% of the time.[13] The majority of patients with positive pharyngeal cultures are asymptomatic. In 3 to 4% of patients infected with *N. gonorrhoeae,* the pharynx is the only site from which the organism is isolated.[13, 14] Although the natural course of the infection in the majority of patients is clearance of the organism with time,[15] the pharynx may serve as a source of transmission[13] and of systemic dissemination.[14] It is therefore important to identify infected patients. Gonococcal pharyngitis should be considered in patients from high-risk populations (homosexuals, prostitutes); patients with history of orogenital contact; those with presence of gram-negative intracellular diplococci on pharyngeal Gram stain; or patients with other symptoms suggestive of genital infection. The organism is exceptionally fragile and requires immediate plating onto selective growth medium and incubation in an atmosphere enriched with CO_2 to achieve optimal growth.

It has been suggested that *Chlamydia trachomatis* and *Mycoplasma pneumoniae* may be important causes of pharyngitis. A study of adult patients with sore throats resulted in serologic evidence of infection by *C. trachomatis* and *M. pneumoniae* in 20.5 and 10.6% of patients,

TABLE 19–2. BREESE NINE-FACTOR STREPTOCOCCAL SCORECARD

	Score		
Symptom/sign	Yes	No	Unknown
Fever (100.5 or more)	4	2	2
Sore throat	4	2	2
Cough	2	4	4
Headache	4	2	2
Abnormal pharynx	4	1	3
Abnormal cervical glands	4	2	3
Age (years)			
5–10		4	
4, 11, 12, 13, 14		3	
3, 15, or more		2	
2 or under		1	
WBC (in thousands per cubic millimeter)			
0–8.4		1	
8.5–10.4		2	
10.5–13.4		3	
13.5–20.4		5	
20.5 or more		6	
Not done		3	
Season			
February, March, April		4	
January, May, December		3	
June, October, November		2	
July, August, September		1	
	Total score: 18–38		
Association of positive culture and score			
<30: 22% of all positive cultures			
>30: 78% of all positive cultures			

Adapted from Breese BB: A simple scorecard for the tentative diagnosis of streptococcal pharyngtis. *Am J Dis Child.* 1977;131:514–517. ©1977, American Medical Association.

respectively.[16] In the same study, evidence of GABH streptococcal infection was found in only 9.1% of patients. The clinical presentation of patients with *M. pneumoniae* does appear to differ from that of those with GABH streptococci, more often having an increased incidence of postnasal drip, hoarseness, and cough.[17]

Since this report, the importance of *Mycoplasma* and *Chlamydia* as causes of pharyngitis has been controversial. The role of the two organisms in pediatric pharyngitis appears to be minimal. A study of pediatric patients with pharyngitis identified *C. trachomatis* and *M. pneumoniae* in only 2 and 5% of patients, respectively.[18]

The importance of these organisms as etiologic agents of pharyngitis in adults has also been disputed. Two studies of adult patients have found *M. pneumoniae* to only rarely be associated with pharyngitis.[19, 20] The role of antibiotic therapy in the management of pharyngitis caused by these organisms is unclear.

Infections by a variety of other bacteria (eg, *Corynebacterium diphtheriae, Arcanobacterium haemolyticum*—formerly *Corynebacterium haemolyticum, Yersinia enterocolitica*) may also cause pharyngitis. Clinical findings often are very similar to those of GABH streptococci. Definitive diagnosis can be made only by culture, although pharyngeal Gram stain may be useful as a screening test.

Many viruses have been associated with sore throat, although this usually is part of a symptom complex including other respiratory symptoms. Sore throat is frequently associated with the flu syndrome of influenza and parainfluenza virus infections. Adenovirus infections may be associated with an isolated pharyngitis. Febrile pharyngitis has also been described as an initial clinical presentation of human immunodeficiency virus infection.[21]

The Epstein-Barr virus is the causative agent of infectious mononucleosis. In early childhood, infectious mononucleosis is often asymptomatic or associated with rashes and respiratory symptoms. In higher socioeconomic groups, individuals are not infected until they are older (15 to 25 years of age). In these patients, infection is more commonly associated with the typical infectious mononucleosis syndrome consisting of fever, sore throat, and lymphadenopathy. The typical clinical course is of an initial prodrome of headache, chills, and myalgia followed by sore throat and fever that gradually resolve over 1 to 2 weeks. The incidence of co-infection by infectious mononucleosis and GABH streptococcal pharyngitis is very low.[22, 23]

LABORATORY TESTING

White Blood Cell Count

No statistically significant difference in white blood cell count (WBC) or percentage of neutrophils of patients with viral compared with bacterial respiratory infections has been found.[24] The likelihood of a positive culture for GABH streptococci does increase with total WBC in symptomatic patients. Breese and Disney[25] found 10% of cultures to be positive for GABH streptococci with a WBC <10,000, 25% with a WBC 10,000 to 15,000, 48% with a WBC of 15,000 to 20,000, and 63% of cultures to be positive with a WBC >20,000.

The differential cell count may help in the presumptive diagnosis of infectious mononucleosis. Typically, the total WBC, percentage of lymphocytes, and percentage of atypical lymphocytes are elevated. The following values are suggestive of infectious mononucleosis: $>50\%$ lymphocytes; $>10\%$ atypical lymphocytes; absolute lymphocyte count $>4500/mm^3$; or atypical lymphocyte count $>1000/mm^3$.[26]

These hematologic findings vary with age, the WBC and absolute lymphocyte count generally being higher in children less than 4 years of age. The percentage of atypical lymphocytes, however, is less in children younger than 4 years of age.[27] The degree of atypical lymphocytosis also varies with the time since onset of infection, peaking during the second week of the disease and then gradually declining.[28] Severe neutropenia ($<500/m^3$) may be seen in any age group.[27]

Unfortunately, peripheral blood smear findings are not sensitive indicators. Aronson and coworkers,[29] in a study of adult patients, found only 4 of 15 heterophil antibody-positive patients to have met the criteria previously noted. Fleisher and colleagues,[30] in a study of 500 university students with monolike illnesses, found a lymphocyte count $>50\%$ and an atypical lymphocyte count $>10\%$ to be very specific (99%), but rather insensitive (39%), when compared with Epstein-Barr virus-specific serologic markers.

Monospot

The Monospot (Ortho Diagnostics) and many of the other rapid slide tests used to screen for infectious mononucleosis are based on the findings of Paul and Bunnell.[31] They observed that sera from patients with infectious mononucleosis agglutinated sheep red blood cells. These antibodies, which bind antigens from phylogenetically unrelated species, are called heterophil antibodies. The Monospot and similar tests correlate well with results obtained by the Paul-Bunnell test[32, 33] and have a sensitivity and specificity of 86 and 99%, respectively.[30] False-negative results may occur early in the course of the illness, prior to the development of heterophil antibodies, as only 70% of infectious mononucleosis patients will have heterophil antibodies present during the first week of the illness and 85 to 90% of patients by the third week.[34] Children <4 years of age also may develop a less intense heterophil response than older patients and may have falsely negative results.[35] False-positive results may occur with lymphoma, leukemia, rubella, pancreatic carcinoma, and hepatitis.[28]

Aronson and coworkers[29] suggested that tests to detect heterophil antibodies be used only for patients with any one of the following findings: axillary adenopathy, posterior auricular adenopathy, inguinal adenopathy, and palatal petechiae. In patients without any of these findings, the likelihood of a positive test result is very small.

Fleisher and colleagues[36] suggested the following guidelines for the proper interpretation of Monospot results:

Positive Monospot and clinical history suggestive of infectious mononucleosis: diagnosis confirmed.
Negative monospot and suggestive clinical history: perform the more-sensitive quantitative tests for anti–Epstein-Barr virus antibodies.
Positive Monospot and clinical history not suggestive of infectious mononucleosis: false-negative test result.

Pharyngeal Gram Stain

Gram stain of pharyngeal secretions has been advocated as an inexpensive test to identify patients infected with streptococcus.[37, 38] Crawford and coworkers[38] studied 472 outpatients with pharyngitis and found a positive Gram stain (defined as gram-positive cocci structurally similar to *Streptococcus pyogenes* associated with leukocytes) to have a sensitivity and specificity of 73 and 96%, respectively. The sensitivity of the Gram stain was found to be correlated with the number of streptococcal colonies found on culture (ie, bacterial burden).

The pharyngeal Gram stain may also identify patients with pharyngitis due to unusual organisms (eg, *Corynebacterium diphtheriae, Arcanobacterium haemolyticum, Yersinia enterocolitica, Neisseria gonorrhoeae*). The sensitivity and specificity of the Gram stain in these cases, however, are unknown.

Culture

Culture of the posterior pharynx has been considered the standard by which the diagnosis of GABH streptococcal pharyngitis is made. Throat culture, however, has several limitations. A single throat culture may be falsely negative in about 10% of cultures[5] and a positive culture alone is unable to distinguish actual infection from colonization of the pharynx. Moreover, 24 to 48 hours is required for culture results to be obtained, delaying treatment.

The site from which the sample is obtained is important. Brien and Bass[39] studied the effect of sample location on GABH streptococcal culture results. Sampling from the tonsillar surface yielded the heaviest growth of organism. Posterior pharyngeal wall samples identified all culture-positive cases but yielded less growth of bacteria than specimens from the tonsillar surface. Sampling from other locations in the throat yielded highly variable culture results.

The culture media routinely used for throat cultures is sheep blood agar. The incubation atmosphere (air, carbon dioxide enriched, anaerobic) and other media additives (generally antibiotics) are not standardized and may produce variable results. Wegner and associates[40] compared a single sheep blood agar culture with the combination of aerobically incubated blood agar and anaerobic trimethoprim-sulfamethoxazole blood agar (SXT) cultures in 755 outpatients with suspected pharyngitis. On day 1, the single blood agar culture detected 151 positive cultures and, on day 2, 189 positive cultures. The two-plate technique found 187 positive cultures on day 1 and 261 positive cultures on day 2. The anaerobic SXT culture detected 94% of all positive cultures. Clearly, it is imperative that the physician know which culture technique is being used and its expected sensitivity.

Group A beta-hemolytic streptococcal colonies are tentatively identified by a surrounding zone of beta-hemolysis. The organism often is presumptively confirmed as GABH streptococci by observing a zone of inhibition around a bacitracin disk placed on the agar. Definitive identification by a variety of techniques, including immunofluorescence, coagglutination, or latex agglutination, should be performed.

Rapid Streptococcal Identification Tests

Tests to identify streptococcal cell wall antigens directly from pharyngeal specimens have been developed. Specifically designed swabs are used to collect the specimen from the tonsillar fossae and posterior pharyngeal wall. The swabs are subjected to chemical or enzymatic treatment to digest the streptococcal cell walls and to release cell wall antigens. The resultant supernatant is incubated with streptococcal-specific antibodies. Antigen-antibody complexes are identified, commonly via latex agglutination or enzyme-linked immunoabsorbant assay. Results are available in 10 minutes to 1 hour. Radetsky and colleagues[41] evaluated ten kits available in 1985 and found none clearly superior.

Manufacturers of commercially available kits report sensitivities of 86 to 96% and specificities of 96 to 99%,[42] but these values may be lower in actual clinical use. When pediatric emergency department patients were evaluated with a rapid latex agglutination test, the sensitivity and specificity of the test were 55% and 90%, respectively.[43] Wegner and coworkers[40] evaluated five rapid test kits and found sensitivities ranging from 31 to 50% and specificities from 95 to 100% (except for one kit with a false-positive rate of 28%). The variations in reported rapid test kit sensitivities and specificities may be due to differences in expertise of personnel performing the test, the incidence of streptococcal pharyngitis, culture techniques and thus yield of throat cultures, and definitions of positive throat cultures. The importance of test sensitivity is demonstrated in Table 19–3. Clearly, in situations in which the

TABLE 19–3. IMPACT OF THE INCIDENCE OF STREPTOCOCCAL PHARYNGITIS AND TEST SENSITIVITY ON THE FALSE-NEGATIVE RATE (%)

Incidence (%)	Sensitivity (%)	Specificity (%)	Probability of False-Negative (%)
5	90	95	0.5
	50	95	2.7
	30	95	3.7
15	90	95	1.8
	50	95	8.5
	30	95	11.5
30	90	95	4.3
	50	95	18.4
	30	95	37.5
50	90	95	9.5
	50	95	34.5
	30	95	42.4

pretest probability of streptococcal pharyngitis is high, decreasing test sensitivity leads to an unacceptably high false-negative rate.

Unfortunately, as previously discussed, false-negative test findings do occur and are not uncommon. Patients with higher colony counts are more likely to be detected than are those with lower colony counts.[43, 44] A low colony count or false-negative rapid strep test does not exclude infection. Gerber and associates[44] found 45% of patients with a negative rapid antigen test to have a rise in streptococcal antibodies, indicating infection rather than colonization. The prior use of antibiotics may also cause a false-negative rapid test result. After 18 to 24 hours of antibiotic therapy, 71 to 83% of initially culture-positive cases have negative rapid test findings.[45]

Pertinent Management Issues

Several investigators have conducted cost-benefit analyses to determine appropriate strategies for the management of sore throat. Tompkins and coworkers[46] in 1977 analyzed three strategies: (1) treat only patients with positive GABH streptococcal throat cultures, (2) treat all patients, and (3) treat no one. They concluded that treatment with oral penicillin is cost-effective if the likelihood of a positive throat culture is >20%. For patients with a probability of a positive throat culture between 5 and 20%, treatment would be given only after a positive culture result.

Throat culture and treatment would be deferred if the probability of a positive culture was <5%. During a GABH streptococcal epidemic, however, treatment would be given to all patients without cultures. This analysis was conducted prior to the availability of rapid streptococcal antigen detection tests. The probabilities of a positive throat culture in this analysis were to be based on the known positive culture rate of the patient population.

Hedges and Lowe[47] extended the study of Tompkins and coworkers[46] and analyzed the following four strategies: (1) treat all patients, (2) treat only patients with positive GABH streptococcal throat cultures, (3) treat patients if an initial screening test finding is positive, and (4) treat all patients with a positive screening test finding and culture all others. The investigators included the costs of rheumatic fever owing to incomplete follow-up (ie, patients with positive culture findings not receiving treatment). They concluded that patients with a high probability of GABH pharyngitis (positive screening test or clinical criteria) should be treated. Those patients with a low probability of GABH pharyngitis should be cultured. Treatment should be based on culture results.

Lieu and colleagues[48] employed decision analysis to evaluate strategies for the use of a rapid latex agglutination test and throat culture in the management of pharyngitis. They had a wide range of test sensitivities and follow-up rates; they concluded that all sore throat patients should have a rapid test performed. Patients with a positive test result would be treated and those with a negative test result would be cultured. Subsequent treatment would then be based on culture results. These workers did not evaluate a strategy that incorporated treatment based on clinical findings. In an earlier study[43] of 255 pediatric emergency department patients, they found the use of a rapid antigen test, in conjunction with throat culture, resulted in 80% of patients with positive culture findings receiving antibiotic treatment compared with only 57% with culture alone.

Centor and associates[49] evaluated management strategies for adult GABH streptococcal pharyngitis incorporating the prior probability of a positive culture based on clinical criteria (see Table 19–1). They recommended treatment, without culture or testing, for patients with a probability of a positive throat culture of >38% (three or four criteria present). For all other patients, a rapid antigen test should be performed. Patients with a negative rapid antigen test finding should be cultured, and those with a positive test should receive antibiotic therapy. The likelihood of patient follow-up for positive cultures should also alter the threshold for treatment (16% for a 0% probability of follow-up).

CONCLUSION

After potentially serious causes of sore throat (epiglottis, retropharyngeal abscess) are eliminated from the diagnosis, and patients at risk for

TABLE 19–4. RECOMMENDED MANAGEMENT STRATEGIES

1. Treat, without testing, patients at high likelihood of GABH streptococcal pharyngitis
   Adult patients: presence of 3 or 4 Centor clinical variables
   Pediatric patients: Breese score >28
2. Patients not meeting criteria for treatment (#1); perform screening test (rapid streptococcal antigen test or pharyngeal Gram stain)
   Screening test positive: treat
   Screening test negative: culture
   Culture positive: treat

unusual etiologies (gonococcal pharyngitis, diphtheria) identified, the probability of infection by GABH streptococci must be determined (Table 19–4). Treatment should be initiated for those patients for whom GABH streptococcal pharyngitis is likely. For patients less likely to have a positive throat culture, a rapid streptococcal antigen test should be performed and treatment initiated for those with a positive result.

All patients with negative rapid antigen test findings must have throat cultures performed and receive treatment if the results are positive. For patients for whom follow-up care is unlikely, a lower threshold is sufficient to initiate treatment.

REFERENCES

1. Catanzaro FJ, Stetson CA, Morris AJ, et al: Symposium on rheumatic fever and heart disease. The role of the streptococcus in the pathogenesis of rheumatic fever. *Am J Med.* 1954;17:749–756.
2. Krober MS, Bass JW, Michels GN: Streptococcal pharyngitis: Placebo-controlled double-blind evaluation of clinical response to penicillin therapy. *JAMA.* 1985;253:1271–1274.
3. Randolph MF, Gerber MA, DeMeo KK, et al: Effect of antibiotic therapy on the clinical course of streptococcal pharyngitis. *J Pediatr.* 1985; 106:870–875.
4. Denny FW, Wannamaker LW, Hahn EO: Comparative effects of penicillin, aureomycin and terramycin on streptococcal tonsillitis and pharyngitis. *Pediatrics.* 1953;11:7–14.
5. Kaplan EL, Top FH, Dudding BA, et al: Diagnosis of streptococcal pharyngitis: Differentiation of active infection from the carrier state in the symptomatic child. *J Infect Dis.* 1971;123:490–501.
6. Schwartz RH, Hayden GF, Wientzen R: Children less than three-years-old with pharyngitis: Are group A streptococci really that uncommon? *Clin Pediatr.* 1986;25:185–188.

7. McCue JD: Group G streptococcal pharyngitis: Analysis of an outbreak at a college. *JAMA.* 1982;248:1333–1336.
8. Turner JC, Hayden GF, Kiselica D, et al: Association of group C β-hemolytic streptococci with endemic pharyngitis among college students. *JAMA.* 1990;264:2644–2647.
9. Centor RM, Witherspoon JM, Dalton HP, et al: The diagnosis of strep throat in the emergency room. *Med Decision Making.* 1981;1:239–246.
10. Wigton RS, Connor JL, Centor RM: Transportability of a decision rule for the diagnosis of streptococcal pharyngitis. *Arch Intern Med.* 1986;146:81–83.
11. Breese BB: A simple scorecard for the tentative diagnosis of streptococcal pharyngitis. *Am J Dis Child.* 1977;131:514–517.
12. Funamura JL, Berkowitz CD: Applicability of a scoring system in the diagnosis of streptococcal pharyngitis. *Clin Pediatr.* 1983;22:622–626.
13. Tikob G, Petersen CS, Ousted M, et al: Localization of gonococci in the anterior oral cavity—A possible reservoir of the gonococcal infection? *Ann Clin Res.* 1985;17:73–75.
14. Wiesner PJ, Tronca E, Bonin P, et al: Clinical spectrum of pharyngeal gonococcal infection. *N Engl J Med.* 1973;288:181–185.
15. Hutt DM, Judson FN: Epidemiology and treatment of oropharyngeal gonorrhea. *Ann Intern Med.* 1986;104:655–658.
16. Komaroff AL, Aronson MD, Pass TM, et al: Serologic evidence of chlamydial and mycoplasmal pharyngitis in adults. *Science.* 1983;222:927–929.
17. Williams WC, Williamson HA, LeFevre ML: The prevalence of *Mycoplasma pneumoniae* in ambulatory patients with nonstreptococcal sore throat. *Fam Med.* 1991;23:117–121.
18. Gerber MA, Randolph MF, Chanatry J, et al: Role of *Chlaymdia trachomatis* and *Mycoplasma pneumoniae* in acute pharyngitis in children. *Diagn Microbiol Infect Dis.* 1987;6:263–265.
19. Rotta J, Duben J, Jedlicka F, et al: Prospective study of pharyngitis: Clinical diagnosis and microbiological profile. *Zentralbl Bakteriol.* 1989;271:532–542.
20. Guthrie RM, Ruoff GE, Rofman BA, et al: Aetiology of acute pharyngitis and clinical response to empirical therapy with erythromycin versus amoxicillin. *Fam Pract.* 1988;5:29–35.
21. Valle SL: Febrile pharyngitis as the primary sign of HIV infection in a cluster of cases linked by sexual contact. *Scand J Infect Dis.* 1987;19:13–17.
22. Merriam SC, Keeling RF: Beta-hemolytic streptococcal pharyngitis: Uncommon in infectious mononucleosis. *South Med J.* 1983;76:575–576.
23. Collins M, Fleisher GR, Fager SS: Incidence of beta hemolytic streptococcal pharyngitis in adolescent with infectious mononucleosis. *J Adol Health Care.* 1984;5:96–100.
24. Nichol KP, Cherry JD: Bacterial-viral interrelations in respiratory infections of children. *N Engl J Med.* 1967;277:667–672.
25. Breese BB, Disney FA: Beta-hemolytic streptococcal infection: The clinical and epidemiologic importance of the number of organisms found in culture. *Am J Dis Child.* 1970;119:18–26.
26. Evans AS: Infectious mononucleosis and related syndromes. *Am J Med Sci.* 1978;276:325–339.
27. Sumaya CV, Ench Y: Epstein-barr virus infectious mononucleosis in chil-

dren. I. Clinical and general laboratory findings. *Pediatrics.* 1985;75:1003–1010.
28. Thompson MP: The diagnosis of mononucleosis in the office laboratory. *Primary Care.* 1986;13:647–655.
29. Aronson MD, Komaroff AL, Pass TM, et al: Heterophil antibody in adults with sore throat. *Ann Intern Med.* 1982;96:505–508.
30. Fleisher GR, Collins M, Fager S: Limitations of available tests for diagnosis of infectious mononucleosis. *J Clin Microbiol.* 1983;17:691–624.
31. Paul JR, Bunnell WW: The presence of heterophile antibodies in infectious mononucleosis. *Am J Med Sci.* 1932;183:90–104.
32. Seitanidis B: A comparison of the monospot with the Paul-Bunnell test in infectious mononucleosis and other diseases. *J Clin Pathol.* 1969;22:321–323.
33. Basson V, Sharp AA: Monospot: a differential slide test for infectious mononucleosis. *J Clin Pathol.* 1969;22:324–325.
34. Chetham MM, Roberts KB: Infectious mononucleosis in adolescents. *Pediatr Ann.* 1991;20:206–213.
35. Sumaya CV, Ench Y: Epstein-Barr virus infectious mononucleosis in children. II. Heterophil antibody and viral-specific responses. *Pediatrics.* 1985;75:1011–1019.
36. Fleisher G, Lennette ET, Henle G: Incidence of heterophil antibody responses in children with infectious mononucleosis. *J Pediatr.* 1979;94:723–728.
37. Hedges JR, Wagner DK: Pharyngeal gram stains in the treatment of sore throats. *J Am Coll Emerg Phys.* 1978;7:229–232.
38. Crawford G, Brancato F, Holmes KK: Streptococcal pharyngitis: Diagnosis by gram stain. *Ann Intern Med.* 1979;90:293–297.
39. Brien JH, Bass JW: Streptococcal pharyngitis: Optimal site for throat culture. *J Pediatr.* 1985;106:781–783.
40. Wegner DL, Witte DL, Schrantz RD: Insensitivity of rapid antigen detection methods and single blood agar plate culture for diagnosing streptococcal pharyngitis. *JAMA.* 1992;267:695–697.
41. Radetsky M, Wheeler RC, Roe MH, et al: Comparative evaluation of kits for rapid diagnosis of group A streptococcal disease. *Pediatr Infect Dis J.* 1985;4:274–281.
42. Rapid Office Diagnostic Test for Streptococcal Pharyngitis. *Med Lett.* 1985;27:49–51.
43. Lieu TA, Fleisher GR, Schwartz JS: Clinical evaluation of a latex agglutination test for streptococcal pharyngitis: Performance and impact on treatment rates. *Pediatr Infect Dis J.* 1988;7:847–854.
44. Gerber MA, Randolph MF, Chanatry J, et al: Antigen detection test for streptococcal pharyngitis: Evaluation of sensitivity with respect to true infections. *J Pediatr.* 1986;108:654–658.
45. Beach PS, Balfour LC, Lucia HL: Group A streptococcal rapid test: Antigen detection after 18–24 hours of penicillin therapy. *Clin Pediatr.* 1989;28:6–10.
46. Tompkins RK, Burnes DC, Cable WE: An analysis of the cost-effectiveness of pharyngitis management and acute rheumatic fever prevention. *Ann Intern Med.* 1977;86:481–492.
47. Hedges JR, Lowe RA: Streptococcal pharyngitis in the emergency department: Analysis of therapeutic strategies. *Am J Emerg Med.* 1986;4:107–115.
48. Lieu TA, Fleisher GR, Schwartz JS: Cost-effectiveness of rapid latex aggluti-

nation testing and throat culture for streptococcal pharyngitis. *Pediatrics.* 1990;85:246–256.
49. Centor RM, Meier FA, Dalton HP: Throat cultures and rapid tests for diagnosis of group A streptococcal pharyngitis in adults, in Sox HC (ed): *Common Diagnostic Tests: Use and Interpretation.* 2nd ed. Philadelphia: American College of Physicians; 1990.

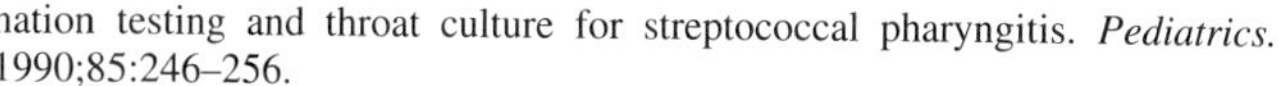

Chapter

Urinary Tract Infection

Raquel L. Gibly

Urinary tract infection (UTI) is one of the most common entities encountered by emergency physicians. In infants, UTIs are seen more commonly in boys than in girls during the first year of life, with a ratio of 1.5:1. In older children, UTI becomes more common in females, with a female-to-male ratio of 10:1 in childhood. By the reproductive years, the ratio increases to 50:1, with approximately 25 to 35% of otherwise healthy women between the ages of 20 and 40 suffering from at least one episode of UTI.[1] After the fifth decade, men and women are equally affected.[2, 3] In men, cystitis and pyelonephritis are rare unless accompanied by underlying anatomic abnormalities.[1]

Patients with indwelling catheters represent a higher-risk population. Almost 100% of these patients will have bacteriuria after 30 days, with the daily rate of infection being 3 to 10%.[4] Pregnant women are also at increased risk for UTI owing to the physiologic changes that occur during pregnancy.

The most common urinary pathogen in all infected individuals is *Escherichia coli.* It is responsible for 80 to 90% of all uncomplicated UTIs.[1, 5] Other Enterobacteriaceae (eg, *Klebsiella, Citrobacter*, *Staphylococcus saprophyticus, Enterococcus,* and *Proteus mirabilis*) are the next most commonly cultured organisms.[2, 5] In sexually active men and women, sexually transmitted diseases such as *Chlamydia trachomatis, Neisseria gonorrhoeae,* and *Trichomonas vaginalis* may also cause urinary symptoms and should be considered. This is especially true for the symptomatic patient with a negative finding on routine bacterial culture, because these aforementioned organisms will not grow on routine urine culture media.

ASYMPTOMATIC PATIENT

Asymptomatic bacteriuria is found in 0.5 to 1% of normal nonpregnant females and in 4 to 7% of pregnant females.[6, 7] The diagnosis is made by culturing more than 10^5 colony forming units (CFUs) of a single pathogen from a clean catch midstream (CCMS) urine specimen in asymptomatic patients. In nonpregnant asymptomatic patients, treatment should be considered only after two positive culture results.[8]

In the asymptomatic pregnant female, one positive culture finding maybe enough to warrant treatment, because UTI in this class of patients has been associated with low-birth-weight infants and higher incidence of prematurity.[9] If untreated, the patient has a 20 to 40% risk of developing a symptomatic UTI.[10]

Owing to factors of aging and hormonal changes, 6 to 33% of females and 11 to 13% of males in the elderly, ambulatory population have asymptomatic bacteriuria.[11] There is no evidence that treatment of asymptomatic bacteriuria in this population will alter outcome. In fact, routine treatment may lead to the development of resistant organisms, so it is not recommended.[4, 12, 13] If the person is institutionalized, asymptomatic bacteriuria increases to 20 to 50% in women and up to 20% in men.[13] Treatment of this class of patient may be beneficial and should be considered.[4, 10]

The presence of asymptomatic bacteriuria in children is 1% in girls and 0.03% in boys. It remains uncertain whether the treatment of these asymptomatic children will decrease the number of symptomatic infections or long-term sequelae. Routine screening and treatment of asymptomatic children is therefore questionable.[14]

SYMPTOMATIC PATIENT

The most common presenting symptom of a lower UTI is dysuria, but only 50 to 60% of women with dysuria have UTIs.[15, 16] External dysuria is the feeling of burning pain caused by the passage of urine over inflamed periurethral or introital tissues. Although this symptom can occur with urethritis, the causes are usually nonurinary, and further genital examination is warranted. Internal dysuria is a more visceral pain that may be constant or occur only during urination. It represents inflammation of the urethra or bladder and may be sensed as a fullness, urgency, or suprapubic pain.[12, 17]

Five factors have been found to be independent predictors of UTI: history of UTI, back pain, pyuria, hematuria, and bacteriuria. The presence of each factor increases the likelihood of infection. When two of these factors are found together, the positive predictive value for infection is 73%. If four or more findings are present, the positive predictive value for infection increases to 88%.[18] If there is accompanying back pain or the patient has systemic complaints such as malaise, nausea, vomiting, or fever, the patient probably has an upper tract infection and may even have accompanying bacteremia and sepsis.

Urinary tract infections are the most frequent cause of sepsis in the elderly population, with a mortality rate for urosepsis of 25%.[11] These patients often have insidious clinical presentations without classic symptoms. Changes in mental status, activity level, or bladder control habits may be the only clues to these infections and clinical suspicion must therefore be high.[20]

Infants also present uncharacteristically, with changes in usual response or feeding or increased irritability being the only sign. Fever is present in up to 49% of cases, so a urine culture should be obtained whenever an infant has an unexplained fever.[2] Because of the difficulty in making the diagnosis in this age group, sepsis is a common finding and accompanies UTI in 21 to 33% of infected neonates.[21]

In males, testicular pain and swelling or lower back or rectal pain may signal epididymitis, orchitis, and prostatitis, all of which can be confused with or accompany UTI. The 4-glass specimen collection technique described next may be helpful in this situation.[22]

DIAGNOSTIC TESTING

In most adults and older children, a properly obtained CCMS (clean catch midstream) urine specimen is adequate to evaluate for a UTI.[23] Catheterization may be necessary in patients who have severe vaginal discharge or who are menstruating, in infants, or in patients physically unable to give a CCMS. The proper technique is described in the chapter on urinalysis.

To obtain a 4-glass specimen in the male patient, the first 5 to 8 mL represents the urethral specimen (VB1). The midstream specimen (VB2) represents bladder, urethral, and renal urine. The prostate is then massaged, and expressed prostatic secretions (EPSs) are then collected at the urethral meatus. Finally, VB3 is collected, which represents the portion of the urine after prostatic massage.[22]

The recommendations for which diagnostic tests to order vary with the age and symptomatology of the patient. The standard is the urine culture in which 10^5 CFUs of a single pathogen is universally considered a positive result. Symptomatic "low-grade" infections have been found with 10^2 to 10^4 CFUs and should be treated.[5]

Other ways of analyzing urine include reagent dipstick and microscopic urinalysis, both of which are quick and inexpensive procedures easily performed by the emergency physician.

In neonates, sensitivity for urinalysis has been found as low as 48%. Cultures should be routinely ordered if UTI is suspected.[24, 25] In older children urine clarity, urine microscopy, and dipstick analysis for leukocyte esterase and nitrites have all been found to be reliable indicators of UTI—with negative predictive values of 99%, up to 100% (if <5 WBC/hpf and no bacteria are visualized), and 98%, respectively.[25–28]

In every symptomatic elderly patient, diagnostic evaluation for a UTI should include urinalysis, Gram stain, and culture and sensitivity (C&S). Blood cultures should be obtained if systemic signs of infection are present.[20] Other sources suggest that in the uncomplicated elderly patient, if urine is clear, a dipstick urinalysis can be performed. If results are negative, the patient can be discharged. This procedure has a sensitivity of 96%.[29] If the urine is cloudy or the dipstick finding is positive, the urine should be sent to the laboratory for microscopic urinalysis and culture.

In the adult, nonpregnant female, the urine dipstick and microscopic urinalysis have both been found to be adequate in assessing lower UTI.[5, 6, 12] In the uncomplicated symptomatic patient, if pyuria, hematuria, or bacteriuria is detected, the patient can be diagnosed with a UTI and treatment may be started without further laboratory tests.[5] If an upper UTI is suspected, a culture should be ordered.[11]

Pyuria, which can be detected on reagent strips and microscopically, is the most valuable variable in predicting UTI and has been found consistently to correlate with a positive culture.[18] Pyuria is often present without bacteriuria.[12] Sensitivity can vary secondary to the bladder dwell time of the urine and the hydration status.[22] In a properly collected specimen, sensitivity can be as high as 98%.[5, 12] In patients with low-grade infections, the sensitivity has been shown to be approximately 80%, and a microscopic examination may be helpful.[30]

Bacteriuria has not been found to be as reliable a test as the leukocyte esterase, with sensitivities only as high as 85%.[22] Direct visualization by microscopic examination is often difficult, especially in low-grade infections, because one may be looking for only one bacterium per high-powered field.

In men, because urinary tract infections occur so rarely, cultures should be always be considered. Follow-up with a urologist should also be arranged.

In the pregnant patient, routine office screening for UTI has been found to be cost-effective in the prevention of symptomatic UTIs.[4] The practice has decreased the incidence of pyelonephritis from 4% in this population to 1 to 2%.[6, 9] Some sources suggest that dipstick urinalysis is not an adequate screening test owing to the severe potential consequences of a missed infection and suggest that microscopy be performed on all urines.[22] Microscopic examination for pyuria has been shown to be 94% sensitive and 95% specific when 5 to 8 WBC/hpf are present.[31]

Tests of cure should be performed only in the complicated case or in upper tract infection. There has been little evidence to support routine follow-up cultures in the asymptomatic patient who was diagnosed with a lower tract infection.[12]

Imaging studies such as urography and ultrasound should be considered in children and adults with recurrent infections of complicating factors.

REFERENCES

1. Hooton TM, Stamm WE: Management of acute uncomplicated urinary tract infection in adults. *Med Clin North Am.* 1991;75:2.
2. Rushton HG: Genitourinary infections, in Kelalis PP, et al (eds): *Clinical Pediatric Urology.* 3rd ed. Philadelphia: WB Saunders; 1992:286–331.
3. Stewart C, Gibly RL, Brillman JC: Infections in the urinary tract and male genitalia, in Brillman JC, Quenzer RW (eds): *Infectious Disease in Emergency Medicine.* Boston: Little, Brown; 1992:645–672.
4. Warren JW: Catheter-associated bacteriuria. *Clin Geriatr Med.* 1992;8:4.
5. Johnson JR, Stamm WE: Urinary tract infections in women: Diagnosis and treatment. *Ann Intern Med.* 1989;111:906–917.
6. Lucas MJ, Cunningham FG: Urinary tract infection in pregnancy. *Clin Obstet Gynecol.* 1993;36:4.
7. Bandy LC: Urinary tract infection, in Gleicher N et al (eds): *Principles of Medical Therapy in Pregnancy.* New York: Plenum Publishing; 1985:403–405.
8. Fihn SD, Stamm WE: Interpretation and comparison of treatment studies for uncomplicated urinary tract infections in women. *Rev Infect Dis.* 1985;7: 468–478.
9. Cunningham FG et al: Renal and urinary tract diseases, in *William's Obstetrics.* 19th ed. Norwalk, CN: Appelton & Lange; 1993:1127–1144.
10. U.S. Preventive Services Task Force: Screening for asymptomatic bacteriuria, hematuria and proteinuria. *Am Fam Phys.* 1990;42:389–395.
11. Mulholland SG: Urinary tract infection. *Clin Geriatr Med.* 1990;6:43–53.
12. Komaroff AL: Urinalysis and urine culture in women with dysuria. *Ann Intern Med.* 1986;104:212–218.
13. Wilkie ME, Almond MK, Marsk FP: Diagnosis and management of urinary tract infection in adults. *Br Med J.* 1992;305:1137–1141.
14. Kemper KJ, Avner ED: The case against screening urinalysis for asymptomatic bacteriuria in children. *Am J Dis Child.* 1992;146:343–346.
15. Nazareth I, King M: Decision making by general practitioners in diagnosis and management of lower urinary tract symptoms in women. *Br Med J.* 1993;306:1103–1106.
16. Leibovici L, Alpert G, et al: A clinical model for diagnosis of urinary tract infection in young women. *Arch Intern Med.* 1989;149:2048–2050.

17. Wyker AW: Standard diagnostic considerations, in Gillenwater JY et al (eds): *Adult and Pediatric Urology.* 2nd ed. St. Louis: CV Mosby; 1991:63–77.
18. Wigton RS, Hoellerich VL, Ornato JP, et al: Use of clinical findings in the diagnosis of urinary tract infection in women. *Arch Intern Med.* 1985; 145:2222–2227.
19. Bauer JD: *Clinical Laboratory Methods.* 9th ed. St. Louis: CV Mosby; 1982:677–735.
20. Rhyne RL, Roche RJ: Infections in the elderly, in Brillman JC, Quenzer RW (eds): *Infectious Disease in Emergency Medicine.* Boston: Little, Brown; 1992:343–365.
21. Stork JE: Urinary tract infection in children. *Adv Pediatr Dis.* 1987;2:115–134.
22. Lowe FC, Brendler CB: Evaluation of the urologic patient, in Walsh PC et al (eds): *Campbell's Urology.* 6th ed. Philadelphia: WB Saunders; 1992:307–330.
23. Walter FG, Knopp RK: Urine sampling in ambulatory women: Midstream clean-catch versus catheterization. *Ann Intern Med.* 1989;18:166–172.
24. Crain EF, Gershel JC: Urinary tract infections in febrile infants younger than 8 weeks of age. *Pediatrics.* 1990;86:363–367.
25. Shaw KN, Hexter D, McGowan KL, et al: Clinical evaluation of a rapid screening test for urinary tract infections in children. *J Pediatr.* 1991; 118:733–736.
26. Vickers D, Ahmad T, Coulthard MG: Diagnosis of urinary tract infection in children: Fresh urine microscopy or culture? *Lancet.* 1991;338:767–770.
27. Phillips G, Fleming LW, Khan I, et al: Urine transparency as an index of absence of infection. *Br J Urol.* 1992;70:191–195.
28. Goldsmith BM, Campos JM: Comparison of urine dipstick, microscopy, and culture for the detection of bacteriuria in children. *Clin Pediatr.* 1990; 29:214–218.
29. Flanagan PG, Davies EA, Rooney PG, et al: Evaluation of four screening tests for bacteriuria in elderly people. *Lancet.* 1989; 1:1117–1119.
30. Kunin CM, White LV, Hua TH: A reassessment of the importance of ''low count'' bacteriuria in young women with acute urinary symptoms. *Ann Intern Med.* 1993;119:454–460.
31. Abyad A: Screening for asymptomatic bacteriuria in pregnancy: Urinalysis vs urine culture. *J Fam Pract.* 1991;33.471–474.

Chapter

The Acute Scrotum

Raymond J. Roberge

When a patient with scrotal pain presents to the emergency department, the emergency physician's foremost concern is the differentiation of ischemic from nonischemic pain, that is, identification or exclusion of testicular torsion as the cause of the patient's symptoms.

The list of disorders that result in scrotal inflammation is not extensive.[1–6] Etiologies of acute scrotal pain include torsion (testicular, appendicular); infectious (orchitis, epididymitis) or cystic formation (hydrocele, spermatocele); trauma (hematoma, fractured testicle); inflammation (Henoch-Schoenlein syndrome); vascular formation (varicocele); and miscellaneous other causes (tumor, inguinal hernia, adrenal hemorrhage, idiopathic scrotal edema). Generally speaking, a well-performed history and physical examination can exclude many, if not most, of these illnesses. In most cases the differential diagnosis is eventually epididymoorchitis vs appendicular or testicular torsion. Because the degree of testicular salvage correlates inversely with the time to presentation and diagnosis (preservation of testicular function is likely to be greatest when symptoms are under 4 to 6 hours' duration),[1, 7] it is essential that the emergency physician formulate a plan for the rapid diagnosis and equally rapid urologic referral in cases of testicular torsion.

Numerous physical findings associated with acute testicular torsion (eg, abrupt onset of pain, scrotal erythema, abnormal testicular lie, testicular elevation, Prehn sign, blue dot sign)[1, 6, 8] have proved too nonspecific to be of diagnostic utility in differentiating torsion from other testicular disorders.[1, 9, 10] Although the physician's consideration of the possibility of testicular torsion is the most important prerequisite for making the diagnosis of torsion, several ancillary tests may be helpful, particularly if the clinical presentation is atypical. Each possesses certain advantages and limitations. In those cases in which the diagnosis of testicular torsion is strongly suspected, the decision to obtain urologic consultation should be immediate and should never await the results of any testing.

URINALYSIS

The differentiation of testicular torsion from infectious causes of testicular pain is clearly an important aspect of the evaluation. Pyuria, demonstrated either by routine urinalysis or qualitatively by leukocyte esterase determination,[11] is a characteristic feature of infectious scrotal disorders such as orchitis and epididymitis and has routinely been cited as useful in the differential diagnosis of testicular torsion.[1, 12] Pyuria has also occasionally been reported in testicular torsion,[9, 13] although in many instances the degree of pyuria has not been documented. Conversely, reports of apyuric orchitis and epididymitis have also surfaced.[10, 13–16] Nonetheless, pyuria in excess of 20 cells per high-power field is unusual with testicular torsion and strongly suggests an infectious etiology.[1]

Urinalysis is a rapid and cost-efficient method of documenting the presence or absence of pyuria and should routinely be performed on all patients presenting with scrotal complaints. The significant overlap of urinary findings demonstrates that the presence or absence of pyuria alone does not reliably differentiate between infectious and noninfectious causes of acute scrotal pathology and must never be relied on to rule in or rule out torsion from the differential diagnosis.

DOPPLER ULTRASONOGRAPHY

Doppler ultrasonography (CDUS) utilizes a hand-held Doppler stethoscope or Doppler flowmeter to assess vascular flow. It is especially well suited for use in the emergency department setting because of its low cost, light weight, noninvasive nature, technical simplicity, and portability.[17–19] It is as effective in young children[20] as in adolescents and adults. The technique involves manually fixing the testis against the anterior scrotal skin, to which an aqueous gel is applied, and then placing the DU probe perpendicular to the long axis of the testis. Arterial vascular sounds of the unaffected testicle are arbitrarily assigned a numerical value of 2+ on a scale of 0 to 4+, and the affected testicle is then compared with the uninvolved side.[21–23] Differences are evaluated in the context of the entire clinical presentation.

Differences in testicular blood flow detected on Doppler auscultation help differentiate disorders such as epididymitis with its increased blood flow (secondary to the hyperemia of infection) from disorders with reduced or absent flow—generally those associated with testicular torsion.[19, 24, 25] Absent or diminished vascular pulsatile sounds of the involved testicle constitute a positive DU test finding[25] and, in the setting of an acute scrotum, support the clinical diagnosis of testicular torsion.[26]

False-negative interpretations of DU arise when torsion occurs at the posterior midtesticular level so that blood flow in the vessels immediately proximal to the torsion is mistakenly identified as arising from the testicle itself.[19] This problem may be circumvented by placing the DU transducer probe at the inferior pole of the testis to ensure evaluation of testicular, rather than spermatic cord, flow.[17, 18] Pulsatile signals arising from an inflamed scrotal wall are also occasionally mistaken as being of testicular origin and may result in a false-negative interpretation.[1] This possibility can be avoided by performing the funicular compression test of Pedersen,[27] wherein the examiner compresses the ipsilateral spermatic cord between two fingers and listens for cessation of pulsatile signals, thereby confirming that the testicular artery, and not the scrotal wall, is the source of flow.[1, 17, 18, 23] A false-negative result can also arise when DU is performed in cases of torsion of greater than 12 hours' duration; in this situation, collateral circulation may have developed and may be confused with testicular flow.[25, 28]

Doppler ultrasonography cannot help to differentiate between orchitis and other high-flow states that require surgical intervention (eg, torsion of a testicular appendage, spontaneously reduced torsion, delayed presentation of torsion, hemorrhagic testicular tumor).[17, 29]

Turnbull and associates[23] have reviewed the literature from a 10-year period and noted that DU demonstrated a sensitivity of 73% in 86 surgically documented cases of testicular torsion. They emphasize, however, that the data from these studies are difficult to interpret because of differing study techniques and lack of surgical confirmation of testicular torsion in many of the reported cases.[23] The positive predictive value of DU has been reported to be 100% by several investigators; this may be the true value of this modality.[17, 19, 20] Doppler ultrasonography may also be of special utility in cases with low probabilities of testicular torsion that cannot be ruled out on clinical grounds alone.[17]

Pending further prospective clinical trails addressing the role of DU in the evaluation of the acute scrotum, it can be stated that although DU alone does not lead to diagnosis of testicular torsion, it does continue to be extremely accurate in demonstrating the status of testicular blood flow.[25] Doppler ultrasonography has the added advantage of not delaying definitive therapy[17] and is useful in documenting the resumption of testicular flow after manual attempts at detorsion in the emergency department, while definitive urologic intervention is awaited.[17]

COLOR DOPPLER ULTRASONOGRAPHY

Color Doppler ultrasonography (CDUS) is a relatively new modality that combines real-time ultrasonographic delineation of anatomic features with display of the temporospatial characteristics of blood flow,[30, 31] thereby combining the strengths of both testicular scintigraphy and conventional sonography.[32] Color Doppler ultrasonography allows the display of color-encoded, differing Doppler flow velocities simultaneously superimposed on real-time, gray-scale images to produce a color flow map.[33, 34] Thus, CDUS is ideally suited for diagnosing scrotal disorders in which evaluation of testicular perfusion is essential to appropriate management.

Although experience with this technique is still limited, clinical studies have demonstrated specificities of 100% and sensitivities ranging from 86 to 100%,[32, 34, 35] equal to those demonstrated with testicular scintigraphy.[36] Color Doppler ultrasonography offers several potential benefits over scintigraphy in that it requires no administration of contrast agents, is more cost-effective, and can be performed in as little as 15 minutes.[33] Compared with scintigraphy, CDUS provides excellent resolution of the scrotal contents, thereby enabling the accurate determination of the presence of scrotal masses, fluid collections, or testicular fractures.[31] Combined with the excellent blood flow data, this anatomic detail avoids the misinterpretation of paratesticular for testicular blood flow that may occur occasionally with scintigraphy.[35] Color Doppler ultrasonography is likewise useful for documenting resumption of testicular arterial flow after spontaneous detorsion and after successful manual detorsion.[34, 35] Additionally, there may be less interobserver variability in interpreting CDUS results than that noted with scintigraphy.[32] False-negative results are uncommon but occasionally are encountered in loose torsions in which vascular flow is not totally compromised,[34] but this situation is noted with scintigraphy as well.[32] Color Doppler ultrasonography may be more difficult to perform in neonates and children,[31] but, as experience with this modality increases, it may become the technique of choice for evaluation of equivocal cases of testicular torsion in both children and adults.

TESTICULAR SCINTIGRAPHY

In 1973, Nadel and coworkers[37] described the use of sodium pertechnetate (^{99m}Tc) in evaluating perfusion of the testes and other scrotal contents. Since that time, numerous studies have demonstrated sensitivities of 80 to 100% and specificities of 86 to 100%[18, 36, 38, 39] for this technique. These have led to its designation as the standard for diagnosing altered blood flow states of scrotal contents.

The technique involves placing the patient supine with his scrotum parallel to the face of a low-energy collimeter/camera and injecting ^{99m}Tc (15 to 20 mCi in an adult and a minimum dose of 5 mCi in children) as a bolus into an antecubital vein.[40] The study then consists of two phases, the radionuclide angiogram, or flow study phase, which delineates the major vascular supply to the testes, and the scrotal scan (static ''blood pool'' image) phase, which demonstrates the degree of tissue perfusion.[41]

In the angiography or flow study phase, six to eight 5-second camera frames are obtained commencing with the first appearance of isotope on the oscilloscope or after 10 seconds, whichever occurs first.[39] These films are scrutinized, and blood flow through the spermatic cord vessels (testicular, deferential, and cremasteric arteries) and extracord vessels is reported as normal, increased, decreased, or absent. Scrotal flow is likewise reported but as a separate entity.[39, 40] In the static blood pool phase, scrotal contents are visualized, and areas of increased, decreased, or absent vascularity are reported.[40]

In cases of torsion, the testicle typically demonstrates a central photopenic defect (''halo sign'')[42] on both phases of the study.[32, 41] Increased radionuclide angiogram perfusion and vascular definition as well as intense increased vascularity on the blood pool phase are the hallmarks of inflammatory states such as epididymitis or abscess.[39] False-negative findings occur with spontaneous detorsion; early or late torsion; small retracted scrotum; small testes; or inflammatory hydrocele.[1, 41–43] False-positive scans may be noted in association with testicular tumor, hydrocele, abscess, or hernia.[42]

Disadvantages of scintigraphy as compared with CDUS include poorer resolution of intrascrotal contents[32, 41]; necessity for performance of the test in the nuclear medicine suite; greater expense[32]; and increased scanning time (up to 2 hours in some instances).[33] Nonetheless, nuclear scintigraphy is a highly accurate test and for the moment remains the standard to which other modalities for the detection of testicular flow are compared.

FUTURE DIRECTIONS: MAGNETIC RESONANCE IMAGING AND SPECTROSCOPY

Magnetic resonance imaging (MRI) is highly accurate in depicting scrotal anatomy[44] and has been found to be highly sensitive and specific in demonstrating both testicular (tumor, cysts, orchitis, trauma, abscess) and extratesticular (epididymitis, spermatoceles, hydroceles, varicoceles) pathology[45, 46] as well as undescended testes.[47] Studies of MRI in a rat model of testicular torsion have demonstrated a characteristic spiral (''whirlpool'') distortion of the fascial planes of the spermatic cord.[48] In addition, ^{31}P magnetic resonance spectroscopy studies in an animal model of testicular torsion have correlated changes in intracellular ATP levels with testicular viability.[49] When compared with other available imaging techniques, MRI offers the advantages of lack of ionizing radiation, short procedure time, exquisite anatomic detail, enhanced fields of view, simplified understanding of images by referring physicians, less dependency on operator technique, and less need for manipulation of the painful scrotum.[44–46, 49] Disadvantages include lack of availability at some institutions, relatively high cost, and degradation of images by patient movement.[45] Thus, although MRI holds much promise, its true value in the diagnosis of testicular torsion awaits human trials.

CONCLUSION

Torsion is a urologic emergency and as such must be evaluated and diagnosed in a timely fashion. Highly suspect presentations warrant immediate urologic referral. The diagnosis of torsion in atypical clinical presentations requires the emergency physician's high index of suspicion coupled with appropriate diagnostic testing. Time considerations, availability, and—increasingly—cost must be taken into account when considering diagnostic tests. Doppler ultrasonography should be carried out at the bedside to evaluate the status of testicular blood flow. Nuclear scintigraphy is still considered the standard test for diagnosing testicular torsion, but increasing experience with CDUS suggests it may be equally efficacious while offering several distinct advantages. Preliminary investigations have suggested a potential role in the future for nuclear MRI in scrotal disorders,[44] including torsion,[40] but definitive recommendations await further clinical trials.

REFERENCES

1. Haynes BE, Bessen HA, Haynes VE: The diagnosis of testicular torsion. *JAMA.* 1983;249:2522–2527.
2. Khan UV, Williams TH, Malek RS: Acute scrotal swelling in Henoch-Schoenlein syndrome. *Urology.* 1977;10:139–141.
3. Ryan PG: Henoch-Schoenlein purpura mimicking testicular torsion (letter). *J R Coll Surg Edinburgh.* 1988;33:107.
4. Giacoia GP, Cravens JD: Neonatal adrenal hemorrhage presenting as scrotal hematoma. *J Urol.* 1990;143:567–568.
5. Evans JP, Snyder HMcC: Idiopathic scrotal edema. *Urology.* 1977;9:549–551.
6. Holland JM, Graham JB, Ignatoff JM: Conservative management of twisted testicular appendages. *J Urol.* 1981;125:213–214.
7. Williamson RCN: Death in the scrotum: Testicular torsion. *N Engl J Med.* 1977;296:338.

8. Carriere JN Jr: Horizontal lie of the testicle: A diagnostic sign in torsion of the testis. *J Urol.* 1972;107:616–617.
9. Ransler CW III, Allen TD: Torsion of the spermatic cord. *Urol Clin North Am.* 1982;9:245–250.
10. Harwood-Nuss AL: Genitourinary disease, in Rosen P, Baker FJ III, Barkin RM, et al (eds). *Emergency Medicine: Concepts and Clinical Practice.* 2nd ed. St. Louis: CV Mosby; 1988:1558–1560.
11. Frank SH: The genitourinary system, in Taylor RB (ed). *Family Medicine: Principles and Practice.* 3rd ed. New York: Springer-Verlag; 1988:298.
12. O'Brien WM, Lynch JW: The acute scrotum. *Am Fam Physician.* 1988;97:239–247.
13. Stage KH, Schoenvogel R, Lewis S: Testicular scanning: Clinical experience with 72 patients. *J Urol.* 1981;125:334–337.
14. Abu-Sleiman R, Ho JE, Gregory JG: Scrotal scanning. Present value and limits of interpretation. *Urology.* 1979;13:326–330.
15. Cass AS, Cass BP, Veeraraghavan K: Immediate exploration of the unilateral acute scrotum in young male subjects. *J Urol.* 1980;124:829–832.
16. Del Villar RG, Ireland GW, Cass AS: Early exploration in acute testicular conditions. *J Urol.* 1972;108:887–888.
17. Bickerstaff KI, Sethia K, Murie JA: Doppler ultrasonography in the diagnosis of acute scrotal pain. *Br J Surg.* 1988;75:238–239.
18. Rodriguez DD, Rodriguez WC, Rivera JJ, et al: Doppler ultrasound versus testicular scanning in the evaluation of the acute scrotum. *J Urol.* 1981;125:343–346.
19. Perri AJ, Slachta GA, Feldman AE, et al: The doppler stethoscope and the diagnosis of the acute scrotum. *J Urol.* 1976;116:598–599.
20. Iuchtman M, Zaireff L, Assa J: Doppler flowmeter in the differential diagnosis of the acute scrotum in children. *J Urol.* 1979;121:221–222.
21. Nasrallah PF, Manzone D, King LR: Falsely negative doppler examinations in testicular torsion. *J Urol.* 1977;118:194–195.
22. Levy BJ: The diagnosis of torsion of the testicle using the Doppler ultrasonic stethoscope. *J Urol.* 1975;113:63–65.
23. Turnbull TJ, Dymoinski JJ: Emergency department use of hand-held doppler ultrasonography. *Am J Emerg Med.* 1989;7:209–215.
24. Harzmann R, Weckerman D: Importance of doppler sonography in urology. *Urol Int.* 1989;45:258–263.
25. Perri AJ, Morlaes JD, Feldman AE, et al: Necrotic testicle with increased blood flow on doppler ultrasonic examination. *Urology.* 1976;8:265–267.
26. Bird K, Rosenfield AT, Taylor JW: Ultrasonography in testicular torsion. *Radiology.* 1983;147:527–534.
27. Haynes BE: Doppler ultrasound failure in testicular torsion. *Ann Emerg Med.* 1984;13:1103–1107.
28. Pedersen JF, Holm HH, Hold T: Torsion of the testis diagnosed by ultrasound. *J Urol.* 1975;113:65–68.
29. Kiviat MD, Ansell JD: Doppler ultrasonic examination (letter). *Urology.* 1976;8:743.
30. Waggoner AD, Perez JE: Principles and physics of doppler. *Cardiol Clin.* 1990;8:173–190.
31. Middleton WD, Melson GL: Testicular ischemia: Color doppler sonographic findings in five patients. *Am J Roentgenol.* 1989;152:1237–1239.

32. Middleton WD, Seigel BA, Melson GL, et al: Acute scrotal disorders: Prospective comparison of color doppler US and testicular scintigraphy. *Radiology.* 1990;177:177–181.
33. Jensen MC, Leee KP, Halls JM, et al: Color doppler sonography in testicular torsion. *J Clin Ultrasound.* 1990;18:446–448.
34. Burks DD, Markey BJ, Durkhard TK, et al: Suspected testicular torsion and ischemia; evaluation with color doppler sonography. *Radiology.* 1990;175:815–821.
35. Lerner RM, Mevorach RA, Huylbert WC, et al: Color doppler US in the evaluation of acute scrotal disease. *Radiology.* 1990;176:355–358.
36. Chen DCP, Holder LE, Melloul M: Radionuclide scrotal imaging; Further experience with 210 new patients. II. results and discussion. *J Nucl Med.* 1983;24:841–853.
37. Nadel NS, Gittler MH, Hahn LC, et al: Preoperative diagnosis of testicular torsion. *Urology.* 1973;1:478–479.
38. Romics I, Wesseler T, Bach K: Scintigraphy for the diagnosis of testicular torsion and differential diagnosis of acute intrascrotal processes. *Int Urol Nephrol.* 1988;20:631–639.
39. Holder LE, Nartire JR, Holmes ER, et al: Testicular radionuclide angiography and static imaging; Anatomy, scintigraphic interpretation and clinical indications. *Radiology.* 1977;125:739–752.
40. Chen DCP, Holder LE, Melloul M: Radionuclide scrotal imaging: Further experience with 210 patients. I. Anatomy, physiology, and methods. *J Nucl Med.* 1983;24:735–742.
41. Lowry PA, Brown WD: Spontaneously reduced testicular torsion. A pitfall in radionuclide scrotal imaging. *Urology.* 1989;33:135–136.
42. Witherington R, Jarrel TS: Torsion of the spermatic cord in adults. *J Urol.* 1990;143:62–63.
43. Fischman AJ, Ahmad M, Chheda H, et al: Reliability of radionuclide scintigraphy for detection of testicular torsion: an animal study. *Eur J Nucl Med.* 1990;16:657–661.
44. Baker LI, Hajek PC, Burkhard TK, et al: MR imaging of the scrotum: Normal anatomy. *Radiology.* 1987;163:89–92.
45. Rholl KS, Lee JKT, Ling D, et al: MR imaging of the scrotum with a high-resolution surface coil. *Radiology.* 1987;163:99–103.
46. Baker LI, Hajaek PC, Burkhard TK, et al: MR imaging of the scrotum: Pathologic conditions. *Radiology.* 1987;163:93–98.
47. Fritschke PJ, Hricak H, Kagan BA, et al: Undescended testis: Value of MR imaging. *Radiology.* 1987;164:169–173.
48. Landa HM, Gylys-Moran VM, Matery RF, et al: Detection of testicular torsion by magnetic resonance imaging in a rat model. *J Urol.* 1988; 140:1178–1180.
49. Tzika AA, Vigneron DB, Hricak H, et al: P-31 MR spectroscopy in assessing testicular torsion: Rat model. *Radiology.* 1989;172:753–757.

Chapter

Urologic Trauma

Michael A. Gibbs and Andrew Peitzman

Injuries to the genitourinary tract occur in 10 to 15% of patients sustaining trauma.[1] Because the presentation of urologic injury can be subtle, it is frequently overlooked during the initial evaluation of the trauma patient, leading to significant morbidity. Although the management of other life-threatening injuries may take precedence, early diagnosis of urologic injury is essential to avoid potentially serious complications.

Hematuria is the most common sign of urologic injury. All patients suffering blunt multisystem trauma and those with penetrating trauma to the back, abdomen, flank, or groin should have a urine sample examined. Because hematuria is often transient and may clear after voiding and following resuscitation with crystalloid, it is critical that the first-voided urine or the first portion of the catheterization specimen be collected.[2, 3]

The diagnostic assessment of urology injury is typically performed in a retrograde fashion, with an initial evaluation of the "lower tract" (external genitalia, urethra, bladder) followed by an evaluation of the "upper tract" (ureters and kidneys). This approach is effective and reduces the risk of iatrogenic injury. Deciding which patients should undergo diagnostic studies can often be a dilemma. The following are potential markers of urologic injury and should prompt a diligent evaluation:

A. Markers of lower tract injury:
   1. Blood at the urethral meatus
   2. Gross hematuria
   3. Inability to pass a Foley catheter
B. Markers of upper tract injury:
   1. Gross hematuria
   2. Hemodynamic instability associated with any degree of hematuria
   3. Penetrating trauma in proximity to the urologic system (lower chest, back, flank, abdomen, or groin) with or without hematuria

URETHRAL TRAUMA

Although urethral trauma is far less common than injury to the kidneys or bladder, it is associated with a high incidence of complications (eg, strictures, impotence, incontinence); therefore, early diagnosis and treatment of urethral injury are essential.[4]

The male urethra is anatomically divided into anterior and posterior segments by the urogenital diaphragm. The anterior urethra is located below the urogenital diaphragm and includes the bulbous and penile urethra. The posterior urethra is within and above the urogenital diaphragm and includes the prostatic and membranous urethra. The posterior urethra is firmly attached to the pubis by the puboprostatic ligament, making it prone to injury following pelvic fractures.

Injuries to the anterior urethra are usually the result of a straddle injury or a direct blow to the perineum. Injuries to the posterior urethra are most often the result of pelvic fractures involving the symphysis or pubic rami. An injury to the posterior urethra should always be suspected in a patient with a pelvic fracture, particularly if the fracture is displaced. Between 5 and 25% of patients with pelvic fractures have an associated urethral injury. Conversely, a pelvic fracture is present in over 95% of patients with an injury to the posterior urethra.[4, 5]

In contrast to the male urethra, the female urethra is not fixed to the pelvis. Increased mobility and shorter length protect it from injury. Urethral trauma in the female patient is exceedingly rare, with only occasional case reports in the literature.[6, 7]

Diagnosis

The patient with a urethral injury typically complains of perineal pain, dysuria, or inability to void. Micturition may cause swelling of the penis and perineum. On physical examination blood at the urethral meatus is the single best indication of urethral trauma.[4, 8] Although perineal discoloration and swelling may be present, it is usually a late finding. Rectal examination may reveal a ''high-riding prostate'' or a tender boggy mass representing extravasated blood and urine. In the female patient, lacerations of the labia and vagina may be associated with urethral injury.

In patients with a suspected urethral injury, urinary catheterization is contraindicated because it increases the incidence of infection, stricture formation, and conversion of a partial urethral transection into a complete one.

The diagnosis of urethral injury is made by retrograde urethrography. Urethrography is indicated in any trauma patient who presents with blood at the urethral meatus or in a patient without blood at the meatus in whom the gentle passage of a urethral catheter is met with resistance. The retrograde urethrogram is performed as follows: (1) an 8-French Foley catheter is gently placed in the urethra and the balloon is inflated in the fossa navicularis with 2 to 3 mL of sterile water. A three-way stopcock connected directly to a syringe may be used as an alternative. (2) Ten to 20 mL of water-soluble contrast material diluted to a 10% solution is *slowly* injected as an anteroposterior (AP) radiograph is taken.[4]

When the urethra is transected, extravasation of contrast material will be seen. In the presence of extravasation, if contrast is seen in the bladder, a partial injury is present. If none is seen a complete transection has occurred. Because urethrography cannot be performed in the female patient, the diagnosis is made clinically if blood is present at the urethral meatus or if a gentle attempt at catheterization is met with resistance.

BLADDER TRAUMA

Bladder injuries are usually the result of motor vehicle crashes or crush injuries to the pelvis. Between 70 and 95% of patients with bladder injuries have associated pelvic fractures. Conversely, between 4 and 8% of patients with pelvic fractures have an associated bladder injury. The fracture types most often associated with bladder injury include pubic arch fractures, symphyseal fractures, and displaced two-part pelvic fractures. A blow to the lower abdomen (as might occur with a steering wheel or seat belt injury) may also cause bladder injury without an associated fracture.[9–14]

Bladder injury can be classified into three categories: (1) partial thickness bladder wall contusions, (2) extraperitoneal rupture, involving a laceration below the pelvic peritoneum, and (3) intraperitoneal rupture, which violates the pelvic peritoneum and communicates with the peritoneal cavity.

Diagnosis

The patient with a bladder injury usually complains of lower abdominal pain. Physical examination may reveal bruising and tenderness of the lower abdomen. Pelvic instability may be noted. Because pelvic fractures alone can produce any or all of these signs and symptoms, a high index of suspicion for a bladder injury is important. Hematuria is always present, although it does not correlate with the degree of injury. A patient with a simple contusion may display gross hematuria, whereas an intraperitoneal rupture may be associated with only microscopic hematuria.[9]

The diagnosis of bladder injury is made by retrograde cystography. Proper technique is essential to avoid false-negative studies.[15–17] Because the natural elasticity of the detrusor muscle tends to approximate the edges of a bladder wall tear, contrast material may not extravasate if the bladder is inadequately distended. Most investigators recommend that 300 to 400 mL of water-soluble contrast material be used to ensure complete distension. After urethral injury has been ruled out, a Foley catheter is gently inserted and contrast material is instilled under gravity. The Foley catheter is then clamped, and an AP radiograph is taken. Next, the bladder is drained and a second AP postdrainage radiograph is performed. This view is important to demonstrate extravasated contrast material situated posteriorly, which be may obscured on the initial film. Using this technique, bladder injuries can be detected with 98% accuracy.

Although an intravenous pyelogram (IVP) can be used to assess the upper urinary tract, this method alone is inadequate to exclude an injury to the bladder.[18] Several studies have shown that the routine abdominopelvic computed tomography (CT) is not a reliable method for evaluating bladder injuries.[19, 20] When accurate imaging of the bladder is desired in patients undergoing abdominal tomography, instill contrast material via a Foley catheter to distend the bladder, clamp the catheter, and then perform the CT.

In cases of bladder contusion, the cystogram demonstrates an intact bladder that may be deformed by a pelvic hematoma, causing the bladder to assume a teardrop appearance or to deviate to one side of the pelvic cavity. In a patient with extraperitoneal rupture, extravasated contrast is confined to the pelvis, whereas a patient with intraperitoneal rupture demonstrates layering of contrast material in the dependent portion of the peritoneal cavity, in the paracolic gutters, between adjacent loops of bowel, or adjacent to the liver and spleen.

URETERAL TRAUMA

Ureteral injuries are rare and usually occur as a result of penetrating trauma. In most case series, over 90% of injuries are the result of gunshot wounds.[21] Rarely blunt trauma causes avulsion of the ureter at either the ureteropelvic or ureterovesical junction.[22–24] Regardless of the mechanism, more than 90% of ureteral injuries are associated with other intraabdominal injuries.

Diagnosis

Injury to the ureter is typically silent, and the diagnosis is usually delayed. Transection of the ureter is painless, with symptoms not developing until extravasated urine produces abdominal pain, inflammation, and swelling. Although hematuria is present in 80 to 90% of cases, it is usually microscopic. Complications of unrecognized ureter injury include urinoma or abscess formation, stricture, hydronephrosis, pyelonephritis, and permanent loss of renal function.[21]

Intravenous pyelography remains the technique of choice for the detection of ureteral injury, with a sensitivity of over 90%.[21] Although the sensitivity of abdominopelvic CT has never been tested in a prospective fashion, there is the potential to miss a ureteral injury between consecutive cross-sectional images. Evaluation of the ureters using IVP should be considered in the following situations: (1) Penetrating trauma in proximity to the ureter (regardless of CT findings). (2) Computed tomography scan suggestive, but not diagnostic, of ureteral injury. In the presence of a ureteral injury the IVP demonstrates extravasation of contrast material or, rarely, an abrupt cutoff of the opacified ureteral lumen.

RENAL TRAUMA

Renal injury can result from either penetrating or blunt trauma. In most case series, 5 to 10% of renal injuries are a consequence of penetrating trauma (stab or gunshot wound), whereas 90 to 95% are a consequence of blunt trauma (motor vehicle crashes, falls, direct blows to the abdomen). For purposes of investigation and staging, these injuries are classified as *class 1* (contusions or subcapsular hematomas); *class 2* (superficial cortical lacerations not involving the medulla or collecting system); *class 3* (deep lacerations extending into medulla or collecting system); or *class 4* (renal vascular pedicle injuries). Between 85 and 90% of all renal injuries are class 1 or 2 and are considered "minor." Five to 10% of renal injuries are class 3 or 4 and are considered "major."[1, 3]

Diagnosis

Patients with renal injury usually complain of abdominal, flank, or back pain. Physical examination may reveal tenderness, rigidity, or ecchymosis of the involved area. A palpable abdominal or flank mass, representing an expanding retroperitoneal hematoma, is seen in rare cases. Decreased bowel sounds may be noted in the patient with secondary ileus. Either microscopic or gross hematuria is usually present, although the degree of hematuria does not correlate with the degree of injury.

The understanding of renal injury and the recommendations for diagnosis and treatment have evolved over the last 2 decades. Most early studies recommended that all patients with blunt abdominal trauma and any degree of hematuria undergo immediate radiologic evaluation for renal injury.[24–26] This recommendation was justified by a small number of patients with ''major'' renal injuries presenting with only microscopic hematuria. A growing body of literature now supports a more selective approach. Pooled data from several independent studies have shown that, in hemodynamically stable blunt trauma patients with microscopic hematuria (>3 to 5 RBC/hpf), the risk of ''major'' renal injury is exceedingly low (approximately 0.05%).[3, 27–35] The majority of these patients have no demonstrable injury or ''minor'' renal injuries that can be managed nonoperatively. Diagnostic studies can be safely withheld in this situation. Depending on the individual patient, a brief period of observation with repeat physical examination and follow-up urinalysis may be indicated.[3] This approach to testing offers significant cost savings because stable patients with microscopic hematuria represent 80 to 90% of all cases. This approach also decreases the potential morbidity associated with intravenous contrast and may expedite the evaluation and management of other injuries.

Current indications for radiologic assessment of suspected renal injury include (1) penetrating trauma in proximity to the genitourinary tract (lower chest, back, flank, or abdomen) with or without hematuria; (2) blunt trauma associated with hypotension (BP <90 mmHg) and any degree of hematuria; many of these patients proceed directly to laparotomy; and (3) blunt trauma and gross hematuria.

Plain Film Radiography

Abdominal radiographs often provide important clues of potential renal injury: (1) fractures of the lower ribs or transverse processes; (2) loss of the renal outline or psoas shadow; (3) scoliosis, concave to the side of injury; and (4) focal ileus over the renal shadow. These findings, however, are neither sensitive nor specific.

Computed Tomography

Contrast-enhanced CT has replaced IVP as the modality of choice for the diagnosis of renal injury.[36–40] Computed tomography offers two important advantages: (1) the severity of renal injury can be more precisely defined and (2) the associated intraabdominal injuries, which are present in 80% of patients with penetrating renal injuries and 20% of patients with blunt renal injuries, can also be detected.[1, 41]

Intravenous Pyelography

Although CT has replaced IVP in most centers as the diagnostic modality of choice of patients with suspected renal injury, the IVP remains a valuable tool in certain situations. In patients who are too unstable to leave the trauma suite and in those being resuscitated for immediate laparotomy, a "one-shot IVP" can provide critical information. This is performed by rapidly injecting water-soluble contrast (2 mL/kg) via a central or peripheral intravenous line and obtaining a single 10-minute postinjection abdominal radiograph. The IVP film can (1) verify the presence (or absence) of two functioning kidneys and (2) demonstrate any major parenchymal disruption or urinary extravasation.[1, 37]

REFERENCES

1. Schneider RE: Genitourinary trauma. *Emerg Med Clin North Am.* 1993;11:137–145.
2. Mendez R: Renal trauma. *J Urol.* 1977;118:698–703.
3. Mee SL, McAninch JW: Indications for radiographic assessment in suspected renal trauma. *Urol Clin North Am.* 1989;16:187.
4. McAninch JW: Traumatic injuries to the urethra. *J Trauma.* 1981;21:291–297.
5. Pontes JE, Pierce JM: Anterior urethral injuries: Four years of experience at the Detroit General Hospital. *J Urol.* 1978;120:563–564.
6. Carter CT, Schafer N: Incidence of urethral disruption in females with traumatic pelvic fractures. *Am J Emerg Med.* 1993;11:218–220.
7. Diekmann-Guiroy B, Young DH: Female urethral injury secondary to blunt pelvic trauma. *Ann Emerg Med.* 1991;20:1376–1378.
8. Devine PC, Devine CJ: Posterior urethral injuries associated with pelvic fractures. *Urology.* 1982;20:467–470.
9. Brosman SA: Trauma of the bladder. *Surg Gynecol Obstet.* 1976;143:605–608.
10. Cass AS: Bladder trauma in the multiple injured patient. *J Urol.* 1976;115:667–669.
11. Corriene JN, Sandler CM: Management of the ruptured bladder: Seven years of experience with 111 cases. *J Trauma.* 1986;26:830–833.
12. Cass AS: Diagnostic studies in bladder rupture. *Urol Clin North Am.* 1989;16:267–273.
13. Clark SS, Pruencio RF: Lower urinary tract injuries associated with pelvic fractures: Diagnosis and management. *Surg Clin North Am.* 1972;52:183–201.
14. Tile M: Pelvic fractures: Operative vs nonoperative treatment. *Ortho Clin North Am.* 1980;11:423–434.
15. Carroll PR, McAninch JW: Major bladder trauma. The accuracy of cystography. *J Urol.* 1983;130:887–888.

16. Cass AS, Ireland GW: Bladder trauma associated with pelvic fractures in severely injured patients. *J Trauma.* 1973;13:205–212.
17. Lieberman AH, Walden TB, Bogash M, et al: Negative cystography with bladder rupture: Presentation of 2 cases and review of the literature. *J Urol.* 1980;123:428–430.
18. Schiff M, Glickman MG, Herter GE: Radiologic procedures for the evaluation of urinary tract trauma, in Roberts JR, Hedges JR (eds): *Clinical Procedures in Emergency Medicine.* Philadelphia: WB Saunders, 1991.
19. Mee SH, McAninch JW, Federle MP: Computerized tomography in bladder rupture: Diagnostic limitations. *J Urol.* 1987;137:207–209.
20. Rehem CG, Mure AJ, O'Malley KF, et al. Blunt traumatic bladder rupture: The role of retrograde cystogram. *Ann Emerg Med.* 1991;20:845–847.
21. Guerriero WG: Ureteral injury. *Urol Clin North Am.* 1989;16:237–248.
22. Boston VE, Smith BT: Bilateral ureter avulsion following closed trauma. *Br J Urol.* 1975;47:149–151.
23. Diokno AC: Avulsion of the proximal ureter secondary to blunt trauma. *J Urol.* 1974;111:412–414.
24. Rao CR: Ureteral avulsion secondary to blunt abdominal injury. *J Urol.* 1973;110:188–190.
25. Bright TC, White K, Peters PC: Significance of hematuria after trauma. *J Urol.* 1978;120:455–456.
26. Cass AS, Luxenberg M, Gleich P, et al: Clinical indications for radiographic evaluation of blunt renal trauma. *J Urol.* 1986;136:370–372.
27. Griffen WO, Belin RP, Ernst CB, et al: Intravenous pyelogram in abdominal trauma. *J Trauma.* 1978;18:287–391.
28. Eastham SA, Wilson TG, Ahlering TE: Radiographic assessment of blunt renal trauma. *J Trauma.* 1991;31:1527–1528.
29. Guice K, Oldham K, Brock E, et al: Hematuria after blunt trauma: When is pyelogram useful? *J Trauma.* 1983;23:305–311.
30. Hardeman SW, Husmann DA, Chin HKW, et al: Blunt urinary tract trauma: identifying those patients who require radiological diagnostic studies. *J Urol.* 1987;138:99–101.
31. Klein S, Johs S, Fuhitani R, et al: Hematuria following blunt abdominal trauma. *Arch Surg.* 1988;123:1173–1176.
32. Mee SL, McAninch JW, Robinson AL, et al: Radiographic assessment of renal trauma: a 10-year prospective study of patient selection. *J Urol.* 1989;141:1095–1098.
33. Nicolaisen GS, McAninch JW, Marshall GA, et al: Renal trauma: re-evaluation of the indications for radiographic assessment. *J Urol.* 1985;133:183–186.
34. Peterson NE, Schylze S: Selective diagnostic uroradiography for trauma. *J Urol.* 1987;137:449–451.
35. Thomason RB, Jullian JS, Mostellar HC, et al: Microscopic hematuria after blunt trauma. Is pyelogram necessary? *Am Surg.* 1989;55:145–150.
36. Bretan PN, McAninch JW, Federle MP, et al: Computerized tomographic staging of renal trauma: 85 consecutive cases. *J Urol.* 1986;136:561–565.
37. Cass AS, Vieira JL: Comparison of IVP and CT findings in patients with suspected severe renal injury. *Urology.* 1987;29:484–487.
38. Lang EK: Intra-abdominal and retroperitoneal organ injuries diagnosed on

dynamic computed tomograms obtained for assessment of renal trauma. *J Trauma.* 1990;30:1161–1168.
39. McAninch JW, Federle MP: Evaluation of renal injuries with computerized tomography. *J Urol.* 1982;128:456–460.
40. Sandler CM, Toombs BD: Computed tomographic evaluation of blunt renal injuries. *Radiology.* 1981;141:461–466.
41. Federle MP: The role of computerized tomography in renal trauma. *Radiology.* 1981;41:455–460.

Chapter

Blunt Abdominal Trauma

David A. Jerrard

The diagnostic accuracy of clinical evaluation alone in detecting significant blunt intraabdominal injury has been cited to range from 42 to 84%.[1–3]

Prior to the introduction of diagnostic peritoneal lavage (DPL) in the mid-1960s, the management of blunt abdominal trauma entailed nothing more than expectant observation, with surgical exploration for cases of hemodynamic deterioration or worsening pain. This strategy resulted in unnecessary morbidity and mortality.[4–6] Computed tomography (CT) scanning, introduced in the 1980s, has supplanted diagnostic peritoneal lavage in some trauma centers, but many argue that reliance on CT alone would result in a lower detection rate for certain types of intra-abdominal injuries or at least would significantly delay diagnosis and appropriate treatment.

DIAGNOSTIC PERITONEAL LAVAGE

Diagnostic peritoneal lavage is an excellent test for demonstrating the presence of intraperitoneal injury.[7, 8] Gomez and coworkers reported that DPL was 96.5% sensitive and 98.1% specific in their evaluation of patients with blunt abdominal trauma.[2] They also noted that DPL was 97.8% accurate in their review of the literature comprising 5000 patients with blunt abdominal trauma.

Criteria

The standard criteria for a positive lavage include the initial aspiration of gross blood or a lavage containing >100,000 RBC/mL or >500 WBC/mL; a lavage amylase of 175 units/dL; or the presence of bile or vegetable matter. Diagnostic peritoneal lavage is considered negative if the lavage fluid contains <50,000 RBC/mL or 100 WBC/mL or has an amylase activity of <75 IU/mL. Similarly, some clinicians have elected to lower their threshold for a positive tap, accepting a count of 50,000 RBC/mL, increasing the sensitivity of the test but yielding to a higher false-positive lavage rate.[9]

Limitations

There are some drawbacks to the use of DPL in blunt abdominal trauma. Standard lavage RBC and WBC counts have failed to identify a significant number of isolated hollow viscus injuries.[11] One reason may be that peritoneal leukocytosis does not usually occur until 3 hours have elapsed since injury, so that a DPL performed earlier may fail to show this abnormality.[9] Marx and colleagues, however, have found lavage alkaline phosphate to be useful in detecting small bowel injury.[10] Similarly, McAnena and coworkers studied lavage amylase elevation and found it to be highly specific for small bowel injury.[11]

If the catheter is inadvertently placed through a pelvic hematoma, DPL may be falsely positive because of diapedesis of blood across the parietal peritoneum, although no intraperitoneal injury exists. False-positive peritoneal lavage is expected to occur in 17 to 50% percent of patients with severe pelvic fractures. In fact, 60% percent of all false-positive DPL results have been noted in patients with pelvic fractures.[13]

A further limitation to the use of DPL is its unreliability in assessing injury to retroperitoneal organs such as ureters, bladder, and kidneys unless significant diapedesis of RBCs has taken place across the peritoneal membrane.[13] Diaphragmatic injuries are also not reliably detected.

Nevertheless, DPL is exceptionally accurate in detecting or excluding intraperitoneal hemorrhage.[4, 5, 10] In addition, its ability to measure the leukocytic and enzymatic response to trauma makes it a valuable adjunct in the diagnosis of intraperitoneal hollow viscus injury. Diagnostic peritoneal lavage is so sensitive in detecting small amounts of blood that it can lead to unnecessary surgery or laparotomy in as many as 25% of patients in whom DPL is the sole diagnostic intervention.[11, 12] At laparotomy, these patients are usually found to have self-limited injury to the liver and spleen, which in retrospect could have been managed nonoperatively. Nontherapeutic laparotomy negatively influences outcome by increasing the frequency and severity of pulmonary complications.[13, 14] The risk of postlaparotomy bowel obstruction is also a real one.[15]

Diagnostic peritoneal lavage is less specific for diaphragmatic injury as well. The diaphragm tends to bleed minimally when injured. If diaphragmatic injury is suspected, the criteron for a positive lavage should be as low as 5000 RBC/mL to maximize detection. Another disadvantage of DPL relative to CT is its inability to visualize the retroperitoneal organs and evaluate their integrity.

CT SCANNING

Computed tomography scanning is the noninvasive counterpart of DPL in the evaluation of blunt abdominal trauma. Unlike DPL, CT can provide visual localization of the injury and give an indication of the severity of injury. For example, the sensitivity and specificity of CT in diagnosing splenic trauma exceeds 95%.[16] Computed tomography may allow patients to avoid unnecessary laparotomy for some splenic injuries that do not require operative intervention.

Generally, for abdominal scanning a 50-mL bolus of full-strength diatrizoate sodium (Renografin-76) is administered intravenously just before the scan is begun. Administration of intravenous contrast medium improves the distinction between viscera and blood or hematoma and allows a better evaluation of the urinary system. Gastrointestinal contrast medium is a dilute solution (1 to 2%) of diatrizoate meglumine (Gastrografin), which is instilled through a nasogastric tube after the stomach has been evacuated—300 to 500 mL administered 30 to 45 minutes before scanning. The volume and timing of administration allow opacification of the duodenum and proximal small bowel as well as the stomach. This effect facilitates differentiation of these opacified organs from hematoma and solid viscera, especially pancreas and spleen. The nasogastric tube should be withdrawn into the esophagus before scanning begins to avoid producing artifact due to radiopaque markings on its side.[17]

Abdominal scanning is helpful in establishing the presence of hemoperitoneum and in estimating the amount of blood present. The pelvis is the most dependent part of the peritoneal cavity, and blood tends to collect there whether an individual is supine or upright. Blood is found in Morrison's pouch in up to 97% of patients with hepatic or splenic injury.[16]

Limitations

Like DPL, CT scanning has certain limitations. The use of contrast material is not without hazard. Allergic reactions as well as aspiration of contrast material have occurred.[18] In addition, failure to wait the necessary 2 hours for the contrast material to adequately opacify the small intestine may result in scans that do not detect hollow viscus injuries.[19, 20]

Patient movement may also be a limiting factor because a patient may be required to be stationary for more than 1 hour.[21, 22] Thus, sedation or paralysis using drugs may be necessary for the patient who is combative (eg, because of head trauma, alcohol, or drugs) with all the attendant risks of these drugs.[21]

Another drawback is the necessity to move the patient from the emergency department to obtain the scan, a distinct risk in the potentially unstable patient.[18, 22, 23] Computed tomography takes significantly longer to perform than DPL, making the patient's absence much more worrisome. Thus, a significant part of the ''golden hour of resuscitation may be used in obtaining a CT scan.''[23]

The interpretation of CT scans is dependent on the level of expertise of the reviewer, and in many hospitals radiologists trained to interpret trauma CT scans are not available on a 24-hour basis. Frame and coworkers[21] and Fabian and coworkers[24] found that the sensitivity of CT scanning for abdominal injury increased from 20 to 40% and from 60 to 85% respectively, when scans were reviewed blindly by ''experienced tomographers.''

COMPUTED TOMOGRAPHY VS DIAGNOSTIC PERITONEAL LAVAGE

Direct visualization of the abdominal contents is considered the standard in determining the presence of intraabdominal injury. It exposes the patient to more potential for morbidity and mortality.[25, 26]

There is little disagreement regarding the diagnostic superiority of CT over DPL in detecting certain injuries, notably those involving the retroperitoneal organs, exclusive of the pancreas and duodenum. In contrast, DPL can assess reliably only the intraperitoneal organs. Of the studies that champion the use of CT over DPL in the evaluation of blunt abdominal trauma, none have used laparotomy to verify CT scan results. Peitzman and coworkers[27] found CT scanning to be 97.6% sensitive, 98.7% specific, and 98.3% accurate in 120 patients who had sustained blunt abdominal trauma. However, of the 42 patients who were found to have intraabdominal injury by CT, only one third underwent laparotomy to confirm CT findings. Similarly, the validity of a negative CT scan was never verified.

In contrast, studies that assert the superiority of DPL over CT have verified the findings by laparotomy. Fabian and associates used both modalities to evaluate 91 patients who had stable vital signs and equivocal abdominal examination findings after sustaining blunt abdominal trauma.[24] In this group, CT was found to be 60% sensitive, 100% specific, and 90% accurate, whereas DPL was found to be 90% sensitive, 100% specific, and 98% accurate. Seven patients with negative CTs but positive DPLs were found upon laparotomy to have four splenic injuries and two hepatic injuries. One ileal injury was missed.

In another prospective study comparing DPL with CT, Frame and coworkers examined 54 patients who had sustained blunt abdominal trauma.[21] Diagnostic peritoneal lavage was positive in all patients with intraabdominal injury, whereas a CT failed to detect six splenic lacerations and three hepatic lacerations. The sensitivity of DPL was 100%, the specificity 92.3%, and the accuracy 92.4%. For CT, the sensitivity was 20%, the specificity 100%, and the accuracy 97.8%. A weakness of this study, however, is that CT interpretations were performed by senior surgical and radiology residents and trauma fellows.

Meyer and coworkers used DPL and CT in a prospective study that examined 301 blunt abdominal trauma patients.[28] In this study, the specificity of both DPL and CT scans was >99%. Diagnostic peritoneal lavage had a sensitivity of 95.9 vs 74.3% for CT in 19 patients with injuries identified at laparotomy. The initial CT scan was falsely negative. Missed were seven splenic lacerations, three liver injuries, three mesenteric injuries, three small bowel lacerations, and three colonic injuries.

Marx and colleagues evaluated 65 patients with blunt abdominal trauma.[22] Computed tomography failed to detect intraabdominal injury in three of the five patients explored. The three missed injuries included a bleeding liver laceration, a splenic laceration, and a partially avulsed gallbladder. Diagnostic peritoneal lavage had detected injury in all five. The sensitivity of the scan was 40% compared with 100% for DPL with the specificity for both being 99%. In this study, a staff radiologist performed the interpretations.

SUMMARY

Claims that CT should supplant DPL in the evaluation of blunt abdominal trauma appear to be premature. Studies that have compared DPL with CT and then proceeded to laparotomy for ultimate confirmation have consistently shown that DPL is more sensitive. Computed tomography often fails to detect significant intraabdominal injury. Diagnostic peritoneal lavage is safe, inexpensive, and accurate and should continue to be the primary diagnostic modality in the evaluation of blunt abdominal trauma. Computed tomography should be used selectively, particularly when retroperitoneal organ injury is suspected. CT should also be done in the hemodynamically stable patient in whom knowledge of the anatomic location of the injury is desired.

REFERENCES

1. Fifer T, Obeid F, Sorensen V, et al: Comparative accuracy of diagnostic peritoneal lavage, liver-spleen scintigraphy, and visceral angiography in blunt abdominal trauma. *Am Surg.* 1989;55:614.
2. Gomez G, Alvarez R, Plascenia G, et al: Diagnostic peritoneal lavage in the management of blunt abdominal trauma: Reassessment. *J Trauma.* 1987;27:1.
3. Olsen W, Redman H, Hildreth D: Abdominal paracentesis and peritoneal lavage in blunt abdominal trauma. *J Trauma.* 1971;11:824–829.
4. Bivins B, Sachatello C, Daugherty M, et al: Diagnostic peritoneal lavage is superior to the clinical evaluation in blunt abdominal trauma. *Am Surg.* 1978;44:637–641.
5. Engrav L, Benjamin C, Strate R, et al: Diagnostic peritoneal lavage in blunt abdominal trauma. *J Trauma.* 1975;15:854–859.
6. Perry J, Strate R: Diagnostic peritoneal lavage in blunt abdominal trauma: Indications and results. *Surgery.* 1972;71:898–901.
7. Smedira N, Schecter W: Blunt abdominal trauma, in Cales R, Keirnan G (eds): *Acute Abdominal Disorders. Emergency Medicine Clinics of North America.* Philadelphia: WB Saunders; 1989:631–641.
8. Fischer R, Beverlin B, Engrav L: Diagnostic peritoneal lavage—Fourteen years and 2,586 patients later. *Am J Surg.* 1978;136:701–704.
9. Root H, Keizer P, Perry J: The clinical and experimental aspects of peritoneal response to injury. *Arch Surg.* 1967;95:531.
10. Marx J, Bar-Or D, Moore E, et al: Utility of lavage alkaline phosphatase in detection of isolated small intestinal injury. *Ann Emerg Med.* 1985;14:49–53.
11. McAnena O, Marx J, Moore E: Contributions of peritoneal lavage enzyme determinations to the management of isolated hollow visceral abdominal injuries. *Ann Emerg Med.* 1991;20:834–837.
12. Pachter H, Hoffstetter S: Open and percutaneous paracentesis and lavage for abdominal trauma. *Arch Surg.* 1981;116:318–319.
13. Soderstrom C, Dupriest R: Pitfalls of peritoneal lavage in blunt abdominal trauma. *Surg Gynecol Obstet.* 1980;151:531–538.
14. Ang J, Hanslits M, Clark R, et al: Computed tomography of abdominal and pelvic trauma. *J Emerg Med.* 1985;3:312.
15. Bell C, Coleridge S: A comparison of diagnostic peritoneal lavage and computed tomography (CT scan) in evaluation of the hemodynamically stable patient with blunt abdominal trauma. *J Emerg Med.* 1992;10:275–280.
16. Federle M, Griffiths B, Minagi H, et al: Splenic trauma: Evaluation with CT. *Radiology.* 1987;162:69–71.
17. Federle M, Jeffrey R: Hemoperitoneum studied by computed tomography. *Radiology.* 1983;148:187–192.
18. Davis R, Shayne J, Max M, et al: The use of computerized axial tomography

versus peritoneal lavage in the evaluation of blunt abdominal trauma: a prospective study. *Surgery.* 1985;98:845–849.

19. Sherck J, Oakes D: Intestinal injuries missed by computed tomography. *J Trauma.* 1990;30:1–5.
20. Ceraldi C, Waxman K: Computerized tomography as an indicator of isolated mesenteric injury: A comparison with peritoneal lavage. *Am Surg.* 1990;56:806–810.
21. Frame S, Browder I, Lang E, et al: Computed tomography versus diagnostic peritoneal lavage: usefulness in immediate diagnosis of blunt abdominal trauma. *Ann Emerg Med.* 1989;18:513–516.
22. Marx J, Moore E, Jorden R, et al: Limitations of computed tomography in the evaluation of acute abdominal trauma: A prospective comparison with diagnostic peritoneal lavage. *J Trauma.* 1985;25:933–937.
23. Davis J, Hoyt D, Mackersie R, et al: Complication in evaluating abdominal trauma: Diagnostic peritoneal lavage versus computerized axial tomography. *J Trauma.* 1990;30:506–509.
24. Fabian T, Mangiante E, White T, et al: A prospective study of 91 patients undergoing both computed tomography and peritoneal lavage following blunt abdominal trauma. *J Trauma.* 1986;26:602–608.
25. Shah R, Max M, Flint L Jr: Negative laparotomy: Morbidity and mortality among 100 patients. *Am Surg.* 1978;44:150–154.
26. Petersen S, Sheldon G: Morbidity of a negative finding at laparotomy in abdominal trauma. *Surg Gynecol Obstet.* 1979;148:23–26.
27. Peitzman A, Makaroun M, Slasky B, et al: Prospective study of computed tomography in initial management of blunt abdominal trauma. *J Trauma.* 1986;26(7):585.
28. Meyer D, Thal E, Weigelt J, et al: Evaluation of computed tomography and diagnostic peritoneal lavage in blunt abdominal trauma. *J Trauma.* 1989;29:1168–1172.

Chapter

Traumatic Aortic Disruption and Aortic Dissection

Allan Doctor

TRAUMATIC AORTIC DISRUPTION

Principles of Investigation

Aortic injury secondary to blunt trauma is thought to be due to rapid deceleration, creating a shearing force that acts at the juncture of mobile and fixed segments of the vessel. These injuries tend to occur at the level of the ligamentum arteriosum, just distal to the origin of the subclavian artery (80%), at the supravalvular portion of the ascending aorta (15%), or at the origin of the great vessels.[1] Given the lethal nature of untreated aortic rupture, rapid diagnosis and treatment are imperative.

Plain Films

All patients sustaining trauma sufficient to cause damage to the thoracic aorta should have a plain film of the chest performed as soon as possible in resuscitation. The following plain film findings are suggestive of aortic injury (Table 24–1).

MEDIASTINAL WIDENING. Extravasation of blood from the vessel lumen initially accumulates adjacent to the descending aorta just inferior to the aortic knob either between the media and intima or between the aorta and parietal pleura. Hematoma formation in this area widens the mediastinal silhouette. This sign is particularly helpful if it is progressive over a short period of time.

Several investigators have formulated quantitative criteria to aid in the recognition of the wide mediastinum. Most believe that if the transverse width of the superior mediastinum is >8 cm it should be considered abnormal.[2] The mediastinal width to chest width (M/C) ratio is determined by dividing the largest width of the mediastinum at the level of the aortic arch by the internal diameter of the thorax at the same level. It was originally suggested that an M/C ratio >0.25 should identify 95% of ruptures with a 25% false-negative rate.[3] This level of reliability has not been borne out in subsequent studies. In fact, in 100 trauma patients without aortic injury, the mean M/C ratio was

TABLE 24–1. SENSITIVITY, SPECIFICITY, AND PREDICTIVE VALUES OF PLAIN FILM (SUPINE AP) FINDINGS INDICATIVE OF AORTIC RUPTURE (%)

	Sensitivity	Specificity	Positive Predictive Value	Negative Predictive Value
Abnormal aortic arch	81	37	22	90
Widened mediastinum[a]	67	45	21	86
Tracheal shift[b]	24	90	36	84
Depressed left main bronchus[c]	4	99	43	82
Left hemothorax	4	98	33	82
Nasogastric tube displaced to right	6	95	22	82
Left apical cap				
With rib fracture	1	95	5	81
Without rib fracture	14	95	39	83
Rib fracture (1–4)	18	84	20	82
Loss of descending contour	74	48	24	89
Negative				96

[a]Subjective impression.
[b]Left tracheal wall to right of the T4 transverse process.
[c]Depressed >40° below horizontal.
Adapted from Mirvis SE: Value of chest radiography in excluding traumatic aortic rupture. *Radiology.* 1987;163:487–493. By permission of the Radiological Society of North America.

demonstrated to be 0.30, and the criteron of an M/C ratio >0.25 resulted in an 87% false-positive rate.[4] Overall, subjective assessment of mediastinal widening appears to be superior to any specific measurements.[5, 6] This is probably due to physicians' noting other specific signs of mediastinal abnormality in addition to assessing mediastinal width.

The supine anteroposterior (AP) view of the chest results in 20% magnification when compared with the erect posteroanterior (PA) view.[6] Thus, a sitting inspiratory view should be obtained if possible. Mediastinal widening reflects hematoma formation regardless of its origin. Causes other than aortic disruption include small mediastinal, intercostal, or great vessel injury and fractures of the upper thoracic spine.

OBSCURED AORTIC KNOB AND AORTIC CONTOUR. The fluid density of a hematoma adjacent to the aortic knob and the descending aorta separates the normally contiguous lung parenchyma from the aortic margin, blurring its borders.

RIGHTWARD DEVIATION OF TRACHEA OR ESOPHAGUS, DEPRESSION OF THE LEFT MAINSTEM BRONCHUS. Even very small paraaortic hematomas will displace adjacent structures in the mediastinum. If a nasogastric tube is present, its displacement, or that of the trachea, to the right of the spinous process of T4 is a sensitive and relatively specific sign of aortic injury.[8] These findings are reliable only if the film is not rotated.

LEFT APICAL EXTRAPLEURAL CAP. There is a potential space between the aortic arch and the parietal pleura on the left into which extravasating blood may travel, producing a smooth thickening of the pleural shadow at the apex of the lung. This sign may be noted prior to widening of the mediastinum but may be present secondary to upper rib fractures or small vessel bleeding.

HEMOTHORAX. If the parietal pleura is disrupted during injury, mediastinal hemorrhage will not be contained and will travel to the pleural space. The presence of massive hemothorax, especially on the left, should thus suggest aortic injury.

FRACTURE OF THE FIRST OR SECOND RIB. Impact severe enough to fracture these ribs suggests a deceleration force sufficient to result in aortic disruption. The incidence of great vessel injury in one series of 121 patients with either first or second rib fractures was only 6.8%.[9]

Paradoxically, these signs are most useful in their absence. In one series the combination of the absence of nasogastric tube deviation, tracheal deviation, loss of aortic knob, and loss of contour of the descending aorta resulted in a 0% chance of aortic rupture.[7] In a larger study, discriminant analysis revealed the combination of a normal aortic arch and the absence of a tracheal shift to be 96% specific and to have a negative predictive value of 82%.[10]

The decision to pursue further evaluation should be based on bedside evaluation combined with knowledge of the mechanism of injury. Plain radiography findings are of limited value as predictors of aortic injury; only 10 to 30% of patients with a suggestive initial chest film and appropriate history are found to have aortic injury.[2, 5, 7, 18]

Special Investigations

Options for further evaluation include aortography, contrast-enhanced CT scanning, and transthoracic or transesophageal echocardiography. Aortography is generally considered to be the standard in the diagnosis of aortic injury. As the technical quality of CT scanning has improved, this means of investigation has become more attractive. Echocardiography has been principally studied in nontraumatic aortic dissection.

Concern about the accuracy of thoracic CT scanning in identifying traumatic aortic rupture stems from the fact that the laceration is often transversely oriented. Computed tomography can easily and reliably demonstrate a mediastinal hematoma or exclude its presence in cases in which plain films are equivocal.[11] In all clinical trials thus far, with a total of 356 patients studied, a completely normal CT scan accurately excluded the presence of aortic injury in all but one patient (a noncontrast study distorted by artifact), but false-positive studies occurred in approximately 30 to 50% of patients.[13–17]

Findings indicative of aortic disruption on contrast-enhanced CT scan include mediastinal hematoma contiguous with the aorta, false aneurysm, irregular aortic contour, divided aortic lumen, or intimal flap.[14] A CT scan of the chest should not be considered reliably negative unless all the signs mentioned previously are absent, good contrast enhancement of the aorta is observed, no interfering artifact is observed, and the films are read by an experienced CT radiologist.[17]

Most trauma centers accept negative aortography rates approaching 90% to exclude traumatic aortic disruption. Aortography often requires prolonged transport and study times and is rarely immediately available when required. Computed tomography is often used in the evaluation of other injuries in the victim of blunt trauma, and the addition of thoracic scanning to CT of the abdomen, pelvis, or head is suggested by its efficiency and lack of additional risk. The decision to exclude potential aortic or great vessel injury on the basis of plain films of the chest or chest CT should be tempered by clinical suspicion of injury and should be made in consultation with the radiologist and trauma surgeon. The decision to send a patient to aortography should be made after prioritizing investigations for other injuries and taking into account the likelihood of correctable intracranial injury, hemodynamic stability, potential abdominal or thoracic injury, and the surgeon's willingness to operate based only on plain film or CT findings.

DISSECTION OF THE THORACIC AORTA

Goals of Investigation

There are three categories of information to be obtained in patients with suspected aortic dissection: confirmation of dissection, ascertainment of ascending aortic involvement, and full demonstration of associated complications. A chest radiograph may lend support to the clinical suspicion of aortic dissection, but it cannot give a decisive answer. Special investigations that can provide some or all of the information include aortography, CT, and transthoracic or transesophageal echocardiography (Table 24–2). Because of the varying availability, time, and transportation required by the tests available, the stability of the patient often ultimately determines test selection (Table 24–3).

Information obtainable about an aortic dissection, aside from confirmation of the diagnosis, must be prioritized by its impact on therapeutic decision making. Classifying the *origin of the dissection* as ascending (DeBakey type 1 or 2 or Stanford type A) or descending (DeBakey type 3 or Stanford type B) places patients into surgical or initial medical management and is therefore the most important information to obtain.

An assessment of *left ventricular function* is a determinant of the outcome of both Stanford A and B dissections and will help guide both the cardiologist and the anesthesiologist in their care of the patient. In the presence of *aortic valve pathology* (eg, bicuspid valve and Marfan syndrome), valve replacement is indicated. If the valve is anatomically normal but made incompetent by the dissection, function can be restored during surgery. Quantification of the severity of regurgitation is of some importance to the anesthesiologist, but most work on the assumption that this risk is present in all cases of ascending dissection. Knowledge of the *sites of tears* and *extent of dissection* enables the surgeon to assess the complexity of the case and plan either reconstruction or graft replacement. Preoperative information about the distal anatomy and precise location of entry and exit sites is given variable importance in the surgical literature. The most crucial anatomic information to be obtained in investigating aortic dissection is involvement of the arch, thus classifying cases into Stanford types A or B. The *involvement of coronary arteries* in the dissection can be determined intraoperatively, and preoperative coronary angiography has been shown not to affect outcome. The *involvement of arch and branch vessels* also can be assessed intraoperatively, and preoperative knowledge in an emergency

TABLE 24–2. INFORMATION AVAILABLE AFTER INVESTIGATION OF SUSPECTED AORTIC DISSECTION

	Angiography	CT Scan	Standard Echo	Color Flow	TE Echo	Color Flow
Anatomic						
Origin of dissection	+	±	−	±	−	±
Aortic valve pathology	+	−	+		+	
Rupture into pericardium	−	+	+		+	
Involvement of arch vessels	+	−	−		−	
Entry/exit sites	+	±	−	±	−	±
Functional						
Aortic regurgitation	+	−	−	+	−	+
Tamponade	−	−	+		+	
Left ventricular function	±	−	+		+	

TABLE 24–3. LOGISTICAL CHARACTERISTICS OF SPECIAL INVESTIGATIONS FOR AORTIC DISSECTION

Angiography	*Disadvantages* Intravenous contrast required Prolonged mobilization of resources Transport of patient Invasive
Computed tomography	*Disadvantages* Intravenous contrast required Transport of patient *Advantages* Usually relatively accessible Once initiated, rapid test
Transthoracic echo	*Disadvantages* Requires in-house cardiologist/fellow Poor quality in obese or emphazematous patients *Advantages* Bedside test Once initiated, rapid test
Transesophageal echo	*Disadvantages* Requires in-house cardiologist/fellow May necessitate sedation or airway management Bronchospasm or AV block (rare) *Advantages* Bedside test Once initiated, rapid test

case is not necessary. The presence of tamponade indicates leakage and impending rupture and is crucial information in the patient who presents with shock.

Plain Films

As noted in the section on blunt injury to the thoracic aorta, a chest radiograph may lend support to clinical suspicion, but although abnormal in 80 to 90% of cases[19] it will seldom aid in decision making. In addition to the signs mentioned in the preceding section, the following signs may aid in the diagnosis of aortic dissection.

1. Change in configuration of the aorta on successive chest films: a

demonstrated short-term change in the aortic contour or width should prompt further investigation.[20]

2. Aortic wall thickening (displacement of intimal calcification): displacement of intimal calcification 6 mm or more from the outer margin of the aortic wall is suggestive of dissection.[20] Two caveats, however, should be borne in mind when looking for this sign. To be certain that the apparent position of an intimal plaque in relation to the outer aspect of the aorta is valid, one must determine that the plaque and the soft-tissue contour are indeed at the same level in the body: a lateral or oblique view may be necessary to confirm this relationship. Intimal calcification may appear displaced if any process causes mediastinal thickening or opacification of the adjacent lung.

Special Investigations

Arteriography

Arteriography has until recently been the investigation of choice. The basic angiographic signs of dissection include demonstration of a false lumen compressing the true lumen and visualization of the intimal flap. The main source of false-positive findings lies in the difficulty of discriminating between a nonfilled false lumen and other causes of a thickened aortic wall. False-negative examinations have been attributed to simultaneous opacification of both channels, projection so that the intimal flap is not tangent to the x-ray beam, and thrombosis of the false channel without compression of the true channel.[37]

The advantages of angiography lie in its potential to demonstrate entry, exit, and full extent of the dissection and any extension into branch vessels. Angiography also allows recognition of aortic incompetence and evaluation of left ventricular function. Its sensitivity has been reported to range from 91 to 100%, with specificities from 94 to 100%.[22, 29]

The preeminence of angiography as the standard of diagnosis has been challenged and, according to many, replaced by transesophageal echocardiography either alone or in combination with dynamic CT scanning.[29, 38] In skilled hands, despite its invasive nature, aortography can be performed with low morbidity and mortality. Of the tests discussed, however, it requires the most mobilization of skilled personnel and movement of the patient from the emergency department. Like CT, it also carries all the risks of intravenous contrast material use.

Computed Tomography

Computed tomography may establish the diagnosis of aortic dissection by demonstrating double channels with an intimal flap or may suggest the diagnosis by demonstrating displaced intimal calcification or a thickened wall if one channel is thrombosed.[23] Dynamic scanning following a bolus of contrast material can demonstrate the relative filling of the true and false channels and thereby increases the likelihood of visualization of the intimal flap.[24] Blood that has leaked into the mediastinum and the pleural or pericardial space can also be detected.[23] Computed tomography scans produced sensitivity ranges from 83 to 100% and specificities from 92 to 100%.[24–28, 37]

Unfortunately, CT scanning is unlikely to reveal information regarding the extent of dissection into branch vessels of the arch or the location of the exit or entry sites. On the one hand, although angiography can reveal this information, CT is much better in discriminating a nonfilling false lumen from wall thickening. On the other hand, CT provides no functional information regarding competence of the aortic valve, left ventricular function, or the presence of tamponade. Although usually logistically less difficult to perform and less invasive than aortography, intravenous contrast agent is used and movement from the emergency department is necessary.

Echocardiography

Transthoracic echocardiography (TTE) is a noninvasive study that can be performed at the bedside. Ultrasound waves are transmitted poorly through bone and air, however, and thus sonographic access to viscera bordering such tissue must be obtained via the "acoustic window" of a fluid-filled or solid organ. For this reason, even with the addition of nonstandard views, only the proximal 2 to 3 cm of the ascending aorta can be visualized by TTE.[21, 22] The descending aorta is not accessible to standard sonography until it enters the abdomen. Although it can provide important anatomic information in cases of proximal dissection regarding aortic valve pathology or rupture into the pericardium, and although it can also provide information regarding left ventricular function, tamponade, and aortic regurgitation (with the addition of Doppler color flow mapping),[30] only 70 to 80% of dissections are recognized using TTE. Moreover, Stanford type B or DeBakey type 2 dissections cannot be recognized.[21, 31] In several papers the sensitivity is reported to be between 70 and 100% and the specificity 90%.[21, 31, 32]

In contrast, transesophageal echocardiography (TEE) is performed with a miniaturized ultrasound transducer, which is placed through the mouth into the esophagus and positioned immediately posterior to the heart. Because the transducer is essentially in the mediastinum without any gas or bone intervening, the full extent of the intrathoracic aorta, its branches, and the heart can be displayed, substantially improving diagnostic accuracy. Entry and exits sites may be identified by recognition of high-velocity jets or turbulent flow with Doppler color flow mapping.[30, 33] Transesophageal scanning is reported to improve the sensitivity of echocardiography to 97 to 99% and the specificity to 98 to 100%.[22, 35]

Limitations of TEE include difficulty in distinguishing intimal thrombus from a thrombosed false channel and the frequent necessity of sedation and its potential hemodynamic and airway complications in an unstable patient. The transesophageal approach must also be used with caution in patients with underlying esophageal disorders. This approach may necessitate intubation in a patient with a tenuous airway. In addition, esophageal intubation with the ultrasound probe may dramatically increase vagal tone (in about 1% of patients), resulting in bronchospasm or transient AV block.[34]

The price of a delayed diagnosis in patients who suffer from aortic dissection is remarkably high. The mortality rate during the first 48 hours of symptoms for patients with unrecognized or untreated Stanford A aortic dissection has been estimated to be 1% per hour.[36] Its most dire consequences—aortic rupture, pericardial tamponade, coronary dissection, and acute aortic regurgitation—are all potentially correctable surgically. Successful intervention, however, is dependent on rapid discrimination between Stanford A and B dissections, location of the communications between the two channels; extent of dissection; and for type A, degree of aortic valve incompetence and leak into the pericardium. Although angiography has been generally accepted as the reference standard in the investigation of aortic dissection, it is gradually being supplanted by newer-generation dynamic CT scanners and TEE with color flow mapping.

REFERENCES

1. Marnocha KE, Maglinte DD: Plain film criteria for excluding aortic rupture in blunt chest trauma. *AJR.* 1985;144:19–21.
2. Marsh DG, Sturm JT: Traumatic aortic rupture: Roentgenographic indications for aortography. *Ann Thoracic Surg.* 1976;21:337–340.
3. Seltzer SE, D'Orsi C, Kirshner R, et al: Traumatic aortic rupture: Plain radiographic findings. *AJR.* 1981;137:1011–1014.
4. Woodring JH, King JG: Determination of normal transverse mediastinal width and mediastinal width to chest width (M/C) ratio in control subjects: Implications for subjects with aortic or brachiocephalic arterial injury. *J Trauma.* 1989;29:1268–1272.
5. Gundry SR, Williams S, Burney RE, et al: Indications for aortography-radiography after blunt chest trauma: A reassessment of the radiographic findings associated with traumatic rupture of the aorta. *Surg Gynecol Obstet.* 1970;131:900–904.
6. Schrob CW, Lawson RB, et al: Aortic injury: Comparison of supine and

upright portable chest films to evaluate the widened mediastinum. *Ann Emerg Med.* 1984;13:896–899.
7. Marhocha KE: Blunt chest trauma and suspected aortic rupture: Reliability of chest radiographic findings. *Ann Emerg Med.* 1985;14:644–649.
8. Tisnado J, et al: A new radiographic sign of acute traumatic rupture of the aorta: Displacement of the NG tube to the right. *Radiology.* 1977;125:603–608.
9. Woodring JH: Fractures of first and second ribs: Predictive value for arterial and bronchial injury. *AJR.* 1982:138;211–215.
10. Mirvis SE: Value of chest radiography in excluding traumatic aortic rupture. *Radiology.* 1987;163:487–493.
11. Heiberg E: CT in aortic trauma. *AJR.* 1983;140:1119–1124.
12. Mirvis SE: Role of CT in excluding major arterial injury after blunt thoracic trauma. *AJR.* 1987;149:601–605.
13. Miller FB, Richardson JD: Role of CT in diagnosis of major arterial injury after blunt thoracic trauma. *Surgery.* 1989;106:596.
14. Egan TJ, Neiman HL, et al: CT in the diagnosis of aortic aneurysm, dissection, or traumatic injury. *Radiology.* 1980;136:141.
15. Ishikaura T, Nakajima Y: The role of CT in traumatic rupture of the thoracic aorta and its proximal branches. *Semin Roentgenol.* 1989;24:38.
16. Fenner MN, Fisher KS, Sergel NL: Evaluation of possible traumatic thoracic injury using aortography and CT. *Am Surg.* 1990;56:497.
17. Agee CK, Metzler MH, Curlhill RJ, et al: CT evaluation to exclude aortic disruption. *J Trauma.* 1992;33:876–881.
18. Kram HB, Appel PL, et al: Diagnosis of traumatic aortic rupture: A 10 year retrospective analysis. *Ann Thorac. Surg.* 1989;47:282.
19. Slater EE, DeSanctis RW: The clinical recognition of dissecting aortic aneurysm. *Am J Med.* 1976;60:625–633.
20. DeScaanctis RW, Eagle KA: Aortic dissection. *Curr Prob Cardiol.* May 1989:231–278.
21. Victor MF: Two-dimensional echocardiographic diagnosis of aortic dissection. *Am J Cardiol.* 1981;48:1155–1163.
22. Erbel R, Daniel W, Visser C, et al: Echocardiography in the diagnosis of aortic dissection. *Lancet.* 1989;1:457–461.
23. Heiberg E, Wolverson M, Sundaram M, et al: CT findings in thoracic aortic dissection. *AJR.* 1981;136:13–17.
24. Godwin JD, Herfkens CG, Federle MP: Evaluation of dissection and aneurysms of the thoracic aorta by conventional and dynamic CT scan. *Radiology.* 1980;136:125–133.
25. Gussenhoven RJ, Taams MA, Roelandt, et al: Transesophageal two-dimensional echocardiography; Its role in solving clinical problems. *J Am Coll Cardiol.* 1986;8:975–979.
26. Thorsen MK, San Dretto MA, Lawson TL, et al: Dissecting aortic aneurysms: Accuracy of computed tomographic diagnosis. *Radiology.* 1983;148:773–778.
27. Moncada R, Salinas M, Curchill R, et al: Diagnosis of dissecting aortic aneurysms by CT. *Lancet.* 1981;136:13–17.
28. Larde D, Bellor C, Vasile N, et al: CT in dissection of the thoracic aorta. *Radiology.* 1980;136:147–151.

29. Treasure T, Raphael MJ: Investigation of suspected dissection of the thoracic aorta. *Lancet.* 1991;338:490–495.
30. Ilicetos S, Nanda NC, Rizzon P, et al: Color Doppler evaluation of aortic dissection. *Circulation.* 1987;75:748–755.
31. Khandheria BK, Tajik AJ, Taylor CL, et al: Aortic dissection: A review of the value and limitations of two-dimensional echocardiography in a six year experience. *J Am Soc Echo.* 1989;2:17–24.
32. Granato JE, Dee P, Gibson RS: Utility of two-dimensional echocardiography in suspected aortic dissection. *Am J Cardiol.* 1985;56:123–129.
33. Hashimoto S, Kumada T, Osakada G, et al: Assessment of transesophageal Doppler echocardiography in dissecting aortic aneurysms. *J Am Coll Cardiol.* 1989;14:1253–1262.
34. Erbel R, Borner N, Stelly D, et al: Detection of aortic dissection by transesophageal echocardiography. *Br Heart J.* 1987;58:45–51.
35. Ballal RS, Nanda NC, Gatewood R, et al: Usefullness of transesophageal echocardiography in assessment of aortic dissection. *Circulation.* 1991;84:1903–1914.
36. Jamieson WR, Munro AI, Miyagishima R, et al: Aortic dissection: Early detection and surgical management. *Can J Surg.* 1982;25:145–149.
37. St. Amour TE, Gutierrez FR, Levitt RG, et al: Diagnosis of type A aortic dissection not demonstrated by angiography. *J Comput Assist Tomog.* 1988;12:963–967.
38. Kotler MN: Is transesophageal echocardiography the new standard for diagnosis for dissecting aortic aneurysms? *J Am Coll Cardiol.* 1989;14:1263–1265.

Chapter

Trauma

David Ellis

Rapid and accurate clinical decisions are imperative in the emergency department (ED) trauma patient. The decision to perform diagnostic tests on trauma patients, however, must take into account the prevalence of the abnormalities being sought and the positive and negative predictive value of the tests ordered in the population being tested. This chapter discusses the rationale that guides diagnostic testing in the trauma patient and the use of the clinical laboratory in the initial evaluation of trauma.

In general terms, traumatic injuries occur by the transfer of energy to the victim. The spectrum of possible injuries reflects the amount, type, and direction of that energy transfer.[1] Diagnostic testing appropriate for the identification, treatment, and management of these injuries should be guided by the history, physical examination, and known injury patterns.

The effective use of time and the team approach have been shown to be essential to the effective management of major trauma. Certain test results (eg, arterial blood gases, urine testing for blood or pregnancy, x-rays) may have important implications for immediate management and should be obtained as quickly as possible, when indicated. Other tests (eg, hematocrit, white blood cell count) reflect premorbid conditions in most cases but may be useful as baselines for the evaluation of future changes.

TO PROTOCOL OR NOT TO PROTOCOL?

Protocols have been developed that designate certain members of the trauma team to obtain and label samples, order diagnostic tests, deliver the samples to the laboratory, and have those results returned to the team in a timely fashion. Drawing samples and ordering diagnostic laboratory tests and radiographs by protocol have several advantages and disadvantages.

Using a protocol ensures that complete information is available as quickly as possible and, most importantly, that it will be available at the time critical management decisions must be made. For example, the indications for blood transfusion or surgery may not be readily apparent on presentation, but when those indications become apparent the steps necessary to administer type-specific blood products or to proceed with anesthesia and surgery must be taken rapidly. Protocols minimize the time required for team members to order specific tests and the wait for test results during the critical initial periods. Furthermore, they also minimize the potential for human error in the omission of tests that might be crucial to management decisions.

On the negative side, ordering by protocol cannot be allowed to take the place of adequate history and physical examination and critical thinking in the clinical setting. Overapplication of protocols can lead not only to unnecessary testing and increased health care costs but also to increased patient morbidity.[2] For example, screening examinations should not be applied in clinical situations in which the likelihood of disease is so low and the test sufficiently nonspecific that testing yields an inappropriate number of false-positive results. This is true, for example, in the utilization of nonspecific tests for cardiac contusion, in which a positive test can lead to unnecessary cardiac monitoring and misappropriation of often limited hospital resources.[3]

Moreover, protocols intended for the victim of major trauma should not be automatically extended to patients who are less severely injured or to those with isolated or limited trauma unless the initial evaluation results in the identification of the potential for more severe injuries. Tests should thus be utilized selectively for the assessment of the specific areas injured. In any case, **necessary interventions in major trauma should not be delayed if the results of diagnostic tests are not available**.[4]

LABORATORY TESTING

A protocol to guide diagnostic laboratory testing in the trauma patient is proposed here. This proposal reflects a stratified approach to the diagnostic workup based on the findings from the history and physical examination and testing protocols currently in use at trauma centers.[1, 4]

Initial Presentation, Admission Uncertain, or Isolated Trauma

Samples Are Obtained but Not Sent Automatically

Blood samples should be obtained at the time intravenous access is established in the ED or prehospital setting or by arterial or venous puncture of the femoral vessels. Nursing and prehospital protocols (eg, three or four red tops, purple top, and blue top) that encourage personnel to obtain blood specimens routinely at initial presentation, but to not automatically send them to the laboratory, effectively help anticipate any testing needs that might arise. Following this practice, the group of patients that eventually does have tests ordered will have a prevalence of injury high enough to justify screening laboratory tests and will minimize false-positive results. In the pediatric patient, special consideration should be given to the use of microtechniques for blood sampling to reduce the amount of blood loss.[5]

Baseline Admission Testing for the Trauma Patient

Complete Blood Count, Electrolytes, Blood Urea Nitrogen, Creatinine, Liver Function Tests, Urinalysis, Pregnancy Testing, Pulse Oximetry

The goal of this level of testing is to provide a baseline assessment of function of the hepatic, pulmonary, hematologic, and urinary systems and in particular to assess the patient's premorbid condition. Although a rationale for obtaining each of these tests can be provided, the yield of these studies and their actual utility in patient management have not yet been systematically evaluated. Studies of injured children and adults have documented a very low yield and utility of a battery of routine tests.[6–8]

The initial *hematocrit* reflects the patient's premorbid condition. It can be expected to fall approximately three points for every unit of blood lost, but this change may not occur for several hours without exogenous fluid replacement. With rapid fluid administration the hematocrit falls quickly. Serial determinations are helpful in monitoring for occult blood loss.

The *white blood cell count* is used as an initial baseline study. Serial determinations (and particularly the appearance of a "shift to the left" or an increase in the number of neutrophils) provide an early clue to infection or an inflammatory response to injury (eg, bowel perforation).

Determinations of *serum electrolytes, BUN, serum creatinine, and glucose* are performed to assess metabolic status and renal function. Unavailability of test results should not delay any necessary diagnostic radiographic studies that require the use of contrast material and should not delay emergency surgery.

Liver function tests are commonly ordered in the admitted trauma patient. Although elevations in enzyme activity may indicate hepatic injury, a lack of elevation does not rule out significant injury. Studies have reported a correlation between hepatic enzyme elevation and injury, but the actual utility of these tests in the trauma patient has not been demonstrated.[9]

The *urine* should be tested with reagent strips, primarily to detect hematuria but also to assess for glycosuria and other abnormalities. Gross hematuria or significant microscopic hematuria in patients with blunt trauma should prompt further radiographic evaluation for renovascular, renal parenchymal, ureteral, or bladder injuries.[10–12] In cases of penetrating trauma or significant acceleration-deceleration forces, or if clinical parameters suggest urinary tract injury,[13] these studies should be performed regardless of the presence or degree of hematuria. If there is a positive dipstick test result for blood or no evidence of red blood cells, the urine can be tested for myoglobin and the serum tested for total creatine kinase, if indicated.

A *urine pregnancy test* should be performed in female trauma patients of childbearing potential. This may minimize the risk of fetal radiation exposure or the administration of potentially fetotoxic medications.

Pulse oximetry is in most cases an adequate measure of oxygenation and can detect rapid decreases in peripheral perfusion and oxygenation. Pulse oximetry may allow the trauma team to avoid arterial blood gas analysis in up to half the cases in which it previously would have been performed, avoiding the associated cost and invasiveness as well as the risks to hospital personnel of needlestick injury.[14]

Testing of the Severely Injured Patient and in Preparation for Surgery

Admission Testing plus Arterial Blood Gases, Electrocardiogram, Coagulation Studies, Blood Bank Specimen, Toxicology Screen

Arterial blood gases reflect important changes in oxygenation, ventilation, and acid-base status. As with the physical examination and other diagnostic tests, serial determinations may be necessary to determine the significance of the results. Roux and associates have advised that in the trauma patient less than 60 years of age, screening of arterial blood gases alone deserves to be a part of routine preoperative laboratory assessment.[15]

Although no data are available on the utility of a routine *electrocardiogram* (ECG) in the trauma patient, it is generally considered a standard of care.

Coagulation studies (prothrombin and partial thromboplastin time) are ordered to detect premorbid abnormalities in the clotting mechanism. It may be necessary to follow these studies with a determination of the bleeding time if concerns are identified. Several studies have shown that the likelihood of significant hemorrhage due to a coagulation disorder is extremely low in adults who have no history or clinical evidence of an increased bleeding risk. Screening for coagulation disorders results in an unacceptable proportion of false-positive results.[16]

In providing a *blood bank specimen*, a ''type-and-screen'' may be chosen over a ''type-and-cross'' when transfusion is not immediately indicated, given its lower cost, its conservation of blood units, and its ability to be rapidly converted to a type-and-cross.[17, 18] O-negative blood (for women) and type-specific uncrossmatched blood must be available in any case for initial transfusions, along with predetermined procedures for rapid delivery of blood from the blood bank to the ED or resuscitation area.[19, 20]

In patients with an altered level of consciousness or a clinical toxidrome, *toxicology screening* can help to identify alcohol and other drugs of abuse that may have contributed to the clinical picture or injury pattern. Toxicology testing may be considered part of the admission screen when mechanisms are in place to counsel or intervene based on the findings of the testing. One should nonetheless keep in mind the limitations of toxicology screening in individuals with significant chronic substance abuse. For example, chronic alcoholics may not show positive blood ethanol levels at ED presentation.[21] The basic ED toxicology screen in trauma patients must at least include determination of serum ethanol level, screening for barbiturates and benzodiazepines, and urine testing for cocaine and amphetamines.

Other Issues

One investigation of *serum amylase determinations* in blunt trauma patients has shown serum amylase to be a very poor predictor of pancreatic or hollow viscus injury, greatly limiting its utility as a screening test.[22]

Through extensive investigation of the natural history of myocardial contusion, it has become evident that the majority of putative cases are clinically benign and that the best predictors of a need for monitoring or treatment are initial ECG abnormalities and shock.[23, 24] This extremely low prevalence of clinically significant injuries means that *cardiac enzymes* have very poor positive and negative predictive values and are thus of little utility as a screening test in trauma.

SUMMARY

Whether a selective approach to diagnostic testing in the trauma patient proves to be of benefit depends on critical evaluations of cost, relative utilization, and effectiveness. The ultimate challenge for emergency medicine and for emergency physicians practicing and teaching in trauma centers is to influence the design of the trauma evaluation process and the practice of their surgical colleagues in the direction of critically evaluated protocols and cost-effective approaches.

REFERENCES

1. McCabe CJ: Early management of visceral nervous system and musculoskeletal injuries, in Burke JF, Boyd RJ (eds): Trauma Management. Chicago: Year Book Medical Publishers; 1988.
2. Kaplan C: Use of the laboratory, in Walker H, Hall WD, Hurst JW (eds): *Clinical Methods: History, Physical, and Laboratory Examinations*, Boston: Butterworths; 1990:40–48.
3. Cachecho R, et al: The clinical significance of myocardial contusion. *J Trauma*. 1992;33:68.
4. Kreis DJ, Gomez GA: *Trauma Management*. Boston: Little, Brown; 1989.
5. Marcus RE (ed): *Trauma in Children*. Rockville, MD: Aspen; 1986.

6. Bryant MS, Tepas JJ, Talbert JL, et al: Impact of emergency room laboratory studies on the ultimate triage and disposition of injured child. *Am Surg.* 1988;54:209.
7. Isaacman DJ, Scarfone RJ, Kost SL, et al: Utility of routine laboratory testing for detecting intra-abdominal injury in the pediatric trauma patient. *Pediatrics.* 1993;92:691.
8. Donaldson VP, Wolfson AB, Heil B: unpublished data.
9. Hennes HM, et al: Elevated liver transaminase levels in children with blunt trauma: A predictor of liver injury. *Pediatrics.* 1990;86:87.
10. Hoffman JR, et al: Use of intravenous pyelography in blunt trauma: A reappraisal. *West J Med.* 1987;146:576.
11. Knudson MM, et al: Hematuria as a predictor of abdominal injury after blunt trauma. *Am J Surg.* 1992;164:482.
12. Fortune JB, et al: Emergency intravenous pyelography in the trauma patient: A reexamination of the indications. *Arch Surg.* 1985;120:1056.
13. Wong L, et al: The role of the IVP in blunt trauma. *J Trauma.* 1988;28:502.
14. Lambert MA, et al: The role of pulse oximetry in the accident and emergency department. *Arch Emerg Med.* 1989;6:211.
15. Roux A, et al: Contribution of preoperative investigations to the anesthetic management of adult trauma patients. *Injury.* 1993;24:17.
16. Suchman AL, et al: Diagnostic uses of the activated thromboplastin time and prothrombin time. *Ann Intern Med.* 1986;104:810.
17. West HC, et al: Immediate prediction of blood requirements in trauma victims. *South Med J.* 1989;82:186.
18. Hooker EA, Miller FB, Hollander JL, et al: Do all trauma patients need early crossmatching for blood? *J Emerg Med.* 1994;12:447.
19. Gervin AS, et al: Resuscitation of trauma patients with type-specific uncrossmatched blood. *J Trauma.* 1984;24:327.
20. Schwab CW, et al: Immediate trauma resuscitation with type O uncrossmatched blood: A two-year prospective experience. *J Trauma.* 1986;26:897.
21. Jurkovich GJ, et al: The effect of acute alcohol intoxication and chronic alcohol abuse on outcome from trauma. *JAMA.* 1993;271:51.
22. Boulanger BR, et al: The clinical significance of acute hyperamylasemia after blunt trauma. *Can J Surg.* 1993;36:63.
23. Miller FB, et al: Myocardial contusion: When can the diagnosis be eliminated? *Arch Surg.* 1989;124:805.
24. McLean RF, et al: Significance of myocardial contusion following blunt chest trauma. *J Trauma.* 1992;33:240.

Chapter

Soft Tissue Infection

Loren Rood

Diagnostic adjuncts for soft tissue infections range from the nonspecific (complete blood count, CBC; erythrocyte sedimentation rate, ESR) to the highly specific (culture and sensitivity, C&S; serology). The value of many of these tests in influencing management is questionable. Even the yield of useful information from the more invasive and specific tests has rarely been addressed in the literature. This chapter reviews the value of several frequently ordered diagnostic adjuncts in the setting of acute soft tissue infections.

WHITE BLOOD CELL COUNT AND TEMPERATURE TO PREDICT BACTEREMIA

Of bacteremic children (age <2 years), 5% will develop invasive infection (meningitis, cellulitis). The white blood cell (WBC) count is frequently used to evaluate for possible bacteremia and sometimes influences therapy. Unfortunately, an elevated WBC count has not been found to correlate with the extent of disease.[1] Bonadio and coworkers reported a 69% sensitivity for WBC >15,000/mm^3 as predictive for "serious bacterial infection."[2] Fleisher and coworkers, in a prospective study of 50 patients with cellulitis (median age of 5 years), found only 12% with a WBC count >15,000.[3] Of those patients, 83% had a fever >38.5°C. There was poor correlation between fever and leukocytosis. When both were present, however, the likelihood of blood cultures yielding *Streptococcus pneumoniae* or *Haemophilus influenzae* increased significantly.

In a retrospective review of 20 patients with cellulitis ages 13 months to 83 years, Goldgeier found that 40% had a WBC count greater than 15,000 and 65% (13/20) had a temperature >38.5°C.[4] No correlation was found between leukocytosis and fever, however. Only 2 of 20 patients had positive blood cultures. Both were febrile, one had a markedly elevated leukocyte count, and the other was on immunosuppressive therapy and leukopenic.

In a prospective study of 50 patients, Hook and colleagues found 6% had leukocytosis and 26% were febrile.[5] Neither of these factors was predictive of later positive cultures (blood, needle aspirate, punch biopsy). A prospective analysis by Sachs also determined that temperature and WBC count are not predictive of positive needle aspirate cultures in patients with cellulitis.[6]

These studies reflect that both fever and leukocytosis do not correlate well with severity of illness from cellulitis. A reasonable approach to utilizing the WBC count in patients with cellulitis would seem to be based on the presence or absence of fever. The data from these studies reveal a lack of consistency in WBC count or fever in patients with cellulitis (Table 26–1).

In a correspondence pertaining to febrile children without a source of infection, Cox and associates cited several studies using WBC count >15,000 to determine bacteremia and reported a sensitivity of 65% and specificity of 72%.[7]

Previous studies in pediatric patients presenting with fever (various etiologies including fever of unknown origin) have revealed evidence of increasing risk of bacteremia with increasing temperature.[8] As indicated, these patients had various sources for their fevers; thus, these data cannot be directly correlated with patients having cellulitis.

Waskerwitz and Berkelhamer studied outpatient bacteremia in children <2 years old with temperature >39.5°C.[9] They found that the physician's assessment was the most useful factor for predicting bacteremia, with the WBC count (positive predictive value 5%, sensitivity 36%) the least useful. They concluded that the WBC count and blood C&S were not essential for effective diagnosis and treatment.

Liu and coworkers evaluated febrile (various etiologies) children for bacteremia.[10] Their findings revealed that a WBC count >15,000 had a positive predictive value of 12%, sensitivity 59%, and specificity 63%.

Unfortunately, no studies could be found specifically evaluating the WBC count and bacteremia in patients with cellulitis. In an isolated patient presenting to an emergency department with cellulitis, however, the literature would appear to support that clinical evidence of toxicity should be the primary criteria for determining aggressiveness of therapy. The literature does not support basing this decision on nonspecific indicators such as WBC count and temperature. In addition, these

TABLE 26–1. LEUKOCYTOSIS IN CELLULITIS

	WBC >15,000 (%)	Temp >38°C (%)	N
Fleisher et al, 1980	12	18	50
Goldgeier, 1983	40	65	20
Hook et al, 1986	6	26	50

parameters do not provide any information as to the bacteriologic etiology of cellulitis.

ERYTHROCYTE SEDIMENTATION RATE

Wyler reviewed 200 patients with ESR >100 and found that infectious etiologies (various sources) accounted for 35% of all cases.[11] Noninfectious inflammatory processes (collagen vascular diseases, arthritides, hypersensitivity reactions, acute myocardial infarction) composed 22% of the study group. Wyler noted that ESR >100 did not have diagnostic specificity.

Hook and coworkers, in the study previously discussed, also looked at the ESR of their patients in relation to fever, leukocytosis, and positive cultures.[5] Of 44 patients with this test performed, 59% had a value of >25 mm/h. As with fever and WBC count, however, an elevated ESR was not predictive of positive culture findings. No other study has critically evaluated the use of the ESR in cellulitis.

This test is frequently used to follow therapy in patients with rheumatologic diseases, osteomyelitis, and septic arthritis. It is often ordered initially in evaluation of patients until these are ruled out by other means (eg, bone scan, MRI). There have not been any definitive studies addressing the ESR in patients with cellulitis. Because of the nonspecific nature of this test, its diagnostic value in cellulitis in probably nil.

BLOOD CULTURES

Multiple investigators have studied the yield of positive blood cultures in cellulitis. Fleisher and coworkers demonstrated 8% positive cultures in their study of 50 patients.[3] There was no comment on whether a positive culture finding altered initial therapy. Among those with isolated extremity involvement, there was only one positive blood culture from the group.

Ginsberg reviewed 101 patients retrospectively.[12] Although the population was somewhat skewed with 18% intravenous (IV) drug abusers, there were no positive cultures of the 27 performed.

The series reviewed by Goldgeier revealed that 18% of the blood cultures were positive (the highest percentage found in the literature for patients with cellulitis).[4] This was a small series, and one of the three positive cultures was believed to be a contaminant.

In another retrospective review of 66 patients with cellulitis, only one blood culture was positive of the 130 performed.[13] The conclusion was that, in afebrile, otherwise healthy adults, blood cultures do not provide information useful in the management of cellulitis.

The aforementioned results are in "all comer" series including all sites of cellulitis. If one specifically studies facial cellulitis in children, a significantly greater yield is noted in cultures. In 1974, Goetz and investigators reported a 100% positive yield of blood cultures in three patients with *H. influenzae* facial cellulitis.[14] In their review of the literature, they found a 79% positive yield of blood cultures in children with this disease. Table 26–2 is adapted from this review article.

Rudoy and Nakashima retrospectively reviewed 78 pediatric patients with *H. influenzae* cellulitis of the extremities and found only a 5% rate of positive blood cultures.[15] It was not noted whether any other organisms were cultured.

Carroll and associates performed a randomized prospective study of outpatient treatment of occult bacteremia.[16] Febrile children less than 24 months old received a full septic-type workup. They were then randomized for empiric outpatient antibiotic therapy or observation. Of the treated patients with positive blood cultures, 80% improved clinically and did not require alteration of therapy. Although this type of study cannot be directly extrapolated to patients with cellulitis, it is apparent that empiric treatment for the most common pathogen will often suffice, and blood cultures will not alter therapy.

Pediatric patients with facial cellulitis typically are more toxic and have a higher incidence of septicemia. These patients often present with a toxic appearance and are frequently admitted for treatment. It is probably prudent to obtain cultures in this subset of cellulitis patients. Obtaining blood cultures does not alter initial management, as these

TABLE 26–2. BLOOD CULTURES AND NEEDLE ASPIRATES IN *H. INFLUENZAE* CELLULITIS

	Positives / Total N	
	Blood	*Aspirate*
Green, 1957	4/6	—
Thilenius, 1959	1/1	—
Feingold, 1965	7/9	—
Medina, 1967	3/3	—
Rapkin, 1972	6/8	—
Minnefor et al, 1972	1/2	1/1
Rasmussen, 1973	1/1	—
Goetz et al, 1974	3/3	2/3

Adapted from Goetz JP, Tafari N, Boxerbaum B: Needle aspiration in *Haemophilus influenzae* type B cellulitis. *Pediatrics.* 1974;54:504.

results typically do not become available for 24 to 48 hours. Patients are treated empirically based on clinical presentation. If clinical indicators warrant a change, antibiotic therapy can be altered based on culture and sensitivity results.

NEEDLE ASPIRATION

Needle aspiration was first reported by Suarez in 1930 while studying lymphangitis.[17] Leading edge needle aspiration of cellulitis lesions for culture was first reported by Minnefor and coworkers in a case of a child with *H. influenzae* cellulitis.[18] Goetz and colleagues published the first series report utilizing needle aspiration in three patients with facial cellulitis.[14] Two of the three patients had positive aspirates, and all three had positive blood cultures. It is Uman and Kunin, however, who are most commonly cited as first describing the procedure.[19] They studied a series of seven patients, three with true cellulitis and four with discrete abscesses.

Since then, needle aspiration has been both praised and condemned as a useful tool in the management of cellulitis. Minor variations in technique are common, and a two-needle cutaneous lavage technique has been reported.[20] Most investigators report poor yields. Table 26–2 demonstrates the poor correlation between aspirates and blood cultures. Fleisher and coworkers had one of the highest yields, with 48% of patients with extremity lesions having aspirate cultures positive for bacterial pathogens.[3] If the patients in their series with facial lesions are included, the yield is 50%.

Hook and colleagues demonstrated only 10% positive aspirates in their study,[5] and Ginsberg reported 12% positive.[12] Goldgeier[4] and Rudoy and Nakashima[15] reported only 5 and 6.4% positive, respectively. Liles and Dall, however, found a 33% positive yield in a retrospective review of 24 adults.[21] Newell and Norden prospectively studied 30 patients and personally performed all aspirates to reduce interinvestigator variance.[22] Their results still demonstrated a low positive yield of 10%. Table 26–3 summarizes the findings of these studies.

Epperly evaluated the yield of aspirates from the leading edge and midpoint of cellulitis lesions in 103 otherwise healthy young adults.[23] He found no difference between the midpoint aspirates (8.6% positive) vs leading edge aspirates (8.7% positive). The overall yield was 14.5% positive aspirates in his study. Epperly concluded that needle aspiration in a young, healthy population is unnecessary and that empiric therapy will suffice. Sachs' study of 25 adults with cellulitis supports this conclusion, stating that needle aspiration is usually not helpful in establishing a bacteriologic diagnosis.[6]

TABLE 26–3. NEEDLE ASPIRATION YIELDS

	% Positive	N
Fleisher et al, 1980	50	50
Ginsberg, 1981	12	101
Goldgeier, 1983	5	20
Hook et al, 1986	10	50
Liles and Dall, 1985	33	24
Newell and Norden, 1988	10	30
Rudoy and Nakashima, 1979	6.4	78

Kielhofner and coworkers specifically addressed the influence of underlying disease states on the yield of needle aspirations in a prospective study with 87 patients.[24] The population included patients with IV drug abuse, diabetes, malignancies, and cardiac disease. The overall rate of positive aspirates was 38%. Of those with positive aspirates, only 7% had positive blood cultures. Table 26–4 lists the underlying disease state and the corresponding percentage of positive aspirates. If the cardiac and healthy patients are excluded, the yield is approximately 61% positive.

As is evident, studies of needle aspiration yields have demonstrated a wide range of positive yields (5 to 50%). The reason for this discrepancy is not readily apparent, although differences in technique (location and depth of needle insertion, volume of fluid injected and aspirated, two-needle lavage), culture methods, and severity of cellulitis could possibly play a role. At best one could expect a 50% positive yield, with better yields possible in compromised patients and pediatric patients with facial cellulitis. In the latter group, however, blood cultures

TABLE 26–4. INFLUENCE OF UNDERLYING DISEASE STATES ON NEEDLE ASPIRATION

Risk Factor	Positive Aspirates (%)
Diabetes mellitus	70.5
IV drug abuse	38.8
Malignancy	100
Cardiac disease	20
None	17

From Kielhofner MA, Brown B, Dall L: Influence of underlying disease process on the utility of cellulitis needle aspirates. *Arch Intern Med.* 1988; 148:2451–2452. ©1988, American Medical Association.

are probably a more sensitive and less traumatic test. In compromised hosts, aspirates may provide useful information if initial empiric therapy fails.[6, 24]

CONSIDERATIONS WITH BITE WOUNDS

Bite wounds have always been the most dreaded wounds with regard to infection. This is the primary reason we tend not to close any wounds less than gaping (the exception being facial wounds). The value of culturing fresh wounds that do not appear clinically infected is questionable. A review article by Martin strongly advocates both aerobic and anaerobic cultures and prophylactic antibiotics even in clinically noninfected wounds.[25] This conservative approach is practiced by many physicians.

Spencer and associates reported on 121 patients with dog bites and recommended a more selective approach to management.[26] In their study, 12% were found to be infected. Two thirds of those yielded positive cultures. Of the remaining 106 without signs of infection, only 18% yielded a potential pathogen. They concluded that the low incidence of pathogenic bacteria in noninfected wounds should preclude the use of routine cultures. Spencer and associates stated that infected wounds should be cultured because of the common occurrence of polymicrobial infections that may require combination therapy. Not addressed is whether all isolates are true pathogens requiring specific antibiotic therapy. Empiric therapy for the most common pathogens and clinical reassessment for response may be a more cost-effective and practical approach.

Baker and Sally studied 322 human bite wounds in children.[27] A total of 75% of the injuries were abrasions, 13% were punctures, and 11% lacerations. None of the abrasions became infected, whereas 38% of the punctures and 37% of the lacerations did become infected. Of significance is that, when good local wound care was rendered by a physician within 12 hours of injury, the overall rate of infection fell from 9% to 1.6%.

Lindsey and coworkers studied 434 human bite wounds in 79 institutionalized patients and compared their course with 803 simple lacerations in the same group.[28] All wounds were treated with local care and closure if necessary. Lindsey and coworkers concluded that human bites do have a higher incidence of infection than simple lacerations, but the increased susceptibility to infection secondary to bites is not significant enough to justify more than observation. Antibiotic therapy can be initiated if infection develops.

CONCLUSIONS

The data suggest that nonspecific tests such as the CBC and ESR do not contribute to the management of patients with cellulitis. These tests have not been found to be predictive of positive cultures.[4–6, 9, 10] Thus, in an outpatient setting, the value of these tests is next to nil.

Needle aspiration and blood cultures likewise have not been found to be consistently helpful (5 to 50% positive yield).[3–6, 12, 15, 21–23] Patients with studies not yielding pathogens are still treated empirically. In pediatric patients with facial cellulitis, blood cultures are preferred over needle aspiration, as they probably are less painful and traumatic to the patient. This subset of patients is at higher risk for septicemia, and more aggressive management is usually indicated. *Staphylococcus* and *Streptococcus* species are the organisms most commonly associated with cellulitis; *Haemophilus influenzae* often is found in pediatric patients with facial cellulitis.[3, 5, 13, 24, 29–31] Review of the literature does not demonstrate frequent recovery of unexpected organisms; therefore, empiric therapy will usually suffice.[22, 23, 32–34] Patients with certain underlying disease states have been shown to have higher yields on needle aspiration.[24]

Bite wounds have been found to have a slightly increased incidence of infection when compared with other simple lacerations. Only clinically infected wounds should be treated with antibiotics,[28] with therapy directed at the most likely pathogen. If treatment fails, wound cultures may then be of value. Prophylactic antibiotics have not been shown to reduce the incidence of infection in the initial management of bite wounds.[27] Early evaluation by a physician and good local wound care remain the best modalities to prevent infection secondary to bite wounds.

REFERENCES

1. Young GP: CBC or not CBC? That is the question. *Ann Emerg Med.* 1986;15:367.
2. Bonadio WA, Smith D, Carmody J: Correlating CBC profile and infectious outcome. *Clin Pediatr.* 1992;31:578.
3. Fleisher G, Ludwig S, Campos J: Cellulitis: Bacterial etiology, clinical features, and laboratory findings. *J Pediatr.* 1980;97:591.
4. Goldgeier MH: The microbial evaluation of acute cellulitis. *Cutis.* 1983;31:649.
5. Hook EW, Hooten TM, Horton CA, et al: Microbiologic evaluation of cutaneous cellulitis in adults. *Arch Intern Med.* 1986;146:295.
6. Sachs MK: The optimum use of needle aspiration in the bacteriologic diagnosis of cellulitis in adults. *Arch Intern Med.* 1990;150:1907.

7. Cox RD, Wagner M, Woolard DJ: Infants and children with fever without source. *Ann Emerg Med.* 1994;23:598.
8. McCarthy PL: Controversies in pediatrics: What tests are indicated for the child under 2 with fever. *Pediatr Rev.* 1979;1:51.
9. Waskerwitz S, Berkelhamer JE: Outpatient bacteremia: Clinical findings in children under two years with initial temperature of 39.5°C or higher. *J Pediatr.* 1981;99:231.
10. Liu CH, Lehan C, Speer ME, et al: Early detection of bacteremia in an outpatient clinic. *Pediatrics.* 1985;75:827.
11. Wyler DJ: Diagnostic implications of markedly elevated erythrocyte sedimentation rate: A reevaluation. *South Med J.* 1977;70:1428.
12. Ginsberg MB: Cellulitis: Analysis of 101 cases and review of the literature. *South Med J.* 1981;74:530.
13. Ho PWL, Pien FD, Hamburg D: Value of cultures in patients with acute cellulitis. *South Med J.* 1979;72:1402.
14. Goetz JP, Tafari N, Boxerbaum B: Needle aspiration in *Hemophilus influenzae* type B cellulitis. *Pediatrics.* 1974;54:504.
15. Rudoy RC, Nakashima G: Diagnostic value of needle aspiration in *Hemophilus influenzae* type B cellulitis. *J Pediatr.* 1979;94:924.
16. Carroll WL, Farrell MK, Singer JI, et al: Treatment of occult bacteremia: A prospective randomized clinical trial. *Pediatrics.* 1983;72:608.
17. Suarez J: A preliminary report on the clinical and bacteriological findings in 60 cases of lymphangitis associated with elephantoid fever in Puerto Rico. *Am J Trop Med.* 1930;10:183.
18. Minnefor AB, Murray JJ, Davis PH: *Hemophilus influenzae* cellulitis of the lower extremity. *Am J Dis Child.* 1972;124:920.
19. Uman SJ, Kunin CM: Needle aspiration in the diagnosis of soft tissue infections. *Arch Intern Med.* 1975;135:959.
20. Wormser GP, Forseter G, Cooper D, et al: Use of a novel technique of cutaneous lavage for diagnosis of Lyme disease associated with erythema migrans. *JAMA.* 1992;268:1311.
21. Liles D, Dall LH: Needle aspiration for diagnosis of cellulitis. *Cutis.* 1985;36:63.
22. Newell PM, Norden CW: Value of needle aspiration in bacteriologic diagnosis of cellulitis in adults. *J Clin Microbiol.* 1988;26:401.
23. Epperly TD: The value of needle aspiration in the management of cellulitis. *J Fam Prac.* 1986;23:337.
24. Kielhofner MA, Brown B, Dall L: Influence of underlying disease process on the utility of cellulitis needle aspirates. *Arch Intern Med.* 1988;148:2451.
25. Martin LT: Human bites. *Postgrad Med.* 1987;81:221.
26. Spencer RC, Matta H, Ferguson DG, et al: Routine culture of dog bites. *Ann Emerg Med.* 1987;16:730.
27. Baker MD, Sally EM: Human bites in children. *Am J Dis Child.* 1987;141:1285.
28. Lindsey D, Christopher M, Hollenbach J, et al: Natural course of the human bite wound. *J Trauma.* 1987;27:45.
29. Yagupsky P: Bacteriologic aspects of skin and soft tissue infections. *Ped Ann.* 1993;93:175.
30. Lindsey D: Soft tissue infections. *Emerg Med Clin North Am.* 1992;10:737.

31. Kahn RM, Goldstein EJC: Common bacterial skin infections. *Postgrad Med.* 1993;93:175.
32. Sigurdsson AF, Gudmundsson S: The etiology of bacterial cellulitis as determined by fine-needle aspiration. *Scand J Infect Dis.* 1989;21:537.
33. Leppard BJ, Seal DV, Colman G, et al: The value of bacteriology and serology in the diagnosis of cellulitis and erysipelas. *Br J Dermatol.* 1985;112:559.
34. Lutomski DM, Trott AT, Runyon JM, et al: Microbiology of adult cellulitis. *J Fam Prac.* 1988;26(1):45.

Chapter

Superficial Foreign Bodies

George L. Ellis and Lynda L. Flom

The possibility of a retained foreign body must be considered in any patient with an acute laceration or a puncture wound as well as in those with more remote (or unrecalled) injury who present with unexplained pain, swelling, or infection or with a chronically draining sinus tract, particularly of the hand or foot. Technical advances have added significantly to the radiologic imaging modalities available to the emergency physician in identifying and locating a suspected retained foreign body. Failure to diagnose a retained foreign body has been reported to be the second leading cause of malpractice litigation against emergency physicians (14%), accounting for 5% of total settlement dollars.[1] In a review of 200 cases of retained foreign bodies, Anderson found that 38% of cases had been missed by the previous treating surgeons.[2]

PLAIN RADIOGRAPHY

In the study by Anderson, 77% of the 75 foreign bodies that were missed on initial evaluation were radiopaque and, therefore, detectable on plain radiography.[2] A plain radiograph, readily available in most emergency departments, should be the initial imaging modality of choice in patients suspected of harboring a retained foreign body. Techniques using small focal spot, small field size, and slight overexposure have led to improved detection. High-resolution mammography film has also proved useful.[3]

Plain radiography is based on differential absorption of x-rays by objects of different densities and atomic numbers.[4] The relative difference in density of the foreign body compared with the surrounding tissues determines whether the foreign object is detectable. The density of soft tissue is in the range of 1.08 gm/cc[5] to 1.5 gm/cc[6]; glass ranged from 2.4 gm/cc to 5.9 gm/cc[6]; the density of plastic is approximately 1.2 gm/cc[5]; wood is generally less dense than soft tissue but varies with the type of wood, the painting of the wood, and the degree to which the wood is saturated with fluid.[7] Metal fragments are radiopaque.[2, 8] Although it has been stated in the literature that aluminum is not radiopaque,[1] aluminum foreign bodies are in fact radiopaque and are well visualized when not superimposed on bone,[9] as would be expected by the fact that the density of aluminum is 2.7 gm/cc.

There has been a widespread misconception as to the radiopacity of *glass* fragments. A number of standard textbooks and references have asserted that glass is invisible or only barely visible unless it contains manganese, iron, lead, or titanium. All glass, including ordinary machine glass, which does not contain lead, is radiopaque.[4, 10] Size and location, however, are factors limiting detection. Fragments as small as 0.5 mm, when unobscured by bone, and fragments as small as 2 mm, when superimposed on bone, are detectable by standard x-rays.[6]

In a chicken leg model, glass fragments that were 2.0, 1.0, and 0.5 mm in size had 99, 83, and 61% average detection rates, respectively.[11] Four-view radiography did not significantly improve detection rates in this model, in which one bone was involved; in a setting involving multiple bones, which may more easily obscure a foreign body (eg, a hand), oblique views may be indicated to ''free'' the foreign body of overlying bone or change the orientation of the foreign body with respect to the radiographic beam.

Wood is often not visible on radiographs. In Anderson's study, only 15% of wooden foreign bodies were identified on standard radiograph.[2] Unfortunately, wooden splinters and thorns are commonly retained foreign bodies. Because most wood is less dense than soft tissues, wooden objects attenuate the x-ray beam less than the surrounding tissue and, therefore, may appear as filling defects. Dense, painted, and water-saturated woods are more radiopaque and therefore create less discernible defects.[7] In the initial hours after injury, radiographs may also reveal wooden foreign bodies by detecting the air trapped within and around the wood. Air around the foreign body may produce a halo effect. Wood becomes less detectible after it has been embedded in soft tissues for 24 to 48 hours owing to absorption of fluid. Even when the foreign body is not seen, however, there are often indirect radiographic signs of a retained foreign body that should be sought. For example, there have been reports of lytic lesions of bone, periosteal reaction of bone, and pseudotumors of soft tissue in cases of retained foreign bodies of the leg.[2] Deep soft tissue swelling is another indirect sign of a retained foreign body.

The density of common *plastics* is similar to that of soft tissues. Plastic fragments, therefore, are generally not detectable on plain films unless accompanied by other contaminants or air or unless they are large enough to cause obvious distortion of normal anatomic detail.[8]

XERORADIOGRAPHY

With the advent of xeroradiography for mammography, radiologists began utilizing this modality for foreign body detection. Xeroradiography utilizes standard x-ray equipment, but the exposure is made on a homogeneously charged, selenium-covered plate. Various electrostatic discharge zones are created between areas of different thickness and density, and photoconduction then attracts the selenium powder. An electrostatic image is thereby created, which is permanently recorded by a special copying process. The borders of the different electrostatic zones are particularly well demonstrated—a phenomenon called edge enhancement. If a small foreign body lies immediately adjacent to bone, it may be incorporated into the excess electrostatic discharge area, thus being obliterated in the resultant xerogram—a situation referred to as "edge wipeout."

A number of studies have demonstrated that, whereas xeroradiography may improve detailed visualization of radiopaque objects, it produces little or no advantage in detecting nonradiopaque materials such as wood or plastic.[5, 12–14] Xeroradiography is not readily available in the emergency department and involves a much larger radiation dose compared with conventional radiographs. It is, therefore, not recommended to use xeroradiography for the detection of foreign bodies.

SONOGRAPHY

The sonographic reflectivity of a foreign body depends on its acoustic impedance. All foreign bodies in soft tissues are seen as hyperechoic foci, with or without acoustic shadow or hyperechoic comet tail. This factor also applies to radiolucent foreign bodies, such as wood and plastic, that are often not detectable on plain films. When the foreign body incites an inflammatory reaction, an adjacent hypoechoic mass can be seen surrounding the hyperechoic focus. The hyperechoic focus caused by the reflectivity of the foreign body is more easily detected within a homogeneous hypoechoic area, such as subcutaneous fat, muscle, or inflammatory tissue.

In a series of 39 patients who presented with a suspected foreign body of the hand in whom standard soft tissue radiographic studies were negative, ultrasonography was found to have a sensitivity and specificity of 95 and 89.5%, respectively.[15]

In an experimental model, utilizing cubes of beef approximately 6 cm on a side, Schlager[1] evaluated the detection of six different types of foreign bodies, including gravel (approximately 4 × 4 mm), plastic (2 × 1 mm), agave cactus spine, metal (1.5-cm section of paper clip), wood (1.5-cm section of Q-tip swab), and glass fragments (none larger than 5 × 5 mm). A "blinded" emergency physician with no formal training in ultrasonography was asked to use a portable ultrasound unit with a 7.5-mHz transducer to determine the presence or absence of foreign body in 120 cubes of meat, 60 of which did and 60 of which did not contain a foreign body. Ultrasound correctly detected 59 of the 60 foreign bodies and recorded one false-positive in the 60 cubes containing no foreign body, yielding a sensitivity and specificity of 98%.[1]

Sonography has been recommended as the study of choice in the evaluation of suspected nonradiopaque superficial foreign bodies.[5, 16] Ultrasound also offers excellent three-dimensional localization that can be used preoperatively or intraoperatively during foreign body retrieval.[17–19] Intraoperative ultrasound has been found superior to fluoroscopy for foreign body localization even when the foreign body is radiopaque. In addition, sonography does not carry the risk of significant irradiation that accompanies fluoroscopically guided removal. Sonography is most helpful in superficial foreign bodies. The best resolution is in the near zone of the transducer. Because gas and bone reflect the sound beam and cause acoustic shadowing, foreign bodies positioned behind gas or bone cannot be visualized.

COMPUTED TOMOGRAPHY

Computed tomography (CT), with density differentiation up to 100 times greater than plain radiography, can aid in the detection of foreign bodies not identified by other imaging modalities. Narrow bone windows are required in cases involving foreign bodies composed of wood, plastic, or other materials having densities similar to normal soft tissue.[20] Computed tomography is able to give a precise location relative to other anatomic structures[21] and is superior to ultrasound in the evaluation of deep foreign bodies or foreign bodies positioned behind air or bone.

Computed tomography does expose the patient to radiation, however, is expensive, and is often not readily available.

MAGNETIC RESONANCE IMAGING

The soft tissues in which a foreign body is embedded are composed primarily of fat or muscle and contain hydrogen atoms that produce a positive signal on MRI. Foreign bodies, however, generally contain little or no free water and so produce a signal void that is easily distinguished from the surrounding soft tissues. Glass, plastic, and wooden foreign bodies produce easily detectable signal voids. Gravel and other specimens containing variable amounts of magnetic material create streak artifacts, thereby obscuring visualization.[14] Because of its expense and lack of ready accessibility, MRI should be used only for cases defying detection by the previously mentioned modalities. Magnetic resonance imaging should not be used for evaluation of metallic foreign bodies located in areas such as the eye or nervous system because their displacement by the magnetic field might cause significant complications.

SUMMARY

Use of the appropriate radiologic imaging modality, along with familiarity with indirect radiologic signs, can help in determining the presence and location of a foreign body (Table 27–1). Plain radiographs should be the initial screening modality for a suspected foreign body. Whereas

TABLE 27–1. ABILITY OF VARIOUS IMAGING MODALITIES TO DETECT FOREIGN BODIES

	Metal	Glass (if ≥2 mm)	Wood	Plastic
Plain radiography	+ + +	+ + +	0/+[a]	0/+
Xeroradiography	+ + +	+ + +	0/+[a]	0/+
Ultrasonography[b]	+ +/+ + +	+ +/+ + +	+ +	+ +
Computed tomography	+ + +	+ + +	+	+
Magnetic resonance imaging	Not used	+ + +	+ + +	+ + +

[a]Dependent on type of wood, air/water content, paint, or other contaminant.

[b]Only for superficial foreign bodies (<3 cm in depth when using 7.5-mHz transducer) not obscured by bone or gas and dependent on size and orientation.

most metal and glass foreign bodies are detectable on radiographs, many foreign bodies including wood and plastic usually are not. Xeroradiography is not recommended for foreign body detection. When a suspected superficial foreign body is not delineated on radiographs, ultrasound should be the next modality of choice. Computed tomography should be reserved for deep foreign bodies, suspected foreign bodies not seen on radiographs or ultrasound, and foreign bodies located behind bone or gas.

REFERENCES

1. Schlager D, Sanders AB, Wiggins D, et al: Ultrasound for detection of foreign bodies. *Ann Emerg Med.* 1991;20:189–191.
2. Anderson M, Newmeyer WL, Kilgore ES Jr: Diagnosis and treatment of retained foreign bodies in the hand. *Am J Surg.* 1982;144:63–67.
3. Kuhns LR, Borlaza GS, Seigel RS, et al: An in vitro comparison of computed tomography, xeroradiography, and radiography in the detection of soft-tissue foreign bodies. *Radiology.* 1979;132:218–219.
4. Felman AH, Fisher MS: The radiographic detection of glass in soft tissue. *Radiology.* 1969;92:1529–1531.
5. Ginsburg MJ, Ellis GL, Flom LL: Detection of soft-tissue foreign bodies by plain radiography, xerography, computed tomography, and ultrasonography. *Ann Emerg Med.* 1990;19:701–703.
6. Tandberg D: Glass in the foot and hand: Will an x-ray film show it? *JAMA.* 1982;248:1872–1874.
7. Mucci B, Stenhouse G: Soft tissue radiography for wooden foreign bodies—A worthwhile exercise? *Injury.* 1985;16:402–404.
8. DeLacey G, Evans R, Sandin B: Penetrating injuries: How easy is it to see glass (and plastic) on radiographs? *Br J Radiol.* 1985;58:27–30.
9. Ellis GL: Are aluminum foreign bodies detectable radiographically? *Am J Emerg Med.* 1993;11:12–13.
10. Pond GD, Lindsey D: Localization of cactus, glass and other foreign bodies in soft tissues. *Ariz Med.* 1977;34:700–702.
11. Courter BJ: Radiographic screening for glass foreign bodies—What does a ''negative'' foreign body series really mean? *Ann Emerg Med.* 1990;19:997–1000.
12. De Flaviis L, Scaglione P, Delbo P, et al: Detection of foreign bodies in soft tissue: Experimental comparison of ultrasonography and xeroradiography. *J Trauma.* 1988;28:400–404.
13. Russell RC, Williamson DA, Sullivan JW, et al: Detection of foreign bodies in the hand. *J Hand Surg.* 1991;16A:2–11.
14. Stair TO: Xeroradiography and foreign bodies. *Am J Emerg Med.* 1983;1:117–118.
15. Crawford R, Matheson AB: Clinical value of ultrasonography in detection and removal of radiolucent foreign bodies. *Injury.* 1989;20:341–343.
16. Oikarinen KS, Nieminen TM, Makarainen H, et al: Visibility of foreign bodies in soft tissue in plain radiographs, computed tomography, magnetic resonance imaging, and ultrasound. *Int J Oral Maxillofac Surg.* 1993;22:119–124.

17. Fornage BD: Preoperative sonographic localization of a migrated transosseous stabilizing wire in the hand. *J Ultrasound Med.* 1987;6:471–473.
18. Fornage BD, Schernberg FL: Sonographic preoperative localization of a foreign body in the hand. *J Ultrasound Med.* 1987;6:217–219.
19. Gooding GAW, Hardiman T, et al: Sonography of the hand and foot in foreign body detection. *J Ultrasound Med.* 1987;6:441–447.
20. Combs AH, Kernek CB, Heck DA: Retained wooden foreign body in the foot detected by computed tomography. *Orthopedics.* 1986;9:1434–1435.
21. Nyska M, Pomeranz S, Porat S: The advantage of computed tomography in locating a foreign body in the foot. *J Trauma.* 1986;26:93–95.

Chapter

Preoperative and Routine Preadmission Chest Radiography and Electrocardiography

Jeffrey Garland

In many institutions, it has long been standard practice to order a battery of routine diagnostic tests on patients prior to surgery or upon hospital admission. These tests are often ordered routinely so as to "expedite patient care." Two of the tests that are most commonly ordered on a routine basis in these settings are the chest roentgenogram and the electrocardiogram (ECG). This chapter reviews the literature on the diagnostic yield and utility of routine preoperative and admission chest radiography and electrocardiography.

For the purposes of this chapter, a routine test will be defined as one that is ordered without a specific indication solely because the patient is to undergo surgery or be admitted to the hospital.

PREOPERATIVE CHEST X-RAYS

The purpose of routine preoperative testing is to predict the likelihood of intraoperative and postoperative complications, with the hope of either avoiding them by delaying surgery or being prepared to manage them more effectively if they occur. Thus, a preoperative test is clinically useful if it can detect conditions that are associated with significant morbidity or mortality but are not easily detected on clinical grounds alone.

It is generally agreed that a preoperative chest x-ray (CXR) should be obtained on all patients with a history of, or active signs or symptoms of, cardiac or pulmonary disease. Most also agree that preoperative CXRs should *not* be ordered routinely when no indications are present.[1, 2] There is controversy, however, as to what, besides the presence of acute or chronic cardiopulmonary disease, constitutes an appropriate indication for preoperative CXR. Some have proposed that age alone is an indication. Recommendations for an age cutoff have ranged from 20 to 60 years. Most of the recommendations based on age are predicated on the fact that there is a higher frequency of unexpected abnormalities uncovered on the preoperative CXR in patients with advanced age.[1–7] Because there is little, if any, evidence that uncovering such abnormalities leads to a change in patient management or, more importantly, to an improvement in patient outcome, the ordering of a CXR based purely on age remains controversial. Overall, because CXR abnormalities are especially common in patients over the age of 60, it is probably reasonable to order a routine CXR at least in this group of patients.

Preoperative CXRs have also been proposed to be useful as baseline studies for later comparison if problems were to arise in the perioperative period. Whereas reviews on the utility of CXRs in this setting have reached mixed conclusions, there is no definitive evidence that they improve outcome.[3, 8–14] It seems reasonable to recommend that preoperative CXRs be ordered only in patients with a history of or acute signs or symptoms of cardiac or pulmonary disease and in patients over the age of 60.

PREOPERATIVE ELECTROCARDIOGRAMS

A second almost universally ordered preoperative test is the ECG. Perhaps the chief concern that surgeons and anesthesiologists have is that an unforeseen asymptomatic cardiac abnormality might become manifest perioperatively and increase the risk of complications. The preoperative ECG might detect such abnormalities so that surgery could be postponed or so that appropriate preparations could be made to deal with complications if they occurred. A number of studies have examined the utility of the preoperative ECG. Although some investigators believe that it has little benefit,[15–17] most agree that, whereas it should not be ordered routinely in *all* patients, as is commonly done, there are times when it is indicated. Generally accepted indications for preoperative electrocardiography include a history of documented heart disease; physical examination findings indicative of cardiac abnormalities; presence of disease that may be associated with unrecognized cardiac abnormalities (eg, hypertension, peripheral vascular disease, diabetes, cardiovascular disease); administration of medications with known cardiac toxicities (eg, antidepressant and antiarrhythmic medications); and proposed surgical procedures known to have a high risk of cardiac complications (eg, intrathoracic, intraperitoneal, aortic, emergency surgery). Under these circumstances the likelihood of finding asymptomatic cardiac disease is clearly increased.[18]

Age alone, in the absence of any of the other risk factors mentioned, is also generally accepted as an indication for preoperative electrocardiography. The consensus is that men over the age of 40 and women over the age of 55 not only have more frequent electrocardiographic abnormalities found but that they have much more frequent complications associated with these abnormalities, thus justifying routine preoperative ECG.[18, 19] In particular, there is a greater likelihood in elderly patients that rhythms other than normal sinus rhythms, or benign premature atrial contractions undetected on physical examination, will be discovered.[20–22] Such rhythms are known to increase the complication rate associated with surgery.[23] Others argue that the risk may not be dramatically increased until about age 60 in both men and women.[24–29]

It has also been proposed that the preoperative ECG be performed as a means of detecting silent myocardial infarction (MI) in patients without risk factors. The occurrence of MI within the previous 6 months has been shown to be a major risk factor for a life-threatening cardiac complication,[23, 30–33] and it has been shown that either postponing surgery or instituting careful intraoperative and postoperative management can decrease the complication rate.[34] Although a preoperative ECG might be able to detect a clinically silent MI, it cannot indicate whether the MI occurred within the past 6 months or earlier than that. Thus, it appears to be of limited utility in this setting.

It has been argued that the preoperative ECG is helpful as a baseline study in patients without other indications and can be used for comparison if perioperative problems occur. There are no data published to support this contention.

A reasonable recommendation, therefore, is that a preoperative ECG be performed in any patient who has a documented history of heart disease, a physical examination showing cardiac abnormalities, or a disease associated with unrecognized cardiac abnormalities; in any patient receiving medications with known cardiac toxicity or undergoing surgical procedures known to have a high risk of cardiac complications; and in all patients over the age of 60.

ADMISSION CHEST X-RAYS

The utility of the routine admission CXR has been studied by a number of investigators, as well as by the United States Department of Health and Human Services, the Canadian Medical Association, and the American College of Radiology, all of which conclude that, in the absence of specific indications, CXRs need not be ordered solely for the reason of hospital admission.[1, 35] The question remains, however, as to what in fact are appropriate indications for an admission CXR. It is clear that one indication is the clinical suspicion of diseases that can be diagnosed and confirmed by CXR, such as congestive heart failure, pneumothorax, pneumonia, or complications of cancer. Age per se has also been proposed as an indication. The consensus is that age is a legitimate indication for admission CXR because of the relatively high prevalence of unexpected pulmonary abnormalities in the older patient. As with preoperative testing, a number of different age cutoffs, ranging from 40 to 65 years of age, have been proposed. Whereas the incidence of unexpected pulmonary abnormalities has been shown to increase with age, obtaining a CXR in these patients has not been shown to improve outcomes. It therefore may be preferable to use a cutoff at the upper limit of those proposed in the literature (eg, 65 years of age).

It has been proposed that admission CXRs are useful in other settings as well. Although they have been proposed to have value as baseline examinations against which future studies can be compared, there is no evidence to support this contention. Similarly, there is no evidence that CXRs in any setting, let alone in the setting of an acute hospitalization, are useful as screening tests for the detection of unexpected findings. In fact, the National Cancer Institute Cooperative Study showed that, to the contrary, at least when it comes to lung cancer, screening CXRs are not useful in improving patient survival. Finally, CXRs have been proposed to be of value for the reassurance provided to the physician as a result of a negative examination finding. Once again, there is no evidence that such reassurance either has a positive effect on patient outcome or is cost-effective.

In summary, admission CXRs should be obtained for patients with clinically suspect acute cardiac and pulmonary disease and should be considered in all elderly patients. They need not be ordered as baseline tests or screening tests or for the purpose of physician reassurance.

ADMISSION ELECTROCARDIOGRAM

The routine admission ECG has been less well studied. Moorman and coworkers[36] in 1985 followed patients admitted to the general medicine service of Duke University Hospital during a 9-month period and found that in 767 patients with no cardiac abnormality (defined as a history of MI, congestive heart failure, palpitations, arrhythmia, or abnormal cardiac physical examinations), the performance of a routine ECG resulted in a change in patient management in only 0.3%. This finding was confirmed in studies done by Hubbell and associates[35] and by Garland and Wolfson.[37] In the latter investigation, the routine admission ECG never resulted in a change in outcome among 247 medical patients who met none of the aforementioned indications for obtaining an admission ECG (Table 28–1).

In Moorman's study, the admission ECG was more often helpful in patients over the age of 65, but this association was of only borderline statistical significance when considered independently of the presence of identified cardiac abnormalities. The study by Garland and Wolfson did not find age to be a useful indication for admission ECG.

The admission ECG has also been proposed as a baseline study that would be likely to be useful in making future patient care decisions.[38–40] However, none of these studies showed that a baseline ECG, ordered without other indications, improved patient outcome. Furthermore, a larger study by Rubenstein and Greenfield, which specifically addressed the utility of the baseline ECG, showed that in 236 patients the absence

TABLE 28–1. PROPOSED CRITERIA FOR OBTAINING AN ADMISSION ELECTROCARDIOGRAM

History of
Coronary artery disease
Arrhythmia
Congestive heart failure
Conduction disturbance
Cor pulmonale
Pericarditis
Cardiomyopathy
Palpitations
Syncope or coma
Symptom complex suggestive of angina or congestive heart failure
Suspected cardiotoxic overdose
Irregular pulse
Pulse >120 or <60
Systolic blood pressure >200 or <90
Diastolic blood pressure >120
Serum potassium >5.7 or <3.0

From Garland JL, Wolfson AB: Routine admission electrocardiography in emergency department patients. *Ann Emerg Med.* 1994; 23:275–280.

of a baseline ECG would not have resulted in an adverse patient outcome.[41] Other investigators have drawn similar conclusions.[42, 43]

The literature thus offers little support for the routine ordering of an ECG purely for the reason of hospital admission. In fact, there is clearly a subset of patients (those not meeting the criteria in Table 28–1) in whom it appears that the ordering of a routine admission ECG can be safely omitted. These proposed indications for ordering an admission ECG, however, have not yet been validated in other settings. For the present, they may have utility in conjunction with the physician's clinical judgment in determining which patients should receive an admission ECG and which should not. The issue of whether age alone should be an indication for ordering an admission ECG remains unsettled.

CONCLUSION

Rough guidelines for the routine ordering of preoperative and preadmission CXR and ECG have been presented here. These are meant to be used only as reference points. They should be combined with the physician's experience and personal judgment in deciding when to order a particular test. In general, these tests are indicated when suggested by the patient's history and physical examination and potentially in all patients over age 65.

REFERENCES

1. Eagel SS, Evens RG, Forrest JV, et al. Efficiency of routine screening and lateral chest radiographs in a hospital based population. *N Engl J Med.* 1974;291:1001–1004.
2. Turnbull JM, Buck C. The value of preoperative screening investigations in otherwise healthy individuals. *Arch Intern Med.* 1987;147:1101–1105.
3. National Study by the Royal College of Radiologists. Pre-operative chest radiology. *Lancet.* 1979;ii:83–86.
4. Catchlove BR, Wilson McL R, Spring S, et al: Routine investigations in elective surgical patients. Their use and cost effectiveness in a teaching hospital. *Med J Aust.* 1979; 2:107–110.
5. Petterson SRF, Janower ML: Is the routine pre-operative chest film of value? *Appl Radiol.* 1977;6:70.
6. Wood RA, Hoekelman RA: Value of the chest X-ray as a screening test for elective surgery in children. *Pediatrics.* 1981;67:447–452.
7. Royal College of Radiologists: Preoperative chest radiology. *Lancet.* 1979;1:83–86.
8. Fowkes FG. The value of routine pre-operative chest X-rays. *Br J Hosp Med.* 1986;35:120–123.

9. Kerr IH: The pre-operative chest X-ray. *Br J Anaesthesia.* 1974;46:558–563.
10. Evison G: Routine pre-operative chest radiography. (letter). *Br Med J* 1976;ii:44.
11. Loder RE: Routine pre-operative chest radiography. 1977 compared with 1955 at Peterborough District General Hospital. *Anaesthesia.* 1978;33:972–974.
12. Milne ENC: Chest radiology in the surgical patient. *Surg Clin North Am.* 1980;60:1503–1518.
13. Seymour DG, Pringle R, Shaw JW: The role of the routine pre-operative chest X-ray in the elderly general surgical patient. *Postgrad Med J.* 1982;58:741–745.
14. Mendelson DS, Khilnani N, Whener LD, et al. Pre-operative chest radiography: Value as a baseline examination for comparison. *Radiology.* 1987;165:341–343.
15. Turnbull JM, Buck C. The value of preoperative screening investigations in otherwise healthy individuals. *Arch Intern Med.* 1987;147:1101–1105.
16. Catchlove BR, Wilson McL, Spring S, et al: Routine investigations in elective surgical patients. *Med J Aust.* 1979;2:107–10.
17. Johnson H, Knee-loli S, Butler TA, et al. Are routine pre-operative laboratory screening tests necessary to evaluate ambulatory surgical patients? *Surgery.* 1988;104:639–645.
18. Goldberger AI, O'Konski M. Utility of the routine electrocardiogram before surgery and on general hospital admission. *Ann Intern Med.* 1986;105:552–557.
19. ACC/AHA Task Force Report: Guidelines for electrocardiography. *J Am Coll Cardiol.* 1992;19:473–481.
20. Ferrer MI. The value of obligatory preoperative electrocardiograms: a survey of 1260 patients. *J Am Med Wom Assoc.* 1978;33:459–464.
21. Patterson RR, Caskie JP, Galloway DJ, et al: The pre-operative electrocardiogram: an assessment. *Scott Med J.* 1983;28:116–118.
22. Elston RA, Taylor DJ: The preoperative electrocardiogram (Letter). *Lancet.* 1984;1:349.
23. Goldman L, Caldera DL, Nussbaum SR, et al. Multifactorial index of cardiac risk in noncardiac surgical procedures. *N Engl J Med.* 1977;297:845–850.
24. Gold BS, Young ML, Kinman JL, et al: The utility of preoperative electrocardiograms in the ambulatory surgical patient. *Arch Intern Med.* 1992;152:301–305.
25. Goldberger AL, O'Konski M: Utility of the routine electrocardiogram before surgery and on general hospital admission. *Ann Intern Med.* 1986;105:552–557.
26. Slive HL (ed): Diagnostic and therapeutic technology assessment: mandatory ECG before elective surgery. *JAMA.* 1983;250:540.
27. Forrer MI: The value of obligatory preoperative electrocardiograms: a survey of 1260 patients. *J Am Med Wom Assoc.* 1978;33:459–469.
28. Rabkin SW, Horne JM: Preoperative electrocardiography. Its cost-effectiveness in detecting abnormalities when a previous tracing exists. *Can Med Assoc J.* 1979;121:301–306.
29. Mckee RF, Scott EM: The value of routine preoperative investigations. *Ann R Coll Surg Engl.* 1987;69:160–162.
30. Mauney FM Jr, Ebort PA, Sabiston DC Jr: Postoperative myocardial in-

farction: a study of predisposing factors, diagnosis and mortality in a high risk group of surgical patients. *Ann Surg*. 1970;172:497–503.
31. Tabhan S, Moffitt EA, Taylor WF, et al: Myocardial infarction after general anesthesia. *JAMA*. 1972;220:1461–1464.
32. Steen PA, Tinker JH, Terhan S: Myocardial reinfarction after anesthesia and surgery. *JAMA*. 1978;239:2566–2570.
33. Von Knorring J: Postoperative myocardial infarction: A prospective study in a risk group of surgical patients. *Surgery*. 1981;90:55–60.
34. Rao TLK, Jacobs KH, EL-Etr AA: Reinfarction following anesthesia in patients with myocardial infarction. *Anesthesiology*. 1983;59:499–605.
35. Hubbell FA, Greenfield S, Tyler JL, et al: The impact of routine admission chest X-ray films on patient care. *N Engl J Med*. 1985;312:209–213.
36. Moorman JR, Hlatky MA, Eddy DM, et al: The yield of the routine admission electrocardiogram: A study in a general medical service. *Ann Intern Med*. 1986;103:590–595.
37. Garland JL, Wolfson AB: Routine admission electrocardiography in emergency department patients. *Ann Emerg Med*. 1994;23:276–280.
38. Fesmire FM, Percy RF, Wears RL: Diagnostic and prognostic importance of comparing the initial to the previous electrocardiogram in patients admitted for suspected acute myocardial infarction. *South Med J*. 1991;84:841–846.
39. Lee TH, Cook EF, Weisberg MC, et al: Impact of the availability of a prior electrocardiogram on the triage of the patient with acute chest pain. *J Gen Intern Med*. 1990;5:381–388.
40. Ziemba SE, Hubbell FA, Fine MJ, et al: Resting electrocardiograms as baseline tests: Impact on the management of elderly patients. *Am J Med*. 1991;91:576–583.
41. Rubenstein LZ, Greenfield S: The baseline ECG in the evaluation of acute cardiac complaints. *JAMA*. 1980;244:2536–2539.
42. Hoffman JR, Igarashi E: Influence of electrocardiographic findings on admission decisions in patients with acute chest pain. *Am J Med*. 1985;79:699–707.
43. Sox HC: The baseline electrocardiogram. *Am J Med*. 1991;91:573–575.

SECTION III
DIAGNOSTIC TESTS

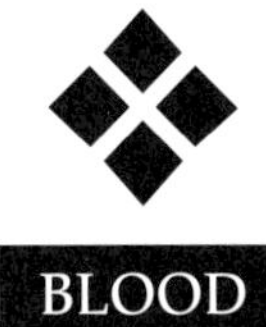

BLOOD

Chapter

Complete Blood Count

Theodore R. Delbridge

The complete blood count (CBC) is the most commonly ordered emergency department (ED) laboratory test.[1] Approximately one fourth to one third of the 100 million patients seen annually in the United States' EDs have a CBC performed.[2, 3] Hematologists have advocated even more frequent performance of the CBC.[4] In fact, the CBC has been viewed by some as an integral component of any physical examination.[5]

COMPONENTS

The CBC report includes hemoglobin (Hgb) concentration, hematocrit (Hct), erythrocyte indices, white blood cell (WBC) count, platelet (Plt) quantification, and evaluation of the peripheral blood smear (PBS). The Hgb concentration is expressed as grams of Hgb per deciliter of blood; the methodology for the determination is generally colorimetric and is precise within $\pm 2\%$.[6] The Hct indicates the fraction of blood volume that is composed of erythrocytes (RBCs); it is reported as a percentage and is more dependent on erythrocyte number than on average cell size.[6–8] The RBC number is determined by direct enumeration or calculated indirectly using Hgb and Hct; normal adult blood contains 5 million (5×10^6) RBCs per microliter, accounting for a total circulating RBC mass of 26 trillion (26×10^{12}) RBCs.[9]

The relative amount of blood plasma affects these parameters. For example, a relative expansion of blood plasma without an equivalent expansion in the number of RBCs, as occurs during pregnancy, results in lower measured RBC parameters, even though the absolute number of RBC has not decreased.

Erythrocyte (ie, RBC) indices can suggest routes for further investigation of disease states,[10] but they are not diagnostic. The mean corpuscular volume (MCV), expressed in femtoliters, is determined by dividing the Hct by the RBC count. The mean corpuscular Hgb (MCH) is the average weight, or content, of Hgb in the RBC sample and is determined by dividing the Hgb concentration by the erythrocyte count; it is reported as picograms Hgb per cell. The mean corpuscular Hgb concentration (MCHC) is the average Hgb concentration in a given volume of packed RBCs. It is determined by dividing the Hgb content by the Hct to yield the weight per 100 mL packed RBCs. The MCHC is reported as a percentage (grams per deciliter). The red blood cell distribution width (RDW) is essentially a mathematic presentation of anisocytosis, which can be seen on the PBS,[11] and represents the coefficient of variation of RBC size.[12] It is normally 11.5 to 14.6%, and it can be normal or high but not low. High RDW values are due to a dimorphic subpopulation of RBCs, often in the presence of a nutritional deficiency, such as iron, folate, or vitamin B12.[9]

The peripheral WBC count is a function of the relative rates of bone marrow and lymphoid leukocyte production, cell margination, and tissue consumption of leukocytes. Therefore, the WBC count may be increased by enhanced marrow and lymphoid production, decreased WBC margination, or decreased tissue migration of cells. The converse is true of leukopenia.

The WBC differential count determines the contribution of neutrophils (PMNs), band forms, lymphocytes, monocytes, basophils, and eosinophils to the total leukocyte count. A number of factors, including age, race, sex, exercise, and smoking, affect the total "normal" WBC and differential counts. Age must be considered when interpreting the differential for pediatric patients. The WBC count peaks in the first 12 hours of life and then declines to normal adult values by age 21 years.[13] Lymphocytes become the predominant cell type soon after birth and are replaced by PMNs by 5 years of age.[14]

It has been noted that in blacks the total WBC count per mm^3 is 1000 to 1200 lower than in nonblacks.[15, 16] Furthermore, 20% of healthy black infants have been found to have an absolute neutrophil count (ANC) less than 1000/mm^3, whereas very few white infants do. In cases of meningitis, black children have significantly lower WBC counts than do white children. Of black children, 23%, compared with 58% of white children, have ANC counts greater than 10,000/mm^3.[17] Furthermore, twice as many black patients as white patients with appendicitis have preoperative WBC counts less than 11,000/mm^3.[18]

During pregnancy the WBC count increases by approximately 1000 mm^3,[19, 20] and cigarette smoking is associated with a WBC increase of 1000 to 1800/mm^3.[21–24]

The normal band:PMN ratio is 0.1:0.3. An increase in this ratio constitutes a "shift to the left," an increase in cell immaturity resulting from a higher bone marrow output of WBCs. Because both PMNs and bands marginate to blood vessel walls in similar proportions, demargination by itself does not alter the circulating band:PMN ratio.[25] Thus, exogenous administration of epinephrine or increased endogenous catecholamine secretion may cause a neutrophilic leukocytosis by demargination but not a higher proportion of bands. In contrast, therapeutic corticosteroid administration not only causes demargination but also increases bone marrow output, resulting in both leukocytosis and more band forms.[13]

In addition to RBC and WBC data, the CBC routinely includes an evaluation of Plts. Platelets are estimated as absent, reduced, adequate, or increased, or they may be specifically quantitated. Thrombocytopenia is present when the Plt count is less than 100,000/mm^3. Normally the Plt : RBC ratio is 1 : 20 (range: 10 to 30).

The PBS, commonly available but often underutilized, may provide useful information in selected ED patients.[26] An examination of RBC morphology identifies cells as normochromic or hypochromic and as macrocytic, normocytic, or microcytic; it thus may narrow the list of potential causes of anemia or indicate a specific etiology.[27] Anisocytosis denotes a variable size of the RBCs. Poikilocytosis indicates cells of variable shape; these include helmet, pear, teardrop, oval, and other shapes, which can result from altered RBC production.[28] Both anisocytosis and poikilocytosis are nonspecific findings found in many blood disorders, but other morphologic variances are more specific for certain disease processes.

Morphologic information about WBCs can also be appreciated by PBS examination. If PMNs with more than five lobes constitute more than 5% of the population, PMN hypersegmentation is said to be present.[28] Atypical lymphocytes, large cells (12 to 16 μm in diameter) with a finely granular cytoplasm and irregular nucleus, may be identified. Other potential findings include Döhle inclusion bodies, (cytoplasmic remnants of free ribosomes), vacuolization (a result of intracellular bacterial degradation), and toxic granulations.

ACCURACY, PRECISION, AND TECHNICAL FACTORS

Complete blood count measurements are affected by a number of factors. The validity of measurements is less for capillary than for venous blood because of interstitial fluid dilution and variations from laminar flow.[6] Fingerstick Hgb measurements can vary by 6% owing to such factors as cold skin and vigorous squeezing. Ear lobe Hgb measurements can be 15% higher than for fingerstick samples.[29] For venous samples, hemoconcentration can occur after 60 seconds of tourniquet application. In addition, hemolysis is frequent with improper technique.

Three anticoagulants are commonly used in blood sample tubes for hematology tests—sodium heparin, trisodium citrate, and tripotassium or disodium ethylenediaminetetra-acetic acid (EDTA). Citrate and EDTA prevent coagulation by precipitating calcium or binding it in a nonionizable form to inhibit activation of the clotting cascade.[9] Blood collection tubes must be adequately filled and the sample exposed to EDTA for at least 20 minutes.[12] Because EDTA prevents Plt clumping, it is the anticoagulant of choice for cell counts. EDTA-preserved blood samples yield valid results for up to 6 hours at room temperature and for 24 hours at 4°C; beyond these times, RBC swelling results in increased MCV and Hct and decreased MHC measurements.[6]

Blood cell counts are now performed almost exclusively by automatic blood cell counters. These instruments rely on colorimetric, electrical, and light-scattering properties to directly measure Hgb, count the number of particles per unit volume, and measure the mean size of particles.[5] All the other parameters are calculated using these three measurements. The Hgb concentration is commonly determined spectrophotometrically, with a precision of ±1 to 2%.[9] Cell populations may be quantitated by suspending the cells in a conductive solution. The cells pass through sized apertures across which an electrical current is applied, and the measured electrical impedance indicates cell numbers and sizes.[12] Light-scattering systems also determine cell numbers after the population of interest is selected by means of chemical reactions that degrade other cells.

White blood cell differential counts are also determined by automated techniques that distinguish leukocytes by cell volume after chemically induced differential cytoplasmic shrinkage.[3] This technique allows quantification of lymphocytes (small cells), monocytes (medium cells), and granulocytes (large cells).

White blood cell counts may be artifactually high if there is incomplete lysis of RBCs prior to WBC measurement or if in vitro Plt clumping occurs.[12, 30] Conversely, a spuriously low WBC count results if there has been inadvertent lysis of WBCs. Similarly, errors in Plt measurement can occur because of preset upper and lower size thresholds.[31] White blood cell or RBC fragments or very microcytic RBCs may be counted as Plts, producing a spuriously high Plt count. Plts clumped in the blood sample, perhaps due to improper collection or anticoagulation, produce a spuriously low Plt count. Likewise, spuriously high MCV measurements may result from RBC rouleau or cold agglutinin presence.[12]

Manual examination of the PBS is also subject to potential error. Estimates of Plt presence vary by as much as 25 to 50% from the actual count.[31] Abnormal estimates should therefore be reevaluated using more accurate counting techniques. The WBC differential count is subject to mechanical errors in preparation and staining of the smear, sampling errors, and errors in interpretation of WBC morphology.[32] In addition, the statistical effects of counting low frequency cells, such as eosinophils, cause the traditional 100-cell manual differential to be poorly reproducible.[33, 32] Thus, the percentage of cells attributed to a particular cell line can differ by as much as 50% in each direction owing to chance variation and the cells selected for counting when the smear is read.[34] Furthermore, the classification of WBCs is often not obvious. When members of the College of American Pathologists were shown a photographed WBC, 50% identified it as a PMN and 50% identified it as a band.[35]

Approximately 50% of WBC differential counts can be considered abnormal on the basis of the relative prevalence of cell types. Only about 10%, however, are abnormal when absolute numbers of cells are considered.[36]

DIAGNOSTIC SENSITIVITY AND SPECIFICITY, PREDICTIVE VALUES, AND UTILITY

The specificity and sensitivity of the CBC, which for other types of laboratory tests may be population independent, depend in many cases on the spectrum of disease to which the CBC is applied. Thus, specificity and sensitivity are somewhat population dependent. Furthermore, results are not reported dichotomously as positive or negative, but rather as a range of values requiring interpretation in light of patients' symptoms and suspected illnesses.

Red Blood Cell Count

The most common RBC-related abnormality is anemia, and the only way to determine whether a patient is anemic is to check a blood count. Although physical findings such as pale mucous membranes are helpful, these are subtle features that have very poor sensitivity and specificity. The recognition of nonemergent anemia should prompt several questions. Among them is whether the anemia is real. Pseudoanemia can be the result of physiologic adjustments, as in distance runner's anemia, or hemodilution, as in overhydration or fluid retention.[9] The morphologic type of anemia is addressed by first-line screening tests, including RBC parameters, leukocyte count and differential, Plt count, reticulocyte count, and evaluation of the PBS.[37] Erythrocyte cell size is used to classify anemia as microcytic, normocytic, or macrocytic and further as hypochromic or normochromic by RBC appearance on the PBS.[9] The appearance of hyperchromia is due to poor light transmission through thicker cells; it is artifactual except in cases of spherocytosis.[9]

An MCV less than 80 often indicates chronic iron deficiency or thalassemia minor. Megaloblastic anemia results in MCV values greater than 100; values greater than 120 are also found in cases of liver disease.[9] The MCHC is rarely below 30% except in cases of severe iron-deficiency anemia. Values greater than 38% are correlated with hereditary spherocytosis; when greater than 40% the MCHC indicates an error in the erythrocyte measurements.[9]

Fragmented RBCs (schistocytes) with thrombocytopenia suggest disseminated intravascular coagulation (DIC) or thrombotic thrombocytopenia purpura (TTP).[38] Pathologic rouleau formation or agglutination is found with elevated plasma fibrinogen, in the presence of cold agglutinins,[39] or in multiple myeloma.

White Blood Cell Count and Differential

The significance of the WBC and differential counts is usually less clear than that of RBC parameters. Infection and inflammation are the two most common causes of leukocytosis, usually accompanied by PMN immaturity (increased bands, ''shift to the left'').[13] Neutrophils are most commonly increased in the presence of bacterial infections, but this may also occur with viral infections and occasionally with parasitic infections.[13] Other causes of PMN elevations include tissue necrosis (eg, cancer, burns, trauma, myocardial infarction); metabolic disorders (eg, renal failure, diabetic ketoacidosis); hemorrhage; hemolysis; and myeloproliferative disorders.[13] Lymphocytic leukocytosis is commonly due to viral infection (eg, Epstein-Barr, hepatitis, varicella, mumps, rubella); chronic infection (eg, syphilis); lymphoproliferative disease; acute lymphocytic leukemia; chronic lymphocytic leukemia; and some bacterial infections (eg, pertussis).

Monocytosis has been associated with lymphoma, myeloproliferative disorders, malignancy, and collagen vascular disorders. Basophilia is associated with chronic granulocytic leukemia and other myeloproliferative disorders. Eosinophilia is associated with parasitic infections, allergies, asthma, and malignancies, such as Hodgkin's disease.

Leukopenia is most commonly due to neutropenia, which can be a poor prognostic sign in cases of overwhelming infection when the pool of stored PMNs is exhausted.[13] Neutropenia can also result from defective marrow production, drug effects, and cytotoxic agents.

Hypersegmented PMNs are typically encountered in cases of megaloblastic anemia,[28, 40] but are also encountered in severe sepsis, uremia, some myeloproliferative disorders, metastic malignancy, and heat stroke.[41]

Use of the White Blood Cell Count in the Evaluation of Abdominal Pain

Blood counts are frequently obtained to aid diagnostic decisions regarding ED patients complaining of abdominal pain. In a retrospective study of 1000 consecutive cases of patients presenting to the ED with complaints of abdominal pain, a CBC was performed in 95%.[42] The WBC count was greater than 10,000/mm^3 in 90% of patients with appendicitis; 78% with acute cholecystitis; 43% with gastroenteritis; 56% with intestinal obstruction; and 31% with abdominal pain of undetermined etiology. Of patients who underwent immediate surgical intervention, those younger than 65 years were more likely to have a WBC count >10,000/mm^3 than those older than 65 years.[42] Thus, although leukocytosis often accompanies diseases requiring surgery, it is also present in those that do not. Normal WBC values are not always reassuring, they are common in the elderly, and they cannot be the determinants of conservative treatment.[42]

The majority of investigations regarding the value of the WBC count in cases of appendicitis have been retrospective, so that evidence regarding its impact on decision making in the ED is indirect. In 312 patients suspected of having appendicitis, leukocytosis (>9000/mm^3 in adults, >15,000/mm^3 in children) had positive predictive values (95% confidence intervals, CI) of 0.46 to 0.64 in adults and 0.1 to 0.65 in children. The negative predictive values of the absence of leukocytosis was 0.84 to 0.96 in adults and 0.60 to 0.83 in children.[43]

In 962 pediatric patients who underwent appendectomy, 84% with histologically proven appendicitis had significant leukocytosis and 88% had a shift to the left. Of those with a normal appendix, 42% had leukocytosis or shift to the left or both.[44]

A prospective analysis of the WBC count when appendicitis was suspected found that 37% of patients with a normal WBC count had histologically proven appendicitis, and 24% with leukocytosis had a normal appendix. The WBC count was at variance with the clinical impression in 39% of patients. In 75% of these cases, the clinical impression was correct. Thus, if undue significance is given to the WBC count when it conflicts with the clinical findings, it is likely to lead to an incorrect course of management in 75% of such cases.[45]

Use of the White Blood Cell Count in the Evaluation of Possible Infection

The WBC count is of limited value when an infection is apparent. Furthermore, it is not very helpful when attempting to identify pediatric patients with occult infections. The positive predictive value of a WBC count ≥15,000/mm^3 has been reported to be 75% for viral infection, 18% for pneumonia, 6% for urinary tract infection, and 0.01% for meningitis in male patients 3 to 24 months old.[46] Although leukocytosis increases the likelihood of occult bacterial infection, even with a left shift viral illness remains much more likely. Furthermore, leukocytosis without an obvious infection source indicates a one in 10,000 chance of occult meningitis. Given the rarity of occult bacterial meningitis, the apparent lack of morbidity associated with gross underdetection of occult pneumonia, and the less invasive, less expensive, and more specific tests for urinary tract infections, clinicians should critically reexamine using the CBC in the young febrile child.[46]

Admission and Preoperative White Blood Cell Count

Blood counts provide little information that affects patient management when obtained routinely prior to medical admission to a hospital or preoperatively. In the case of routine medical preadmission testing, the hematocrit was reported to be abnormal in 8%. Diagnostic and therapeutic management changes were made in only 2.2% of patients (95% CI, 0 to 4.6%).[47] Routine WBC counts were abnormal in 13%, but, although this led to additional testing in 79% of those patients, no treatment changes resulted.[47] Additionally, 62% of all abnormal findings were never acknowledged in the patient's record.[47] In contrast, 49.6% of CBCs specifically obtained as part of a diagnostic evaluation were abnormal.[15]

A preoperative CBC is indicated if physical findings suggest the presence of anemia; if there is abnormal bleeding; if a primary hematologic disorder is suspected or known; if systemic disease associated with anemia (eg, malignancy, chronic renal failure) is present; if there is history of chemotherapy; or if a concurrent infection is present.[27, 48–51] Preoperative CBCs have been reported to be unindicated for 48% of cases in which they were obtained, detecting abnormalities in only 0.2% of patients, none of which were clinically significant.[51] Only 10% of obtained Plt counts are indicated; unsuspected abnormalities occur in only 0.5% of patients and are not clinically significant.[51] In patients who are otherwise well and will be undergoing surgical procedures in which bleeding is expected to be minimal, a CBC is not necessary for management through surgery.

On the average, manual differentials are obtained on every 1.6 CBCs,[3] yet most add little to the information obtained from the history and physical examination and total leukocyte count.[52, 53] When availability of PBS examination was limited, no adverse effect on patient management was noted. Furthermore, all the PBS examinations then requested were potentially helpful for diagnosis or management; 60% of them were related to RBC morphology and not to WBCs.[3] Reportedly, 60% of differential counts are without indication, including those in patients with febrile illness, nonpeptic abdominal illness, respiratory infection, genitourinary infection, local infection, chronic disease, bleeding diathesis, adenopathy, or follow-up of a previously abnormal test.[54] Clinically indicated differentials are abnormal in approximately 37% of cases, whereas 13% of "case-finding" differentials are abnormal.[54]

The WBC differential is most helpful in the diagnostic workup of a patient with a newly suspected infection; fever and normal WBC count; suspected disease associated with secondary abnormalities of the cell lines if the results of the tests will affect diagnostic or treatment decisions; or suspected primary hematologic disorder.[54, 55] The leukocyte differential count does not exclude sepsis when the suspicion is high nor confirm it when suspicion is low.[54, 55]

COST AND UTILITY

The cost of each CBC is approximately $10 to 25.[2, 56, 57, 57a] Charges to the patient for a CBC that includes differential, the most costly part of the examination, and Plt count often exceed $100. In some institutions, the charge for a stat CBC is greater than $150.[57, 57a]

Compared with the costs of many tests utilized in the ED, the cost of a CBC is quite low. However, less expensive items compose an important share of physician-generated healthcare costs.[58, 59] The cost of the CBC is not only that of the test itself but also includes the cost of further actions impelled by abnormal results. When a group of physicians including emergency physicians was given one of two patient vignettes, 19% made a decision for hospital admission, while many opted for outpatient treatment based solely on the WBC count.[60]

A prospective evaluation of the utility of the CBC when evaluating female ED patients with lower abdominal pain found that CBC results prompted correct management decisions in only 1% of patients. Complete blood count results also prompted incorrect decisions in 1% of patients. In the remaining 98%, knowing the CBC result did not change the planned diagnostic or therapeutic course.[61]

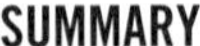

SUMMARY

Complete blood counts are obtained in one fourth to one third of the approximately 100 million ED patients in the United States each year. Directly and indirectly, through resulting decisions for further tests or hospital admission, CBCs compose a significant health care expense. The utility of a test in specific situations depends on its ability to contribute information and on whether the results enable the clinician to cross a diagnostic or therapeutic threshold.[29] Currently, there is a paucity of data to support the use of the CBC in the majority of the ED patients for whom it is obtained. For patients with such illnesses as appendicitis, the CBC is at best supportive and may actually prompt erroneous alterations in management course. The CBC is not useful as an indicator of occult illness, given the many patients who have abnormal results but no serious illnesses. In ED patients overall, leukocytosis $\geq$12,500/mm^3 has been reported to have a positive predictive value for bacterial illness of 26%; PMNs $>$10,000/mm^3 or bands $>$500/mm^3 have a positive predictive value of 33%.[2] It has been calculated that, to obtain a single WBC result that affects patient management, costs in excess of $10,000 must be incurred for tests that have no impact.[2] Furthermore, changes in care based on CBC results may be incorrect in as many as 50% of cases.[2]

In the ED setting the CBC is generally both insensitive and nonspecific, usually does not alter management,[1] and may actually lead the unwary clinician *away* from the correct diagnosis. The widespread routine use of the CBC in the ED setting should continue to be critically reexamined.

REFERENCES

1. Yeung MC, Ferreira P, Frohlich J, et al: The effects of age, smoking and alcohol on routine laboratory tests. *Am J Clin Pathol.* 1981;75:320.
2. Callaham M: Inaccuracy and expense of the leukocyte count in making urgent clinical decisions. *Ann Emerg Med.* 1986;15:774–781.
3. Edelman BB, Groleau GA, Barish RA: Use of a mildly restrictive administrative protocol to reduce orders for manual blood film examination from the emergency department. *J Emerg Med.* 1990;8:1–13.
4. Hamilton P: Routine diagnostic testing. *Lancet.* 1989;2:1528.
5. Gabuzda TG: The diagnosis of anemia. *Del Med J.* 1982;54:527–536.
6. Navari RM et al: The peripheral blood smear in heat stroke—An aid to diagnosis. *Ala J Med Sci.* 1983;20:137–140.
7. Larkin EC, Watson-Williams EJ: Alcohol and the blood. *Med Clin North Am.* 1984;68:105–120.
8. Wintrobe MM: Erythrocytes in man. *Medicine.* 1930;9:195.

9. Gaillard HM, Hamilton GC: Hemoglobin/hematocrit and other erthrocyte parameters. *Emerg Med Clin North Am.* 1986;4:15–40.
10. Winkel P, Statland BE: The acute effect of cigarette smoking on the concentrations of blood leukocyte types in healthy young women. *Am J Clin Pathol.* 1981;75:781.
11. Rich EC, Crowson TW, Connelly DP: Effectiveness of differential leukocyte count in case finding in the ambulatory care setting. *JAMA.* 1983;249:633.
12. Poh S: Shigellosis: A clue to early diagnosis. *Pediatrics.* 1967;39:119.
13. Wenz B, Genhis P, Canova C, et al: The clinical utility of the leukocyte differential in emergency medicine. *Am J Clin Pathol.* 1986;86:298–303.
14. Wasserman M, Levinstein M, Keller E, et al: Utility of fever, white blood cells, and differential count in predicting bacterial infections in the elderly. *J Am Geriatr Soc.* 1989;37:537–543.
15. Caramihai E, Karayalcin G, Aballi A, et al: Leukocyte count differences in healthy white and black children 1 to 5 years of age. *J Pediatr.* 1975;86:251.
16. Karayalcin G, Rosner F, Sawitsky A: Pseudoneutropenia in Negroes: A normal phenomenon. *NY State Med J.* 1972;72:1815.
17. Rumke CL, Bezemer PD, Kuik DJ: Normal values and least significant differences for differential leukocyte counts. *J Chron Dis.* 1975;28:661–668.
18. Hyman P, Westring DW: Leucocytosis in acute appendicitis: Observed racial difference. *JAMA.* 1974;229:1630.
19. Efrati P, Presently B, Margalith M, et al: Leukocytes of normal pregnant women. *Obstet Gynecol.* 1964;23:429.
20. Oski FA, et al: Leukocytic inclusions—Dohle bodies associated with platelet abnormality (the May-Hegglin anomaly). *Blood.* 1962;6:657–667.
21. Bain BJ, England JM: Normal hematological values: sex difference in neutrophil count. *Br Med J.* 1975;1:306.
22. Helman N, and Rubenstein LS: The effect of age, sex and smoking on erythrocytes and leukocytes. *Am J Clin Pathol.* 1975;63:35.
23. Wesson SK, Mercado T, Austin M, et al: Percentage and absolute differential counts on 119 healthy US Navy midshipmen (letter). *Lancet.* 1980;1:552.
24. Wintrobe MM et al: *Clinical Hematology.* 8th ed. Philadelphia: Lea & Febiger; 1981.
25. Boggs DR, Winkelstein A: *White Cell Manual.* Philadelphia: FA Davis; 1981.
26. Clodfelter RL: The peripheral smear. *Emerg Med Clin North Am.* 1986;4:59–74.
27. Wallerstein RO: Role of the laboratory in the diagnosis of anemia. *JAMA.* 1976;236:490–493.
28. Herbert V: Megaloblastic anemias, in Beeson P, McDermott W (eds): *Textbook of Medicine.* 14th ed. Philadelphia: WB Saunders; 1975.
29. Sox HC: Probability theory in the use of diagnostic tests: An introduction to critical study of the literature. *Ann Intern Med.* 1986;104:60–66.
30. Simmons A: *Technical Hematology.* 3rd ed. Philadelphia: JB Lippincott; 1980.
31. Hamilton GC: Platelet count. *Emerg Med Clin North Am.* 1986;4:75–85.
32. Roberts GT, El Badawi SB: Red blood cell distribution width index in some hematologic diseases. *Am J Clin Pathol.* 1985;83:222–226.
33. Dutcher TF: Leukocyte differentials: Are they worth the effort? *Clin Lab Med.* 1984;4:71–87.

34. Barnett CW: The unavoidable error in the differential count of the leukocytes of the blood. *J Clin Invest.* 1933;12:77–85.
35. Bacus JW: The observer error in peripheral blood cell classification. *Am J Clin Pathol.* 1973;59:223–230.
36. Werman HA, Brown CG: White blood cell count and differential count. *Emerg Med Clin North Am.* 1986;4:41–58.
37. Kellermeyer RW: General principles of the evaluation and therapy of anemia. *Med Clin North Am.* 1984;68:533.
38. Bick RL: D.I.C. and related syndromes: Etiology, pathophysiology, diagnosis and management. *Am J Hematol.* 1978;5:265–282.
39. Axlson JA, LoBuglio JA: Immune hemolytic anemia. *Med Clin North Am.* 1980;64:597–606.
40. Chanarin I: Investigation and management of megaloblastic anemia. *Clin Haematol.* 1976;21:747–754.
41. Murphy J, Henry JB: Effective utilization of clinical laboratories. *Hum Pathol.* 1978;9:625–633.
42. Brewer RJ, Golden GT, Hitch DC, et al: Abdominal pain: An analysis of 1000 consecutive cases in a university hospital emergency room. *Am J Surg.* 1976;131:219.
43. Miskowiak J, Burewarth F: The white cell count in acute appendicitis: A prospective blind study. *Dan Med Bull.* 1982;29:210.
44. Lansden FT: Acute appendicitis in children. *Am J Surg.* 1963;106:938.
45. Bolton JP, Craven ER, Croft RJ, et al: An assessment of the value of the white cell count in the management of suspected acute appendicitis. *Br J Surg.* 1975;62:906.
46. Kramer MS, Tange SM, Mills EL, et al: Role of the complete blood count in detecting occult focal bacterial infection in the young child. *J Epidemiol Commun Health.* 1993;46:349–356.
47. Hubbell FA, Frye EB, Akin BV, et al: Routine admission laboratory testing for general medicine patients. *Med Care.* 1988;26:619–630.
48. Dallman PR: Manifestations of iron deficiency. *Semin Hematol.* 1982;19:19–30.
49. Donald WD, Winkler CH: The leukocyte response in patients with shigellosis. *J Pediatr.* 1960;56:61.
50. Friedell GH: Anaemia in cancer. *Lancet.* 1965;1:356–359.
51. Kaplan EB, Sheiner LB, Boeckmann AJ, et al: The usefulness of preoperative laboratory screening. *JAMA.* 1985;253:3576–3581.
52. Sadowitz PD, Oski FA: Differences in polymorphonuclear cell counts between healthy white and black infants: Response to meningitis. *J Pediatr.* 1983;72:405–407.
53. Weitzman M: Diagnostic utility of white blood cell and differential cell counts. *Am J Dis Child.* 1975;129:1183–1189.
54. Rich EL, Crowson TW, Connelly DP: Effectiveness of differential leukocyte count in case finding in the ambulatory care setting. *JAMA.* 1983;249:633.
55. Shapiro MF, Greenfield S: The complete blood count and leukocyte differential count. *Ann Intern Med.* 1987;106:65–74.
56. Karas SJ: *Guidelines for Cost Containment in Emergency Medicine.* Dallas, *Am Coll Emerg Phys.* 1983.
57. University of Pittsburgh Medical Center Hematology Laboratory. Personal communication. 1994.

57a. Todd, JK: Childhood infections: Diagnostic value of peripheral white blood cell and differential cell counts. *Am J Dis Child.* 1974;127:810.
58. Fineberg HV: Clinical chemistries: The high cost of low cost diagnostic tests, in Altman SH, Blendon R (eds): *Medical Technology: The Culprit Behind Health Care Costs?* publication (PHS) 79-3216. Washington, DC: U.S. Dept. of Health, Education and Welfare, 1979;144–165.
59. Moloney TW, Rogers DE: Medical technology: A different view of the contentious debate over costs. *N Engl J Med.* 1979;301:1413–1429.
60. Badgett RG, Hansen CJ, Rogers CS: Clinical usage of the leukocyte count in emergency room decision making. *J Gen Intern Med.* 1990;5:198–202.
61. Silver BE, Patterson JW, Kulic MA, et al: The effect of CBC results on the ED management of women with lower abdominal pain. *Acad Emerg Med.* 1994;1:A65.

Chapter

Arterial Blood Gas Analysis

Linda Carpenter and Vincent P. Verdile

Arterial blood gas (ABG) analysis is the study of choice for evaluating the acid-base and respiratory status of the acutely ill or injured patient. Because ABG analysis is a test commonly ordered within the emergency department (ED), the emergency physician must be familiar with its indications and its limitations and with the interpretation of test results in a variety of clinical situations.

In a typical university hospital, the charges for a simple ABG analysis (pH, pO_2, pCO_2, HCO_3^-, and O_2 saturation) can approach $200.

Oxygen (O_2) is absorbed by the lungs from ambient air or supplemental sources and carried in the blood to cells, where it is needed for cellular metabolism. The majority of oxygen is transported bound to the hemoglobin in red blood cells; a small and usually clinically insignificant amount is dissolved in plasma. Carbon dioxide (CO_2), the end product of cellular combustion, diffuses out of the cells and is carried by the blood to the lungs, where it is released into the environment. Like oxygen, some CO_2 is transported by red blood cells and by plasma, but, unlike oxygen, the majority of CO_2 is transported dissolved in plasma.

The partial pressure of oxygen in ambient air at sea level is approximately 150 mmHg. Oxygen diffuses from the alveoli to the pulmonary capillary blood, where it is exchanged for CO_2. Oxygen diffuses at about one twentieth the rate of CO_2. The alveolar gas equation quantifies the relationship between alveolar partial pressure of oxygen (P_{AO_2}) and partial pressure of CO_2 (Pa_{CO_2}).

$$P_{AO_2} = F_{IO_2}\ (P_{atm} - P_{H20}) - (P_{ACO_2}/0.8)$$

Unlike oxygen, carbon dioxide readily diffuses across the capillary-alveolar membrane. The arterial pCO_2 is thus identical to the alveolar pCO_2 and directly reflects alveolar ventilation.

SAMPLE ACQUISITION

Several guidelines should be followed when obtaining a sample. If possible, the patient should be exposed to a constant inspired oxygen concentration (F_{IO_2}) for 15 to 20 minutes prior to obtaining the sample.[1] The radial, brachial, and femoral arteries are commonly utilized vessels. Prior to cannulation of the radial artery, the Allen test should be completed to assess the patency of the collateral circulation of the palmar arch. The patient is asked to open and close the fist forcefully several times. The examiner first occludes both the radial and ulnar arteries and then releases pressure from the ulnar artery. If the palmar arch is intact the hand's normal color should return promptly on both the ulnar and radial sides of the palm. If the test indicates a lack of adequate collateral circulation, the sample should not be obtained from that wrist and the contralateral wrist should be tested.

A small (22 to 25)-gauge needle minimizes patient discomfort when obtaining the sample. Test results do not appear to be affected by needle size or the need to aspirate to obtain the sample.[2] A local anesthetic such as 1% lidocaine can also be injected dermally at the puncture site to minimize pain. Care must be taken to avoid making a large wheal with local anesthetic because this might interfere with or obscure palpation of the radial pulse. A heparinized syringe must be used to prevent clotting of the specimen. Once the needle is withdrawn pressure should be immediately applied at the puncture site for several minutes. Potential complications from arterial puncture include bleeding, hematoma formation, thrombosis, and infection.

Rapid transport of the sample to the laboratory for prompt analysis is mandatory to ensure accurate results. If transport or analysis is to be delayed more than 20 minutes, it is recommended that the sample be placed on ice to decrease cellular metabolism and resulting changes in pO_2 and pCO_2 values.[3]

A blood sample from a warmed hand vein has pH and pCO_2 values similar to those of arterial blood.[4] It is recommended that the puncture site be warmed to 45°C for 10 to 15 minutes prior to obtaining the sample.[1, 5] In addition, in the neonate, capillary blood samples are often used for analysis of pH and $Pa\text{CO}_2$. Indwelling arterial catheters can also be used when obtaining a specimen. One must be careful to draw up and discard the amount of standing fluid in the heparinized line to avoid erroneous test results.

SPECIMEN ANALYSIS

Modern blood gas analyzers are equipped with three electrodes for measuring pH, $p\text{CO}_2$, and $p\text{O}_2$. Severinghaus and glass/calomel electrodes measure the potential difference between the sample and standard solutions to determine $Pa\text{CO}_2$ and pH values, respectively.[1] The $Pa\text{O}_2$ value is obtained by measuring the current created by the reduction of oxygen in the sample.[5] Most clinical laboratories use fully automatic blood gas analyzers that have the capacity to measure not only pH, $p\text{CO}_2$, and $p\text{O}_2$ but also Na^+, K^+, Ca^{2+}, and Hct. These instruments can then use these measured values to calculate values for HCO_3^-, base excess, oxygen saturation, hemoglobin concentration, and alveolar-arterial (A-a) oxygen gradient.[6] Direct measurement of oxygen saturation is made with the use of a cooximeter. Generally speaking, contemporary blood gas analyzers are highly accurate devices.[6]

SOURCES OF MEASUREMENT ERRORS

Delay in Transport or Analysis

As noted previously, rapid transport and analysis are mandatory to ensure accurate blood gas results. The sample should be placed on ice to slow cell metabolism if a delay of more than 20 minutes is anticipated before analysis can be performed. This recommendation is based on the results of several studies that have shown that there is a significant decrease in the $p\text{O}_2$ and pH and a significant increase in the $p\text{CO}_2$, when blood gas samples are kept at room temperature longer than 20 to 30 minutes.[3, 7]

Heparin

Heparin is used to prevent clotting of the blood sample prior to analysis. If liquid heparin is present in the blood gas syringe, the excess should be expelled before the specimen is drawn, leaving just enough liquid to coat the syringe barrel and fill the needle dead space. More than this amount can result in alterations of blood gas measurements. Excessive heparin in the syringe causes a significant decrease in pCO_2, HCO_3^-, and base excess values.[8–10]

Air Bubbles

Care should also be taken to avoid the introduction of air bubbles into the sample. Air bubble volumes as small as 5 to 10% of the specimen volume have been shown to result in significant increases in the pO_2 value[7, 11] and decreases in the pCO_2 value.[11] The size of the air bubble does not correlate with the rate of change of the pO_2 and pCO_2. Thus, complete evacuation of air bubbles from the blood gas specimen is necessary to prevent substantial errors in sample analysis.

Temperature

Arterial blood gas analysis is normally performed at 37°C. For every °C difference between the patient's body temperature and the temperature at which the sample is analyzed, the PaO_2 and $PaCO_2$ vary by 7 and 3%, respectively.[5, 12] Most analyzers are capable of reports of temperature-corrected ABG values. The changes in ABG values due to temperature differences are not, however, usually considered clinically significant if the patient's temperature is between 35 and 39°C.[12, 13] The current consensus appears to be that temperature correction is not necessary, and arterial blood should be uniformly reported at 37°C.[4]

Leukocytosis

Cellular metabolism is responsible for the increase in pCO_2 and decrease in pO_2 that become evident when the blood sample is allowed to remain at room temperature for a prolonged period. Intuitively, one might then conclude that in states in which there is an increased cell count (eg, leukemia, thrombocytosis) a much greater fall in the pO_2 value would occur when the blood sample is kept at room temperature. A study by Hess and coworkers did conclude that the pO_2 value fell at a significantly faster rate in patients with leukocytosis or thrombocytosis compared with control subjects, resulting in the phenomenon of pseudohypoxemia.[14]

RANGE OF NORMAL AND INTERPRETATION OF ARTERIAL BLOOD GAS RESULTS

Oxygen

The normal $Pa{O_2}$ values for healthy adults at sea level range from 80 to 100 mmHg. Values less than 80 mmHg are generally said to indicate hypoxemia. The arterial $p{O_2}$ *decreases* with advancing age. Estimates of the normal $Pa{O_2}$ in the older population can be made by the use of several formulas. One simple formula for $Pa{O_2}$ estimation in patients between the ages of 60 and 80 years is $Pa{O_2} = 80 - (\text{age} - 60)$.[1] Supplemental oxygen normally increases the $Pa{O_2}$. In healthy individuals, the normal $Pa{O_2}$ must be at least equal to the inspired $Fi{O_2}$ multiplied by 500.[12]

The oxygen saturation (O_2 sat) reflects the ratio of oxyhemoglobin to total hemoglobin, with an O_2 sat of 95 to 100% considered normal. The oxyhemoglobin dissociation curve illustrates the relationship between the arterial $p{O_2}$ and the O_2 sat. As reflected in the sigmoidal shape of the curve, large changes in $Pa{O_2}$ may result in only small changes in the percent saturation. This is an important consideration for clinicians who use pulse oximetry and O_2 sat as their only guides in assessing a patient's respiratory function.

Alveolar-Arterial Gradient

The accepted range of the normal A-a gradient is 5 to 20 mmHg. An increased A-a gradient results from impaired oxygen exchange between the alveoli and the blood, for example, in pulmonary embolism. The A-a gradient, however, normally increases with age and when healthy subjects breathe 100% O_2.[15, 16] It has been proposed that the a/A ratio may be more useful than the A-a gradient because it is subject to less variation with increasing $Fi{O_2}$ concentrations.[1, 17] The normal a/A ratio is greater than 0.75.

Carbon Dioxide

The accepted range of normal values for $Pa{CO_2}$ is 35 to 45 mmHg. Healthy women, however, have $Pa{CO_2}$ values that are consistently and significantly lower than those of age-matched healthy men.[16] An increase in minute ventilation is directly reflected by a decrease in the $Pa{CO_2}$ value. Hypercapnia reflects inadequate ventilation even though the minute ventilation may be low, high, or normal. Hypercapnia may result from respiratory center dysfunction, neuromuscular disorders, or increased work of breathing and significant fatigue.

Chronic hypercapnia, which is seen frequently in patients with chronic pulmonary disease, can be distinguished from acute hypercapnia by the fact that the pH is relatively normal. This finding is due to a compensatory elevation of the measured bicarbonate value.

Acid-Base Status

The normal range of the arterial pH is 7.35 to 7.45. Acidemia is defined as an arterial pH less than 7.35 and alkalemia as a pH greater than 7.45. Acidosis or alkalosis may be secondary to a respiratory, metabolic, or mixed process. Respiratory acidosis exists when the pco_2 is elevated and the pH is low. The underlying processes precipitating respiratory alkalosis are many, but the basic problem is the patient's enhanced ability to eliminate CO_2 (hyperventilation). This problem results in a low pco_2 level and a high pH. When respiratory acidosis or alkalosis exists, metabolic compensation by the kidneys occurs in an attempt to restore the pH. This result is accomplished by retaining or excreting HCO_3^- as appropriate.

Metabolic disturbances, such as lactic acidosis, diabetic ketoacidosis, and severe diarrhea, can result in a low pH and low HCO_3^-, leading to a metabolic acidosis. Elevation of the serum HCO_3^- and pH by prolonged vomiting or excessive diuretic use can result in metabolic alkalosis. The body attempts to maintain a normal pH during these metabolic disturbances by increasing or decreasing the pco_2 through changes in the respiratory rate or volume.

Table 30–1 summarizes the anticipated physiologic changes that occur with the various acid-base disturbances.

SPECIFIC INDICATIONS FOR OBTAINING ARTERIAL BLOOD GASES IN THE EMERGENCY DEPARTMENT

Asthma

The need for ABG evaluation in patients with asthma has been challenged. In cases of mild airway obstruction, there is usually a respiratory alkalosis because of hyperventilation. There may also be mild hypoxemia. With moderate airway obstruction, the CO_2 is usually in the low to low-normal range, and hypoxemia may be more prominent. In severe airway obstruction, the CO_2 is normal or higher than normal, and hypoxemia is usually quite significant.

TABLE 30–1. NORMAL COMPENSATORY RESPONSES IN ACID-BASE DISORDERS

Metabolic acidosis
For each 1.0 mmol/L decrease in HCO_3^-, the pCO_2 decreases by 1–1.5 mmHg
Metabolic alkalosis
For each 1.0 mmol/L increase in HCO_3^-, the pCO_2 increases by 0.25–1.0 mmHg
Respiratory acidosis, acute
For each 10 mmHg increase in pCO_2, the HCO_3^- increases by 1.0 mmol/L and pH decreases by 0.08
Respiratory acidosis, chronic
For each 10 mmHg increase in pCO_2, the HCO_3^- increases by 4.0 mmol/L
Respiratory alkalosis, acute
For each 10 mmHg decrease in pCO_2, the HCO_3^- decreases by 2.0–4.0 mmol/L and pH increases by 0.0228
Respiratory alkalosis, chronic
For each 10 mmHg decrease in pCO_2, the HCO_3^- decreases by 2.0–5.0 mmol/L

Adapted from Narins RG, Gardner LB: Simple acid-base disturbances. *Med Clin North Am.* 1981;65(2):321–345.

The most common blood gas pattern in an acute asthmatic attack is hypoxemia and respiratory alkalosis. Only in very extreme degrees of obstruction does respiratory acidosis occur.[18] Studies comparing ABGs with pulmonary function testing have shown that ABG values do not correlate with the severity of an attack. Peak expiratory flow rate (PEFR), however, does correlate with the severity of the asthma attack.[19] Hypercarbia or acidosis becomes evident only if the PEFR is less than about 25% of predicted. Although many clinicians still routinely obtain ABGs during the evaluation of a patient with an asthma attack, these data suggest that this practice is unwarranted.

Chronic Obstructive Pulmonary Disease

Arterial blood gases are important to determine the degree of hypoxemia or hypercarbia and acid-base status in the patient with chronic obstructive pulmonary disease (COPD). Emerman and coworkers found a correlation between spirometric data and ABGs in an effort to reduce the need for obtaining ABGs in this patient population. They concluded that hypoxemia and hypercarbia were common findings in patients with

COPD and that spirometry (FEV_1) did not correlate well with the severity of the exacerbation.[20] Thus, ABG analysis remains an important diagnostic tool in this patient population and is instrumental to clinical decision making.

Pulmonary Embolism

Arterial blood gases are mandatory in the evaluation of the patient with suspected pulmonary embolism (PE). Nonetheless, 10 to 15% of patients with documented PE have a po_2 value of >80 mmHg. Thus, an important role of the ABG is in determining the A-a gradient, which is the most sensitive indicator of PE. The combination of an increased A-a gradient and a decreased $paco_2$ has a 98% sensitivity for detecting PE. Conversely, a normal A-a gradient and a normal $paco_2$ are strong evidence against the diagnosis of PE.[21]

Artificial Ventilation

Arterial blood gases are imperative with intubated patients to evaluate the effectiveness of oxygenation and ventilation. Although pulse oximetry can provide an estimate of oxygenation, baseline measurements of pco_2 and po_2 are highly advisable to provide a baseline for monitoring.

ALTERNATIVES TO ARTERIAL BLOOD GASES

The PEFR can be measured simply and inexpensively in the ED. As noted previously, peak flow measurements correlate well with the severity of an asthma attack. Serial measurements can also be used to evaluate a patient's response to therapy and to determine whether hospital admission is necessary. The disposable peak flow devices have decreased significantly the need for ABG evaluation in the asthmatic individual.

Pulse oximetry is a simple, inexpensive, and noninvasive method for evaluating O_2 sat. Although po_2 values can change significantly with minimal changes in the O_2 sat, the pulse oximeter provides a quick and reasonably accurate estimate of oxygenation status.

REFERENCES

1. Ventriglia WJ: Arterial blood gases. *Emerg Med Clin North Am.* 1986;4:235–249.

2. Bageant RA: Variations in arterial blood gas measurements due to sampling techniques. *Res Care.* 1975;20:565–570.
3. Nanji AA, Whitlow KJ: Technical communications: Is it necessary to transport arterial blood samples on ice for pH and gas analysis? *Int Can Anaesth Soc J.* 1984;31:568–571.
4. Hansen JE: Arterial blood gases. *Clin Chest Med.* 1989;10:227–237.
5. Fleisher M, Schwartz MK: Blood gas analysis and acid-base balance, in Sonnenwirth AC, Jarett L (eds.): *Gradwohl's Clinical Laboratory Methods and Diagnosis.* St. Louis: CV Mosby, 1980.
6. Barth E, Muller-Plathe O, Haeckel R, et al: Multicenter evaluation of the blood gas-electrolyte-analyser "BGE." *Eur J Clin Chem Clin Biochem.* 1991;29:281–292.
7. Madiedo G, Sciacca R, Hause L: Air bubbles and temperature effect on blood gas analysis. *Int J Clin Pathol.* 1980;33:864–867.
8. Ordog GJ, Wasserberger J, Balasubramamiam S: Effects of heparin on arterial blood gases. *Ann Emerg Med.* 1985;143:233–238.
9. Goodwin NM, Schreiber MB: Effects of anticoagulants on acid-base and blood gas estimations. *Crit Care Med.* 1979;7:473–474.
10. Hutchinson AS, Ralston SH, Dryburgh FJ, et al: Too much heparin: Possible source of error in blood gas analysis. *Br Med J.* 1983;287:1131–1132.
11. Biswas CK, Ramos JM, Agroyannis B, et al: Blood gas analysis: Effect of air bubbles in syringe and delay in estimation. *Br Med J.* 1982;284:923–927.
12. Shapiro BA, Cane RD: Interpretation of blood gases, in Shoemaker WC, Ayres S, Grenrik A, et al. (eds.): *Textbook of Critical Care Medicine.* Philadelphia: WB Saunders Co, 1989;305–311.
13. Rose CC, Wolfson AB: Respiratory physiology. *Emerg Clin North Am.* 1989;7:187–204.
14. Hess CE, Nichols AB, Hunt WB, et al: Pseudohypoxemia secondary to leukemia and thrombocytosis. *N Engl J Med.* 1979;301:361–363.
15. Tobin MJ: Respiratory monitoring in the intensive care unit. *Am Rev Respir Dis.* 1988;138:1625–1642.
16. Andrews JL, Copeland BE, Salah RM, et al: Arterial blood gas standards for healthy young nonsmoking subjects. *Am J Clin Pathol.* 1981;75:773–780.
17. Gilbert R, Auchincloss JH, Kuppinger M, et al: Stability of the arterial/alveolar oxygen partial pressure ratio. Effects of low ventilation/perfusion regions. *Crit Care Med.* 1979;7:267–272.
18. McFadden ER, Lyons HA: Arterial-blood gas tension in asthma. *N Engl J Med.* 1968;278:1027–1032.
19. Martin TG, Elenbaas RM, Pingleton SH: Use of peak expiratory flow rates to eliminate unnecessary arterial blood gases in acute asthma. *Ann Emerg Med.* 1982;11:31–34.
20. Emerman CL, Connors AF, Lukens TW, et al: Relationship between arterial blood gases and spirometry in acute exacerbations of chronic obstructive pulmonary disease. *Ann Emerg Med.* 1989;18:523–527.
21. Cvitanic O, Marino PL: Improved use of arterial blood gas analysis in suspected pulmonary embolism. *Chest.* 1989;95:48–51.

Chapter

Serum Electrolyte Determination

Clifton W. Callaway

Homeostasis of electrolyte concentrations is critical for maintenance of cellular function throughout the body. Ratios of the intracellular to extracellular concentrations of sodium (Na) and potassium (K) determine transmembrane electrical potentials and drive transport of other molecules. Bicarbonate (HCO_3) is the principal buffer for hydrogen ions, maintaining physiologic pH in the optimum range for many enzymatic reactions. Along with HCO_3, chloride (Cl) ions balance the electrical charge of Na and K. Isolated changes in HCO_3 and Cl, therefore, reflect the presence of other unmeasured anions. Because of these central roles in cellular metabolism, electrolyte abnormalities can be life threatening. Although intracellular electrolyte concentrations are not usually measured, extracellular electrolyte concentrations are frequently measured in serum.

Electrolyte abnormalities occur in many diseases and clinical situations and with many pharmacologic interventions. Consequently, measurement of serum electrolytes has little specificity as a diagnostic test. The primary motivation for ordering electrolytes is to guide further therapy in a clinical situation in which electrolyte abnormalities are suspected. In a few instances, such as altered mental status in hyponatremia and ECG changes in hyper- or hypokalemia, the clinical effects of the electrolyte abnormality are evident, and a diagnostic approach is required to determine the primary etiology of that abnormality. Most often, historical data rather than further testing support a particular diagnosis. This chapter describes the pathophysiologic features of particular electrolyte disturbances and reviews the clinical criteria proposed for ordering serum electrolytes in the emergency department.

SERUM SODIUM

Pseudohyponatremia

Sodium concentration is measured in serum. Because Na is dissolved only in the aqueous phase of serum, nonaqueous, volume-occupying constituents of serum that are Na poor will decrease the apparent concentration of sodium.[1] This situation occurs in hyperlipidemia and hyperproteinemia, in which the aqueous concentration of Na and serum osmolality are normal. Centrifugation of the serum sample in hyperlipidemia provides a better estimate of Na concentration. Alternatively, aqueous Na concentration can be calculated if serum protein or lipid concentrations are known:

$$[Na]_{serum} \text{ decreases } 0.002 \times [\text{plasma lipid (in mg/dL)}]$$

$$[Na]_{serum} \text{ decreases } 0.25 \times [\text{serum protein (in g/dL)} - 8]$$

Osmotically active molecules that do not cross cell membranes, such as glucose and mannitol, draw water out of the intracellular compartment to equalize osmotic gradients. The dilution of serum by these fluid shifts can produce hyponatremia. In contrast, serum Na is normal in uremia because urea passes freely into the intracellular compartment. The degree of hyponatremia is predicted as follows: $[Na]_{serum}$ decreases 1.6 mEq/L per 100 mg/dL increase in glucose or mannitol.

Hyponatremia

True hyponatremia reflects a hypotonic serum and requires an outside source of hypotonic fluid. Decreased serum Na occurs in patients with decreased, increased, or normal extracellular fluid volume (Table 31–1).[1, 2] Partial replacement of Na-containing fluid losses by drinking pure water or by administering hypotonic intravenous fluids produces hypovolemic hyponatremia. Water retention stimulated by decreased intravascular volume or decreased cardiac output produces hypervolemic hyponatremia, such as in congestive heart failure and cirrhotic or nephrotic hypoalbuminemia. Isovolemic hyponatremia occurs in the syndrome of inappropriate antidiuretic hormone secretion (SIADH), hypokalemia, and psychogenic polydipsia.

Clinical features of hyponatremia include mental status changes, lethargy, muscle cramps, seizures, and coma.[2] The central nervous system effects result from the development of cerebral edema as extracellular fluid shifts into the intracellular space. Because the intracellular osmolality can adjust slowly to prevent edema, the rate at which hyponatremia develops determines the severity of symptoms. Nevertheless, serum Na <120 mEq/L should prompt immediate treatment. Increasing serum Na by <0.5 mEq/L/hr in chronic hyponatremia reduces the incidence of central pontine myelinolysis and other adverse side effects.[3]

Hypernatremia

Hypernatremia represents a deficit of body water relative to body Na and is associated with hyperosmolality. The etiology of hypernatremia

TABLE 31–1. CAUSES OF HYPONATREMIA

Sodium loss (urine Na decreased)
Vomiting
Diarrhea
Nasogastric or ostomy drainage
Sodium loss (urine Na increased)
Diuretics
Adrenal insufficiency
Nephropathies
Water excess (urine Na variable)
SIADH
Reset hypothalamic osmotic receptors (sick cell syndrome)
Hypothyroidism
Congestive heart failure
Cirrhosis
Nephrotic syndrome
Renal insufficiency
Hypokalemia
Psychogenic polydipsia
Drugs
Hypoglycemic agents: chlorpropamide, tolbutamide
Antineoplastic agents: cyclophosphamide, vincristine
Sedatives: barbiturates, morphine
Psychotropic agents: thioridazine, thiothixene, amitriptyline, fluphenazine
Others: clofibrate, nicotine, oxytocin

usually is evident from history. Causes include uncompensated losses of hypotonic fluids, hypertonic fluid administration, and defects in the renal handling of sodium excretion.[1, 2] These clinical syndromes are classified by the apparent extracellular fluid volume into hypovolemic, isovolemic, and hypervolemic. The free water deficit can be calculated from the serum Na concentration by the following formula:

$$H_2O \text{ deficit} = \text{volume of total body water} \times ([\text{serum Na}] - [\text{normal serum Na}])/[\text{serum Na}]$$

or

$$H_2O \text{ deficit} = 0.6 \times (\text{weight in kg}) \times ([\text{serum Na}] - 140)/140$$

Hypovolemic hypernatremia develops from unreplaced hypotonic fluid loss, including urinary, gastrointestinal, and insensible loss. Hypovolemia stimulates Na retention, resulting in a low (<20 mEq/L) urinary Na. Isovolemic hypernatremia results from net loss of free water with preservation of the intravascular volume. Replacement of hypotonic insensible or gastrointestinal losses with isotonic fluids produces isovolemic hypernatremia. Diabetes insipidus, intrinsic renal disease, hypercalcemia, hypokalemia, and certain drugs (lithium, demeclocycline, methoxyflurane) can impair renal concentrating mechanisms with similar results. Hypervolemic hypernatremia can result from either iatrogenic volume expansion or mineralocorticoid excess. The resultant hypervolemia suppresses ADH release. Thus, dilute urine is excreted until serum Na increases to 145 to 148 mEq/L.[1]

The clinical features of hypernatremia result from cerebral dehydration.[2] Signs and symptoms include mental status changes, muscle twitching, seizures, and coma. With severe or rapid cerebral dehydration, the shrunken brain places traction on the bridging veins, predisposing the patient to subarachnoid hemorrhage or venous thrombosis. As with hyponatremia, hypernatremia that develops gradually allows adjustment of intracellular osmolality to prevent cerebral dehydration.

SERUM POTASSIUM

Hypokalemia

Hypokalemia develops either from redistribution of K or from depletion of body potassium stores (Table 31–2).[4] The extracellular fluid contains approximately 70 mEq K in a 70-kg adult, whereas the intracellular compartment contains approximately 4200 mEq potassium.[1] Redistribution of serum K into the intracellular compartment lowers the serum K, although total body K may be normal. Potassium depletion via gastrointestinal or skin losses stimulates renal K conservation and is associated with urinary K excretion of less than 20 mEq/day. Because inappropriate potassium wasting occurs when the kidney is stimulated to conserve sodium, accurate assessment of renal potassium handling requires adequate sodium delivery to the distal nephron (urinary sodium excretion of at least 100 mEq/d).

Hypokalemia may result in muscle weakness, ileus, and characteristic ECG changes.[4] The ECG typically shows flattening or inversion of T waves with serum K levels less than 3.0 mEq/L. Depression of ST segments and prominent U waves may appear. Arrhythmias including premature atrial contractions, premature ventricular contraction, AV nodal conduction defects, and atrial tachycardia increase with hypokalemia. Correction of even mild hypokalemia can require hundreds of milliequivalents of K because serum K equilibrates with intracellular stores.

TABLE 31–2. CAUSES OF HYPOKALEMIA

Redistribution
Alkalosis
Insulin therapy
Vitamin B12 therapy
Barium poisoning
Familial periodic paralysis
Extrarenal losses (urine K<20 mEq/d)
Inadequate intake
Vomiting
Diarrhea
Nasogastric or ostomy drainage
Renal losses (urine K>20 mEq/d)
Primary hyperaldosteronism
Secondary hyperaldosteronism
(hypovolemia, cirrhosis, heart failure, nephrosis, GI bleeding, magnesium depletion)
Glucocorticoid excess (endogenous or exogenous)
Renal tubular acidosis, proximal and distal
Bartter's syndrome
Liddle syndrome
Hyperreninemic states (eg, renal artery stenosis)

Pseudohyperkalemia

Potassium is released from the cellular components of blood during clotting. Thus, serum K concentration is slightly higher than plasma K concentration. This difference is usually small (0.5 mEq/L or less) but increases in hypercellular states, such as thrombocytosis and leukocytosis. Artifactual hyperkalemia also occurs when intracellular K is released by hemolysis in the test tube or when tissue is made ischemic by prolonged tourniquet application during phlebotomy.[1] Because repeat testing of samples might delay treatment of a life-threatening disorder if suspected pseudohyperkalemia was in fact true hyperkalemia, an ECG should be examined for changes whenever high serum K is detected.

Hyperkalemia

Serum K increases by greater stores of K or by redistribution of intracellular K into the extracellular space (Table 31–3).[4] Potassium intake may exceed urinary clearance in renal insufficiency or in syndromes with impaired mineralocorticoid secretion or action. Leakage of

TABLE 31–3. CAUSES OF HYPERKALEMIA

Excessive intake
Renal insufficiency
Potassium-sparing diuretics
Deficiency in renin-angiotensin-aldosterone renal axis
Glucocorticoid deficiency
Primary hypoaldosteronism
Addison's disease
Congenital adrenal hypoplasia
Intrinsic renal disease
Hyporeninemic hypoaldosteronism
Angiotensin-converting enzyme inhibitors
Acidosis
Tissue destruction
(rhabdomyolysis, tumor lysis, burns, GI bleeding, hemolysis)
Hyperkalemic familial periodic paralysis
Drugs
Digoxin and cardiac glycosides, succinylcholine, glucagon, arginine, lead, beta-blockers, methyldopa, nonsteroidal antinflammatory drugs

intracellular K into the extracellular compartment is promoted by acidosis, insulin deficiency, tissue necrosis, and certain drugs.

Hyperkalemia produces muscle weakness and characteristic ECG changes.[4] With increasing serum K, T-wave amplitude increases in precordial leads. Further increases prolong the PR interval and widen the QRS complex. Eventually, the S wave and T wave may merge, producing a wide-complex tachycardia that resembles a sine wave. This terminal arrhythmia occurs as serum K approaches or exceeds 10 mEq/L.

SERUM ANIONS

Bicarbonate

Decreased serum HCO_3 reflects metabolic acidosis. Three mechanisms can produce hypobicarbonatemia.[5] First, an endogenous or exogenous acid titrates the serum pool of HCO_3. In this situation, the Na salt of the acid replaces $NaHCO_3$, producing an elevated anion gap acidosis. Second, gastrointestinal HCO_3 is lost during voluminous diarrhea or drainage of other HCO_3-rich secretions. The kidney retains NaCl to maintain volume, producing hyperchloremic, non–anion gap acidosis.

Third, renal failure or renal tubular acidosis can promote retention of acids or impair production of HCO_3.

Increased $NaHCO_3$ represents a metabolic alkalosis. Hyperbicarbonatemia develops when the kidney is stimulated to retain HCO_3 and excess HCO_3 is available.[5] Volume depletion results in a "volume-contraction metabolic alkalosis," as Na is avidly retained by the kidney, and H and K are preferentially excreted. Alternatively, loss of gastrointestinal acid during protracted vomiting can leave unneutralized HCO_3. Administration of exogenous HCO_3 or other alkalis metabolized to HCO_3 (lactate, citrate, gluconate) can overwhelm renal HCO_3 clearance. Renal retention of HCO_3 also is stimulated by hypokalemia, hypercapnia, hyperaldosteronism, and hypoparathyroidism.

Chloride

Serum Cl balances the electrical charge of serum cations along with HCO_3. Consequently, serum cation concentration and the presence of other anions affect serum Cl concentration.[6] Hyperchloremia occurs with hypernatremia, low anion gap state, or normal anion gap metabolic acidosis (hypobicarbonatemia). Hypochloremia occurs with metabolic alkalosis (hyperbicarbonatemia).

ANION GAP

The anion gap is measured as the difference between the primary serum cation (Na) and the primary measured anions (Cl and HCO_3): $[Na] - ([Cl] + [HCO_3])$.[7] This difference is normally 8 to 12 mEq/L, reflecting the presence of unmeasured anions including proteins. An increase in the anion gap indicates the presence of anions other than Cl and HCO_3. This situation usually results from administration of an exogenous acid with a nonchloride salt. Causes of an elevated anion gap are listed in Table 31–4.

Decreased anion gaps occur in several situations.[7] The unmeasured anions may be reduced, as in hypoalbuminemia. Alternatively, if cations other than sodium are present, the measured anions will be elevated to maintain neutrality. Thus, hypermagnesemia, hypercalcemia, or lithium toxicity is associated with low anion gaps. The presence of other halides interferes with serum Cl determination in many assays. Bromide, for example, produces stronger signals in colorimetric assays, spuriously elevating the estimation of serum Cl and lowering the calculated anion gap. Pseudohyponatremia will lower the anion gap artifactually.

TABLE 31–4. ELEVATED ANION GAP

Endogenous anions
Renal failure (salts of organic acids accumulate)
Lactic acidosis
Ketoacidosis
Exogenous anions
Salicylates
Ethylene glycol (metabolized to glycolate)
Methanol (metabolized to formate)
Paraldehyde (metabolized to acetate)
Sodium salt of anion with impaired metabolism to bicarbonate (citrate, acetate, lactate)

RECOMMENDATIONS FOR ORDERING ELECTROLYTES

Electrolytes are perhaps the second most common laboratory test ordered for emergency department patients (the first being the complete blood count). Patient charges in 1994 for emergent serum electrolytes range from $30 to $40 per electrolyte. Panels of the basic electrolytes consequently cost $120 to $160 in patient charges. Because these panels are so frequently ordered, serum electrolytes constitute a large fraction of the total expenditures for testing in emergency departments.[8] These facts have prompted several groups to examine the clinical indications for ordering this laboratory test.

Indications for ordering electrolytes in the ED have been proposed (Table 31–5).[9] Among emergency department patients for whom electrolytes were ordered, criteria for predicting the presence of clinically significant abnormalities have been identified (Table 31–6).[10] These criteria were prospectively validated in a separate series of patients for whom electrolytes were ordered, and the tests had a sensitivity of 94%.[11] A separate examination in older (age >55) patients also revealed a sensitivity of 95%.[12] Both studies asserted that no clinical mishap would have resulted from delayed recognition of the false-negative cases. Both series revealed, however, that the criteria had low specificity (24% and 10%) for identifying electrolyte abnormalities. These criteria may, therefore, eliminate the need for electrolyte measurement in a subset of patients for whom little clinical suspicion of abnormality exists.

Routine Electrolytes

Few data support the practice of ordering electrolyte panels as a routine screening test. Reviews emphasize the low yield of routine

TABLE 31–5. INDICATIONS FOR ORDERING ELECTROLYTES

Critically ill
Fluid loss
Fluid gain
New or changing fluid shifts
Toxic ingestions
Specific symptoms or signs of electrolyte disturbance
Mental status changes
Muscle weakness
ECG changes
GI disturbances
Diuretic use
New-onset hypertension (screen for hyperaldosteronism)

From Checchio LM, Comb AJ: Electrolytes, BUN, creatinine: Who's at risk? *Ann Emerg Med.* 1986;15:363–366.

laboratory testing in patients being admitted for medical or surgical services.[13] Surveys of physician motives indicate that serum electrolyte abnormalities are suspected in most patients for whom these studies are ordered.[14] Electrolyte abnormalities not suspected from the clinical setting are rare. In several series, admission testing revealed electrolyte abnormalities in 4 to 10% of patients.[13] Very few of these abnormalities result in significant changes of therapeutic management. Prospective evaluation revealed that the routine admission testing of all patients actually increases the cost of hospitalization without any measurable effect on care.[15] Admission electrolyte panels may be useful in guiding fluid and electrolyte therapy in the hospital.[16] Thus, the yield of abnormal results may not accurately reflect the value of panels.

TABLE 31–6. CLINICAL CRITERIA FOR SIGNIFICANT ABNORMALITIES

Poor oral intake
Vomiting
Chronic hypertension
Diuretic use
Recent seizure
Muscle weakness
Age 65 or older
Alcoholism
Abnormal mental status
Recent history of electrolyte abnormality

From Lowe RA, Wood AB, Burney RE, et al: Rational ordering of serum electrolytes: Development of clinical criteria. *Ann Emerg Med.* 1987;16:260–269.

Electrolytes in Trauma

The laboratory examination of trauma patients frequently includes electrolyte panels. A random sample of adult trauma patients revealed that 2% had abnormal Na and 8% had abnormal K levels.[17] Pediatric trauma patients have similarly low incidences of abnormal Na (3 to 8%) and abnormal K levels (0 to 14%).[18, 19] In contrast, serum HCO_3 was decreased in all pediatric trauma patients examined, probably reflecting lactic acidosis.[18] These studies suggested that electrolytes are not critical for the initial evaluation of trauma patients. The vigorous fluid resuscitation that these patients frequently receive, however, does require monitoring of electrolytes.

Electrolytes in Seizures

Electrolyte abnormalities are an infrequent cause of seizures. Unless the history suggests an abnormality, electrolytes can be omitted from the examination of patients with an *established seizure disorder*.[20] Abnormal Na, K, or Cl levels were noted in 4 to 7% of patients, although these abnormalities were not related to the seizure. In contrast, metabolic acidosis is common and expected after a seizure. In adults with *new-onset seizures*, clinically significant electrolyte abnormalities were found in 6% of patients, and hyponatremia was the etiology for seizures in 2% of patients.[21] These investigators note that electrolyte abnormalities are poorly predicted from history and suggest that electrolytes be measured routinely in new-onset seizures. In the pediatric age group, electrolytes are examined in most children with new-onset nonfebrile seizures and less often in patients with febrile seizures.[22] Abnormal Na was noted in only 2 to 3% of these children, although clinically insignificant hyperkalemia was noted in 14 to 17%. Although an uncommon cause of seizures, electrolyte abnormalities should be considered in new-onset seizures.

SUMMARY

In summary, unexpected electrolyte abnormalities are infrequent. In screening of medical patients, evaluation of trauma, and evaluation of seizures, abnormalities are detected in 5 to 10% of patients, but clinically significant abnormalities appear to be much less frequent. Ordering of electrolytes to screen for unexpected abnormalities may be reduced by developing clinical criteria to predict electrolyte disturbances. Current criteria have sensitivities of 94 to 95%. Monitoring of electrolytes is appropriate during fluid therapy. This type of monitoring may remain the most common indication for ordering electrolytes in the emergency department.

REFERENCES

1. Narins RG, Jones ER, Stom MC, et al: Diagnostic strategies in disorders of fluid, electrolyte and acid-base homeostasis. *Am J Med.* 1982;72:496–520.
2. Janz T: Sodium. *Emerg Med Clin North Am.* 1986;4:115–130.
3. Cluitmans FHM, Meinders AE: Management of severe hyponatremia: Rapid or slow correction? *Am J Med.* 1990;88:161–166.
4. Martin ML, Hamilton R, West MF: Potassium. *Emerg Med Clin North Am.* 1986;4:131–144.
5. Jehle D, Harchelroad F: Bicarbonate. *Emerg Med Clin North Am.* 1986;4:145–173.
6. Baltarowich LL: Chloride. *Emerg Med Clin North Am.* 1986; 4:175–183.
7. Emmett M, Narins RG: Clinical use of the anion gap. *Medicine.* 1977;56:38–54.
8. Karas S: Cost containment in emergency medicine. *JAMA.* 1980;243:1356–1359.
9. Checchio LM, Como AJ: Electrolytes, BUN, creatinine: Who's at risk? *Ann Emerg Med.* 1986;15:363–366.
10. Lowe RA, Wood AB, Burney RE, et al: Rational ordering of serum electrolytes: Development of clinical criteria. *Ann Emerg Med.* 1987;16:260–269.
11. Lowe RA, Arst HF, Ellis BK: Rational ordering of electrolytes in the emergency department. *Ann Emerg Med.* 1991;20:16–21.
12. Singal BM, Hedges JR, Succop PA: Prediction of electrolyte abnormalities in elderly emergency patients. *Ann Emerg Med.* 1991;20:964–968.
13. Cebul RD, Beck JR: Biochemical profiles: Applications in ambulatory screening and preadmission testing of adults. *Ann Intern Med.* 1987;106:403–413.
14. Murata GH, Muranaka E, Ellrody AG: Laboratory testing on admission to a teaching service: Expectations and outcomes of serum electrolytes. *Mt Sinai J Med NY.* 1984;51:141–147.
15. Durbridge TC, Edwards F, Edwards RG, et al: Evaluation of benefits of screening tests done immediately on admission to hospital. *Clin Chem.* 1976; 22:968–971.
16. Singal BM, Hedges JR, Succop PA: Efficacy of the stat serum electrolyte panel in the management of older emergency patients. *Med Decision Making.* 1992;12:52–59.
17. Roux A, Lourens L, Richards E: Contribution of preoperative investigations to the anaesthetic management of adult trauma patients. *Injury.* 1993;24:17–20.
18. Ford EG, Karamanoukian HL, McGrath N, et al: Emergency center laboratory evaluation of pediatric trauma victims. *Am Surg.* 1990;56:752–757.
19. Isaacman DJ, Scarfone RJ, Kost SI, et al: Utility of routine laboratory

testing for detecting intra-abdominal injury in the pediatric trauma patient. *Pediatrics*. 1993;92:691–694.
20. Eisner RF, Trunbull TL, Howes DS, et al: Efficacy of a ''standard'' seizure workup in the emergency department. *Ann Emerg Med*. 1986;15:33–39.
21. Henneman PL, DeRoos F, Lewis RJ: Determining the need for admission in patients with new-onset seizures. *Ann Emerg Med*. 1994;24:1108–1114.
22. Nypaver MM, Reynolds SL, Tanz RR, et al: Emergency department laboratory evaluation of children with seizures: dogma or dilemma? *Pediatr Emerg Care*. 1992;8:13–16.

Chapter

Blood Urea Nitrogen and Creatinine

Owen T. Traynor

The assessments of the blood urea nitrogen (BUN) and creatinine are among the most commonly ordered laboratory tests in the emergency department. To draw valid conclusions from test results, the clinician should have an understanding of the physiology of nitrogen and creatinine metabolism, an appreciation of the methodology used to measure each analyte, and a knowledge of the clinical settings in which abnormalities are likely to occur.

PHYSIOLOGY

Urea is the breakdown product of protein catabolism in the liver, and the production of urea is proportional to hepatic protein load. Increased dietary protein, gastrointestinal hemorrhage, catabolic states (eg, fever, infection, trauma, other stress states), and use of medications that inhibit anabolic metabolism (eg, tetracyclines and glucocorticoids) result in an increased protein load.[1] Urea production depends not only on adequate protein substrate but also on a healthy functioning liver.

The kidney is responsible for nearly all of urea elimination from the body. Approximately 40% of filtered urea is resorbed when urine flow exceeds 2 mL/min. As urine flow decreases, even more of the filtered urea is absorbed.[2] Thus, any condition that results in a decreased glomerular filtration rate (GFR) or decreased effective circulating blood volume results in increased resorption of urea and a rise in the BUN.

Creatinine is the breakdown product of creatine, the chief storage source of the high energy phosphates utilized by muscle cells. Creatine spontaneously breaks down irreversibly into creatinine. Approximately 2% of the body's creatine degrades into creatinine every 24 hours.[1] The only significant source of creatinine is muscle; it is not consumed in any metabolic pathways and is eliminated almost entirely by the kidneys. Like urea, creatinine is filtered at the glomerulus; there is no resorption in the tubules. Although there is some net tubular secretion, creatinine clearance approximates the GFR. Creatinine excretion is also largely independent of urine flow. Because the only significant source of creatinine is the body's muscle mass and creatinine clearance approximates the GFR, the creatinine level is a better indicator of renal function than the BUN.

The BUN is influenced by many extrarenal factors, so it is difficult to assess renal function without simultaneously measuring the serum creatinine. In fact, the ratio of BUN to creatinine, in concert with the absolute values of BUN and creatinine, can provide important information. The BUN increases out of proportion to the creatinine in low urine flow states, resulting in an elevation in the normal BUN:creatinine ratio. This effect occurs because urea absorption rises when urine flow decreases, whereas creatinine does not undergo resorption. Thus, an elevated BUN:creatinine ratio is found with both prerenal and postrenal azotemia. The BUN:creatinine ratio may also be altered when there is either an increase or a decrease in protein load.

MEASUREMENT METHODOLOGY

There are several methods of quantifying the amount of urea or creatinine present in a sample. Serum, and not whole blood, is actually used for analysis. The blood should be collected in a red-top tube and analyzed within 3 hours. If there is to be a delay in running the tests, the samples should be refrigerated and warmed to room temperature prior to analysis.[1]

One of two techniques is commonly employed for quantification of serum urea. The first involves enzymatic degradation of urea using a urease, producing carbonic acid and ammonia. The ammonia can then be quantified by reaction with alpha-ketoglutaric acid to produce a photometrically quantifiable product. Alternatively, an ammonia electrode may be utilized. The second technique involves reaction of the sample with diacetyl, resulting in a product that can be measured photometrically.[1]

There are several methods used to quantify the amount of creatinine in serum. The Jaffe reaction, perhaps the oldest method, is still frequently employed. Creatinine reacts with picric acid to produce a red solution. The color change is proportional to the amount of creatinine present. Unfortunately, other compounds react with picric acid to produce similar color changes. Some modifications have been made to increase the specificity of the Jaffe reaction. Newer methods have also been developed, reacting creatinine with various substances to produce a colorimetric product. An enzymatic process, similar to the technique used for urea analysis, is also available.

CLINICAL CORRELATION

Normal Values

BUN		
Birth–1 y	4–16 mg/dL	SI: 1.4–5.7 μmol/L
1–40 y	5–20 mg/dL	SI: 1.8–7.1 μmol/L
Slight gradual increase with age over 40 years		
Creatinine		
1–5 y	0.3–0.5 mg/dL	SI: 27–44 μmol/L
5–10 y	0.5–0.8 mg/dL	SI: 44–71 μmol/L
Adult males	Up to 1.2 mg/dL	SI: Up to 106 μmol/L
Adult females	Up to 1.1 mg/dL	SI: Up to 97 μmol/L
The BUN: creatinine ratio averages 8–15:1		

Causes of an Elevated Blood Urea Nitrogen[1, 2]

An elevated BUN may be found when there is an increased protein load or when there is a decreased renal clearance.

Causes of increased protein load include

- Increased dietary protein or hyperalimentation
- Catabolic states, such as multiple trauma, infection, fever, stress
- Use of medications that inhibit anabolic metabolism, such as tetracyclines and glucocorticoids
- Gastrointestinal bleeding.

Causes of decreased renal clearance include

- Prerenal etiology, such as in shock, dehydration, congestive heart failure, and renal artery stenosis
- Postrenal etiology, such as in urinary tract obstruction

- Renal dysfunction, such as acute tubular necrosis, renal vein thrombosis, glomerular disease, and acute interstitial nephritis.

Causes of a Decreased Blood Urea Nitrogen[1, 2]

A decreased BUN may be found when there is a decreased protein load or an increased renal clearance of urea.

Causes of a decreased protein load include

- Low dietary protein
- Decreased nitrogen metabolism secondary to hepatic disease.

Causes of increased renal clearance include

- Syndrome of inappropriate antidiuretic hormone (SIADH)
- Overhydration or water intoxication
- Increased GFR in pregnancy.

Causes of an Elevated Creatinine[1, 2]

An elevated creatinine level occurs when there is decreased renal clearance or increased creatinine load.

Causes of decreased renal clearance include

- Renal dysfunction, such as acute tubular necrosis, renal vein thrombosis, glomerular disease, and acute interstitial nephritis
- Prerenal etiology, such as in shock, dehydration, congestive heart failure, and renal artery stenosis
- Postrenal etiology, such as in urinary tract obstruction.

Causes of an increased creatinine load include

- Massive trauma
- Muscle wasting diseases and rhabdomyolysis
- Exogenous creatinine from ingestion of large amounts of meat; this may cause a transient elevation in serum creatinine levels.

There are also factitious causes of elevated creatinine, caused by substances that react with the test reagents as follows:

- Ketones
- Glucose
- Pyruvate
- Uric acid
- Barbiturates
- Penicillins
- Cephalosporins.

Causes of a Decreased Creatinine[1, 2]

A decreased creatinine occurs when there is a decreased creatinine load.

Causes of decreased creatinine load include

- Small stature
- Decreased muscle mass caused by debilitation or end stage muscle wasting diseases
- Reduced creatine production caused by severe hepatic disease and a low protein diet.

Causes of an Elevated Blood Urea Nitrogen:Creatinine Ratio[1, 2]

The BUN:creatinine ratio is elevated when there is an increased protein load (etiology previously noted) or during low urine flow states secondary to prerenal or postrenal etiology (as previously noted).

Causes of a Decreased Blood Urea Nitrogen:Creatinine Ratio[1, 2]

The BUN : creatinine ratio is reduced when there is a decreased protein load, an increased renal clearance of urea, or an increased creatinine production (etiology as previously noted).

INDICATIONS FOR ORDERING BLOOD UREA NITROGEN AND CREATININE

Both the BUN and creatinine levels are influenced by many factors, reducing their specificity. In addition, >50% of the nephrons must be dysfunctional before there is an effect on the measured serum urea or creatinine levels. Thus, BUN and creatinine are not sensitive tests in the context of mild renal disease. The maximum usefulness of these tests depends on clinical correlation. The recommended indications are based largely on the prior likelihood of disease.

Measurements of BUN and creatinine are indicated when there is historical information or physical examination findings that suggest renal dysfunction. Patients who are to receive intravenous contrast agents may benefit from BUN and creatinine determinations to prevent giving a dye load to patients with occult renal disease. Patients who are suspected of having SIADH or water intoxication also may benefit from these laboratory studies.[3]

Ordering the BUN without serum creatinine is not commonly done but may be indicated for calculating the serum osmolarity. The BUN may also help one decide whether emergent dialysis is indicated in a patient with chronic renal failure.[3]

Ordering a creatinine level without a BUN is also uncommon. It may be indicated in the evaluation of the patient with a history of chronic renal insufficiency in attempting to investigate an acute deterioration in renal function.[3]

SUMMARY

Measurements of the BUN and creatinine are commonly performed emergency department diagnostic tests. Their chief use is in evaluating renal function. They lack both specificity and sensitivity and are best ordered when there is a high prior likelihood of renal disease. Intelligent ordering of these tests will provide the maximum patient benefit and reduced health care costs.

REFERENCES

1. Lyman JL: Blood urea nitrogen and creatinine. *Emerg Med Clin North Am.* 1986;4:223–233.
2. Baum N, Dichoso CC, Carlton CE: Blood urea nitrogen and serum creatinine. *Urology.* 1975;V:583–588.
3. Chechio LM, Como AJ: Electrolytes, BUN, creatinine: Who's at risk? *Ann Emerg Med.* 1986;15:363–366.

Chapter

Glucose Testing

Steven J. White

Glucose testing is one of the most commonly performed laboratory and bedside chemical analyses.[1] Because of the myriad conditions that can affect glucose homeostasis, the wide range and subtlety of presenting symptoms, and the potentially devastating consequences of either extreme of blood glucose level, a liberal approach to glucose testing is warranted. Even in some studies seeking to limit inordinate testing, for new-onset seizures[2] and for dizziness,[3] glucose has emerged as an analyte worth measuring. Criteria for ordering serum glucose levels are listed in Table 33–1.

Historically, the urgency of treating potential hypoglycemia has overridden the need for laboratory confirmation because to delay therapy risked irreversible CNS damage.[4] The empiric administration of 25 g of D50 (50% glucose) was long a standard of care for the treatment of unexplained alteration in mental status.[5, 6] This standard has been incorporated into many emergency medical service protocols as well. By necessity, such an approach overtreats for hypoglycemia. It has been suspected that hypertonic glucose solutions may increase ischemic neuronal damage.[7, 8] Because many of the neurologic manifestations of ischemia and hypoxia are clinically indistinguishable from those of hypoglycemia, the empiric use of glucose for altered mental status may be ill advised.

With the advent of practical bedside testing methods, the standard of care for possible hypoglycemia has shifted to one of treatment guided by bedside glucose testing and confirmed by laboratory testing. Bedside testing has been extended to include prehospital testing at the scene and in the ambulance.[9]

METHODS OF MEASUREMENT

Perhaps the first qualitative test for glucose was the observation by early Hindu physicians that ants were attracted to the discarded urine of patients who formed skin "boils."[10] More sophisticated and quantifiable methods have since evolved.

TABLE 33–1. GENERAL INDICATIONS FOR BLOOD GLUCOSE TESTING

1. Altered level of consciousness (ALOC)
   Even in cases where the ALOC appears to be explained by other causes, the contribution of concomitant hypoglycemia should be explored (eg, hypoglycemia as a precipitant of trauma); includes dizziness, confusion, and combativeness as well as depressed level of arousal
2. Seizure
   Glucose is perhaps the only analyte of value in the routine workup of new-onset seizure disorder, and bedside analysis should be performed in all patients presenting to the emergency department with recent seizure
3. Focal neurologic deficit
   Hypoglycemic hemiplegia is well recognized; watershed areas of decreased blood supply are more sensitive to low blood glucose levels and may manifest as a strokelike picture
4. Symptomatic patient with known or suspected diabetes
   Poor glucose control can accompany any number of conditions, medical or surgical; therapy will be guided by blood glucose; many agents are known to interact with oral hypoglycemia medications, leading to hypoglycemia
5. DKA/hyperosmolar state
   Fluid/electrolyte and insulin therapy will be guided by glucose measurements
6. Ingestion/overdose/medication
   Aspirin, iron, ethanol, beta-agonists—can cause hypoglycemia, especially in children
   Oral hypoglycemia agents (sulfonylureas), insulin
7. CSF/synovial/pleural fluid analysis
   Simultaneous measurement of blood glucose is required
8. Other—hypothermia, adrenal/pituitary endocrinopathies, high-dose steroids, sepsis, glycogen storage diseases, starvation, liver failure, renal failure, posthyperalimentation, posthemodialysis, pancreatic disease, major trauma, critical illness, Reye's syndrome, myocardial infarction

Modified from Pointer JE: Glucose analysis: Indications for ordering and alternatives to the laboratory. *Ann Emerg Med.* 1986;15:372–376.

Sample Acquisition and Preparation

Serum/Plasma/Whole Blood

Normal reference values for serum are 70 to 110 mg/dL.[11] In patients with normal hematocrit values, whole blood values (ie, those obtained by bedside methods) are about 15% lower than plasma and serum values, which are about 60 to 95 mg/dL.

Blood glucose can be measured in capillary, arterial, or venous blood. Most emergency department and prehospital measurements are performed on venous blood, often when intravenous lines are started. The concentration of glucose is highest in the arterial circulation; the glucose level falls as it is extracted from the capillary bed and reaches a minimum in venous blood. If the venous circulation is slowed by leaving the tourniquet in place, as may occur with difficult intravenous (IV) placement, venous measurements fall even further, by as much as 25 mg/dL after 6 minutes of tourniquet occlusion.[12]

Glucose concentration in capillaries is intermediate between that of arterial and venous blood, with values about 10 to 20 mg/dL higher than those in venous blood.[13] Warming of the extremity increases capillary flow and "arterializes" the sample, resulting in higher glucose concentration. Conversely, cooling the extremity results in lower glucose concentrations. Good fingerstick technique dictates avoiding the more sensitive volar pulp areas and using the thumb or fourth finger because of a superior capillary blood supply. The second drop of capillary blood from the fingerstick should be used for reagent strip analysis.[13]

Aspiration of a sample from a functioning IV line, even one containing 5% glucose (D5), has been shown to give valid results with respect to glucose testing.[14] The recommended technique is to stop the infusion for about 2 minutes prior to applying the venous tourniquet and to discard the first 5 mL of aspirate.

Glucose samples can be submitted to the clinical laboratory without additives (in a syringe, red-top tube, or red/gray-speckled–top tube) to yield serum samples or in green-top (sodium/lithium/ammonium heparin salts) or gray-top (sodium fluoride/potassium oxalate) tubes for plasma samples. Selection of the type of sample tube is generally governed by the associated tests being run in addition to glucose.

Glucose undergoes glycolysis by both red and white blood cells, resulting in an artifactual lowering of the glucose measurement. The rate of in vitro glucose consumption is approximately 5%/h at body temperature but can be as rapid as 40% over 3 hours.[12] Glycolysis can be prevented by promptly (within 30 minutes) separating the cellular components from the serum fraction, by cooling the sample, or by using sodium fluoride/potassium oxalate–containing sample tubes (gray-top). The use of gray-top tubes, however, prevents the measurement of sodium or other analytes. In addition, fluoride may deactivate the glucose oxidase reagent test strip used for bedside testing,[15] causing falsely low glucose measurements. Therefore, if gray-top tubes containing fluoride are employed by the paramedics to permit more accurate glucose determination "after-the-fact" of prehospital treatment, it is important not to perform glucose-oxidase test strip determination on such samples.

Fingerstick Specimens

Reagent test strips can be divided into two broad categories: those that require rinsing prior to interpretation and those that are blotted but not rinsed. Reagent strips in the first category are Dextrostix, Visidex, and Glucoscan. Of these, only Visidex is designed specifically for visual interpretation. Others are designed for use with reflectance spectrometry. The reagent pad is exposed to a drop of blood for 60 seconds, rinsed with water, and then read immediately against a comparison scale or by reflectance spectrometer.

Reagent strips in the second category include Visidex II and Chemstrip bG. The reagent pad is exposed to a drop of blood for 30 seconds (Visidex II) or 60 seconds (Chemstrip bG), blotted dry with cotton, and developed for an additional 60 seconds (Chemstrip bG) or 90 seconds (Visidex II). It is then read either by visual comparison or reflectance spectrometer. For visual readings higher than 400, an additional minute is allowed for developing. Whereas the timing of the first interval (from blood exposure to blotting) is critical for accurate readings, the timing of the second interval (development time) is less so. Beyond 30 seconds of development time, there is little change in the visual reading.

The reading of a reacted Chemstrip bG has been claimed to be stable for up to 7 days if maintained in a desiccated-like environment.[16, 17] Cox and coworkers tested the stability of 268 reacted Chemstrip bG reagent strips from 67 diabetic patients, however, and found significant decreases in measured glucose even only 1 day after initial exposure.[18] The change was most pronounced for hyperglycemic readings and probably not clinically significant for the hypoglycemic readings. As a quality assurance tool, prehospital reagent strips can be reread in the emergency department, either by visual comparison or reflectance spectrometry.

For emergency department and prehospital use, visual interpretation is adequate for initial treatment considerations. Strips that do not require rinsing are most suitable for prehospital use. Cotton is the recommended blotting agent for such strips. When gauze is employed, it can abrade the reagent pad of the test strip and may render it unreadable subsequently by reflectance spectrometry.

INTERPRETATION OF RESULTS

Hypoglycemia

Although a laboratory diagnosis of hypoglycemia depends on demonstrating a "below normal value of glucose" (ie, ≤70 mg/dL for serum or ≤160 mg/dL for whole blood), the clinical expression of hypoglycemia is quite variable and influenced by such factors as rapidity of onset, patient age and sex, dietary history, physical activity, coexisting disease states, and medication. Thus, some patients can be asymptomatic at a level of 35 mg/dL, whereas others can exhibit signs of adrenergic excess at "normal" levels.[19] To make a diagnosis of hypoglycemia, therefore, the clinical presentation must be correlated with laboratory values and, if warranted, response to treatment.

The visual interpretation of reagent test strips deserves mention because the primary emergency department and prehospital use of such strips is to diagnose hypoglycemia and to limit empiric glucose administration. Most comparative studies have found good correlation between reagent strip and laboratory values,[20–22] with correlation coefficients >.95. More to the point for emergency department and field use is the negative predictive value for hypoglycemia, that is, the probability that a test result interpreted as negative for hypoglycemia truly excludes hypoglycemia. To falsely miss hypoglycemia can have dire consequences. In a prehospital study of 182 patients tested by either Chemstrip bG or Visidex II, Lavery and colleagues found a negative predictive value of 98%, using ≤60 mg/mL as a visual and laboratory cutoff for hypoglycemia.[9] Some 33 patients were diagnosed with hypoglycemia (study prevalence of hypoglycemia = 18%); two of the 33 patients were incorrectly diagnosed as euglycemic by reagent strip, with values of 70 and 90 mg/dL.[9] Other studies, one with nine hypoglycemic patients out of a total of 62 (15% prevalence)[23] and the other with 35 hypoglycemic patients out of a total of 73 (47% prevalence),[24] reported no missed hypoglycemic cases, although both methods suffered from flaws. Using a more liberal cutoff of 80 to 120 to initiate treatment in highly symptomatic patients will increase identification of such patients; treating such patients is unlikely to result in severe hyperglycemia.

Hyperglycemia

In conjunction with classic symptoms of polydipsia, polyuria, polyphagia, and weight loss, diabetes mellitus can be diagnosed in the emergency department by a fasting blood glucose >140 mg/dL or a random blood sugar ≥200 mg/dL.[25] Diabetes mellitus is the most common cause of hyperglycemia, but blood glucose can also be markedly elevated in patients with critical illnesses, such as myocardial infarction, sepsis, multiple trauma, shock, major burns, CNS hemorrhage, and liver disease; in patients who are pregnant; in those who take corticosteroids; and in those with intoxication by carbon monoxide, salicylates, or theophylline. Laboratory serum glucose measurements should guide therapy in terms of fluid, electrolyte, and insulin requirements.

Bedside reagent strips have a limited role in the emergency department beyond excluding hypoglycemia and monitoring the response of hyperglycemia to insulin and fluid therapy to prevent hypoglycemic overshoot.

Hyperglycemic reagent-strip readings can be helpful in guiding appropriate prehospital therapy, but may underestimate the degree of hyperglycemia because visual scales end at 800 mg/dL and reflectance meter scales are calibrated to 400 mg/dL.

SOURCES OF ERROR

Most errors in glucose determination on tube blood samples arise from improper sample preparation and handling. Delays in sample pickup and delivery allow for continued glycolysis in vitro. Similar problems arise when samples are placed in a warm environment, such as under a lamp, because warm temperatures accelerate glycolysis. Although prompt separation of cellular elements from plasma prevents glycolysis, the separation must be complete; serum separator tubes may increase the time of contact with cells.[26] In vitro glycolysis is accelerated by abnormal increases in the white or red blood cell count, and artifactual hypoglycemia has been observed in leukemia, leukemoid reactions,[27] and polycythemia vera.[28] Even the use of fluoride/oxalate tubes may not prevent this enhanced glycolysis. In fact, some investigators have questioned the efficacy of fluoride/oxalate tubes as antiglycolytic agents even in normal samples, citing a 510% decrease in measured glucose values over the first hour.[29] Another potential error can result from the failure of laboratory personnel to recognize grossly lipemic specimens, resulting in the ultracentrifugation of triglycerides from the sample and artifactually low glucose measurement.[30]

Although most such errors result in artifactual hypoglycemia, the blood glucose level can be falsely elevated as well. With marked leukocytosis, increased sample viscosity after cell lysis (performed prior to autoanalysis of whole blood) can result in erroneously high glucose levels.[31]

Table 33–2 summarizes some of the errors associated with glucose reagent strip use. Most arise from improper sample preparation or improper technique. In addition, values from reagent strip testing are whole blood values and are thus influenced by the hematocrit. In one report, glucose values estimated by reagent strip averaged 18% higher than plasma measurements when the hematocrit was <35%; conversely, the reagent strip measured 40% lower than plasma when the hematocrit was >50%.[30] Because a hematocrit value is often unavailable at the time of initial reagent strip testing, caution is advised in a patient who may be anemic and has a falsely euglycemic reading. Fingerstick capillary measurements may underestimate blood glucose in patients in shock.[32]

Drugs can interfere with blood glucose laboratory testing and, because

TABLE 33–2. CAUSES OF REAGENT STRIP ERRORS

Use of outdated strips
  Manufacturer recommends use within 1 year of purchase
Use of improperly stored strips
  Chemstrip bG showed decrement of 60% after 8 weeks of storage in a sealed container at room temperature
Insufficient blood on strip
  Common error if blood is tested from fingersticks or from IV catheter hub
Blood removed from strip too soon
Strip damaged by vigorous wiping
  Often follows use of gauze as a blotting agent
Strip cut in half
  Common prehospital practice to conserve resources
Determination performed at too-low ambient temperature
  Particular problem for field work
Use of gray-top tube for reagent strip testing
  Fluoride may inactivate reagent system
Residual cleansing alcohol on fingertip

Adapted from Horwitz DL: Factitious and artifactual hypoglycemia. *Endocrin Met Clin North Am.* 1989;18:203–210.

TABLE 33–3. DRUG EFFECTS ON GLUCOSE TESTING

Drugs that increase glucose values (via glucose oxidase method)
  Acetaminophen
  Caffeine
  Isoniazid
  Salicylate
  Salicylamide

Drugs that decrease glucose values (via glucose oxidase method)
  Ascorbic acid
  L-Dopa
  Iproniazid
  Methyldopa
  Oxyphenbutazone
  Tetracycline
  Tolbutamide

From Siest G, Galteau M: *Drug Effects on Laboratory Test Results: Analytical Interferences and Pharmacological Effects.* Littleton, MA: PSG Publishing; 1988;248–252.

the same enzyme system is used, presumably with glucose reagent strips as well.[33] These drugs and their effects on glucose testing are listed in Table 33–3.

COST CONSIDERATIONS

The cost of performing glucose analysis in the clinical laboratory is nominal. Including phlebotomy charges, sample tubes, fixed charges for instrumentation, reagents, and technician time, Pointer reported a cost of $2.32 per analysis. If the glucose was part of a panel of tests (eg, SMA-6), the cost was estimated at $3.02 per analysis (1986 dollars).[15] The cost for glucose reagent strip analysis, even by reflectance spectrometry, is less than $1.00. In prehospital care, the cost of glucose reagent strips must be compared with the cost of empirically using glucose. The cost of a 50-mL ampule of 50% glucose is $1.32; the cost of a Chemstrip bG is $0.76 per strip. Potential saving in a large emergency medicine system might exceed $3000 per year.

REFERENCES

1. McConnell TS, Berger PR, Dayton HH, et al: Professional review of laboratory utilization. *Hum Pathol*. 1982;13:399–403.
2. Turnbull TL, Vanden-Hoek TL, Howes DS, et al: Utility of laboratory studies in the emergency department patient with new-onset seizure. *Ann Emerg Med*. 1990;19:373–377.
3. Herr RD, Zun L, Mathews JJ: A directed approach to the dizzy patient. *Ann Emerg Med*. 1989;18:664–672.
4. Posner JB: The comatose patient. *JAMA*. 1975;233:1313–1314.
5. Plum F, Posner JB (eds): *The Diagnosis of Stupor and Coma*. 3rd ed. Philadelphia: FA Davis; 1980:352.
6. Henry GL: Coma and altered states of consciousness, in Tintinalli JE, Krome RL, Ruiz E (eds): *Emergency Medicine—A Comprehensive Study Guide*. 3rd ed. New York: McGraw-Hill; 1992:151.
7. Browning RG, Olson DW, Stueven HA, et al: 50% dextrose: Antidote or toxin? *Ann Emerg Med*. 1990;19:683–687.
8. Lanier WL, Strangland KJ, Scheithauer BW, et al: The effects of dextrose infusion and head position on neurologic outcome after complete cerebral ischemia in primates: Examination of a model. *Anesthesiology*. 1987;66:39–48.
9. Lavery RF, Allegra JR, Cody RP, et al: A prospective evaluation of glucose reagent teststrips in the prehospital setting. *Am J Emerg Med*. 1991;9:304–308.
10. Sobrenes JR, Sherwin JE: Carbohydrates, in Tilton RC, Balows A, Hohnadel

DC, et al (eds): *Clinical Laboratory Medicine*. St. Louis: Mosby–Year Book; 1992:119–124.

11. Tilton RC, Balows A, Hohnadel DC, et al (eds): Appendix A: Chemistry reference intervals, in *Clinical Laboratory Medicine*. St. Louis: Mosby–Year Book; 1992: A2–A11.
12. McMillen JM: Blood glucose, in Walker HK, Hall WD, Hurst JW (eds): *Clinical Methods—The History, Physical, and Laboratory Examinations*. 3rd ed. Boston: Butterworths; 1989:662–665.
13. Pane GA, Epstein FB: Glucose. *Emerg Clin North Am*. 1986;4:193–205.
14. Herr RD, Bossart PJ, Blaylock RC, et al: Intravenous catheter aspiration for obtaining basic analytes during intravenous infusion. *Ann Emerg Med*. 1990;19:789–792.
15. Pointer JE: Glucose analysis: Indications for ordering and alternatives to the laboratory. *Ann Emerg Med*. 1986;15:372–376.
16. Kubilis P, Rosenbloom AL, Cimino P, et al: Stability of reacted reagent strips (Chemstrips) for blood glucose determinations. *Diabetes Care*. 1981;4:412–413.
17. Freeman C: The stability of Chemstrip bG used in conjunction with Accu-Chek bG. *Diabetes Educ*. 1986;12:28–29.
18. Cox D, Herrman J, Snyder A, et al: Stability of reacted Chemstrip bG. *Diab Care*. 1988;11:288–291.
19. Ragland G: Hypoglycemia, in Tintinalli JE, Krome RL, Ruiz E (eds): *Emergency Medicine. A Comprehensive Study Guide*. 3rd ed. New York: McGraw-Hill; 1992:727–734.
20. Holloway R, Eichold S, Hoff C: Home glucose monitoring systems. A field trial of Chemstrip bG. *Ala J Med Sci*. 1983;20:383–386.
21. Clements RS, Keane NA, Kirk KA, et al: Comparison of various methods for rapid glucose estimation. *Diab Care*. 1981;4:392–395.
22. Frindik JP, Kassner DA, Pirkle DA, et al: Comparison of Visdex and Chemstrip bG with Beckman Glucose Analyzer determination of blood glucose. *Diab Care*. 1983;6:536–539.
23. Yealy DM, Hogya PT, Paris PM, et al: Prehospital glucose estimation using reagent strips (Abstract). *Prehosp Disaster Med*. 1989;4:63.
24. Pepe PM, Ginger VF, Ritter RA: Prehospital detection of hypoglycemia (Abstract). *Prehosp Disaster Med*. 1990;5:313.
25. Ravel R (ed): Tests for diabetes and hypoglycemia, in *Clinical Laboratory Medicine—Clinical Application of Laboratory Data*. 4th ed. Chicago: Year Book Medical Publishers; 1984:334–350.
26. Horwitz DL: Factitious and artifactual hypoglycemia. *Endocrin Met Clin North Am*. 1989;18:203–210.
27. Field JB, Williams HE: Artifactual hypoglycemia associated with leukemia. *N Engl J Med*. 1961;265:946–948.
28. Arem R, Jeang MK, Blevins TC, et al: Polycythemia rubra vera artifactual hypoglycemia. *Arch Intern Med*. 1982;142:2199–2201.
29. Savolainen K, Viitala A, Puhakainen E, et al: Problems with the use of whole blood as a sample material in novel direct glucose analyzers. *Scand J Clin Lab Invest*. 1990;50:221–223.
30. Labib M, Digger T, Perks D: Reagent-strip glucose methods and haematocrit. *Lancet*. 1990;335:973–974.

31. Steinbach G, Osswald U, Maier V: Rare error in glucose determination in hemolysate. *Clin Chem.* 1991;37:590.
32. Atkin SH, Dasmahapatra A, Jaker MA, et al: Fingerstick glucose determination in shock. *Ann Intern Med.* 1991;114:1020–1024.
33. Siest G, Galteau M: *Drug Effects on Laboratory Test Results: Analytical Interferences and Pharmacological Effects.* Littleton, MA: PSG Publishing; 1988:248–252.

Chapter

Liver Function Tests

Louis Lambiase and Christopher Forsmark

The term liver function test is really a misnomer. Commonly applied it refers to the measurement of the serum activity of alkaline phosphate (AP), aspartate aminotransferase (AST), alanine aminotransferase (ALT), bilirubin, and lactate dehydrogenase (LDH). These enzymes do not, however, measure hepatic function; they only indicate some level of hepatic damage or inflammation. One may assess function either indirectly (by looking for the sequelae of diminished liver function such as coagulopathy due to decreased production of vitamin K–dependent clotting factors or hypoalbuminemia) or directly (by tests such as the lidocaine clearance of indocyanine green).

The emergency practitioner is most interested in the detection of acute disease, appropriate triage, and institution of treatment. An understanding of these enzyme measurements and their interpretation and limitations can help achieve these goals. This chapter focuses on these enzymes, the tissues in which they originate, and a few of the disease states in which their measurement might prove helpful in the emergency department (ED) setting. No panel of liver tests will in and of itself make a diagnosis. These tests need to be used to support a diagnosis already entertained after examination of the patient rather than as a screen for liver disease.

BILIRUBIN

Bilirubin is a product of red blood cell catabolism. When senescent erythrocytes are removed from the circulation by the reticuloendothelial system, hemoglobin is degraded to heme. The heme molecules undergo a series of oxidations that disrupt the heme ring, forming biliverdin and, after reduction at the center methylidene bridge, bilirubin. Bilirubin has a low solubility in serum and is transported quickly via albumin to the liver. In the rough endoplasmic reticulum of the hepatocyte, the bilirubin undergoes conjugation with two glucuronic acid moieties. The bilirubin conjugate is then excreted via the bile into the intestine. In the intestine bilirubin diglyceride is acted on by intestinal glucuronidases. The bilirubin is broken down further into urobilinogen and excreted in the feces. The kidney plays a role in eliminating bilirubin when excretion into the intestine is hampered by obstruction of the biliary tree or hepatic disease.[1]

The level of bilirubin in the serum represents a balance between production and excretion.[2] Bilirubin measurement is usually expressed as the total amount (conjugated and unconjugated forms) and the direct (conjugated) amount.

Distinguishing between direct and indirect hyperbilirubinemia can be useful in determining the cause of jaundice. Indirect hyperbilirubinemia, indicating mainly a predominance of unconjugated bilirubin, occurs when the indirect or unconjugated fraction is >1.2 mg/dL and the direct or conjugated component is <20% of the total. Direct hyperbilirubinemia, indicating a predominance of the conjugated fraction, is said to occur in the reverse situation, ie, when the indirect portion is <20% of the total.[2]

The cause of indirect hyperbilirubinemia is usually hemolysis or a defect in hepatitic conjugation of bilirubin, due to either a preexisting enzyme defect or severe damage to hepatocytes that compromises their ability to conjugate bilirubin. The differential diagnosis of indirect hyperbilirubinemia is listed in Table 34–1. Of particular note is the fact that hemolysis causing indirect hyperbilirubinemia can accompany a variety of systemic diseases, including acute infection, hemolytic anemia, and Wilson disease.[1, 2]

Direct hyperbilirubinemia is caused by either bile duct obstruction or hepatocellular damage that allows conjugation but not secretion of bile (cholestasis). The differential diagnosis is listed in Table 34–2. The bilirubin alone does not distinguish between obstructive or hepatocellu-

TABLE 34–1. CAUSES OF UNCONJUGATED HYPERBILIRUBINEMIA

Hemolysis	Crigler-Najjar's syndrome
Physiologic jaundice of infancy	Gilbert's syndrome
Breast milk	Congestive heart failure
Shunt hyperbilirubinemia	Severe hepatic failure

TABLE 34–2. CAUSES OF DIRECT HYPERBILIRUBINEMIA

Bile duct obstruction	Drug reaction
Dubin-Johnson's syndrome	Hepatitis
Rotor syndrome	Hepatocellular necrosis

lar jaundice. The clinician must use other means to come to a diagnosis.[2–4]

Serum bilirubin level is not a sensitive indicator of hepatitic dysfunction because there can be mild-to-moderate hepatocellular damage or transient common bile duct obstruction in the presence of a normal serum bilirubin level. The liver's capacity to conjugate and excrete bilirubin is several times greater than the daily pigment load.[2]

There have been no controlled studies correlating the level of the total bilirubin and the cause of jaundice. Likewise, few studies have examined the level of bilirubin as a prognostic indicator. In several instances, it may be helpful. In most patients with viral hepatitis the magnitude of the elevation of total bilirubin correlates with the hepatocellular damage and the length of recuperation. In patients with fulminant hepatitis a bilirubin level of 5 mg/dL or greater is associated with a worse prognosis.[2, 5] In patients with sclerosing cholangitis, a precipitous increase in bilirubin may signal the development of bacterial cholangitis of biliary tumor. Aside from these limited cases, however, the magnitude of the bilirubin elevation gives no specific diagnostic or prognostic information.

ALKALINE PHOSPHATE

Alkaline phosphate (AP) refers to a group of enzymes that hydrolyze, at an alkaline pH, organic phosphoesters to an alcohol and inorganic phosphate. It is clinically useful to think of the group as a single entity.[6]

Alkaline phosphatase is found in a variety of tissues, including hepatic canaliculi, small intestine, bone, kidney, white blood cells, and placenta. The AP activity that is normally present in serum is derived mainly from the liver and bone and, in certain cases, from the small intestine.[2, 6]

Elevated levels of serum AP may be either physiologic or pathologic (Table 34–3). The rapid bone growth of childhood is associated with a tripling of the serum AP. Late in pregnancy the placenta causes an elevated serum level that usually returns to normal by the 20th day post partum. Bone disease, including fractures and Paget's disease, also causes elevations.[2, 6, 7]

TABLE 34–3. CAUSES OF ELEVATED ALKALINE PHOSPHATASE

Bone growth	Myocardial infarction
Pregnancy	Acute hepatitis
Aging	Cirrhosis
Osteoblastic lesions	Cholestasis
Gastrointestinal ulceration	

The main causes of a rise in serum AP level of hepatic origin are obstructions of the biliary tree, cholestatic hepatitis, space-occupying lesions of diffuse infiltration of the liver, adverse drug reactions, and canalicular obstruction in hepatitis. In patients with biliary tree obstruction of cholestasis, the AP is elevated out of proportion to the aminotransferases.[2, 6–8] Whereas the magnitude of elevation of the AP is not specific for any disease state, the highest elevations are present in common bile duct obstruction or infiltrating disease of the liver (eg, lymphoma, tuberculosis, sarcoidosis).

In some diseases that do not involve the liver there appears to be increased AP of hepatic origin in the serum. These include Hodgkin's disease and myeloid metaplasia. Infusion of albumin intravenously may also provoke a rise that persists for several days. The mechanism of this increase is poorly understood.[2, 9]

AMINOTRANSFERASES

The aminotransferases (formerly known as transaminases) are indicators of hepatic injury and hepatocyte necrosis. The most common clinically measured enzymes are alanine aminotransferase (ALT) and aspartate aminotransferase (AST). They were formerly called serum glutamate pyruvate transaminase (SGPT) and serum glutamate oxaloacetic transaminase (SGOT), respectively. These enzymes catalyze the transfer of an alpha amino group from alanine to an alpha keto group of alpha-ketoglutarate. This results in the formation of pyruvate and oxaloacetate.[2, 6]

Aspartate aminotransferase (AST) is present in the mitochondria and cytosol of the cells of a variety of tissues, including heart, skeletal muscle, kidney, brain, and liver. It was first used clinically as a marker of myocardial infarction. Aspartate aminotransferase is also elevated in liver disease, rhabdomyolysis, and musculoskeletal trauma. There may falsely elevated measurements of AST in patients undergoing treatment with opiates and erythromycin. Contamination of specimens with cal-

TABLE 34–4. CAUSES OF ELEVATED AMINOTRANSFERASES

Myocardial infarction	Obstructive jaundice
Pericarditis	Shock
Congestive heart failure	Acute pancreatitis
Hepatitis	Muscular dystrophy
Infectious mononucleosis	Renal infarction
Cirrhosis	Shock

Adapted from Bozzuto TM: *Emerg Med Clin North Am.* 1986;4(2):329–343.

cium-containing dust (eg, because of construction) has also been reported as falsely elevated levels.[2, 6, 8]

Alanine aminotransferase (ALT) is present mainly in the cytosol of hepatocytes, and thus its elevation tends to be more specific for liver cell damage. The ALT tends to be elevated in the same setting as the AST, but the levels are less in patients with myocardial necrosis, cirrhosis, and chronic hepatitis. In rhabdomyolysis, elevations are trivial compared with those of creatinine kinase or of AST. The ALT is usually greater than the AST in acute hepatitis and extensive hepatic necrosis. Table 34–4 lists the causes of elevated aminotransferases.[2, 6, 8]

Much has been written with regard to the height and pattern of elevation of the aminotransferases and the clues they may provide about the nature of the liver disease. A few general guidelines apply:

1. Elevations up to eight times as normal are not diagnostic of any particular disorder. The highest levels occur in disorders that cause extensive hepatocellular necrosis, including acute hepatitis, hepatic ischemia due to shock or congestive heart failure; and after exposure to hepatotoxins such as *Amanita phalloides*. In these cases the AST and ALT can reach into the thousands.[2]
2. In obstructive jaundice, cirrhosis, and alcoholic liver disease the aminotransferase levels are seldom greater than 500 units.[2, 10]
3. The correlation between extent of hepatic damage and the serum elevation of these enzymes is poor.[4]
4. There is no prognostic significance to the height of enzyme elevation in acute hepatitis; patients with aminotransferase levels greater than 1000 units routinely recover without long-term sequelae.[2, 6]
5. The AST/ALT ratio has little importance outside of alcoholic liver disease. If the ALT is less than 300, an AST/ALT ratio greater than 2 is highly suggestive of alcoholic liver disease. Alcoholics have a deficiency of the enzyme pyridoxal 5′-phosphate, which is more necessary for the synthesis of ALT than for AST. The relatively low serum ALT activity in patients with alcoholic liver disease reflects this relative decrease in synthesis of the enzyme.[2, 10]

LACTATE DEHYDROGENASE

Lactate dehydrogenase (LDH) is a cytosolic enzyme widely dispersed in tissues throughout the body. It catalyzes lactate + NAD to pyruvate + NADH and plays an important role in carbohydrate catabolism. Serum LDH activity is composed of five isoenzymes (named LD-1 through LD-5, based on electrophoretic migration speed), with the liver-specific isoenzyme LD-5 migrating the slowest. Normally, the predominant serum LDH activity is from erythrocytes. The primary value of LDH measurement is in detecting tissue necrosis.[2, 6]

The pattern of isoenzyme elevation may be helpful in pinpointing the cause of elevation. In myocardial infarction, megaloblastic anemia, hemolysis, and muscular dystrophy, the LD-1 is greater than LD-2, which is the opposite of the normal pattern.[6] Lactate dehydrogenase is a very nonspecific indicator of hepatocellular damage and plays a limited role in the diagnosis of liver disease.[2] Table 34–5 lists the causes of increased LDH.

LABORATORY EVALUATIONS OF HEPATIC DISEASE

The Jaundiced Patient

When a patient presents to the ED with jaundice, it is most important to distinguish biliary obstruction from hepatocellular causes of jaundice because the therapeutic approach and prognosis differ greatly. Liver enzymes can be of great help in making that distinction, but as with all tests they need confirmation both with history and physical examination and other laboratory and imaging studies.

The hallmark of obstructive jaundice is an elevated AP level.[3] Whereas 75% of patients with prolonged cholestasis of either hepatocellular or obstructive organ have a greater than fourfold elevation of the

TABLE 34–5. CAUSES OF ELEVATED LACTATE DEHYDROGENASE

Myocardial infarction	Infectious mononucleosis
Pulmonary infarction	Hepatitis
Megaloblastic anemia	Obstructive jaundice
Sickle cell anemia	Metastatic cancer
Acute leukemia	Hepatic trauma
Lymphoma	Muscular dystrophy

Adapted from Bozzuto TM: *Emerg Med Clin North Am.* 1986;4(2)329–343.

ALP, the AP is elevated much more significantly than the aminotransferase in obstructive jaundice. This pattern is unfortunately not specific because several drugs including phenytoin and erythromycin estolate can cause cholestasis biochemically similar to bile duct obstruction.[2, 3, 6] Patients with common bile duct stones and bile duct obstruction may also have marked elevations of aminotransferase in addition to elevations of AP.[2] Thus, one must confirm the suspicion of bile duct obstruction with appropriate radiographic evidence of biliary obstruction, using either ultrasound or computed tomography (CT).

In some mild cases, there may be confusion as to the origin of an elevated AP level. The measurement of AP isoenzymes is one method of determining whether the elevation is of bone or hepatic origin. Detection of the hepatic isoenzyme, which is heat-stable as opposed to the heat-labile bone isoenzyme, has been used as a way of determining the source. Subsequent analyses have called the accuracy of this approach into question[9, 11] because in practice the isoenzymes are difficult to separate and their measurement is often inaccurate. Thus, measurement of AP isoenzymes is not helpful in clinical decision making.[9, 11] The most useful confirmation of elevated hepatic AP is measurement of the enzyme 5′-nucleotidase or gamma-glutamyl peptidase, which is present in liver but not in bone.[2]

Aminotransferases may be helpful in distinguishing obstructive from hepatocellular jaundice. In bile duct obstruction, levels of these enzymes are not usually greater than 300 to 400 units, whereas in patients with acute hepatitis they are often much higher.[3] Lower levels are, however, not specific for biliary obstruction; for example, in alcoholic hepatitis the levels are also usually less than 400 units.[10]

Patients with acute viral hepatitis may become jaundiced, and they often present with markedly elevated aminotransferases. These elevations, although suggesting the possibility of viral hepatitis, do not help with triage or diagnosis. Samples for viral serologies (hepatitis B surface antigen and antibody, hepatitis C antibody, and hepatitis A IgM antibody) should be drawn in the ED. These aid in the follow-up of the patient, but they do not convey prognostic information. The decision to admit a patient with acute hepatitis should be based on clinical grounds (dehydration or encephalopathy) or on laboratory evidence of diminished hepatitic synthetic abilities (prolonged PT or decreased albumin).[6]

Although the pattern of liver test abnormality can be helpful in the evaluation of the jaundiced patient and in corroborating a clinical diagnosis, further testing is always required to rule out biliary tract obstruction. As a general rule, all jaundiced patients and all patients with biliary tract disease require a noninvasive imaging study such as ultrasound to look for biliary ductal dilation. This is of fundamental importance because rapid therapy (IV antibiotics and ductal decompression) is often required to prevent morbidity and mortality due to cholangitis in patients with acute ductal obstruction.

Hepatic Trauma

Bilirubin is not a reliable indicator of serious hepatitic trauma. Lactate dehydrogenase, although frequently greater than 1400 units 8 to 12 hours after injury, is so widely distributed that traumatic injury to any tissue may precipitate a rise and is thus insensitive for liver damage. Elevated levels of AST or ALT may be helpful in deciding whether there is a likelihood of hepatic injury. In adult patients with blunt abdominal trauma, an AST or ALT level greater than 130 units correlates highly with a serious hepatic injury and suggests the need for CT scanning or more invasive testing.[12] In the pediatric population the cutoff levels appear to be an AST of 200 units and an ALT of 100 units.[13] Whether these tests are of actual utility in these settings is open to question, however.

Toxin Ingestion

Many ingested drugs and toxins may have an effect on the liver and cause hepatocellular disease. They include solvents such as carbon tetrachloride and mineral spirits, mycotoxins such as aflatoxin and toxic plant products, and certain medications. It is beyond the scope of this chapter to review all hepatic manifestations of poisoning, but a detailed medication, exposure, and ingestion history should be obtained from all patients with undiagnosed liver enzyme abnormalities. Some common hepatotoxins are listed in Table 34–6. We concentrate on two particular types of poisoning as prototypes for the ED practitioner.

Acetaminophen is a commonly used analgesic with few side effects. When ingested in doses of greater than 6 g a day, however, it may cause marked hepatitic necrosis and lead to fulminant hepatic failure. Toxicity occurs when, with ingestion of large doses, the binding capacity

TABLE 34–6. COMMON HEPATOTOXINS

Acetaminophen	Tetracycline
α-Amanitin	Dimethylnitrosamine
Ethanol	Rifampin
Methotrexate	Phenytoin
Yellow phosphorus	Amiodarone

of hepatic glutathione is overwhelmed and drug metabolism proceeds through a secondary pathway. Accumulated metabolites then cause damage to the hepatocytes.[14–16]

The typical clinical scenario involves a single massive dose taken as a suicide attempt, although multiple smaller doses, particularly after alcohol ingestion, can cause lethal damage. Jaundice does not usually appear until 3 to 5 days after ingestion, and even then the bilirubin level is seldom elevated above 4 mg/dL.[15, 17] Aminotransferases may be normal during the acute phase but may soar into the 20,000 unit range several days afterward.[15, 16]

Amanita phalloides is a mushroom species that grows in oak wood in late summer through early winter. It contains toxins that cause severe damage to the liver, kidney, and brain. Much like acetaminophen poisoning, *Amanita* toxicity appears at first with gastroenterologic disturbances, primarily severe diarrhea. These symptoms resolve before hepatocellular damage and renal failure are apparent. As with acetaminophen toxicity, the aminotransferases may be markedly elevated with relatively less elevation in bilirubin. The prognosis is poor, with half of all cases being fatal.[18]

Reye's Syndrome

Reye's syndrome, or acute encephalopathy with fatty degeneration of the viscera, is a true pediatric emergency. It is not uncommon, occurring in about 200 to 400 cases a year with a fatality rate of 25 to 40%. Clinically, there is a prodrome consisting of a febrile renal illness. After a recovery period of less than a week there is abrupt onset of vomiting. Delirium and stupor with seizures and coma begin soon after. The patient is typically anicteric, but hepatomegaly may be found on examination.[19]

The aminotransferases are usually elevated, with levels greater than 100 units. Serum bilirubin is usually normal, but LDH may be elevated owing to muscle damage. Serum ammonia concentration should also be checked as it is often elevated and has prognostic implications.[19]

CONCLUSION

Biochemical measurements of hepatic enzymes may be helpful in the diagnosis of certain disease states. However, they are often nonspecific and offer only general clues to the nature of the hepatic injury. They are no substitute for a thorough history and careful physical examination. The low specificity of these tests limits their use in routine screening. Their only utility in the ED is in supporting a diagnosis that is suspected before they are ordered and in helping the clinician decide on the need for urgent noninvasive imaging studies.

REFERENCES

1. Billing BH: Bilirubin metabolism, in Schiff L, Schiff ER (eds): *Diseases of the Liver*. Philadelphia: JB Lippincott; 1987:103.
2. Kaplan MM: Laboratory tests, in Schiff L, Schiff ER (eds): *Diseases of the Liver*. Philadelphia: JB Lippincott; 1987:219.
3. Schiff L: Jaundice: A clinical approach, in Schiff L, Schiff ER (eds): *Diseases of the Liver*. Philadelphia: JB Lippincott; 1987:209.
4. Sherlock S: Biochemical investigation in liver disease; Some correlation with hepatic histology. *J Pathol Bacteriol*. 1946;24:835.
5. Hardison WG, Lee FL: Prognosis in acute liver disease of the alcoholic patient. *N Engl J Med*. 1976;275:61.
6. Bozzuto TM: Other enzymes. Creatinine phosphokinase, lactate dehydrogenase, serum glutamic oxaloacetate transaminase, serum glutamic pyruvate transaminase, and alkaline phosphatase. *Emerg Med Clin North Am*. 1986;4:329.
7. Wallach J: *Interpretations of Diagnostic Tests: A Handbook Synopsis of Laboratory Medicine*. Boston: Little, Brown and Company; 1978:53.
8. Wallach J: *Interpretations of Diagnostic Tests: A Handbook Synopsis of Laboratory Medicine*. Boston: Little, Brown and Company; 1978:57.
9. Kaplan M: Alkaline phosphatase. *Gastroenterology*. 1977;62:452.
10. Cohen JA, Kaplan MM: The SGOT/SGPT ratio—An indicator of alcoholic liver disease. *Dig Dis Sci*. 1979;24:835.
11. Winkelmen J: The clinical usefulness of alkaline phosphatase isoenzyme determination. *J Clin Pathol*. 1972;57:625.
12. Sahdev P, Garramore RR, Schwartz RJ: Evaluation of liver function tests in screening for intraabdominal injuries. *Ann Emerg Med*. 1991;20:838.
13. Oldham KT et al: Blunt hepatic injury and elevated hepatic enzymes: A clinical correlation in children. *J Pediatr Surg*. 1984;19:457.
14. Bass NM, Ochner RK: Drug induced liver disease, in Zakim D, Boyer TD (eds): *Hepatology: A Textbook of Liver Disease*. Philadelphia: WB Saunders; 1990:754.
15. Prescott LF et al: Plasma paracetamol half life and necrosis in patients with paracetamol overdosage. *Lancet*. 1971;1:519.
16. Prescott LF et al: Successful treatment of severe paracetamol overdosage. *Lancet*. 1978;1:588.
17. Zimmerman HJ, Maddrey WC: Toxic and drug induced hepatitis, in Schiff L, Schiff ER (eds): *Diseases of the Liver*. Philadelphia: JB Lippincott; 1987:591.
18. Klein AS et al: Amanita poisoning: treatment and the role of liver transplantation. *Am J Med*. 1989;86:187.
19. Balistreri WF, Schubert WK: Liver disease in infancy and childhood, in Schiff L, Schiff ER (eds): *Diseases of the Liver*. Philadelphia: JB Lippincott; 1987:1337.

Chapter

Serum Calcium

James M. Kelley

As the body's most plentiful cation, calcium is utilized in numerous physiologic processes. It participates in platelet aggregation, is a cofactor in the clotting process, and promotes leukocyte function. Calcium also plays a key role in hormone secretion, neurotransmitter release, and depolarization of nerve, smooth muscle, and myocardial cells.[1–3]

The largest part of total body calcium is the extravascular component, composed primarily of the mineralized matrix of bone.[2] The intravascular space contains calcium in three forms. A protein-bound form, primarily albumin, accounts for 40% of the total serum calcium. Five to 15% of serum calcium is complexed with phosphate, bicarbonate, citrate, and oxalate. The free or ionized form constitutes the final 45 to 55% of total serum calcium.[4]

These fractions can be altered by changes in the blood pH and serum protein levels. Alkalemia, as induced by hyperventilation, vomiting, or rapid administration of intravenous bicarbonate, causes increased binding of calcium and a resultant decrease in the serum ionized calcium. It is estimated that each 0.1 increase in pH units causes a 1.7 mg/dL (0.42 mmol/L) decrease in the serum ionized calcium. Changes in serum albumin also affect the serum calcium concentration. For every decrease in serum albumin of 1 g/dL there is a concomitant fall in the total serum calcium of 0.8 mg/dL.[2, 4] Interestingly, changes in other serum proteins (eg, elevated paraproteins in multiple myeloma) rarely cause a change in the total serum calcium.

ASSESSING CALCIUM STATUS

The decision to order a serum calcium level in the emergency department is best aided by a knowledge of the test and of the clinical signs, symptoms, and outcomes one might expect in a patient with an altered serum calcium level.

Although the total serum calcium is most commonly measured, it is most helpful clinically to obtain an ionized calcium measurement because the ionized form is the physiologically active component. In fact, several studies have documented that the total serum calcium level (which requires knowledge of the patient's serum albumin concentration for accurate interpretation) correlates poorly with the serum ionized level.[6, 7] The additional cost to the patient of obtaining an ionized serum calcium rather than a total serum calcium and serum albumin is in the range of only $10 to $15.

When measured by an ion-selective electrode, the normal range for serum ionized calcium is 3.6 to 5.6 mg/dL,[7] although reference values differ among laboratories (1.13 to 1.32 mmol/L).

Laboratory results can be subject to errors of sampling and storage. It has been suggested that the use of a tourniquet affects measured pH and calcium. McMullen and coworkers, however, reported no effect on ionized calcium when a tourniquet was used.[8] Anticoagulants used in sample collection can also cause errors in calcium determination. It is thus important to use a standard amount of heparin or citrate anticoagulant in order to avoid spuriously low calcium determinations due to binding of calcium, sample coagulation, or dilutional effects of the anticoagulant.[9, 10] The sample should be stored on ice to prevent the accumulation of lactic acid secondary to continuing metabolic activity. There is also a theoretic concern that rapid infusion of albumin-containing plasma expanders may lower the serum ionized calcium.[11]

Without a clinical suspicion or symptoms, the indiscriminate testing of serum calcium in the emergency department may be of little value. In fact, in one study in which serum ionized calcium was measured routinely in asymptomatic patients who had known malignancy, the presence of an elevated serum ionized calcium level had no apparent bearing on prognosis or clinical condition.[12]

HYPERCALCEMIA

As with other metabolic and electrolyte abnormalities, the signs and symptoms of hypercalcemia are often nonspecific. The rate of rise of serum calcium and duration of the condition are major determinants of whether there are clinical manifestations.[1–3, 13]

Hypercalcemia can cause symptoms in multiple organ systems. The central nervous system responds with a depressed level of consciousness and depressed reflexes. The kidneys demonstrate a renal concentrating defect with polyuria, polydipsia, and dehydration. The gastrointestinal system displays nausea, vomiting, constipation, or dysphagia. The cardiac effects of hypercalcemia include varying degrees of heart block, ventricular arrhythmia, potentiation of digitalis toxicity, and especially a shortened Q-T interval on the electrocardiogram.[1, 14]

Chief among the causes of hypercalcemia are hyperparathyroidism and certain malignancies, including breast carcinoma, lung adenocarcinoma, renal cell carcinoma, squamous cell carcinoma, transitional cell carcinoma, multiple myeloma, and lymphoma. Therefore, in the emergency department a serum calcium level might best be determined in the patient with suspected hyperparathyroidism or malignancy and accompanying symptoms.

HYPOCALCEMIA

As with hypercalcemia, the symptoms of hypocalcemia depend to a degree on the rate of change of the serum calcium concentration.[13] In a small study, Sorrell and Rosen observed that a serum ionized calcium level of <2.5 mg/dL was the threshold for the development of symptoms.[7] In the emergency department, the measurement of serum calcium might be better limited to individuals who demonstrate clinical signs or symptoms or those who have a predisposing risk.

The cardinal sign of symptomatic hypocalcemia is neuromuscular excitability. This may be manifested in a range of symptoms including paresthesia, muscle cramping, carpopedal spasm, laryngospasm, and tonic-clonic seizure. Cardiac signs of hypocalcemia include decreased cardiac contractility (manifested rarely as heart failure) and a prolonged Q-T interval and terminal T-wave inversion on the electrocardiogram.[3, 13] Nonspecific psychiatric symptoms may develop including irritability, anxiety, depression, and confusion. The classic bedside signs of hypocalcemia, Chvostek and Trousseau signs, may be absent in about one third of patients; conversely, Chvostek sign is present in only about 10% of normal individuals.[9]

There are many causes of hypocalcemia to consider. Identifying those patients at greatest risk for symptomatic hypocalcemia can simplify the decision to assess serum calcium in the emergency department. Those at greatest risk for hypocalcemia are postoperative neck surgery patients, low birth weight or premature neonates of diabetic mothers, patients given intravenous phosphate or bicarbonate, patients on anticonvulsant therapy, patients receiving massive quantities of transfused blood, and those with renal failure. Hypocalcemia can also be associated with respiratory alkalosis and hypoalbuminemia. An additional group of patients at risk are those predisposed to hypomagnesemia (eg, alcoholics, patients on diuretic therapy) because hypomagnesemia can cause a refractory hypocalcemia.

To justify ordering a serum calcium in the emergency department, thought must be given to the patient's symptoms and predisposing risks. Ordering ''routine'' laboratory studies without symptoms or risk factors is likely to have a low yield. Given the costs inherent in emergency department evaluation, patients may be best served by the application of high-yield criteria, such as symptoms, signs, and risk factors before a serum calcium determination is ordered.

REFERENCES

1. Jansen CL: Fluid and electrolyte balance, in Rosen P (ed): *Emergency Medicine*. 3rd ed. St. Louis: CV Mosby; 1992:2132–2176.
2. Wolfson AB, Feldman HI: Disorders of calcium and magnesium metabolism, in Wolfson AB (ed): *Endocrine and Metabolic Emergencies*. New York: Churchill Livingstone; 1990:45–59.
3. DeRubertis FR: Hypocalcemia: Etiology and management. *Hospital Med.* March 1985:88–118.
4. Kleerekoper M, Rao DS: Hypercalcemia and hypocalcemia, in Callaham ML (ed): *Current Therapy in Emergency Medicine*. Toronto: BC Decker; 1987:729–731.
5. Lynch RE: Ionized calcium: Pediatric perspective. *Pediatr Clin North Am.* 1990; 37:373–389.
6. Forman DT, Lorenzo L: Ionized calcium: Its significance and clinical usefulness. *Ann Clin Lab Sci.* 1991;21:297–304.
7. Sorell M, Rosen JF: Ionized calcium: Serum levels during symptomatic hypocalcemia. *J Pediatr.* 1975;87:67–70.
8. McMullan AD, Burns J, Paterson CR: Venepuncture for calcium assays: Should we still avoid the tourniquet? *Postgrad Med J.* 1990;66:547–548.
9. Juan D: Hypocalcemia: Differential diagnosis and mechanisms. *Arch Intern Med.* 1979;139:1166–1171.
10. Sachs C et al: Anticoagulant-induced preanalytical errors in ionized calcium determination on blood. *Scand J Clin Invest.* 1989;49:647–651.
11. Thode B et al: Comparison of serum total calcium, albumin-corrected total calcium, and ionized calcium in 1213 patients with suspected calcium disorders. *Scand J Clin Invest.* 1989;49:217–223.
12. Riancho JA, Arjona R, Sanz J: Is the routine measurement of ionized calcium worthwhile in patients with cancer? *Postgrad Med J.* 1991;67:350–353.
13. Lafferty FW: Differential diagnosis of hypercalcemia. *J Bone Mineral Res.* 1991;6(suppl 2):51–59.
14. Douglas PS et al: Extreme hypercalcemia and electrocardiographic changes. *Am J Cardiol.* 1984;54:674–675.

Chapter

Serum Magnesium Determination

Kaveh Ilkhanipour

Magnesium serves as an important cofactor in numerous bodily chemical reactions, including all those involving energy transfer with ATP.[1] It also plays important roles in cardiac and muscle contractions as well as in fat, carbohydrate, and protein metabolism.

Magnesium is the fourth most plentiful cation and the second most abundant intracellular cation in the body. Only 1% of the total body magnesium content is found in the extracellular (serum) space. Serum magnesium is further partitioned into three fractions. Fifty-five percent is found in the ionized or free state, 30% is protein bound, and 15% is chelated with other anions.

The kidney is the primary regulator of magnesium balance. Magnesium is retained in response to deficiency, and excess magnesium is excreted promptly. Persistent hypermagnesemia is very unusual in the presence of normal renal function.[2] Diuretic drug use increases urinary magnesium excretion and has been identified as one of the leading causes of hypomagnesemia.[7–9] Magnesium requirements double during pregnancy and are even greater in magnesium wasting conditions such as ethanol abuse.[4, 14–16]

ASSESSING MAGNESIUM STATUS

The test most commonly used to assess the body's magnesium status is the total serum magnesium concentration. This level represents all three fractions of magnesium found in the serum. A number of investigators have found poor correlation between serum levels and tissue concentrations of magnesium.[7, 9, 17–19] Because 99% of body magnesium is contained in the intracellular compartment,[7, 17, 18] intracellular magnesium levels probably reflect total body magnesium status more accurately. Magnesium retention tests have been recommended as more accurate identifiers of patients with total body magnesium deficiency.[20]

Efforts have been lately directed at measuring free (ionized) intracellular magnesium concentrations, which may better reflect cellular magnesium status.[21–23] Zaloga and colleagues[24] found that normal serum magnesium concentrations essentially rule out normal ultrafilterable (ionized) hypo- or hypermagnesemia in critically ill patients. Low and high total serum magnesium concentrations, however, correlated poorly with ultrafilterable magnesium status.

Low serum magnesium concentrations usually imply total body magnesium deficiency.[25, 26] Intracellular magnesium depletion may be present, however, when serum magnesium levels are normal.[27, 28] Currently, there is no single laboratory test that can reliably establish clinically significant magnesium deficiency. Because there appears to be a poor relationship between the easily measurable serum magnesium concentration and tissue or total body magnesium status, some investigators have recommended empiric treatment with magnesium supplements based on the presence of high-risk criteria for hypomagnesemia.[29, 30] In this setting, a serum creatinine level would be useful if there is any concern regarding renal function. An elevated serum creatinine level greatly increases the risk of causing hypermagnesemia through acute magnesium supplementation. If there is no suspicion of compromised renal function, empiric magnesium supplementation could be started simply on the basis of risk factors associated with clinically significant hypomagnesemia. Serum magnesium levels might then be measured if the patient is to receive multiple doses or prolonged infusion of magnesium in the emergency department.

HYPOMAGNESEMIA

Table 36–1 lists the most commonly used units in which magnesium concentration is expressed, with the corresponding clinical magnesium status. Given the poor correlation of currently measurable serum magnesium concentrations with the presence of total body magnesium depletion, identification of clinical predictors of total body magnesium depletion could aid in the selection of those patients who might benefit most from empiric magnesium supplementation in the emergency department.

There are many causes of hypomagnesemia in the patient presenting to the emergency department (ED). There are four major high-risk criteria that are relatively common and easily identifiable on clinical presentation.

Individuals on *diuretic therapy* represent one class of patients who are at risk for clinically significant hypomagnesemia. Furosemide and thiazide diuretics have been closely linked to hypomagnesemia, hypokalemia, and increased risk of ventricular ectopy.[31, 32] Wester[33] demonstrated a significant prevalence of muscle magnesium deficiency among

TABLE 36–1. MAGNESIUM MEASUREMENTS

Description	mmol/L	mEq/L	mg/dL
Severe hypomagnesemia	0.5	1.0	1.2
Lower limit of normal	0.75	1.5	1.8
Upper limit of normal	1.0	2.0	2.4
Symptomatic hypermagnesemia (mild)	1.5	3.0	3.6
Symptomatic hypermagnesemia (severe)	2.5	5.0	6.0
Possibly fatal levels	5.0	10.0	12.0

From Sachter JJ: Magnesium in the 1990s: Implications for acute care. *Top Emerg Med.* 1992;14(1):23–50.

297 patients with congestive heart failure on long-term diuretic therapy. Potassium-sparing diuretics have been shown to increase tissue levels of both potassium and magnesium significantly when compared with simple potassium supplementation in patients who are receiving conventional diuretics.[34]

Alcohol abuse, both acute and chronic, has been shown to be associated with hypomagnesemia.[35, 36] Lim and Jacob[36] demonstrated that more than 50% of alcoholics had tissue magnesium deficiency in the setting of normal serum magnesium concentrations. The magnesium deficiency seen in alcohol abusers is due to poor nutrition and decreased magnesium intake as well as to increased renal magnesium wasting.[37]

The current literature points to a strong relationship between ischemic heart disease and hypomagnesemia.[38, 39] Current data appear to implicate rises in catecholamine levels during myocardial ischemia or infarction as a cause of magnesium depletion.[40] A number of studies have investigated the apparent beneficial effect of empiric treatment with supplemental magnesium in patients with suspected myocardial infarction. Horner[41] summarized the results of these studies using a meta-analytic approach and found an overall reduction in mortality of 54% when magnesium supplementation was compared with placebo.

The final group of patients who are predisposed to clinical significant hypomagnesemia are those with *ventricular arrhythmias*. Dysrhythmias associated with magnesium deficiency and potentially responsive to magnesium therapy include those secondary to alcohol withdrawal,[42] congestive heart failure,[43] digoxin toxicity,[44, 45] and acute myocardial infarction.[45] Magnesium administration also appears to be effective in terminating torsades de pointes (polymorphous ventricular tachycardia).[46]

In conclusion, because empiric magnesium supplementation in the

ED appears to be safe and beneficial in the high-risk clinical scenarios described here, there appears to be little need to measure the serum magnesium prior to initiating such therapy. This practice appears not to be justified. The only exception to this rule is in the setting of suspected renal insufficiency, in which measurement of the serum creatinine level would help to guide magnesium supplementation.

HYPERMAGNESEMIA

Hypermagnesemia is a rare occurrence in the ED patient. An exhaustive search of the literature by Sachter[30] that encompassed 7000 citations over the past 25 years found no cases of clinically significant hypermagnesemia in the absence of concomitant renal insufficiency or increased exogenous intake.

The normal kidney can excrete 6 g (500 mEq) of excess elemental magnesium per day. Hypermagnesemia usually will not develop until glomerular filtration rate declines to 30 mL/min. Magnesium concentrations >3.5 mg/dL are usually only seen when the creatinine clearance is <10 mL/min.[47–49]

Overuse of magnesium-containing antacids constitutes the most common cause of drug-induced hypermagnesemia.[50] Patients who abuse magnesium-containing laxatives and cathartics may also become hypermagnesemic,[47–49] but typically only if they become dehydrated or have underlying renal insufficiency. A study of 102 patients receiving repeated doses of magnesium-containing cathartics found 12 with magnesium levels of >3.5 mg/dL[51]; no serious adverse consequences were reported, however.

Magnesium toxicity, unlike magnesium deficiency, is associated with specific signs and symptoms that correlate roughly with measured magnesium levels. Nausea, vomiting, and cutaneous flushing occur at levels of 3 mg/dL. Hyperreflexia and drowsiness are seen at concentrations of 4 mg/dL and QRS widening and PR prolongation occur at 5 mg/dL. Respiratory depression and apnea become a risk when levels reach 10 mg/dL. Complete heart block has been reported at concentrations of 15 mg/dL. Elevated serum magnesium concentrations probably reflect total body magnesium stores. Magnesium supplementation is thus unnecessary and potentially risky when the serum level is elevated.

CONCLUSION

Measurement of the serum magnesium level is helpful in establishing a diagnosis of hypermagnesemia when it is suggested by associated signs and symptoms of magnesium toxicity. Underlying renal insufficiency and abuse of magnesium-containing products increase the likelihood of hypermagnesemia, but these are of little therapeutic significance without concurrent evidence of magnesium toxicity.

REFERENCES

1. Graber TW, Yee AS, Baker FJ: Magnesium: Physiology, clinical disorders, and therapy. *Ann Emerg Med.* 1981;10:49.
2. Beyenbach KW: Unresolved questions of renal magnesium homeostasis. *Magnesium.* 1986; suppl:234–247.
3. Seelig MS: Requirement of magnesium by normal adults: Summary and analysis of published data. *Am J Clin Nutr.* 1964;14:242.
4. Seelig MS: Magnesium Deficiency in the Pathogenesis of Disease: Early Roots of Cardiovascular, Skeletal, and Renal Abnormalities. New York: Plenum; 1980.
5. Sos J: An investigation into nutritional factors of experimental cardiopathy, in Bajunz E, Rona G (eds): *Electrolytes and Cardiovascular Disease: Fundamental Aspects.* Baltimore: Williams & Wilkins; 1965:161–180.
6. Selye H: *The Pluricausal Cardiomyopathies.* Springfield, IL: Charles C Thomas; 1961.
7. Dyckner T, Wester PO: Intracellular magnesium loss after diuretic administration. *Drugs.* 1984;28:161–166.
8. Sheehan J, White A: Diuretic-associated hypomagnesemia. *Br Med J.* 1982;285:1157–1159.
9. Ryan MP: Diuretics and potassium/magnesium depletion. *Am J Med.* 1987;82:38–46.
10. Seelig MS: Possible roles of magnesium in disorders of the aged, in Regelson W, Sinex FM (eds): *Intervention in the Aging Process, Part A: Quantitation, Epidemiology, Clinical Research.* New York: Alan R. Liss; 1983:279–305.
11. Johansson G: Magnesium metabolism: Studies in health, primary hyperparathyroidism and renal stone disease. *Scand J Urol Nephrol.* 1979;51:1–47.
12. Mountabealabeis TD: Effects of aging, chronic disease, and multiple supplements on magnesium requirements. *Magnesium.* 1987;6:5–11.
13. Viv SC, Love AHG: Nutritional status of institutionalized and non-institutionalized aged in Belfast. *Am J Clin Nutr.* 1979;32:1934–1947.
14. Kalbfleisch JM, Lindeman RD, Ginn HE, et al: Effects of ethanol administration on urinary excretion of magnesium and other electrolytes in alcoholic and normal subjects. *J Clin Invest.* 1963;42:1471–1475.
15. McCollister RJ, Prasad AS, Doe RP, et al: Normal renal magnesium clearance and the effect of water lading, chlorthiazide and ethanol on magnesium clearance. *J Lab Clin Med.* 1958;52:928.
16. McCollister RJ, Flink ED, Lewis MD: Urinary excretion of magnesium in man following the ingestion of alcohol. *Am J Clin Nutr.* 1963;12:415–420.
17. Reinhart RA, Marx JJ, Broste SJ, et al: Myocardial magnesium: Relationship to laboratory and clinical variables in patients undergoing cardiac surgery. *J Am Coll Cardiol.* 1991;17:651–656.

18. Reinhart RA, Marx JJ, Haas RG, et al: Intracellular magnesium of mononuclear cells from venous blood of clinically normal subjects. *Clin Chim Acta.* 1987;167:187–195.
19. Elin RJ, Hosseini JM: Magnesium content of mononuclear blood cells. *Clin Chem.* 1985;31:377–380.
20. Ryzen E, Elbaum N, Singer FR, et al: Parenteral magnesium tolerance testing in the evaluation of magnesium deficiency. *Magnesium.* 1985;4:137–147.
21. Blatter LA, McGuigan JAS: Estimation of the upper limit of the free magnesium concentration measured with Mg-sensitive microelectrodes in ferret ventricular muscle. *Magnesium.* 1988;7:154–165.
22. Raju B, Murphy E, Levy LA, et al: A fluorescent indicator for measuring cytosolic free magnesium. *Am J Physiol.* 1989;256:C540–C548.
23. Tsien RY: Intracellular measurements of ion activities. *Annu Rev Biophys Bioeng.* 1983;12:91–116.
24. Zaloga GP, Wilkens R, Tourville J, et al: A simple method for determining physiologically active calcium and magnesium concentrations in critically ill patients. *Crit Care Med.* 1987;9:813–816.
25. Hollifield JW: Thiazide treatment of systemic hypertension: Effects on serum magnesium and ventricular ectopic activity. *Am J Cardiol.* 1989;63:22G–25G.
26. Rude RK: Physiology of magnesium metabolism and the important role of magnesium in potassium deficiency. *Am J Cardiol.* 1989;63:31G–34G.
27. Ryzen E, Wagers PW, Singer FR, et al: Magnesium deficiency in a medical ICU population. *Crit Care Med.* 1985;13:19–21.
28. Whang R, Flink E, Dyckner T, et al: Magnesium depletion as a cause of refractory potassium repletion. *Arch Intern Med.* 1985;145:1686–1689.
29. Groopman DS, Powers RD: High-yield criteria have predictive value for hypomagnesemia in ED patients. *Ann Emerg Med.* 1991;20:457.
30. Sachter JJ: Magnesium in the 1990's: Implications for acute care. *Top Emerg Med.* 1992;14:23–50.
31. Dyckner T, Wester PO: Ventricular extrasystoles and intracellular electrolytes before and after potassium and magnesium infusion in patients on diuretic treatment. *Am Heart J.* 1979;97:12–18.
32. Hollifield JW: Potassium and magnesium abnormalities: Diuretics and arrhythmias in hypertension. *Am J Med.* 1984;77:28–32.
33. Wester PO: Diuretic treatment and magnesium losses. *Acta Med Scand.* 1981;647:145–152.
34. Dyckner T, Wester PO: Potassium/magnesium depletion in patients with cardiovascular disease. *Am J Med.* 1987;82:11–17.
35. Sullivan JF: Serum magnesium in chronic alcoholics. *Lancet.* 1962;2:802–803.
36. Lim P, Jacob E: Magnesium status of alcoholic patients. *Metabolism.* 1972;21:1045–1049.
37. McCollister RJ, Flink EB, Lewis M: Urinary excretion of magnesium following ingestion of alcohol. *Am J Clin Nutr.* 1963;12:415–419.
38. Karppanen H: Epidemiological studies on the relationship between magnesium intake and cardiovascular diseases. *Artery.* 1981;9:190–199.
39. Abraham AS, Eylath U, Weinstein M, et al: Serum magnesium levels in patients with acute myocardial infarction. *N Engl J Med.* 1977;296:862–863.
40. Fink ED, Brick JE, Shane E: Alterations in long-chain free fatty acids and

magnesium concentration in acute myocardial infarction. *Arch Intern Med.* 1981;141:441–443.
41. Horner SM: Efficacy of intravenous magnesium in acute myocardial infarction in reducing arrhythmias and mortality: Meta-analysis of magnesium in acute myocardial infarction. *Circulation.* 1992;3:774–779.
42. Flink EB: Magnesium deficiency in alcoholism. *Alcohol Clin Exp Res.* 1986;10:590–594.
43. Iseri LT, Alexander LC, McCaughey RS, et al: Water and electrolyte content of cardiac and skeletal muscle in heart failure and myocardial infarction. *Am Heart J.* 1952;43:215–227.
44. Whang R, Oei TO, Watanabe A: Frequency of hypomagnesemia in hospitalized patients receiving digitalis. *Arch Intern Med.* 1985;145:655–656.
45. Ghani MF, Smith JR: The effectiveness of magnesium chloride in the treatment of ventricular due to digitalis intoxication. *Am Heart J.* 1974;88:621–626.
46. Tzivoni D, Bania S, Schuger C, et al: Treatment of torsade de pointes with magnesium sulfate. *Circulation.* 1988;77:392–397.
47. Gren J, Woolf A: Hypermagnesemia associated with catharsis in a salicylate-intoxicated patient with anorexia nervosa. *Ann Emerg Med.* 1989;18:200–203.
48. Jone J, Heiselman D, Dougherty J, et al: Cathartic-induced magnesium toxicity during overdose management. *Ann Emerg Med.* 1986;15:1214–1218.
49. Woodard JA, Shannon M, Lacouture PG, et al: Serum magnesium concentration after repetitive magnesium cathartic administration. *Am J Emerg Med.* 1990;8:297–300.
50. Mordes JP, Walker WC: Excess magnesium. *Pharmacol Rev.* 1978;29:273–300.
51. Weber CA, Santiago RM: Hypermagnesemia. A potential complication during treatment of theophylline intoxication with oral activated charcoal and magnesium containing cathartics. *Chest.* 1989;95:56–59.

Chapter

Muscle Enzymes and Myoglobin

Gerhard C. Senula

This chapter reviews the causes of elevated serum muscle enzymes and myoglobin and the use of these tests for the evaluation of skeletal muscle disorders in the emergency department. The measurement of these same proteins for the evaluation of cardiac disorders is discussed in Chapter 7.

Elevations in serum aldolase, creatine phosphokinase (CK), aminotransferase, and dehydrogenase characterize the response to a variety of diseases and conditions affecting skeletal muscle and other tissues in which these proteins are found. The term "muscle enzyme" is used in this chapter, but it is recognized that none of these enzymes is completely specific for muscle pathology. Creatine phosphokinase is the most commonly measured serum muscle enzyme and the most important for the emergency physician to understand. The measurement of other muscle enzymes adds little useful information to that more reliably and easily obtained by measuring CK.

Myoglobin is a monomeric oxygen binding protein found in skeletal and cardiac muscle. Like serum muscle enzymes, small amounts of myoglobin are present in the serum and urine of normal subjects. In the setting of muscle damage, myoglobin is released from cells, allowing elevated serum and urine levels to serve as a nonspecific indicator of muscle injury.

CREATINE PHOSPHOKINASE

Creatine phosphokinase is a dimeric enzyme whose physiologic role is to maintain adequate intracellular concentrations of ATP. Large amounts are present in tissues that consume large quantities of energy (skeletal muscle, cardiac muscle, and brain). Creatine phosphokinase consists of two subunits, each of which may be type M or type B. Three CK isoenzymes, identified by their electrophoretic migration patterns, are therefore possible: CK-MM, CK-MB, and CK-BB. Normal mature skeletal muscle CK consists predominantly of the CK-MM isoenzyme, along with small amounts of CK-MB. The isoenzyme CK-BB is primarily found in brain. Cardiac muscle is the chief source of CK-MB, accounting for 15 to 50% of total activity in cardiac muscle.[1, 2] The MM isoenzyme accounts for nearly all serum CK activity in the normal rested state, with the MB isoenzyme accounting for less than 3 to 4% of total serum activity.[3, 4]

Exactly what is a "normal" baseline serum CK value depends on the population being tested. Individuals with greater muscle mass[5] and those who exercise vigorously tend to have higher baseline serum CK values.[6] Basal values in normal subjects also tend to vary with age, race, and sex.[6–8] Serum CK initially increases with age but declines in the geriatric population,[6–8] probably owing to decreased activity and decreased muscle mass. Blacks have higher levels than whites.[6, 8] For reasons not totally explained by differences in muscle mass, CK levels are slightly lower in females than in males.[6, 8] Although serum CK values may be influenced by these factors, any changes are generally mild and rarely

TABLE 37–1. CAUSES OF ELEVATED SERUM CK

1. Rhabdomyolysis (Table 37–2)	6. GI diseases
2. Cardiac disease (Table 37–3)	Colonic infarction
3. Acute neurologic disorders	Metastatic colon cancer
Subarachnoid hemorrhage	7. Psychotic patients
Stroke	8. Various tumors
Head injury	9. Miscellaneous
Neoplasms	Collagen vascular diseases
Meningitis	Sarcoidosis
Encephalitis	Radiotherapy
Seizures	Shock
Coma	Eclampsia
Reye's syndrome	Pancreatitis, pancreatic carcinoma
4. Postpartum women	Urologic procedures
5. Pulmonary	Sleep deprivation
Acute pneumonia	Dissecting aneurysm
Acute pulmonary embolism	Tick paralysis
Pulmonary infarction	Motor neuron disease
Lung cancer	

Data from Joy et al,[8] Perkoff,[30] and Nevins et al.[31]

mimic clinically significant muscle pathology in the emergency department.

The causes of an elevated serum CK are shown in Table 37–1. Although CK is relatively specific for muscle disease, several other conditions may result in elevated CK levels. In a simple clinical situation involving one organ or tissue type, interpretation of an elevated level should not present problems, and tissue specificity should be high. In the case of multiple organ disease, interpretation may be difficult. If multiple organ disease is present but clinically unsuspected, erroneous interpretations may be made. These principles must be remembered when evaluating any patient with an elevated serum enzyme level.

ISOENZYMES OF CREATINE PHOSPHOKINASE

The MB and BB isoenzymes of CK were originally thought to be specific for cardiac muscle and brain, respectively. Several other conditions, however, have been associated with serum increases in these isoenzymes in which the source is probably not heart or brain. In vitro, animal and fetal studies have shown that embryonic skeletal muscle initially synthesizes the B subunit and later switches to primarily the M subunit, resulting in varying ratios of the three isoenzymes throughout development.[2,4] It is hypothesized that muscle damage or disease results in regenerative efforts and immature muscle elements, which revert to fetal patterns of isoenzyme synthesis.[9–11] This may explain the observation that serum CK-MB is sometimes found in pathologic conditions involving organs other than the heart (Table 37–2). The theory may also apply to cardiac muscle because data have shown that muscle from normal left ventricles contains mostly CK-MM and very little CK-MB,[12]

TABLE 37–2. CAUSES OF ELEVATED SERUM CK-MB

Myocardial Conditions
- Myocardial infarction/ischemia
- Myocarditis
- Dilated cardiomyopathies
- Pericarditis
- Cardiac trauma

Skeletal Muscle Conditions
- Muscle trauma
- Muscular dystrophy
- Polymyositis/dermatomyositis
- Electrical injuries
- Viral myositis
- Typhoid myositis
- Muscle ischemia
- Vigorous/sustained exercise

Miscellaneous
- Hypothermia
- Hyperthermia
- GI surgery
- Lung tumors
- Reye's syndrome
- Long-term dialysis
- Subarachnoid hemorrhage
- Hypothyroidism
- Burns
- Miscellaneous myopathies
- Newborns, infants, children
- Myasthenic syndromes and other neuromyopathies
- Acromegalic myopathy
- Acute neurologic disorders
- Hepatic encephalopathy
- Delirium tremens
- Peripartum period
- Fetal distress

Data from Shahangian et al[1]; Lee and Goldman[2]; Noakes[6]; Nanji[9]; Arenas et al[10]; Larca et al[11]; McBride et al[13]; Russell et al[14]; and Siegel and Dawson.[15]

whereas diseased myocardium contains increased amounts of CK-MB.[12] The isoenzyme response of cardiac and skeletal muscle to various disease states needs further study.

Because most CK in skeletal muscle consists of the MM isoenzyme, skeletal muscle injury results primarily in serum elevations of CK-MM. In addition to strenuous exercise, several noncardiac conditions have been associated with an elevated serum CK-MB level in which the isoenzyme is probably released from skeletal muscle (Table 37–2). Shahangian and coworkers[1] retrospectively studied patients with burns (thermal or electric) or blunt trauma without evidence of myocardial injury. Fifty seven percent of the burn and trauma patients had an elevated CK-MB, and 30% of these patients had >10% CK-MB in the serum. Burn and trauma patients had 5 to 9% CK-MB in the serum, whereas a comparison group of MI patients had 21% serum CK-MB. These investigators concluded that serum CK-MB was not a specific marker for myocardial injury in burn and trauma patients. McBride and colleagues found an elevated serum CK-MB in 42% of electrically injured patients with no evidence of myocardial damage.[13] Increased MB isoenzyme was found in skeletal muscle biopsy specimens and was believed to be the source of serum CK-MB.[13] The majority of studies of rhabdomyolysis do not report isoenzyme analysis. Nevertheless, reports of rhabdomyolysis due to viral myositis,[9] muscle ischemia,[14] and alcohol[15] have also been associated with an elevated serum CK-MB in the absence of apparent cardiac injury. Arenas and colleagues[10] studied patients with various myopathies and found that elevated serum CK-MB activities correlated with regenerative histologic features on muscle biopsy. The emergency physician must be aware that serum CK-MB elevations lose specificity for myocardial injury in some clinical situations.

Serum CK-BB is generally not elevated in diseases of skeletal or cardiac muscle. One exception has been the observation of CK-BB in the muscle of trained runners[6] and in sera after strenuous exercise.[6] Otherwise, elevations have not been reported in those with myopathic disease.[10] Acute neurologic conditions are the most common cause of elevated serum CK-BB.

MUSCLE ENZYMES AND EXERCISE

Multiple serum muscle enzymes as well as serum myoglobin[6, 16] are elevated by preceding exercise, with serum CK having the greatest percent increase.[6] Difficulties may arise because the serum activities of those enzymes known to increase with exercise (CK, LDH, and AST) are also used as diagnostic markers for acute myocardial infarction.

Moreover, it has been clearly shown that even the "cardiac" isoenzymes of CK and LDH may be elevated after prolonged exercise in patients with no clinical, electrocardiographic, or scintigraphic evidence of myocardial infarction.[6] Skeletal muscle biopsy findings have shown that CK-MB levels are elevated by training and prolonged exercise to levels usually found in cardiac muscle, suggesting that the source of the MB isoenzyme is actually skeletal muscle.[6] Because the exercise-related increase in serum enzymes, especially CK, closely mimics the enzymatic changes seen with an acute myocardial infarction, the interpretation of elevated serum muscle enzyme levels must be made cautiously in the physically active patient.[6]

TESTS FOR RHABDOMYOLYSIS, MYOGLOBINURIA, AND MYOGLOBINEMIA: SENSITIVITY AND SPECIFICITY

Because the complications of rhabdomyolysis can be minimized with timely treatment, and the ultimate prognosis is good,[17–19] a rapid, sensitive, specific, and preferably cost-effective diagnostic strategy is needed in the emergency department. Although some cases of rhabdomyolysis are obvious at presentation, the clinical picture may be subtle or misleading, and the sensitivity of the history and physical examination is generally poor.[18–20] Various classes of muscle cell components (eg, enzyme, myoglobin, creatinine, purine, electrolyte) are released with rhabdomyolysis. Altered levels of serum electrolytes, uric acid, and creatinine have been found to be insensitive[20] and nonspecific markers of muscle injury.[20] Of the enzymes, CK is considered to be the most sensitive[20, 21] and is the most frequently used biochemical marker of rhabdomyolysis.[20, 22, 23] Numerous reports exist in which well-documented rhabdomyolysis was associated with minimally elevated or normal serum levels of LDH or SGOT.[14, 24, 25] Furthermore, when muscle enzymes other than CK are elevated, the degree is almost universally less than that concurrently observed with CK.[14, 16, 24, 25] Lactate dehydrogenase and the aminotransferases are much less specific than CK for muscle pathology. Thus, whereas studies designed to compare the relative sensitivities of various muscle enzymes are lacking, an elevated CK level in an appropriate clinical setting has effectively become the standard for rhabdomyolysis.

The kinetics of serum CK elevations after a muscle insult are well suited for diagnostic purposes. Released CK has an apparent serum half-life of approximately 1.5 days.[20, 24] Elevations in total CK are generally detected at presentation in patients with muscle injury. Serum CK elevations occur within several hours after a sufficient muscle insult, a situation similar to an acute myocardial infarction. Ongoing injury results in persistent elevations. These characteristics make serum CK very likely to be elevated at presentation to the emergency department in a patient with significant muscle injury of recent onset.

Serum myoglobin is elevated by rhabdomyolysis but peaks much earlier than CK. This characteristic suggests that myoglobin may actually be more sensitive than CK in the first few hours after a muscle insult. Released myoglobin is rapidly excreted in the urine with an elimination half-life of about 1 to 3 hours,[20, 26] making myoglobinemia and myoglobinuria only transiently present. This explains the observation that myoglobinuria is frequently absent by the time patients present for treatment.[20, 27] Thus, even though sensitive assays for myoglobin are available, making very early detection of muscle injury possible, overall they are less sensitive than serum CK because of the characteristics of myoglobin elimination and the usual timing of patient presentation.[18, 20, 27]

Both serum CK and serum myoglobin increase in the setting of myocardial damage, and thus their specificity is limited in patients with rhabdomyolysis and potential cardiac conditions. Levels of CK seen in rhabdomyolysis are often much higher than those typically seen in myocardial infarction.[18–20] Massively elevated serum CK levels probably cannot be explained by myocardial necrosis alone and should stimulate a search for other sources, with special attention given to skeletal muscle.

MYOGLOBIN AND PIGMENTURIA

Both myoglobin and hemoglobin can produce red or brown pigmenturia (Table 37–3). When hemoglobin is released from erythrocytes,

TABLE 37–3. DIFFERENTIAL DIAGNOSIS OF BROWN / RED PIGMENTURIA

	Gross Hematuria	Myoglobinuria/ Rhabdomyolysis	Hemoglobinuria/ Hemolysis
Microscopic RBCs	+	–[a]	–
Dipstick (*o*-toluidine)	+	+	+
Serum color	Normal	Normal	Pink
Serum CK	Normal	Elevated	Normal
Serum myoglobin	Normal	Elevated	Normal
Urine myoglobin	Normal	Elevated	Normal

[a]Hematuria is frequently seen in patients with rhabdomyolysis.

it is bound to serum haptoglobin until the binding capacity is exceeded. Unbound free hemoglobin is poorly filtered in the glomerulus because of its molecular size. Thus, free and bound hemoglobin readily accumulate with hemolysis, rendering the serum pink in color. In contrast, serum myoglobin is largely unbound, easily excreted in the urine, and probably cannot accumulate in sufficient amounts for visible pigmentemia to occur.* Significant hemolysis as well as rhabdomyolysis may produce visible pigmenturia, but concurrent pink serum suggests the presence of hemolysis with hemoglobinuria.

Visible myoglobinuria must also be distinguished from gross hematuria. Pigmenturia due to myoglobin will generally produce a positive ortho-toluidine test for urinary heme pigments with concurrent microscopy revealing few or no erythrocytes. Therefore, red or brown ortho-toluidine–positive urine without microscopic hematuria along with clear serum strongly suggests rhabdomyolysis and myoglobinuria. Because the ortho-toluidine dipstick does not distinguish between hemoglobin and myoglobin, myoglobinuria cannot be confirmed or excluded by dipstick alone in the presence of significant hematuria or hemoglobinuria. Hematuria is commonly associated with rhabdomyolysis, whereas significant hemolysis with hemoglobinuria is not.[20, 22] When hematuria is found during a search for myoglobin, direct measurement of myoglobin must be used to confirm or exclude myoglobinuria.

PREDICTING RENAL FAILURE IN PATIENTS WITH RHABDOMYOLYSIS

Myoglobinuric renal failure is not a rare event,[18–20, 22, 27] and, depending on the study, investigators have found that anywhere from 10 to 43% of patients with rhabdomyolysis develop this complication.[19, 20, 22, 23, 28] Few studies have addressed the problem of which patients with rhabdomyolysis will possibly have complications. Many investigators believe that hypotension, dehydration, and acidemia predispose the patient to the development of myoglobinuric renal failure.[17, 22, 27, 29] The concept that a correlation should exist between the amount and severity of myocyte injury and the development of complications, especially renal failure, is appealing. It is common to assume that the amount of underlying skeletal muscle damage correlates with serum levels of

---

*Although theoretically possible, gross myoglobinemia has not been reported, even in anuric patients. For enough myoglobin to be present in serum, vast amounts of muscle would need to be destroyed. Such an insult would simultaneously release large amounts of potassium, in all likelihood causing fatal hyperkalemia.[19, 26]

released muscle cell contents,[29] especially CK and myoglobin. In the setting of myocardial infarction, echocardiography and nuclear scintigraphy allow independent quantification of the amount of myocardial damage, and correlations with serum CK levels are well established. Currently, no practical tool exists for the accurate quantification of skeletal muscle injury; thus, any correlation is speculative. Some retrospective data address the relationship between serum markers of skeletal muscle injury and renal failure. A largely retrospective study of 87 episodes of rhabdomyolysis found that detectable myoglobinuria at presentation and serum CK did not correlate with the occurrence of acute renal failure.[20] Two other retrospective studies of 157 and 30 rhabdomyolysis patients, however, found that high serum CK levels did correlate with the development of renal failure.[22, 27] A fourth retrospective study found that high serum CK values correlated with a poor response of renal failure to forced alkaline diuresis therapy.[29] No prospective study has assessed the relationship between serum CK values or serum or urine myoglobin levels and development of renal failure in a population of rhabdomyolysis patients. The problem is important, because the renal failure associated with rhabdomyolysis is believed to be largely preventable with early, aggressive therapy.[17–19]

SUMMARY

Although serum CK is elevated in a variety of diseases, the emergency physician will utilize it primarily in the setting of acute skeletal or cardiac muscle disease. Rhabdomyolysis with acute renal failure probably occurs more frequently than suspected. Because the prognosis for renal recovery is good with early therapy, prompt recognition of this condition by the emergency physician is important. Serum CK is currently the most sensitive and specific screening test for rhabdomyolysis available to the emergency physician, and its liberal use should be encouraged whenever skeletal muscle disease is suspected and whenever unexpected renal failure is discovered. The measurement of myoglobin in serum or urine is complementary to that of serum CK, and it may assume greater significance as more sensitive and rapid tests are developed in the future. In any event, a high index of suspicion for significant muscle disease is needed because the history and physical examination are poor screening tools.

In a patient population with a high incidence of myocardial infarction, CK-MB is a highly specific marker for myocardial necrosis. In other patient groups, however, it is much less specific. Emergency physicians must be aware of this situation, especially as rapid assays for the MB isoenzyme become more widely available in the emergency department.

REFERENCES

1. Shahangian S, Ash KO, Walhstrom NO, et al: Creatine kinase and lactate dehydrogenase isoenzymes in serum of patients suffering burns, blunt trauma, or myocardial infarction. *Clin Chem.* 1984;30:1332–1338.
2. Lee TH, Goldman L: Serum enzyme assays in the diagnosis of acute myocardial infarction. *Ann Intern Med.* 1986;105:221–233.
3. Lott JA, Stang JM: Serum enzymes and isoenzymes in the diagnosis and differential diagnosis of myocardial ischemia and necrosis. *Clin Chem.* 1980;26:1241–1250.
4. Lott JA: Serum enzyme determinations in the diagnosis of acute myocardial infarction: An update. *Hum Pathol.* 1984;15:706–716.
5. Garcia W: Elevated creatine phosphokinase levels associated with large muscle mass. *JAMA.* 1974;228:1395–1396.
6. Noakes TD: Effect of exercise on serum enzyme activities in humans. *Sports Med.* 1987;4:245–267.
7. Lott JA, Stand JM: Differential diagnosis of patients with abnormal serum creatine kinase isoenzymes. *Clin Lab Med.* 1989;9:627–642.
8. Joy JL, Riser JB, Oh SJ: Rational approach to asymptomatic creatine kinase elevation. *Ala J Med Sci.* 1988;25:147–150.
9. Nanji AA: Serum creatine kinase isoenzymes: A review. *Muscle Nerve.* 1983;6:83–90.
10. Arenas J, Diaz V, Liras G, et al: Activities of creatine kinase and its isoenzymes in serum in various skeletal muscle disorders. *Clin Chem.* 1988;34:2460–2462.
11. Larca LJ, Coppola JT, Honig S: Creatine kinase MB isoenzyme in dermatomyositis: A noncardiac source. *Ann Intern Med.* 1981;94:341–343.
12. Ingwall JS, Kramer MF, Fifer MA, et al: The creatine kinase system in normal and diseased human myocardium. *N Engl J Med.* 1985;313:1050–1054.
13. McBride JW, Labrosse KR, McCoy HG, et al: Is serum creatine kinase-MB in electrically injured patients predictive of myocardial injury? *JAMA.* 1986;255:764–768.
14. Russell SM, Bleiweiss S, Brownlow K, et al: Ischemic rhabdomyolysis and creatine phosphokinase isoenzymes, a diagnostic pitfall. *JAMA.* 1976; 235:632–633.
15. Siegel AJ, Dawson DM: Peripheral source of MB band of creatine kinase in alcoholic rhabdomyolysis, nonspecificity of MB isoenzyme for myocardial injury in undiluted serum samples. *JAMA.* 1980;244:580–582.
16. Demos MA, Gitin EL: Acute exertional rhabdomyolysis. *Arch Intern Med.* 1974;133:233–239.
17. Better OS, Stein JH: Early management of shock and prophylaxis of acute renal failure in traumatic rhabdomyolysis. *N Engl J Med.* 1990;322:825–829.
18. Koffler A, Friedler RM, Massry SG: Acute renal failure due to nontraumatic rhabdomyolysis. *Ann Intern Med.* 1976;85:23–28.
19. Grossman RA, Hamilton RW, Morse BM, et al: Nontraumatic rhabdomyolysis and acute renal failure. *N Engl J Med.* 1974;291:807–811.
20. Gabow PA, Kaehny WD, Kelleher SP: The spectrum of rhabdomyolysis. *Medicine.* 1982;61:141–152.
21. Hess JW, MacDonald RP, Frederick RJ, et al: Serum creatine phosphokinase

(CPK) activity in disorders of heart and skeletal muscle. *Ann Intern Med.* 1964;61:1015–1028.
22. Ward MW: Factors predictive of acute renal failure in rhabdomyolysis. *Arch Intern Med.* 1988;148:1553–1557.
23. Akmal M, Valdin JR, McCarron MM, et al: Rhabdomyolysis with and without acute renal failure in patients with phencyclidine intoxication. *Am J Nephrol.* 1981;1:91–96.
24. Rubin RB, Neugarten J: Cocaine-induced rhabdomyolysis masquerading as myocardial ischemia. *Am J Med.* 1989;86:551–553.
25. Wrenn KD, Oschner I: Rhabdomyolysis induced by a caffeine overdose. *Ann Emerg Med.* 1989;18:94–97.
26. Knochel JP: Rhabdomyolysis and myoglobinuria. *Semin Nephrol.* 1981;1:75–86.
27. Cadnapaphornchai P, Taher S, McDonald FD: Acute drug-associated rhabdomyolysis: An examination of its diverse renal manifestations and complications. *Am J Med Sci.* 1980;280:66–72.
28. Curry SC, Chang D, Conner D: Drug- and toxin-induced rhabdomyolysis. *Ann Emerg Med.* 1989;18:1068–1084.
29. Eneas JF, Schoenfeld PY, Humphreys MH: The effect of infusion of mannitol-sodium bicarbonate on the clinical course of myoglobinuria. *Arch Intern Med.* 1979;139:801–805.
30. Perkoff GT: Demonstration of creatine phosphokinase in human lung tissue. *Arch Intern Med.* 1968;122:326–328.
31. Nevins MA, Saran M, Bright M, et al: Pitfalls in interpreting serum creatine phosphokinase activity. *JAMA.* 1973;224:1382–1387.

Chapter

Amylase and Lipase

Alan K. Hodgdon and David C. Seaberg

Serum amylase and lipase levels are commonly ordered in the emergency department evaluation of abdominal pain. Specifically, these tests are frequently used to determine if the pancreas should be implicated in the etiology. Although the pancreas has high concentrations of both amylase and lipase, the serum levels of these enzymes are neither particularly sensitive nor specific for pancreatic disease.

AMYLASE

The amylases act on starch to split alpha-1,4-glucosidic bonds. They are found primarily in the salivary glands and pancreas, although small

TABLE 38–1. CAUSES OF HYPERAMYLASEMIA OR HYPERAMYLASURIA

1. Pancreatic disease
2. Salivary gland disease
3. Intraabdominal disorders
   - Peptic ulcer disease
   - Intestinal obstruction/infarction
   - Cholecystitis/choledocholithiasis
   - Acute appendicitis
4. Renal insufficiency
5. Diabetic ketoacidosis
6. Ruptured ectopic pregnancy
7. Prostatic disease
8. Cerebral trauma
9. Aortic aneurysm with dissection
10. Tumors—lung, ovary, salivary gland

amounts are also found in the small intestine, large intestine, prostate, ovary, skeletal muscle, and fallopian tube. There are many causes of elevated amylase levels in the serum and, because amylase is freely filtered at the glomerulus, in the urine (Table 38–1).

Serum amylase has been generally regarded as the single most important practical diagnostic test in acute pancreatitis. In acute pancreatitis, serum amylase usually begins to rise within 2 to 6 hours of the onset of symptoms, reaching a peak level of four to six times normal in 12 to 72 hours. The level then falls rapidly, usually to normal levels by 3 to 5 days. Levels that persist beyond 1 week should raise the possibility of a complication, such as pseudocyst or phlegmon.[9] Rarely, normalization of the amylase level occurs very rapidly, indicating early resolution of the disease or, less often, extensive destruction of the pancreas with cessation of pancreatic amylase production. Occasionally, pancreatitis can occur with normal amylase levels. This is most frequently seen in chronic pancreatitis, where it is presumed that the pancreas has too few functional exocrine cells to be able to produce an increased serum amylase level, even with acute inflammation of the pancreas. Reported sensitivities of serum amylase as a test for acute pancreatitis vary from 45 to 95%.[10] The magnitude of the elevation of serum enzyme activity is not related to the severity of pancreatic involvement[5]; the greater the rise, the greater the probability of acute pancreatitis.[12] This lack of any amylase response proportional to injury is the reason the absolute value of amylase holds no prognostic value and is not part of Ranson's criteria for severe pancreatitis (Table 38–2).

The specificity of serum amylase as a test for acute pancreatitis is low because a number of other acute disorders can elevate amylase to

TABLE 38–2. RANSON'S CRITERIA*

Time of Admission
- Age > 55 years
- Blood glucose > 200 mg/dL (in patients without diabetes mellitus)
- WBC > 16,000/mm^3
- Serum SGOT > 250 U/dL
- Serum LDH > 350 U/L

During Initial 48 Hours of Admission
- Hematocrit fall > 10%
- BUN rise > 5 mg/dl
- Serum calcium < 8 mg/dL
- Arterial Po_2 < 60 mm Hg
- Base deficit > 4 mEq/L
- Estimated fluid sequestration > 6 L

*Patients with three or more criteria at admission or at 48 hours have prognoses of "serious illness" (ie, an ICU stay greater than 7 days) or "death." These are defined by Ranson as an ICU stay greater than 7 days or death.

From Ranson JHC, Rifkind KM, Roses DF, et al: Prognostic signs and the role of operative management in acute pancreatitis. *Surg Gynecol Obstet.* 1974;139:69–81. By permission of Surgery, Gynecology and Obstetrics now known as the Journal of the American College of Surgeons.

high levels. Although normally only about 25% of the serum amylase is eliminated by the kidney, in renal insufficiency serum amylase levels can increase by up to twofold, usually in proportion to the extent of renal impairment.[12] In addition, tumors of the lung, ovary, prostate, and salivary gland can elevate amylase levels to as high as 50 times normal.

Biliary tract disease such as cholecystitis can cause up to fourfold elevations in the serum amylase activity, owing to either primary or secondary pancreatic involvement. Numerous other intraabdominal problems such as peritonitis, acute appendicitis, peptic ulcer disease, and intestinal obstruction can be associated with high amylase levels. Such increases may be due to leakage of amylase from the intestinal wall into the peritoneal cavity where it is absorbed into the circulation.[12] In ruptured ectopic pregnancy, hyperamylasemia may derive from the damaged fallopian tube. Dissecting aortic aneurysm can also produce elevated serum amylase levels by an unknown mechanism.

In diabetic ketoacidosis, elevations of serum amylase up to fourfold normal can be found in as many as 80% of patients.[12] The mechanism is unknown, but hyperamylasemia occurs most frequently when blood glucose concentration exceeds 500 mg/dL and the onset of ketoacidosis is relatively acute. Acidosis from a variety of etiologies can be associated with elevated serum amylase levels. In one study of ICU patients without evidence of pancreatitis, 30% of patients with a pH of <7.20 had amylase values at least twice that of normal.

Serum amylase consists primarily of two separate types of isoenzymes: pancreatic (p-type) and salivary (s-type). In normal serum, total amylase consists of approximately 40% p-type and 60% s-type.[4] Attempts to measure these independently to clarify a diagnosis have not met with great success, mainly because of problems with specificity. Although an elevation in p-type amylase may suggest a pancreatic source, cases of pancreatitis have been reported with elevation of only the s-type isoenzyme. The isoenzyme issue is complicated by the fact that the isoenzymes have different half-lives and that the percentages of each enzyme in plasma may vary considerably. Even with elevations of the p-type amylase, the test cannot differentiate between pancreatitis and other abdominal disorders, such as perforated ulcer. The best reason to order isoenzyme tests is that the p-type enzyme remains elevated in cases of acute pancreatitis for 10 to 14 days. This finding is in contrast to the total amylase, which often returns to normal within 1 week in uncomplicated pancreatitis.

Because renal excretion of amylase depends on adequate renal function, urinary excretion of amylase correlates with creatinine clearance. In acute pancreatitis, however, there is an increased clearance of amylase compared with creatinine due to the rather limited proximal tubular reabsorption of the freely filtered enzyme. Because urinary amylase may be elevated more frequently, reach higher levels, and persist for longer periods than the serum amylase, the ratio of urinary clearance of amylase compared with that of creatinine is sometimes helpful when serum amylase is normal or equivocal and the diagnosis of pancreatitis is still being considered.

Determination of this clearance ratio involves simultaneous collection of one serum and urine sample and does not require a timed specimen because the units cancel. Normal values range between 2 and 5%, whereas values in acute pancreatitis are often >8%. Caution should be observed in the interpretation of this result, however, because elevated ratios have also been seen in patients with burns, renal insufficiency, ketoacidosis, and other disease processes. In addition, some studies have noted normal amylase-creatinine clearance ratios in patients with proven pancreatitis.[1, 3] The amylase/creatinine clearance ratio is calculated as follows:

$$\text{Ratio} = \frac{\text{urine amylase} \times \text{serum creatinine}}{\text{serum amylase} \times \text{urine creatinine}}$$

This test is rarely ordered in the emergency department setting.

LIPASE

Human lipase is a 48,000-dalton glycoprotein that exists in a single form without isomers. It requires a coenzyme, colipase, to perform its function of hydrolyzing glycerol esters from long-chain fatty acids. The serum lipase level is considered more specific for pancreatic damage than is the amylase level because the pancreas is the only major source of lipase.[7] There is no urinary excretion of lipase. During acute pancreatic inflammation, serum lipase activity rises slightly later than amylase but may stay elevated for longer periods (10 to 14 days).[12] For these reasons, the two assays often complement each other in the diagnosis of acute pancreatitis.

When evaluated, the sensitivity and specificity of the serum lipase have been subject to the same wide variations as those of the serum amylase, with the sensitivity averaging 75 to 80% and the specificity about 70%.[8] In general, lipase has a sensitivity about 10% less than that of the serum amylase, but its specificity is greater by about 20 to 30%. Although the lipase level is not elevated in several conditions that cause hyperamylasemia (eg, salivary gland disease, macroamylasemia, diabetic ketoacidosis, acidosis), it shares with the serum amylase the disadvantage of being elevated in many of the same diseases that one would most like to differentiate from acute pancreatitis (intestinal obstruction, intestinal perforation, acute cholecystitis, choledocholithiasis, and mesenteric infarction).[6]

Studies now suggest that increasing the upper limits of normal of both serum amylase and lipase levels may improve their diagnostic utility in acute pancreatitis. In a study by Steinberg and colleagues,[11] serum samples from 29 patients with acute pancreatitis, 237 patients with acute abdominal pain judged to be of extrapancreatic origin, and 50 normal subjects were obtained. Total amylase levels, pancreatic isoamylase levels (p-isoenzyme), and lipase activities were measured. Both the normal upper limit and a "best cutoff level" of approximately 1.7 times the conventional upper limit of normal for the total serum amylase level were used in the evaluation. The best cutoff level was obtained by graphing sensitivity vs specificity and choosing the line with the highest numerical efficiency (the highest sensitivity and specificity). Using the normal upper limit, the total serum amylase had a sensitivity of 95% and a specificity of 87% for acute pancreatitis. Using the best cutoff level, the specificity increased to nearly 99% with a negligible decrease in sensitivity. Despite using the best cutoff level for each of the tests, none of the tests offered a clear advantage over the traditional measurement of total serum amylase.[2, 11]

OTHER LABORATORY TESTS

Several newer laboratory tests have been proposed and evaluated to provide laboratory confirmation of pancreatic inflammation. Such tests include serum immunoreactive trypsinogen/trypsin, C-reactive protein, pancreatic ribonuclease, deoxyribonuclease, methemalbumin, and phospholipase A2. None of these has sufficient advantages over serum amylase and lipase measurement to recommend routine use.

CONCLUSION

The laboratory test most widely employed to support the diagnosis of acute pancreatitis is still the total serum amylase level. A normal value is sufficiently unusual in cases of acute pancreatitis that the diagnosis should be questioned if the amylase level is not elevated. If a patient presents a few days after the onset, peak levels may be missed. In addition, many other intra- and extraabdominal diseases cause an elevation of the serum amylase. Amylase isoenzymes and urinary amylase/creatinine clearance ratios have not been shown to add much in terms of sensitivity or specificity. Lipase levels, although more specific for pancreatic disease, still cannot reliably differentiate pancreatitis from other abdominal disorders. Employing higher upper limits of normal for both serum amylase and lipase may increase the specificity for diagnosing pancreatitis. Currently, however, amylase and lipase levels can offer only supporting evidence that must be combined with either a strong clinical suspicion or imaging (sonogram or computerized tomography) evidence of pancreatic pathology if the full extent of pancreatic disease is to be diagnosed and treated.

REFERENCES

1. Durr HK, Bode JC, Lankisch PG, et al: Amylase-creatinine clearance ratio in pancreatitis (letter). *N Engl J Med.* 1977;296:635.
2. Eckfeldt JH, Leatherman JW, Levitt MD: High prevalence of hyperamylasemia in patients with acidemia. *Ann Intern Med.* 1986;104:362–368.
3. Farrar WH, Calkins WG: Sensitivity of the amylase-creatinine clearance ratio in acute pancreatitis. *Arch Intern Med.* 1978;138:958–962.
4. Geokas MC, Baltaxe HA, Banks PA, et al: Acute pancreatitis. *Ann Intern Med.* 1985;103:86–100.
5. Geokas MC, Van Lancker JL, Kadell BM, et al: Acute pancreatitis. *Ann Intern Med.* 1972;76:105–117.
6. Hodgdon AK, Wolfson AB: Pancreatitis. *Emerg Med Clin North Am.* 1990;8:873–885.
7. Moosa AR: Diagnostic tests and procedures in acute pancreatitis. *N Engl J Med.* 1984;311:639–643.

8. Ravel R: Pancreatic function, in Ravel R (ed): *Clinical Laboratory Medicine*. Chicago: Year Book Medical Publishers; 1989:453–460.
9. Salt WB, Schenker S: Amylase—Its clinical significance: A review of the literature. *Medicine*. 1976;55:269–281.
10. Speicher CE, Smith JW: Pancreatic subproblems, in Speicher CE, Smith JW (eds): *Choosing Effective Laboratory Tests*. Philadelphia: WB Saunders; 1983:231–240.
11. Steinberg WM, Goldstein SS, Davis ND, et al: Diagnostic assays in acute pancreatitis. *Ann Intern Med*. 1985;102:576–582.
12. Tietz NW: Digestive enzymes of pancreatic origin, in Tietz NW (ed): *Textbook of Clinical Chemistry*. Philadelphia: WB Saunders; 1986:724–740.
13. Ranson JHC, Rifkind KM, Roses DF, et al: Prognostic signs and the role of operative management in acute pancreatitis. *Surg Gynecol Obstet*. 1974; 139:69–81.

Chapter

Erythrocyte Sedimentation Rate

Bruce A. MacLeod

The erythrocyte sedimentation rate (ESR) is a laboratory test, introduced in 1918 by Fahraeus,[1] which measures the distance in millimeters that erythrocytes fall in 1 hour. It is an index of the suspension stability of red blood cells (RBCs) in citrated blood. The sedimentation rate of the RBCs depends on the difference in specific gravity between the RBCs and the plasma. The rate of the fall of the RBCs, or ESR, depends primarily on the concentration of fibrinogen and, to a lesser extent, alpha- and gamma-globulin in plasma.

Normally, as isolated RBCs settle in plasma, the rate of fall is limited by the surface area of the RBCs in relation to the plasma flow upward against the descending RBCs. Erythrocytes will form rouleaux, aligning themselves along a single axis, thus reducing the surface area, increasing the weight, and increasing the rate of descent through the plasma.

Red blood cells will not normally aggregate into rouleaux because of negative charges on the cell membranes. Serum globulins nullify the negative charge on the erythrocytes, allowing for more rouleau formation and more rapid ESR.

The ESR is rapid in syndromes associated with changes in serum globulins, especially in disorders in which the levels of serum fibrinogen or alpha-globulins are increased.

In defining the factors that influence the ESR, investigators[2, 3] have found that not only the size of the rouleaux and the quantity of the macromolecules but also the colloidal state of the plasma affects the ESR. A complete understanding of the mechanics of erythrocyte aggregation and sedimentation remains to be elucidated.

METHOD TO MEASURE THE ERYTHROCYTE SEDIMENTATION RATE

There are many methods to measure the ESR but the current standard is the Westergren method first developed in 1920.[4] To determine the ESR using the Westergren method, the blood sample and sodium citrate are mixed at room temperature within 2 hours of the blood being drawn. The sample is placed in a glass tube and the ESR is measured over a 1-hour period. There are a number of potentially confounding mechanical, environmental, and technical factors.[5–7] It is important to establish the reliability of the test within a given institution to confidently interpret the results of the test.

ERYTHROCYTE SEDIMENTATION RATE IN THE EMERGENCY DEPARTMENT

The ESR is a diagnostic test that is simple and inexpensive. It is used to obtain three types of information: the presence or absence of disease, the progression or improvement of an already recognized disease, and the response to therapy.[8] In the emergency department the clinician is most concerned with identifying the presence or absence of disease.

The sensitivity of a clinical test can be identified when all patients with a positive test undergo a definitive procedure or test to confirm the presence of the disease. The specificity can be calculated when all patients, with or without an abnormal ESR, undergo a definitive procedure or test to confirm or disprove the presence of the disease. There have been few studies of the ESR that would allow for the enumeration of the specificity.[9] The positive predicative value of abnormal ESR, which can be calculated from the positive test results, has been identified in a number of clinical entities.

A patient's age, gender, comorbid disease, and medication must be considered when the ESR is abnormal. Women have a higher baseline ESR than men.[10] An unexplained elevated ESR in the absence of other findings may simply reflect advanced age.[11–14] Many disease entities that raise the ESR have been identified and might confound the decision process when trying to diagnose other disease processes. Medications such as antiinflammatory agents and cortisone can lower the ESR,[15] whereas medications such as heparin[16] and oral contraceptives[17] can raise the sedimentation rate. A normal ESR does not exclude organic disease.[18, 19]

Temporal Arteritis and Polymyalgia Rheumatica

Temporal arteritis (giant cell arteritis) and polymyalgia rheumatica are related syndromes that can occur alone or together. Most investigators have found that patients with temporal arteritis almost always have an elevated ESR.[20, 21] These studies may have underestimated the false-negative rate, however, because patients with normal ESR values were not likely to undergo a biopsy.[22] Reviews of patients with the diagnosis of temporal arteritis based on clinical grounds have found up to 22% of patients with normal ESR.[23] Wong and Korn[24] found that the lack of an elevation of the ESR did not correlate with a milder clinical course. The most consistent laboratory abnormality in polymyalgia rheumatica is an ESR >50, and often >100.[25]

If there is a low clinical suspicion of temporal arteritis (TA), a normal ESR lowers the likelihood of TA to <1%.[26] If there is a high clinical suspicion, treatment should be initiated in spite of a normal ESR. Realizing that the elevation in the ESR may be from a comorbid disease, a temporal artery biopsy finding will confirm the diagnosis.

In TA or giant cell arteritis, even in the absence of overt clinical symptoms of recurrent disease, an elevated ESR appears to be a measure of disease activity and sufficient evidence to justify increasing the dose of steroids.[27]

Infections

Any infectious process may accelerate the ESR. The ESR is slow to rise over the first few days of an infectious process and is slower to return to normal than an elevated temperature or leukocytosis.[28]

The ESR has been recommended to aid in the diagnosis of a number of infectious processes. In 1937, Bannick and coworkers[29] reported that an elevated ESR was associated with ruptured appendicitis and pelvic inflammatory disease. Steihm and Damrosch[30] proposed a low ESR as part of a prognostic variable for meningococcemia in pediatric patients. Schulak and Raycheck[31] reported that 85 to 100% of the patients with infections in the lumbar disk space have elevated ESR. Hematogenous septic arthritis in adults has been reported to be associated with an increased ESR in 95%.[32] Ninety three percent of the admitted patients with bacterial endocarditis were found to have elevated ESRs.[33]

However, other investigators have found the ESR to be less helpful. Banyai and Anderson showed that a normal ESR does not exclude pulmonary tuberculosis.[34] The ESR is of little use in the diagnosis and management of pediatric patients with suspected bacteriemia or neonatal sepsis.[35] In pediatric patients with acute refusals to walk who had bacterial infections, Callanan found that only 72% had ESRs >40 mm/h.[36] Collert[37] found that only 76% of patients with hematogenous osteomyelitis had an accelerated ESR >50 mm/h. The ESR is not helpful in patients with suspected subacute hematogenous osteomyelitis (Brodie's abscess).[38] There has been conflicting support for the use of the ESR in evaluating febrile drug abusers.[39, 40]

Erythrocyte sedimentation rate may be used to follow the course of a disease as the inflammatory process resolves. Adequate surgical drainage of an abscess is indicated by an elevated ESR returning to normal levels.[41, 42]

Malignancy

Medical lore has long been that the ESR is a criterion for metastatic carcinoma and for following patients with malignancies such as Hodgkin's lymphoma. No studies substantiate these teachings.[43] Rafnsson and coworkers[44] found that an elevated ESR does not destine a patient to be diagnosed with a carcinoma. Peyman[45] found that a markedly elevated ESR does not distinguish among the patients with metastases. The ESR does not appear to be an effective diagnostic adjunct for identifying occult malignancies.[46, 47]

"Sickness" Index

Some investigators have suggested that, because a number of disease processes may cause elevations in the ESR, it may be more useful as a "sickness index" particularly if the ESR is markedly elevated (>100 mm/h).[48] Fincher and Page,[49] in their study of 1000 clinic outpatients, reported a specificity of 99% and a positive predictive value of 90% for a markedly elevated ESR. The most common cause for the markedly elevated ESR was infection followed by malignant neoplasm, renal disease, and inflammatory process.

RECOMMENDATIONS FOR USE OF THE ERYTHROCYTE SEDIMENTATION RATE

The ESR is a simple laboratory test with poorly understood physicochemical mechanics. In the emergency department, the clinician is most concerned with establishing the presence or absence of disease. The ESR is not useful in screening asymptomatic patients or patients with nonspecific complaints in the emergency department. For the patient with a low likelihood of TA, a low ESR can effectively rule out the disease. The role of the ESR in the diagnosis of an infectious process is limited and should be interpreted in light of the clinical presentation. Patients with elevations in the ESR without evidence of disease in the history and physical examination can be managed with adequate follow-up care. The patient with a markedly elevated ESR (>100 mm/h), however, warrants a careful and judicious examination and workup.

REFERENCES

1. Fahraeus R: The suspension-stability of the blood. *Acta Med Scand.* 1921;55:1–228.
2. Ropes MW, Rossmeisl E, Bauer W: The relationship between ESR and plasma proteins. *J Clin Invest.* 1939;18:791–798.
3. Kernick D, Jay AW, Rowlands S, et al: Experiments on rouleaux formation. *Can J Physiol Pharmacol.* 1973;5:155–160.
4. Westergren A: The technique of the red cell sedimentation reaction. *Am Rev Tuberc.* 1926;14:94–101.
5. Ham TH, Curtis FC: Sedimentation rate of erythrocytes; Influence of technical erythrocytic and plasma factors and quantitative comparisons of five commonly used sedimentation methods. *Medicine.* 1971;50:1–27.
6. Kernick D, Jay AW, Rowlands S, et al: Experiments on rouleaux formation. *Can J Physiol Pharmacol.* 1973;5:155–160.
7. Miale JB: *Laboratory Medicine: Hematology.* St. Louis: CV Mosby; 1972:468–475.
8. Bedell SE, Bush BT: Erythrocyte sedimentation rate: From folklore to facts. *Am J Med.* 1985;78:1001–1009.
9. Sox HC, Liang MH: The erythrocyte sedimentation rate: Guidelines for rational use. *Ann Intern Med.* 1986;104:515–523.
10. Lawrence JS: *Assessment of the Activity of Disease.* New York: Paul B. Hoeber;1961.
11. Talkers R: Erythrocyte sedimentation rate/zeta sedimentation rate. *Emerg Med Clin North Am.* 1986;4:87–93.
12. Zacharski LR, Kyle RA: Significance of extreme elevation of erythrocyte sedimentation rate. *JAMA.* 1967;202:264–266.
13. Hart GD, Soots M, Sullivan J: Significance of extreme elevation of erythrocyte sedimentation rate. *Appl Ther.* 1970;12:12–13.
14. Bouchet H, Dupoisot H, Laoussadi S, et al: Erythrocyte sedimentation rate of healthy subjects—Chronological aspects. *Chronobiol Int.* 1986;3:179–187.
15. Lascari AD: The erythrocyte sedimentation rate. *Pediatr Clin North Am.* 1972;19:1113–1121.
16. Penchas S: Heparin and the ESR. *Arch Intern Med.* 1978;138:1865–1866.

17. Burton JL: Effect of oral contraceptives on erythrocyte sedimentation rate in healthy young women. *Br Med J.* 1967;3:214–215.
18. Bedell SE, Bush BT: Erythrocyte sedimentation rate: From folklore to facts. *Am J Med.* 1985;78:1001–1009.
19. Talkers R: Erythrocyte sedimentation rate/zeta sedimentation rate. *Emerg Med Clin North Am.* 1986;4:87–93.
20. Hamilton CR, Shelley WM, Tumulty PA: Giant cell arteritis: including temporal arteritis and polymyalgia rheumatica. *Medicine.* 1971;50:1–27.
21. Goodman BW: Temporal arteritis. *Am J Med.* 1979;67:839–852.
22. Sox HC, Liang MH: The erythrocyte sedimentation rate: Guidelines for rational use. *Ann Intern Med.* 1986;104:515–523.
23. Ellis ME, Ralston S: The ESR in the diagnosis and management of the polymyalgia rheumatica/giant cell arteritis syndrome. *Ann Rheum Dis.* 1983;42:168–170.
24. Wong RL, Korn JH: Temporal arteritis without an elevated erythrocyte sedimentation rate: Case report and review of the literature. *Am J Med.* 1986;80:959–964.
25. Bedell SE, Bush BT: Erythrocyte sedimentation rate: From folklore to facts. *Am J Med.* 1985;78:1001–1009.
26. Sox HC, Liang MH: The erythrocyte sedimentation rate: Guidelines for rational use. *Ann Intern Med.* 1986;104:515–523.
27. Beevers DG, Harpur JE, Turk KAD: Giant cell arteritis—The need for prolonged treatment. *J Chronic Dis.* 1973;26:571–584.
28. Wintrobe MM: The erythrocyte sedimentation rate. *Int Clin.* 1936;2:34–61.
29. Bannick EG, Gregg RO, Guernsey CM: The erythrocyte sedimentation rate. *JAMA.* 1937;109:1257–1262.
30. Steihm ER, Damrosch ES: Factors in prognosis of meningococcal infection. *J Pediatr.* 1982;68:457.
31. Schulak DJ, Raycheck JM, et al: The erythrocyte sedimentation rate in orthopedic patients. *Clin Orthop.* 1982;167:197–202.
32. Kelly PJ, Martin WH, et al: Bacterial arteritis of the hip in the adult. *J Bone Joint Surg.* 1965;47A:1005–1018.
33. Ford Von Reyn C et al: Infective endocarditis: An analysis based on strict case definitions. *Ann Intern Med.* 1981;94:505–518.
34. Banyai AL, Anderson SV: Erythrocyte sedimentation test in tuberculosis. *Arch Intern Med.* 1930;46:787–796.
35. Singer JI, Buchino JJ, Chabali R: Selected laboratory in pediatric emergency care. *Emerg Med Clin North Am.* 1982;4:377–396.
36. Callanan DL: Causes of refusal to walk in childhood. *South Med J.* 1982;75:20.
37. Collert S: Osteomyelitis of the spine. *Acta Orthop Scand.* 1977;48:283–290.
38. Kelly PJ, Martin WH, et al: Bacterial arteritis of the hip in the adult. *J Bone Joint Surg.* 1965;47A:1005–1018.
39. Marantz PR et al: Inability to predict diagnosis in febrile intravenous drug abusers. *Ann Intern Med.* 1987;106:823–828.
40. Gallagher EJ, Gennis P, Brooks F: Clinical use of the erythrocyte sedimentation rate in the evaluation of febrile intravenous drug abusers. *Ann Emerg Med.* 1993;22:776–780.
41. Zacharski LR, Kyle RA: Significance of extreme elevation of erythrocyte sedimentation rate. *JAMA.* 1967;202:264–266.

42. Hart GD, Soots M, Sullivan J: Significance of extreme elevation of erythrocyte sedimentation rate. *Appl Ther.* 1970;12:12–13.
43. Bedell SE, Bush BT: Erythrocyte sedimentation rate: From folklore to facts. *Am J Med.* 1985;78:1001–1009.
44. Rafnsson V et al: Erythrocyte sedimentation rate in a population sample of women, with special reference to its clinical and prognostic significance. *Acta Med Scand.* 1979;206:207–214.
45. Peyman MA: The effect of malignant disease on the erythrocyte sedimentation rate. *Br J Cancer.* 1962;16:56–71.
46. Bedell SE, Bush BT: Erythrocyte sedimentation rate: From folklore to facts. *Am J Med.* 1985;78:1001–1009.
47. Sox HC, Liang MH: The erythrocyte sedimentation rate: Guidelines for rational use. *Ann Intern Med.* 1986;104:515–523.
48. Bedell SE, Bush BT: Erythrocyte sedimentation rate: From folklore to facts. *Am J Med.* 1985;78:1001–1009.
49. Fincher RME, Page MI: Clinical significance of extreme elevation of the erythrocyte sedimentation rate. *Arch Intern Med.* 1986;146:1581–1583.

Chapter

Prothrombin Time and Partial Thromboplastin Time

James G. Adams and Laurence Katz

The functioning of the coagulation cascade is reflected in the prothrombin time (PT) and partial thromboplastin time (PTT). This chapter discusses the clinical circumstances in which it is useful to measure PT and PTT in the emergency department (ED) patient.

THE COAGULATION CASCADE

The coagulation cascade comprises two components, the extrinsic and intrinsic pathways, which converge to form the common pathway (Fig. 40–1). The extrinsic pathway, which includes factor VII and tissue factor, is initiated by tissue thromboplastin. The thromboplastic complex, with activated factor VII and calcium, is central in initiating the common pathway. The common pathway can also be activated through

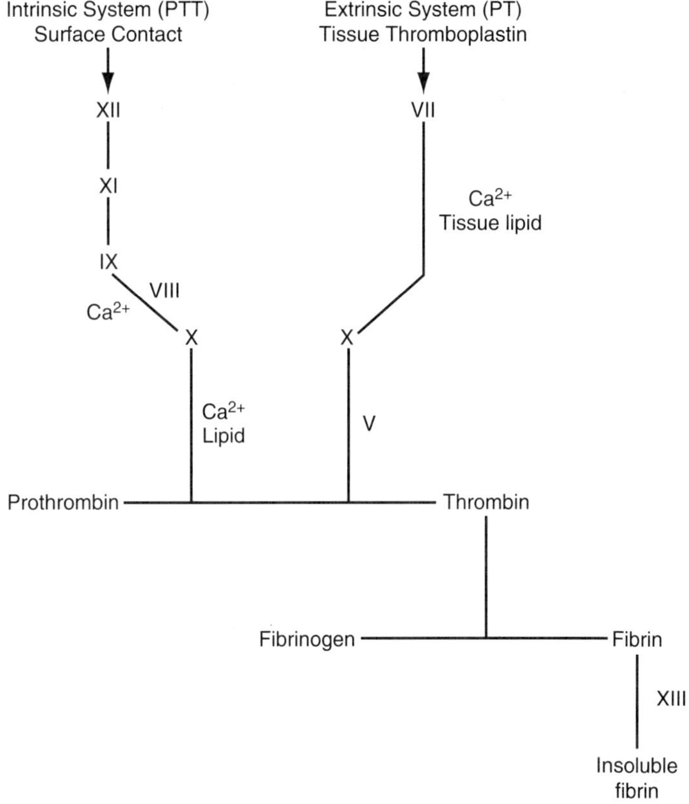

FIGURE 40–1. Simplified outline of blood coagulation pathways.

the intrinsic pathway, a cascade of factors XII, XI, IX, and VIII. This is triggered by negatively charged particles such as collagen, sebum, and glass. Activation of the common pathway, comprised of factors X, V, II (prothrombin), and fibroinogen, results in formation of a blood clot.

Prothrombin Time

The PT reflects the function of the extrinsic pathway. This test most specifically assesses the activity of factor VII, in which synthesis in the liver is vitamin K dependent. An abnormal PT thus yields information about warfarin use, vitamin K absorption, and synthetic capacity of the liver. Heparin has little effect on the PT in therapeutic doses. When heparin and warfarin are given together, however, there is an additive effect on the PT. One should wait for 5 hours after an intravenous heparin bolus or 12 to 24 hours after subcutaneous administration before obtaining a PT. The effect of heparin can be reversed by administering protamine. The administration of vitamin K can reverse the effect of warfarin, but there is a lag phase of 12 to 24 hours before significant amounts of coagulation factors can be synthesized. Antibiotics, such as cefoperazone, cefamandole, and moxalactam, have been identified as causes of a prolonged PT. This effect is also reversible by administration of vitamin K.

The PT has virtually 100% sensitivity in the detection of severe and moderate factor VII deficiency (<5% of normal and 5 to 25% of normal, respectively). Functional decreases in factor VII activity are the result of defects more proximal in the coagulation cascade. Actual deficiency of factor VII can occur with hepatic dysfunction, malabsorption, or malnutrition but only in the presence of advanced disease.

The PT is performed by adding tissue thromboplastin with phospholipid (''complete thromboplastin'') and calcium to the patient's plasma. The time to formation of a fibrin clot is measured. Defects in the intrinsic system do not affect the PT because the complete thromboplastin activates the extrinsic system and bypasses the intrinsic pathway. Severe deficiencies in fibrinogen, however, do prolong the PT because fibrin is necessary to produce the clot. The fibrinogen level must be <100 mg/100 mL (reference range: 200 to 400 mg/100 mL) before the PT is affected. False-positive test results can occur with underfilling of the tube or with improper specimen handling.[1]

International Normalized Ratio

The International Normalized Ratio (INR)[13] was developed in order to standardize reports of coagulation status and anticoagulant effect despite the variations in the PT. These variations occur with the use of different thromboplastin preparations at different institutions and at different times within the same institutions. The INR is calculated as follows: the measured PT is divided by the mean normal PT value, and the ratio is raised to the c power. The c power is the International Sensitivity Index identified for the particular thromboplastin utilized in the assay.

$$\text{INR} = (\text{Measured PT}/\text{Mean Normal PT})^{c}$$

Partial Thromboplastin Time

The PTT assesses the intrinsic pathway. It is determined by measuring the time it takes for a fibrin clot to form in the patient's platelet-poor citrated plasma after calcium and an activating agent have been added. The test is sensitive to any coagulation factor deficiency within the intrinsic system. The only abnormality detected by the PT and not detected by the activated PTT is isolated factor VII deficiency. False-positive PTT results may occur in patients with polycythemia because the elevated hematocrit in a fixed volume creates a relative deficiency of plasma and therefore less clotting factors in a given volume of blood. Conversely, false-negative results can be obtained when a minor deficiency of one clotting factor is masked by high levels of another.

SCREENING

The PT and PTT are easily obtained, relatively inexpensive, accurate, and commonly performed. They have little utility in screening asymptomatic individuals for occult bleeding disorders because the frequency of asymptomatic coagulopathies is so low. In fact, the prevalence of asymptomatic coagulopathies is so low that false-positive test results outnumber true-positive results when obtained for general screening.[2, 3] Kaplan and coworkers found the frequency of abnormalities in asymptomatic patients who were screened preoperatively to be 0%.[4]

Robbins and Rose retrospectively reviewed all abnormal PTT measurements from 1000 consecutive tests performed. They found either that the abnormal results were clinically insignificant or that the patients with prolonged PTT had known risk factors. They suggested that the test added little unsuspected clinical information.[5] Nevertheless, numerous studies have demonstrated that the PT and PTT continue to be commonly ordered despite the lack of clinical indications. The Medical Necessity Project of the Blue Cross and Blue Shield Association of

America has developed a comprehensive set of guidelines for the use of these tests. These guidelines have been endorsed by the American College of Physicians (Table 40–1).[6,7]

DETECTION OF BLEEDING DISORDERS

A careful and thorough history and physical examination are sensitive methods of screening for bleeding disorders. The PT and PTT are not indicated for the detection of coagulopathy in patients with neither history nor physical evidence of abnormal bleeding or liver disease. This indication holds true for both preoperative patients and medical patients.[8] Table 40–2 summarizes the important historical information to be obtained. The physical assessment should concentrate on evidence of bleeding, to be noted on examination of the skin, mucous membranes, and optic fundi.

The PTT and PT as well as the platelet count and bleeding time are indicated studies for all patients in whom there is clinical suspicion of coagulation defect. Specific abnormalities on these tests direct the

TABLE 40–1. APPROPRIATENESS CRITERIA FOR THE USE OF THE PROTHROMBIN TIME AND PARTIAL THROMBOPLASTIN TIME

Clinical Evaluation
Evidence of liver disease
History of malabsorption
History of malnutrition
Prior to procedures that may disrupt the coagulation cascade (eg, cardiopulmonary bypass)
Clinical history unavailable prior to procedure
Evaluation of Abnormal Bleeding
Evidence of abnormal bleeding by history (eg, excessive or spontaneous bleeding)
Evidence of abnormal bleeding on physical examination (eg, unexplained petechia or purpura)
Anticoagulant Use
Recent or current use of heparin or warfarin; use of subcutaneous, low-dose heparin does not routinely need to be monitored
Evaluation of Abnormal Coagulation
Suspected or proven thromboembolism
Suspected or proven disseminated intravascular coagulation

Used with permission, from Erban SB, Kinman JL, Schwartz JS: Routine use of the prothrombin and partial thromboplastin times. *JAMA*. 1989;262:2428–2432. Copyright 1989, American Medical Association.

TABLE 40–2. PATIENT HISTORY AND THE EVALUATION OF BLEEDING DISORDERS

Personal or family history of known bleeding disorder
Personal or family history of prolonged bleeding after an injury, dental extraction, or other surgical procedure
Personal or family history of frequent or severe nosebleeds or spontaneous bleeding at other sites
Personal history of liver disease, malabsorption, or malnutrition
Recent use of anticoagulants

From Rapaport SI: Preoperative hemostatic evaluation: Which tests, if any? *Blood.* 1983;61:229–231. With permission.

practitioner to specific segments of the coagulation system. Abnormal results can be due to congenital coagulation disorder, acquired coagulation disorder, or anticoagulant therapy (Tables 40–3 and 40–4).[11] A normal PTT and PT effectively rule out abnormality of the coagulation cascade.

Patients with acute or chronic liver dysfunction (eg, hepatitis and cirrhosis) should have PT and PTT measurement performed. These tests are important indicators of the synthetic capacity of the liver and can guide admission decisions.

A history of easy or excessive bruising, bleeding from mucous membranes, or prolonged bleeding after minor trauma or invasive procedures suggests the presence of a coagulation defect.[9] This may be either congenital or acquired. A child with isolated recurrent epistaxis, for

TABLE 40–3. CAUSES OF PROLONGED PROTHROMBIN TIME

Hereditary deficiencies in factors VII and X as well as deficiencies in factor V, prothrombin, and fibrinogen
Vitamin K deficiency (decreased factors II, VII, IX, X)
Warfarin use
Liver disease
Disseminated intravascular coagulation
Hypofibrinogenemia and dysfibrinogenemia
Therapeutic fibrinolysis
Heparin
Factor inhibitors
Artifactual (in patients with polycythemia)

From Samly AH (ed): *Textbook of Diagnostic Medicine.* Philadelphia: Lea & Febiger; 1987:111. With permission.

TABLE 40–4. CAUSES OF PROLONGED PTT

Deficiency of one or more factors involved in intrinsic and common pathway: prekallikrein; HMW kininogen; factors XII, XI, X, IX, VII, and V; prothrombin; and fibrinogen
Coagulation factor inhibitors, lupus anticoagulant
Fibrin split products
Heparin administration

From Samly AH (ed): *Textbook of Diagnostic Medicine.* Philadelphia: Lea & Febiger; 1987:111. With permission.

example, may have a mild bleeding disorder, such as mild hemophilia or a variant of von Willebrand's disease,[10] and should be tested.

Among congenital disorders, hemophilia A (classic hemophilia), due to congenital deficiency of functional factor VIII, is an entity relatively commonly encountered in the ED. The PTT is prolonged, but test results of platelet function are normal. Hemophilia B (Christmas disease) is due to deficiency of factor IX and gives similar test results. The two conditions can be differentiated only by specialized testing for the specific factors involved. In contrast, von Willebrand's disease is due to decreased platelet aggregation and adherence. Although it is not fundamentally a disorder of clotting factors, factor VIII activity is decreased and the PTT is prolonged in this condition.

Bleeding disorders can also be acquired. Disseminated intravascular coagulation can result from endogenous activation of the coagulation cascade by trauma, endotoxin, hemolysis, or other conditions that may expose the blood to tissue thromboplastic components. Generally, the PT and PTT are both prolonged, and the platelet count is low. Further investigation reveals a fibrinolytic state, manifested by low fibrinogen levels and elevated fibrin split products.

Coagulopathy can also result from vitamin K deficiency, leading to decreased synthesis of factors II, VII, IX, and X. Similarly, severe liver disease can result in impaired production of all coagulation factors except factor VIII.

The anticoagulant properties of heparin are derived from its inhibition of the conversion of prothrombin to thrombin. The anticoagulant effect has an immediate onset. The effect of warfarin, in contrast, is not noted for at least 1 to 2 days. This compound affects prothrombin and factors V and VII. Increased sensitivity to anticoagulant drugs may be noted in patients who have liver disease or are poorly nourished or who are receiving aspirin or broad-spectrum antibiotic. The latter interferes with intestinal bacterial flora, which are important in the production of vitamin K (a component of prothrombin and factor VII).[12]

Patients with bleeding disorders of unknown cause present a diagnostic challenge. A common impediment to correct diagnosis is transfusion with blood products prior to diagnostic testing. Thus, if there is any question of abnormal bleeding, a citrate-anticoagulant blood tube, an EDTA-anticoagulated tube, and a non–anticoagulated serum tube should be obtained before transfusion in case coagulation studies are needed. The citrated tube should be kept refrigerated.

Fresh frozen plasma contains all of the noncellular coagulation factors and is therefore the treatment of choice for unknown bleeding disorders with prolonged PT or PTT. It contains only 1 unit of activity per milliliter, and large volumes are thus required to correct significant factor deficiencies. Far better is the use of precise replacement factor if a specific coagulation deficiency is known. In the most common factor disorder, hemophilia A, the PTT is not prolonged until factor VIII levels are <30 to 35% of normal.

INVASIVE PROCEDURES

Every patient who will need an invasive procedure, whether it is surgery, central line, or lumbar puncture, must first be evaluated from a clinical standpoint for evidence of a bleeding disorder. A history of a familial bleeding disorder, excessive bleeding after dental procedures, easy bruising, hematemesis, epistaxis, hemoptysis, or gastrointestinal bleeding must be elicited. Physical examination that reveals ecchymosis, petechia, purpura, angioma, telangiectasia, or hematoma may suggest a bleeding disorder. Hepatomegaly, splenomegaly, jaundice, ascites, and abdominal venous distension may be associated with liver disease. The clinical evaluation is the most important indicator for the risk of hemorrhagic complications after an invasive procedure.

SUMMARY

- A thorough history and physical examination are the most important means of detecting congenital and acquired coagulopathies.
- The PT and PTT are indicated in the clinical circumstances as outlined in Table 40–1.
- Heparin therapy should be monitored with activated PTT measurements.
- Warfarin therapy should be monitored with PT measurements. Emergency department patients who are taking warfarin should generally have PT measured.
- A prolonged PT and normal PTT suggest factor VII deficiency.

- A prolonged PTT and normal PT suggest deficiency of factor VIII, IX, XI, or XII or von Willebrand's disease.
- Prolongation of both the PT and PTT results from deficiency of fibrinogen or factor II, V, or X.

REFERENCES

1. National Committee for Clinical Laboratory Standards: Collection, Transport and Preparation of Blood Specimens for Laboratory Specimens for Coagulation Testing and Performance of Coagulation Assays. Approved Guidelines. NCCLS document H21-A. Villanova, PA: NCCLS; 1986.
2. Suchman AL, Griner PF: Diagnostic uses of the activated partial thromboplastin time and prothrombin time. *Ann Intern Med.* 1986;104:810–816.
3. Eisenberg JM, Clarke JR, Sussman SA: Prothrombin and partial thromboplastin times as preoperative screening tests. *Arch Surg.* 1982;117:48–51.
4. Kaplan EB, Sheiner LB, Boeckmann AJ, et al: The usefulness of preoperative laboratory screening. *JAMA.* 1985;253:3576–3581.
5. Robbins JA, Rose SD: Partial thromboplastin time as a screening test. *Ann Intern Med.* 1979;90:796–797.
6. Erban SB, Kinman JL, Schwartz JS: Routine use of the prothrombin and partial thromboplastin times. *JAMA.* 1989;262:2428–2432.
7. Sox HC (ed): *Common Diagnostic Tests: Use and Interpretation.* Philadelphia, PA: American College of Physicians; 1987:350–351.
8. Rohrer MJ, Michelotti MC, Nahrwold DL: A prospective evaluation of the efficacy of preoperative coagulation testing. *Ann Surg.* 1988;208:554–557.
9. Taylor RE, Blatt PM: Clinical evaluation of the patient with bruising and bleeding. *J Am Acad Dermatol.* 1981;4:348–368.
10. Kiley V, Stuart JJ, Johnson CA: Coagulation studies in children with isolated recurrent epistaxis. *J Pediatr.* 1982;100:579–581.
11. Coleman RW, Hirsh J, Marder VJ, et al. (eds): *Hemostasis and Thrombosis: Basic Principles and Clinical Practice.* 2nd ed. Philadelphia: JB Lippincott; 1987.
12. Raskob GE, Carter CJ, Hull RD: Anticoagulant therapy for venous thromboembolism, in Coller BS (ed): *Progress in Hemostasis and Thrombosis.* Vol 9. Philadelphia: WB Saunders; 1989.
13. Hirsch J, Poller L: The International Normalized Ratio. *Arch Intern Med.* 1994;154:282–288.

Chapter

Toxicology Laboratory Testing

Thomas G. Martin

The history and clinical examination are often inadequate for optimal management of acutely poisoned patients. The history of ingestion may be unreliable because the patient is incapacitated or intentionally misrepresenting the exposure.[1] Other patients mislead the physician by misnaming a drug, eg, calling a bottle of acetaminophen "aspirin." The physical examination may be deceptively benign when a toxin is ingested with delayed effects. Thus, toxicology laboratory testing is often essential in providing high-quality care in the emergency department. Toxicology laboratory tests consist of qualitative or quantitative analyses. Toxicology screens or panels are groups of these tests that vary in breadth from basic to comprehensive. Appropriate use of these expensive resources is essential to the emergency physician, requiring knowledge of the general indications, capabilities, limitations, and costs of the tests.

INDICATIONS FOR ORDERING TOXICOLOGY TESTS

General indications for ordering toxicology screens are listed in Table 41–1. Many studies have determined the utility of toxicology laboratory analysis in acutely poisoned patients.[2, 3] The results of these studies must be interpreted cautiously because they have concentrated primarily on change in therapy or discovery of unsuspected toxins.

AVAILABILITY TO CLINICIANS

Toxicology laboratory tests that should be available in every emergency department are listed in Table 41–2. The American Association of Poison Control Centers (AAPCC) has published a list of the 12 most common substance categories causing fatal poisonings.[4] The four most common substance categories—analgesics, antidepressants, sedative hypnotics, and "street" drugs—accounted for >60% of the deaths in all 12 categories. The tests listed in Table 41–2 allow for the identification of many intentional poisonings, including the top four categories.

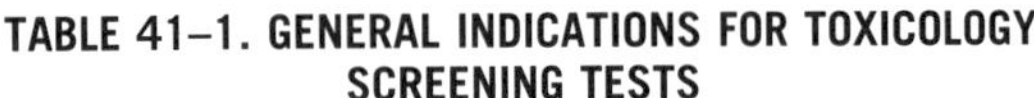

TABLE 41–1. GENERAL INDICATIONS FOR TOXICOLOGY SCREENING TESTS

To verify the presence or absence of a toxin
To identify indications for specific toxicologic therapy
To identify patients suspected of substance abuse
To identify patients at risk of acute drug withdrawal
To avoid the use of unnecessary diagnostic procedures

QUALITATIVE VS QUANTITATIVE TESTS

Qualitative analysis is useful only to identify the presence of a substance. Qualitative tests are often not useful for substances that are used therapeutically because they do not distinguish between therapeutic and toxic concentrations. Qualitative analysis is also not useful when a substance has been taken for a long period. Regional toxicology treatment centers must be prepared to manage unusual poisonings and so must have a wider variety of toxicologic laboratory tests available.[5]

Some poisons are considered ''time bombs'' because an initial benign clinical presentation does not portend the potentially severe adverse effects. When time bombs are identified early and treatment started promptly, the serious adverse effects may be prevented or minimized. Examples include acetaminophen, *Amanita phalloides*, arsenic, chlorinated hydrocarbon, ethylene glycol, lead, lithium, mercury, monoamine oxidase inhibitor, methanol, paraquat, and sustained-release preparations. Quantitative analysis can help to identify significant exposures to these time bombs and facilitate early therapy.

The results of toxicology laboratory tests may identify indications or contraindications for specific therapies. Specific antidote, multiple doses

TABLE 41–2. MINIMUM STAT TOXICOLOGY LABORATORY TESTS FOR ALL EMERGENCY DEPARTMENTS

Quantitative

Acetaminophen, barbiturate, carbamazepine, carboxyhemoglobin, digoxin, ethanol, ethylene glycol, iron, isopropanol, lithium, methanol, methemoglobin, phenytoin, salicylate, theophylline, tricyclic antidepressant

Qualitative

Acetaminophen, amphetamine, barbiturate, benzodiazepine, cocaine, opiate, phencyclidine, phenothiazine, salicylate of activated charcoal, hemodialysis, hemoperfusion, and alkalization of blood or urine are examples of specific therapies. Quantitative levels are usually required to determine when these specific therapies are indicated.

TEST RESULT RESPONSE TIMES

Emergency physicians usually require rapid results from toxicology laboratory tests. When toxicology screens results are not available for 24 hours, they can still confirm a clinical diagnosis but will usually be too late to suggest specific therapy or to guide the proper use of other diagnostic tests. Shorter laboratory turnaround times are often more costly and may be impractical for small hospitals. The use of outside reference laboratories for toxicology laboratory testing can be an acceptable alternative. Regional toxicology treatment centers must ensure that turnaround times are appropriately short for a variety of toxicology tests. For many occupational or environmental poisonings timing is not as critical.

SPECIMEN COLLECTION

Most toxicology laboratories request both urine and blood specimens for toxicology screening. Urine specimens are easier to extract drugs from and more often contain identifiable drug or metabolite than do blood specimens. Acidic drugs are more easily identified in the serum and basic drugs in the urine. Urine toxin quantitation is often of limited value in emergency medicine. One exception is heavy metal intoxication. The usual quantitative toxicology tests pertinent to emergency medicine requires a blood specimen.

Some laboratories routinely request gastric specimens for toxicology screens. Gastric specimens may be valuable when the time from ingestion is very short or the parent drug is rapidly metabolized. Gastric specimens collected soon after the toxic ingestion have high concentrations of the parent drug. Gastric specimens are more difficult to extract, and some laboratories are simply not prepared to analyze them. Gastric analysis may be useful in cases of mushroom poisoning or nonpharmaceutical ingestions in which techniques for biologic fluid analysis are not available. Most pharmaceutical agents can be measured in the blood or urine, making gastric analysis unnecessary in most drug overdoses.

Saliva and breath specimens are used to test for the presence of certain toxins, such as ethanol. Breath alcohol (ethanol) correlates well with blood concentrations.[6] Breath alcohol analyzers have been used by law enforcement agencies for years. The accuracy of breath alcohol analysis is limited by recent alcohol ingestion, alcohol containing emesis, or belching.[7] Salivary ethanol levels also correlate well with blood alcohol levels but are subject to the same limitations.[8] A colorimetric dipstick assay and a device for measuring ethanol in the saliva have been successfully developed.[9, 10]

ANALYTICAL PROCEDURES

Spot test, spectroscopy, immunoassay, radioimmunoassay, and chromatography are commonly employed analytical procedures. The *spot test* relies on a color change resulting from the interaction between a toxin and the reagent. Spot tests are fast, inexpensive, and easy to perform but have only fair sensitivity and specificity. *Spectroscopy* relies on matching the pattern of peak absorbance of monochromatic wavelength light with known patterns of absorbance. Spectroscopy has better specificity than spot tests. *Immunoassays* rely on the competitive binding of antibodies to drugs along with enzyme fluorescent light scattering or radioactive tags.[11] Generally, immunoassays have good sensitivity and specificity and are fast and easy to perform but are moderately expensive.[12–15] The *radioimmunoassay* is expensive and time consuming but very sensitive. *Chromatography* relies on different rates of migration of compounds within two different media. Chromatographic procedures include thin layer chromatography (TLC), high-performance liquid chromatography (HPLC), and gas liquid chromatography (GLC or GC) alone, or combined with mass spectroscopy (GCMS). Thin layer chromatographic techniques are time consuming and require highly trained technicians but otherwise are inexpensive and sensitive. High-performance liquid chromatographic and GC methods are expensive and time consuming but have good sensitivity and specificity. Gas chromatography/mass spectroscopic analyses are very expensive and time consuming and require great expertise but are very specific and sensitive.

APPROPRIATE UTILIZATION OF TEST RESULTS

Most emergency physicians and medical toxicologists would agree that not all suspected poisoning victims need comprehensive toxicology laboratory screening to make the correct diagnosis or to guide appropriate therapy. In fact, a number of studies have concluded that routine comprehensive toxicology laboratory testing is not cost-effective in emergency departments and trauma centers.[16] A limited battery of toxicology laboratory tests is useful in most poisoned patients. Comprehensive toxicology screening is indicated frequently enough that it should be available quickly in all emergency departments. Some hospitals have developed a small panel of blood and urine toxicology laboratory tests as a basic screening for suicidal or intoxicated patients. An example of such a panel for suicidal patients would be quantitative blood tests for ethanol, acetaminophen, and tricyclic antidepressant (TCA) and qualitative urine screens for drugs of abuse. Salicylate and acetaminophen analyses are recommended in poisoning victims because they are widely available and commonly implicated in serious suicide attempts. Although the incidence of an unsuspected acetaminophen poisoning is quite low, the test is inexpensive and the medicolegal consequences of a missed diagnosis are potentially severe.[17] A qualitative screen for the commonly prescribed pain killer, propoxyphene and its cardiotoxic metabolite norpropoxyphene, is desirable. A qualitative screen for diphenhydramine, the most commonly used over-the-counter sleeping aid, would be very desirable but is currently unavailable. The tests for acetaminophen, salicylate, and TCA could be omitted in recreationally intoxicated patients.

Tricyclic antidepressant analysis is recommended because TCAs are frequently prescribed to severely depressed patients who are prone to suicidal ingestions. A qualitative TCA analysis is not acceptable because it does not distinguish between levels in the therapeutic range and levels in the toxic range. Only a quantitative or semiquantitative TCA analysis is useful. A semiquantitative TCA test would be sufficient for clinical use but some toxicology laboratories are more comfortable with a quantitative procedure. Following an acute ingestion, a TCA level greater than 1000 ng/mL is associated with a high risk of serious toxicity.[18] Many would routinely admit any TCA poisoned patient with a level greater than 1000 ng/mL to the ICU for cardiac monitoring and systemic alkalinization.

When a poisoning is suspected and the initial toxicology screen is negative, a comprehensive drug screen is warranted. Criteria for comprehensive drug screening in the emergency department are unexplained abnormalities such as acidosis, altered level of consciousness,[19] arrhythmia, hypertension, hypotension, or seizure. Routine use of comprehensive drug screens is usually both unnecessary and quite costly.

Routine screening for the drugs of abuse is recommended in patients with self-induced poisoning. Substance abuse is very common in these patients, and drug withdrawal frequently complicates their recovery. Sometimes a positive screen for a substance of abuse is the first hint that acute withdrawal will occur as the patient emerges from coma. Ethanol levels and urine screens for drugs of abuse can be used to confirm drug abuse in other emergency department patients such as those suspected of seeking drugs. The popularity of substances of abuse may vary between regions, which may require customization of substance abuse screens.

INFORMED CONSENT

Suicidal patients by definition forfeit their right to informed consent for procedures that pertain to the diagnosis or treatment of the suicidal act. All other emergency department patients do have the right to give informed consent for toxicology laboratory testing. Although the general consent that a patient signs when registering for an emergency department visit suffices for most emergency laboratory testing, it may not be sufficient for toxicology laboratory testing. Emergency physicians should be aware that the results of some toxicology laboratory tests can be used against the patient. For example, the result of medical blood ethanol test may be subpoenaed by police as evidence in driving under the influence (DUI) cases. Similarly, an employer may use the results of substances abuse screens to discipline employees. Some would argue that proper informed consent for emergency patients would include the information that the results of the tests could be used against them. A conservative approach would be to perform substance abuse screening only when there are appropriate medical indications and not simply to confirm the suspicion of substance abuse. Examples of appropriate medical indications for substance abuse screening are evaluating an altered level of consciousness, evaluating suspected drug-seeking behavior, and predicting a withdrawal reaction during hospitalization. Some employers will severely penalize employees caught using illicit drugs, including marijuana. Because medical indications for marijuana screen are rare, some laboratories have removed this substance from their routine toxicology screens. Because of these concerns, a prudent policy would be not to screen for drugs of abuse unless medically warranted or unless specific informed consent has been obtained.

INACCURACY OF TOXICOLOGY LABORATORY ANALYSIS

Ideally, toxicology laboratory testing should have high degrees of sensitivity, specificity, and accuracy. Frequent false-positive and false-negative laboratory results significantly reduce the utility of toxicology laboratory tests. The College of American Pathologists (CAP) accredits clinical laboratories and requires participation in interlaboratory comparison surveys that are not proficiency tests.[20] Historically, toxicology laboratories have generally performed poorly in blind proficiency tests, often with high false-positive and false-negative rates.[21–23] Some have criticized these studies because the drug concentrations were based on detection limits for substance abuse, not those for poisoning victims. In one study of poisoned patients, the results were not much better than in the proficiency tests.[24] In the poisoned patient study, the laboratories only identified drugs responsible for the poisoning 50 to 70% of the time and the concentrations varied up to 10-fold. Most of the older proficiency studies are flawed by many methodologic deficiencies.[25] The Department of Health and Human Services has developed standards for proficiency testing and requires successful performance for laboratories to obtain their certification. The Clinical Laboratory Improvement Amendments of 1988 (CLIA'88) contain rules for proficiency testing.[26]

TOXICODYNAMIC VARIABILITY

Even when the serum levels can be measured with great accuracy, their clinical usefulness may be limited. Toxicodynamics are the relationships between toxicity and serum levels. For many toxins there is a high degree of toxicodynamic variability. A given drug may be associated with different degrees of toxicity in different patients. Toxicodynamic variability is also increased when the time from ingestion is not taken into account. The formation of toxic metabolites, development of tachyphylaxis, and involvement of secondary messengers are other causes. Despite the numerous causes of variability, quantitative levels can be useful in selected cases.

PITFALLS OF ROUTINE TOXICOLOGY LABORATORY TESTING

"Negative toxicology screen" is meaningless unless one knows exactly what tests were performed in the particular case. Toxicology screens vary tremendously between institutions. Some hospitals routinely perform a comprehensive battery of tests, whereas others perform a limited set. Many common drugs are not detected in routine toxicology screens (Table 41–3). Unless one is certain that the suspected toxin can be detected, the toxicology laboratory should be told what toxins are suspected. The laboratory technician could notify the physician when the suspected toxin cannot be identified with the tests that were ordered. The list of identifiable compounds varies widely from one institution to another. Each toxicology laboratory should provide for its clinical staff

TABLE 41–3. COMMON POISONS NOT DETECTED WITH ROUTINE TOXICOLOGY SCREENING TESTS

Anticholinergics (diphenhydramine)	Iron
Antipsychotics	Isoniazid
Beta blockers	Lithium
Calcium channel blockers	LSD
Carbon monoxide	Metals (arsenic, lead, mercury)
Clonidine	Monoamine oxidase inhibitors
Cyanide	Organophosphates
Digoxin	Selective serotonin reuptake inhibitors
Fentanyl and analogs	Toxic alcohols
Hydrocarbons	Venoms
Hypoglycemic agents	

a list of compounds identifiable by its basic toxicology screen. This practice is not feasible for comprehensive toxicology tests sometimes capable of identifying thousands of drugs. Rather than stating "the toxicology screen was negative," the laboratory personnel should either list the pertinent negatives or describe the method used.

False-positive and false-negative test results can be problematic but may be anticipated by an astute clinician. Compounds with similar structures often cross-react or otherwise lead to a similar test result. A false-positive result occurs when nontoxic compounds cross-react with toxic compounds. Cyclobenzaprines have a tricyclic ring structure and will cross react with TCA immunoassay reagents. Cyclobenzaprine poisoning is rarely as severe as a TCA poisoning can be. Diphenhydramine, chlorpromazine, mesoridazine, and thioridazine are other common causes of false-positive TCA results. False-positives for salicylate may result from diflunisal because of structural similarities.[27]

Cross-reactivity of metabolites or analogs with the parent compound may actually be beneficial. The cross-reactivity of many sympathomimetic amines in immunoassays has been called a flaw by some but recognized as an advantage by others.[28] In fact, cross-reactivity of analogs in immunoassays for drugs of abuse is now expected by clinicians. Immunoassays for morphine may be positive following use of codeine or paregoric. Morphine is a metabolite of codeine and paregoric contains 10% morphine. A phencyclidine (PCP) analog, phenylcyclohexylpyrrolidine (PHP), is popular because it is not detected by radioimmunoassay or TLC tests for PCP.[29] Certain barbiturates such as hexobarbital, methohexital, mephobarbital, thiamylal, and thiopental are considered to give false-negative results because they do not cross-react in the barbiturate immunoassay. Drug screens may be positive for amphetamines when monoamine oxidase inhibitors (MAOIs) such as phenylzene or selegiline are used in therapeutic amounts. This is not a false-positive finding but is due to the production of amphetamine as a metabolite. Although cross-reactivity may lead to false-positives, it also increases the sensitivity of a screen by detecting analogs and metabolites.

Critical errors may occur when toxicologic test results are given without units or in a unit that the clinician is not accustomed to using. Acetaminophen, ethylene glycol, methanol, and salicylate are examples of toxins in which reported units vary within regions. The criteria for ethanol blocking therapy and hemodialysis with ethylene glycol poisoning are levels >25 and >50 mg/dL, respectively. An ethylene glycol level of 5 gm/L is equivalent to 500 mg/dL. One may fail to order appropriate therapy when informed that the ethylene glycol level was "5" unless the units "gm/L" were known or recognized!

Calculation of the osmolal gap is frequently used to help diagnose a toxic alcohol ingestion and guide specific therapy in lieu of specific levels. Renal failure can falsely increase the osmolal gap and potentially lead to unnecessary interventions.[30] A false-negative osmolal gap could delay diagnosis and specific therapies and markedly enhance morbidity and mortality. Measuring osmolality by vapor point elevation may lead to a false-negative osmolal gap owing to evaporation of volatile substances such as methanol. When relying on the osmolal gap to guide initial therapy, emergency physicians must be certain that their laboratory employs the freezing point depression method to determine osmolality.

Certain routine analytic tests provide important information in acutely poisoned patients. These tests may also produce false-positive or false-negative results. For example, the total iron binding capacity is often falsely elevated in acute iron poisoning[31] due to inadequate amounts of magnesium carbonate in the assay[32] or interference by deferoxamine.[33]

Chemicals contained in blood collection tubes may interfere with toxicology laboratory analysis (eg, citrate in blue tops, EDTA in lavender tops, lithium heparin in green tops, and oxalate in gray tops).[34, 35] These problems may be avoided by careful adherence to the instructions for specimen handling supplied by the toxicology laboratory.

Several toxins or antidotes interfere with pulse oximetry tests for oxygen saturation. Carbon monoxide forms carboxyhemoglobin in the blood, which falsely elevates the cutaneous oxygen saturation.[36] Both methemoglobin and its antidote, methylene blue, have been shown to interfere with cutaneous oxygen saturations.[37, 38]

SUMMARY

Toxicology laboratory testing is an invaluable tool for the emergency physician when used appropriately. Routine comprehensive toxicology screening is not cost-effective but selective toxicology laboratory analysis can be. Emergency physicians should be familiar with the list of drugs identifiable by the routine toxicology screens at their hospital. When uncertain as to whether the suspected toxin may be identified by your toxicology laboratory, tell them what toxins you are looking for. Laboratory personnel will suggest alternatives when the tests you have ordered will not answer your questions. Consultation with the nearest regional poison information center or a medical toxicologist should be considered when there is a question as to the necessity for or interpretation of toxicology laboratory analysis.

REFERENCES

1. Yaron M, Lowenstein S, Koziol-McLain J, et al: Do overdose patients lie about what drugs they took? (Abstract) *Ann Emerg Med.* 1992;21:662–663.
2. Kellermann AL, Fihn SD, LoGerto JP, et al: Impact of drug screening in suspected overdose. *Ann Emerg Med.* 1987;16:1206–1216.
3. Rygnestad T, Berg J: Evaluation of benefits of drug analysis in the routine clinical management of acute self poisoning. *J Toxicol Clin Toxicol.* 1984;22:51–61.
4. Litovitz TL, Holm KC, Bailey KM, et al: 1991 Annual Report of the American Association of Poison Control Centers National Data Collection System. *Am J Emerg Med.* 1992;10:452–505.
5. American Academy of Clinical Toxicology Facility Assessment Guidelines for Regional Toxicology Treatment Centers. *J Toxicol Clin Toxicol.* 1993;31:209–217.
6. Gibb KA, Yee AS, Martin SD: Accuracy and usefulness for a breath alcohol analyzer. *Ann Emerg Med.* 1984;13:516–520.
7. Gibb K: Screen alcohol levels, toxicology screen, and use of the breath alcohol analyzer. *Ann Emerg Med.* 1986;15:349–353.
8. Jones AW: Inter and intra individual variation on the saliva/blood alcohol rates during ethanol metabolism in man. *Clin Chem.* 1979;25:1394–1398.
9. Tu GC, Kapur B, Israel Y: Characteristics of a new urine, serum, and saliva alcohol reagent strip. *Alcoholism.* 1992;16:222–227.
10. Christopher TA, Zeccardi JA: Evaluation of the Q.E.D. saliva alcohol test: A new, rapid, accurate device for measuring ethanol in saliva. *Ann Emerg Med.* 1992;21:1135–1137.
11. Wisdom GB: Enzyme-immunoassay. *Clin Chem.* 1976;22:1243–1255.
12. Simpson D, Jarvie DR, Heyworth R: An evaluation of six methods for the detection of drugs of abuse in urine. *Ann Clin Biochem.* 1989;26:172–181.
13. Caplan YH, Levine B: Abbot phencyclidine and barbiturates abused drug assays: Evaluation and comparison of ADx FPIA, TDx FPIA, EMIT, and GC/MS methods. *J Anal Toxicol.* 1989;13:289–292.
14. Schwartz JG, Zollars PR, Okorodudu AO, et al: Accuracy of common drug screen tests. *Am J Emerg Med.* 1991;9:166–170.
15. Przekop MA, Manno JE, Kunsman GW, et al: Evaluation of the Abbott ADx

amphetamine/methamphetamine II abused drug assay: Comparison to TDx, EMIT, and GC/MS methods. *J Anal Toxicol.* 1991;15:323–326.

16. Clark RF, Harchelroad F: Toxicology screening of the trauma patient: A changing profile. *Ann Emerg Med.* 1991;20:151–153.
17. Ashbourne JF, Olson KR, Khayam-Bashi H: Value of rapid screening for acetaminophen in all patients with intentional drug overdose. *Ann Emerg Med.* 1989;18:1035–1038.
18. Boehnert MT, Lovejoy FH: Value of the QRS duration versus the serum drug level in predicting seizures and ventricular arrhythmias after an acute overdose of tricyclic antidepressants. *N Engl J Med.* 1985;313:474–479.
19. Helliwell M, Hampel G, Sinclair E, et al: Value of emergency toxicological investigations in differential diagnosis of coma. *Br Med J.* 1979;2:819–821.
20. Hamlin W: Proficiency testing as a regulatory device: A CAP prospective. *Clin Chem.* 1992;38:1234–1236.
21. Jain NC, Sneath TC, Budd RD: Blind proficiency testing in urine drug screening: The need for an effective quality control program. *J Anal Toxicol.* 1977;1:142–146.
22. Mason MF: Some realities and results of proficiency of laboratories performing toxicological analysis. *J Anal Toxicol.* 1981;5:201–208.
23. Hansen JH, Caudill SP, Boone J: Crisis in drug testing: Results of CDC blind study. *JAMA.* 1985;253:2382–2387.
24. Ingelfinger JA, Isakson G, Shine D, et al: Reliability of the toxic screen in drug overdose. *Clin Pharmacol Ther.* 1981;29:570–575.
25. McCoy HG: Proficiency testing of drug analysis laboratories. (Letter) *J Occup Med.* 1991;33:428–429.
26. Jenny RW, Jackson KY: Evaluation of the rigor and appropriateness of CLIA'88 toxicology proficiency testing standards. *Clin Chem.* 1992;38:496–500.
27. Bessen HA, Smilkstein MJ, Kulig KW, et al: Difunisal overdose causing falsely elevated serum salicylate levels. (Abstract) *Vet Hum Toxicol.* 1986;28:475–476.
28. Warner M: Jumping to conclusions; The perceived inaccuracy of drug-screening tests has raised questions about their suitability for routine drug testing. *Anal Chem.* 1987;59:521A–522A.
29. Budd RD: Mass screening and confirmation of phencyclidine (PCP) in urine by radioimmunoassay/TLC. *J Toxicol Clin Toxicol.* 1981;18:85–90.
30. Sklar AH, Linas SL: The osmolal gap in renal failure. *Ann Intern Med.* 1983;94:841–842.
31. Burkhart KK, Kulig KW, Hammond KB, et al: The rise in the total iron-binding capacity after iron overload. *Ann Emerg Med.* 1991;20:532–535.
32. Tenenbein M, Yatsoff RW: The total iron-binding capacity in iron poisoning: Is it useful? *Am J Dis Child.* 1991;145:437–439.
33. Bentur Y, St. Louis P, Klein J, et al: Misinterpretation of iron-binding capacity in the presence of deferoxamine. *J Pediatr.* 1991;118:139–142.
34. Smith JC, Lewis S, Holbrook J, et al: Effect of heparin and citrate on measured concentrations of various analytes in plasma. *Clin Chem.* 1987;33:814–816.
35. Dorian P, Sellers EM, Reed KL: Spurious detection of a high serum imipramine level due to coating of Vacutainer stopper. *Can Med Assoc J.* 1982;127:509–510.

36. Barker SJ, Tremper KK: The effect of carbon monoxide on pulse oximetry and transcutaneous PO_2. *Anesthesiology*. 1987;66:677–679.
37. Watcha MF, Connor MT, Hing AV: Pulse oximetry in methemoglobinemia. *Am J Dis Child*. 1989;143:845–847.
38. Eisenkraft JB: Methylene blue and pulse oximetry readings: Spuriouser and spuriouser! (Letter) *Anesthesiology*. 1988;68:171–172.

Chapter

Type, Screen, and Crossmatch

Laurence Katz and James Kelley

In 1992 alone, over 12 million units of blood products were transfused in the United States, 57% being packed RBCs, 27% platelets, 10% fresh frozen plasma, and 6% cryoprecipitate. Even so, over half of all blood products prescribed were believed to be inappropriately utilized,[3] primarily because physicians lacked an understanding of the types of blood components available and the indications for their administration.

Blood transfusions are frequently administered in the emergency department as life-saving procedures. Blood and blood products are required most commonly for volume resuscitation, symptomatic anemia, or coagulopathy. Knowledge of the types of blood components, the indications for their use, and the risks of transfusion are vital if the emergency physician is to ensure that transfusions are used appropriately and safely.

Blood is the ideal fluid for volume resuscitation because it has both an oxygen-carrying capacity and a relatively high oncotic pressure. The increased delivery of oxygenated blood reduces ischemia to vital organs, and oncotic pressure allows the blood to stay longer in the circulation compared with crystalloids. Blood is not used for all volume resuscitation because of limitations of cost and availability and because of its inherent risks.

In general, anemia should be corrected when the patient is symptomatic or when there is a potential for serious sequelae from uncorrected anemia. What degree of anemia requires a transfusion is controversial. Likewise, the amount of blood that should be given for any given degree of anemia has not been standardized.

Uncontrolled hemorrhage may be a consequence of a coagulopathy.

Identification of causative agents or of deficiencies in certain blood components will help direct specific transfusion therapy if necessary.

INDICATIONS FOR TRANSFUSION

There are no established guidelines for when blood should be used for volume resuscitation in trauma cases. Gervin[4] recommends an initial infusion of 3000 mL crystalloid infusion to stabilize vital signs. If vital signs stabilize with crystalloids, the hemoglobin level is used to determine the need for transfusion. If 3 L of crystalloid has failed to stabilize the patient, blood is administered.

These recommendations are based on estimated blood loss. Class I hemorrhagic shock (<15% blood loss) produces no alterations in vital signs or outcome. Class II hemorrhagic shock (20 to 25% blood loss) causes an increased heart rate but no change in blood pressure or perfusion. Class III hemorrhagic shock (30 to 40% blood loss) causes decreased blood pressure and increased heart rate. Class IV hemorrhagic shock is reflected by altered mental status as well as altered vital signs. Class III hemorrhagic shock represents a 1000 to 2500 mL blood loss, depending on the patient's weight.[5] Replacement of more than 30% of blood volume by crystalloid is associated with increased mortality.[6] The emergency physician must also recognize the potential need for blood in patients undergoing operations such as thoracotomy and pelvic surgery.

There is no agreement on the hemoglobin level below which transfusion is necessary. Young patients can tolerate levels of 7 g/dL with little difficulty and few complications.[7] A study investigating the need for blood in patients with hemoglobin of 8 g/dL showed no benefit from transfusion if the patient was adequately fluid resuscitated.[8] Patients with cardiac disease frequently receive transfusions to maintain a hemoglobin above 10 g/dL. Hemoglobin levels below 8 g/dL increase resting cardiac output significantly, increasing the risk of ischemia in myocardium[9] because of the tenuous balance between oxygen supply and demand. The rate of development of anemia is also important when determining the need for a transfusion. Patients with chronic renal failure commonly have chronic anemia and tolerate very low levels well, whereas other patients who develop anemia acutely from bleeding or hemolysis may deteriorate rapidly if the same level of anemia is not promptly corrected.

Blood loss may be the result of a coagulopathy. Hereditary coagulopathies usually require replacement of specific blood factors, whereas acquired diseases such as disseminated intravascular coagulation (DIC) and liver dysfunction generally require correction of the underlying illness, as well as replacement of blood components.

Because many of the blood components possess the same risks as blood transfusions, they also must be administered only for specific indications. Massive blood replacement (usually greater than 10 units) is associated with an acquired coagulopathy that is usually due to a combination of platelet dysfunction and low-grade DIC from the patient's underlying disease. Replacement of platelets and supplementation of deficient clotting factors usually stabilizes the bleeding disorder.

ORDERING BLOOD

Blood type is determined by the surface antigens (agglutinogens) on RBCs. The major blood groups A and B have corresponding surface antigens, whereas blood group O has neither antigen. Type O blood is the most frequently banked blood (47%), followed by A (41%), B (9%), and AB (3%).[10] Preformed antibodies (agglutinins) related to each blood group occur naturally and are thought to arise through a combination of environmental exposure and genetic determination.

Transfusion reactions occur when similar group antigens (agglutinogens) and antibodies (agglutinins) are mixed. When recipient antibodies interact with donor surface RBC antigens, there is agglutination or hemolysis of donor RBCs. Destruction of donor RBCs defines a major transfusion reaction. A minor transfusion reaction occurs when recipient RBCs are destroyed by donor antibodies. Minor reactions are infrequent because the recipient's blood volume dilutes the titer of donor antibodies and because whole blood is currently given infrequently.

A blood screen ("typescreen") evaluates RBCs for Rh factor and other antigens such as Kell, Duffy, Kidd, and MNS. Reaction to blood antigens such as Rh factor does not usually occur on the first exposure to a mismatch because there are no preformed antibodies to Rh. To generate a response, the patient must have been sensitized by a previous transfusion.

Crossmatching determines the compatibility of the donor and recipient blood by determining autoantibodies and cold agglutinins that are not detected by the blood screen.

Before blood can be available for transfusion, there is often a relatively short but definite delay. To perform a type and crossmatch requires 45 minutes, restricting the availability of that unit of blood to one patient during that time period. Typed and screened blood can be ready for use in 25 minutes. Uncrossmatched type-specific blood takes less than 15 minutes to prepare, whereas uncrossmatched O-negative blood (universal donor) can be available in less than 5 minutes.

Which method of blood processing should be requested is dictated by the clinical situation. A trauma patient who is exsanguinating should receive uncrossmatched O-negative blood, whereas a patient in shock who temporarily stabilizes with crystalloids is more likely to benefit from type-specific blood. When a patient is to be transfused prophylactically (eg, preoperatively), a full type and crossmatch provide the lowest risk of transfusion reaction. Other blood components require between 5 (platelets) and 40 minutes (fresh frozen plasma) to prepare.

BLOOD COMPONENTS

Fresh whole blood can either be stored in a preservative or separated to provide various blood components. The volume of one unit of collected donor whole blood is about 450 mL. Whole blood can be stored at 4°C for 21 days, although the various components, especially platelets and clotting factors, become nonfunctional after 24 hours. The hemoglobin concentration of whole blood is 12 to 14 g/dL and can raise the recipient's hemoglobin level by approximately 1 g/dL per unit administered. A type and crossmatch is usually required prior to transfusion. Whole blood is indicated for patients who require massive transfusion for stabilization of hemorrhagic shock or those who require exchange transfusion. The risk of whole blood transfusion is higher than that of other blood products because it carries the combined risk of all the individual components as well as antibodies.[11]

The volume of a unit of *packed red blood cells* (PRBCs) is 250 to 280 mL. Packed red blood cells can be stored for 35 days at 4°C. They contain a small amount of plasma that can be removed by washing or freezing techniques. The process is expensive and time consuming but enables the blood to be stored indefinitely and decreases the risk of transfusion reaction, especially in patients who require frequent or multiple transfusions. The hemoglobin concentration of PRBCs is 23 to 26 g/dL and can be expected to raise the recipient's hemoglobin approximately 3 g/dL per unit. A type and crossmatch is the preferred method for requesting this blood component. Packed red blood cells are the most commonly utilized blood component for correcting shock and anemia because of ease of storage, availability, and high hemoglobin concentration. Frozen or washed PRBCs are indicated for patients who have had a previous febrile, nonhemolytic reaction to blood, usually from leukocyte antigens, IgA, or other agglutinins.

Platelets have a volume of 30 mL per unit and can be stored at 22°C for 5 days. Each unit contains 10^{10} platelets per cubic millimeter and can raise the platelet count 5000 to 10,000/mm^3. Patients should be typed for platelets if possible, but it is not essential for a successful transfusion.

A unit of *fresh frozen plasma* (FFP) has a volume of 250 mL and can be stored at −18°C for 1 year. Once a unit of FFP is thawed, it must be used within 24 hours or it will be ineffective. The thawing process takes 40 minutes. Fresh frozen plasma contains coagulation factors, albumin, and plasma protein fractions. Patients requiring FFP should be typed to assure ABO compatibility. Fresh frozen plasma is indicated for coagulopathies. Each unit raises coagulation factors an average of 2 to 3%. Fresh frozen plasma is also used to raise circulating oncotic pressure to mobilize extravascular fluid into the intravascular space.

Cryoprecipitate provides a concentrated quantity of factor VIII (60 to 120 u/unit) as well as factor XIII, fibrinogen, and von Willebrand factor. Cryoprecipitate is collected from single donor plasma. Cryoprecipitate volume is 10 to 25 mL per unit and is stored at −18°C for up to 1 year. Patients should be typed and screened before receiving this product. Cryoprecipitate is indicated for bleeding from hemophilia A (factor VIII deficiency), von Willebrand's disease, and conditions with decreased fibrinogen and bleeding such as DIC or complications of thrombolytics. Ten to 50 u/kg are usually required to correct bleeding caused by a deficiency in these factors.

Factor VIII provides a much higher concentration of factor than FFP or cryoprecipitate. Factor VIII is derived from multiple plasma donors and therefore carries a higher risk of hepatitis and HIV. The concentration of factor varies per unit and is marked on the bag. Ten to 50 μ/kg are required to control bleeding.

Factor IX concentrate is used almost exclusively for patients with hemophilia B. It also provides the vitamin K–dependent factors of the extrinsic pathway. The preparation is collected from multiple plasma donors and carries a nearly 100% risk of hepatitis, thus limiting its widespread use. Ten to 50 μ/kg are required for adequate hemostasis.

Genetically engineered factors VIII and IX are now available and eliminate the inherent risks of pooled products.

COMPLICATIONS OF TRANSFUSION

Blood transfusion is associated with a very low mortality rate (1/100,000). Complications of transfusion can be divided into two broad categories, hemolytic and nonhemolytic.

Hemolytic reactions occur in 1/600 transfusions and are primarily a result of clerical error[12] in the blood bank (53%) or in patient care areas where appropriately typed blood is administered to the wrong patient (29%). As noted previously, hemolytic reactions are divided into major or minor. Both can be manifested by fever, chills, low back pain, or discomfort at the intravenous site. These symptoms can progress to chest pain, shortness of breath, hemodynamic instability, DIC, renal

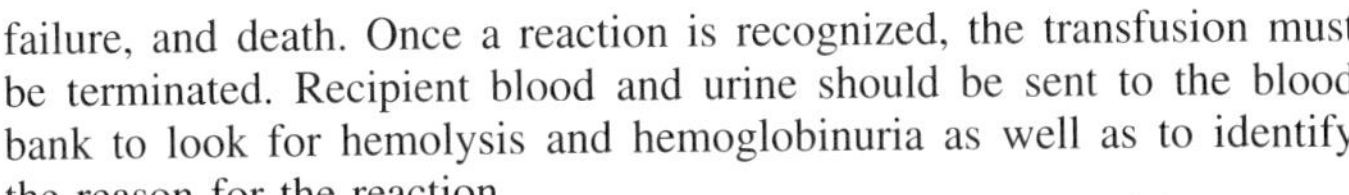

failure, and death. Once a reaction is recognized, the transfusion must be terminated. Recipient blood and urine should be sent to the blood bank to look for hemolysis and hemoglobinuria as well as to identify the reason for the reaction.

Nonhemolytic reactions occur more frequently (2 to 10%) and have multiple etiologies.[13] Reactions occur most commonly as a result of allergic reactions to WBCs or proteins in the blood product and cause a range of symptoms from hives and bronchospasm to life-threatening airway edema and circulatory collapse. Therapy involves terminating the transfusion and administering epinephrine, antihistamine, H_2-blocker, or steroid as needed. Patients with a history of multiple transfusions, allergic reactions to transfusions, or IgA deficiency are at increased risk for reactions and should receive IgA-deficient washed RBCs to reduce the chance of another reaction.

Certain physical properties of donated blood can cause complications. Blood with a long shelf life may have elevated levels of potassium, acid, and ammonia. Large quantities of transfused blood may increase recipient citrate levels and result in hypocalcemia or citrate-mediated direct cardiac toxicity. Large quantities of rapidly infused blood may also lead to hypothermia or coagulopathy. The coagulopathy is caused by a combination of dilution of coagulation factors, platelet dysfunction, and tissue destruction resulting from the patient's underlying disease.

Bacteria and viral infections can be transmitted by transfusion. Gram-negative rods are the most commonly transmitted bacteria.[12] Transfusing blood over more than 4 hours can also increase the risk of bacterial infection from the infused blood. Non-A, non-B hepatitis is transmitted by transfusion at a rate of 1/500 units of blood. Hepatitis C is a marker of non-A, non-B hepatitis; new techniques may further reduce the transmission of this virus. Human immunodeficiency virus (HIV) is the virus responsible for AIDS and is transmitted in 1/250,000 to 1/1,000,000 units of transfused blood. Concentrated multiple-donor pooled blood products currently carry the highest risk of transmitting HIV.

Delayed transfusion reactions can occur days to weeks after the transfusion. The reaction is usually self-limited and manifested by a slow rise in indirect bilirubin with a drop in hemoglobin and haptoglobin. This reaction is the result of the recipient's production of a nonagglutinating antibody and is more frequently seen in multigravid or multiply transfused patients.

Care must also be taken in administering blood. Patients with tenuous fluid status can develop pulmonary edema as a result of the fluid load. Blood transfused with D5W in the same line can result in hemolysis, whereas blood mixed with lactated Ringer solution may form microemboli. Therefore, blood should be transfused with normal saline to reduce complications.

SUMMARY

An awareness of the blood products available for transfusion assists the physician in choosing the appropriate blood product mandated by the clinical situation. Knowledge of the procedures, limitations, and potential errors in blood preparations should guide blood-requesting practices and reduce complications. The risk of blood transfusions must be known so that a risk-benefit ratio can be assessed for each transfusion. This information will also aid the patient in making informed decisions with regard to receiving blood. Intelligent prescribing of blood transfusions will assure appropriate, safe, and effective utilization of blood products.

REFERENCES

1. Maluf N: History of blood transfusion. *J Hist Med Allied Sci.* 1954;9:59.
2. Landsteiner K: Zur Kenntris der Antifermentativen. Lytischen and Agglutinierenden Wirkugen des blut. *Zentralbl Bakteriol.* 1900;27:357.
3. Mozes B, Epstein M, Ben-Bassat I: Evaluation of the appropriateness of blood and blood product transfusion using preset criteria. *Transfusion.* 1989;29:473–476.
4. Gervin AS: Transfusion, autotransfusion, and blood substitutes, in Maatox K, Moore E, Feliciano D (eds): *Trauma.* 2nd ed. New York: Appleton and Lange;1988:165–180.
5. Pruitt B, Mancrief J, Mason A: Effect of Buffered Saline Solutions upon Blood Volume of Man after Acute Hemorrhage. Annual research progress report. San Antonio, TX: Institute of Surgical Research, 1965.
6. Rush B, Eiseman B: Limits of non-colloid solution replacement in experimental hemorrhagic shock. *Ann Surg.* 1967;165:977.
7. Tremper K, Friedman E, Levine E: The preoperative treatment of severely anemic patients with perfluorochemical oxygen transport fluid. *N Engl J Med.* 1982;307:277.
8. Dietrich R, Conrad S, Herbur C: The cardiovascular and metabolic response to red blood cell transfusion in critically ill volume resuscitated nonsurgical patients. *Crit Care Med.* 1990;18:940.
9. Peterdorf R, Adams R, Braunwald E, et al: *Anemia, Principles of Internal Medicine.* 10th ed. New York: McGraw-Hill; 1983.
10. Guyton A: *Textbook of Medical Physiology.* 6th ed. Philadelphia: WB Saunders; 1981.
11. Milner L, Butcher K: Transfusion reactions reported after transfusion of RBCs and of whole blood. *Transfusion.* 1978;18:493.
12. FDA. Records on transfusion fatalities 1979–1985.
13. Baker R, Moinichen B, Nyhus L: Transfusion reactions. *Ann Surg.* 1969;169:684.

Chapter 43 Uric Acid Level

Scott Jolley

Uric acid levels are of limited if any utility in the emergency department. Uric acid levels are neither sensitive nor specific for the diagnosis of gout.[4] The majority of uric acid disorders are not life threatening.

Pathologic conditions associated with altered uric acid levels are divided into four major categories: essential hyperuricemia (overproduction or underexcretory states); renal underexcretion; increased nucleic acid turnover; and enzymatic defects in the purine metabolic pathway. The causes of an elevated serum uric acid level are listed in Table 43–1.

Normal ranges of serum uric acid for men and women are listed in Table 43–2. Hyperuricemia is defined as the concentration of monosodium urate necessary to saturate human plasma. At a serum pH of 7.40 and a temperature of 37°C, this occurs at a uric acid level of 7 mg/dL in men and 6.0 mg/dL in women.

A multitude of factors influences the serum uric acid concentration. These factors include hydration status, renal function, and dietary intake of purines. Drugs affecting secretion at the distal tubule and those causing destruction of ATP may falsely elevate levels. Those most commonly implicated are nicotinic acid, aspirin, alcohol, pyrazinamide,

TABLE 43–1. CAUSES OF HYPERURICEMIA

Essential hyperuricemia
Overproduction
Underexcretion
Renal retention
Renal failure
Drugs
Poisons: lead, alcohol
Organic aciduria: acetoacetate, lactate
Endocrinopathy: hypothyroidism, hyperparathyroidism
Increased turnover of nucleic acid
Myeloproliferative disorders
Chemotherapy: leukemia, lymphoma
Enzymatic defects
Hypoxanthine-guanine phosphoribosyl transferase
Complete: Lesch-Nyhan syndrome
Partial
Abnormal phosphoribosyl pyrophosphate synthetase

TABLE 43–2. REFERENCE LEVELS

Male	3.5–7.2 mg/dL
Female	2.6–7.0 mg/dL

Based upon the uricase method.

ethambutol, ketone, lactic acid, triglyceride, and, most commonly, thiazide diuretics.

The use of the serum uric acid level to detect asymptomatic hyperuricemia was reported on by Campion and coworkers, who found that the incidence of new cases of gouty arthritis was low: 4.9% per year for those with levels above 9 mg/dL, 0.5% for levels of 7.0 to 8.9 mg/dL, and 0.1% for levels <7.0 mg/dL.[7] These data complement those of other studies that have shown no independent predictive value of an elevated uric acid level for the development of either significant renal disease or coronary artery disease.[2, 3, 5, 6]

Although it is the most important risk factor for the development of gout,[7] a single blood level is neither sensitive nor specific for the presence of disease. Halder and colleagues found that, in their patients who had arthrocentesis-documented gout, 38% had uric acids levels less than 7 mg/dL.[8] Although an elevated uric acid level has been included as one of 11 criteria for the diagnosis of gout,[1] the diagnostic standard remains joint aspiration with demonstration of sodium urate crystals.

Gouty arthritis is clearly a disease that can cause great suffering to patients. However, a single emergency department uric acid level is of no use in making the diagnosis of gout nor has it been shown to be of any use as a screening test for gout or other diseases.

REFERENCES

1. Wallace SO, Robinson H, et al: Preliminary criteria for the classification of the acute arthritis of primary gout. *Arth Rheum.* 1977;20:895–900.
2. Roubenoff R: Gout and hyperuricemia. *Rheum Dis Clin North Am.* 1990;16:539–550.
3. Hall AP, Barry PE, et al: Epidemiology of gout and hyperuricemia. *Am J Med.* 1967;42:27–37.
4. McCarty DJ: Gout without hyperuricemia. *JAMA.* 1994;271:302–303.
5. Brand FN, McGee DL, et al: Hyperuricemia as a risk factor of coronary heart disease: The Framingham Study. *Am J Epidemiol.* 1985;121:11–18.
6. Fessel WJ: Renal outcomes of gout and hyperuricemia. *Am J Med.* 1979;67:74–82.
7. Campion EW, Glynn RJ, et al: Asymptomatic hyperuricemia in the Normative Aging Study. *Am J Med.* 1987;82:421–426.
8. Hadler NM, Frank WA, et al: Acute polyarticular gout. *Am J Med.* 1974;56:715–719.

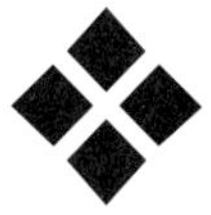

OTHER FLUIDS

Chapter

Urinalysis—Dipstick and Microscopic Examination

William Angelos

Urinalysis is a simple, inexpensive, and noninvasive emergency department (ED) test that can be used to assess the genitourinary tract, to gauge roughly the state of hydration, and, when negative, to suggest that a patient's complaint may be due to a nonrenal cause. The urinalysis can be helpful in the ED evaluation of patients with urinary tract infection, hypertension, preeclampsia, rhabdomyolysis, multiple trauma, and renal calculi.

It is important for the clinician to be aware of the limitations of the urinalysis. Having a small laboratory in the ED for evaluation by the physician can be a time-saving measure, but the results should be confirmed in the hospital laboratory, which is under the rigid quality control required by Joint Commission on Accreditation of Hospitals.

URINE COLLECTION AND TRANSPORT

Proper specimen collection and transport are essential to obtain reliable results. Studies have shown that a randomly obtained urine specimen is frequently contaminated and inaccurate and thus is not a recommended way of collecting urine.[1] There are four main methods of collecting urine: percutaneous suprapubic aspiration, midstream clean catch, bladder catheterization, and urine bag.

Suprapubic aspiration is the most accurate method and avoids contamination.[2] Although the procedure is invasive, it is safe and is associated with very few complications. Because of the high pelvic position of the bladder in neonates and infants, it is frequently employed in workups of septic patients. Aspiration has an extremely low complication rate in this patient population.

The midstream *clean catch* specimen provides a reliable urine specimen if performed correctly. In males, the foreskin should be retracted and the urethral meatus cleaned with an antiseptic solution. In females, the procedure requires an assistant or the patient to spread the labial folds apart to avoid vaginal contamination.

The use of *bladder catheterization* reduces vaginal contamination. There is a risk of introducing an iatrogenic infection with catheterization; an acceptable postcatheterization infection rate is 2 to 4%.[3] Bladder catheterization is preferred over midstream clean catch collection when vaginal infection is present, in the menstruating female, in urinary retention, and when previous results are confusing or doubtful.[4]

Urine is occasionally collected in a *urine bag* for routine urinalysis in the young child. The bag is applied to the perineum after that area has been cleansed with an antiseptic solution. There is a high incidence of fecal contamination, so multiple attempts may be needed to obtain an adequate specimen.

Once the urine is collected, the specimen should be transported to the laboratory with minimal delay. By 2 hours, the formed elements (cells and casts) in the urine break down and become unrecognizable on microscopic examination. In one study, white blood cell degradation worsened with increasing urine pH, decreasing osmolarity, and increasing temperature.[5] Urine that cannot be examined within 2 hours should be either refrigerated or discarded.

The urine is evaluated by both dipstick and microscopic examination.

DIPSTICK

Urine dipstick testing (generally including 6 to 10 semiquantitative readings) is fairly sensitive and specific but does have some important limitations.

Color

The color of the urine can be the first clue to the presence of renal disease or may indicate that a dye or drug has been ingested. Hemoglobin or red blood cells often make the urine red or smokey. Cloudy urine can indicate pyuria or crystalluria. Table 44–1 lists different urine colors and associated clinical conditions.

pH

A random urine pH has a range between 4.5 and 8.5 and is usually of little diagnostic value. The dipstick has two color indicators, methyl

TABLE 44–1. URINE COLORS

Color	Association
Colorless	Dilute urine, diabetes mellitus, diabetes insipidus
Milky white	Chyluria, phosphate crystals, pyuria
Yellow	Normal, quinacrine, riboflavin, atabrine
Amber	Pyridium, concentrated urine, sulfasalizine
Blue, blue green	Methylene blue, amitriptyline, triamterene, biliverdin
Red	Hematuria, myoglobinuria, hemoglobinuria, rifampin, phenolphthalein, phenytoin, adriamycin, anthocyanin (pigment in beets and blackberries)
Red-brown	Urobilinogen, bilirubin, porphyria, desferrioxamine, phenothiazines, metronidazole, nitrofurantoin, chloroquine, primaquine
Brown-black	Melanin, alkaptonuria, senna, cascara, rhubarb

red and bromthymol blue, that can indicate the pH in a range from 5.0 to 9.0. Although urine is usually acidic, it may be alkaline after a meal. Citrate ingestion causes an alkaline urine, whereas cranberries and protein can produce an acidic urine. A highly alkaline urine pH suggests urinary tract infection with a urea-splitting organism such as *Proteus* or *Escherichia coli.*

Serial urine pH monitoring can be used to gauge the effectiveness of measures to alkalinize the urine as an adjunct in the treatment of certain overdoses such as salicylates and phenobarbital.

Specific Gravity

The reaction that occurs on the dipstick measurement of urinary specific gravity is based on the pKa change of treated electrolytes on the strip related to the cation concentration in the urine. The dipstick specific gravity correlated well with hydrometer reading and refractometry in one study.[6] A refractometer should be used if a more accurate reading is required. The specific gravity of urine ranges from 1.001 to 1.040. A specific gravity >1.040 is associated with the administration of iodinated contrast media or mannitol. The specific gravity is usually elevated in volume-depleted states and decreased in volume-repleted states. The use of the dipstick for specific gravity has a limited clinical role.

Protein

Normal individuals excrete 50 to 150 mg of protein in a 24-hour period. Strenuous exercise and fever may increase this rate to 300 mg/

24 h. In proteinuric states, albumin, globulin, and Tamm-Horsfall protein are the most commonly found in the urine. On dipstick testing, protein (predominantly albumin) in the urine reacts with tetrabromophenol impregnated on the strip. Tetrabromophenol is yellow and changes in color from yellow to green to dark blue as the urine protein concentration increases. It reliably detects protein concentrations greater than 30 mg/dL.

The dipstick test is more sensitive to albumin than globulins. Thus, Bence Jones proteinuria may be missed by the dipstick. Dilute urine (specific gravity <1.010) may also be responsible for false-negative results. False-positive results can occur with radiographic contrast media, alkaline urine, or high-dose penicillin therapy.

If proteinuria is suspected but the dipstick result is negative, an acid precipitation test should be performed. The sulfosalicylic acid test (performed by adding eight drops of 20% sulfosalicylic acid to 2 mL of urine) is more sensitive than the dipstick and can detect as little as 5 mg/dL of protein. A positive test result is indicated by urine turbidity after the acid is added. False-positive findings occur with radiographic contrast media, penicillins, and sulfonylurea drugs. An alkaline urine may cause a false-negative result.

Blood

Normal urine contains no red blood cells. Although microscopic hematuria can occur after vigorous exercise, blood in the urine should be considered pathologic until proved otherwise. The dipstick is very sensitive in detecting heme pigments. False-negative results can occur with inadequate sample mixing, conditions with an elevated pH and high specific gravity, and high urinary vitamin C urine levels.[4] False-positive results can occur if the urine is contaminated with povidone-iodine.[7]

Red blood cells, myoglobin, and hemoglobin all react with orthotoluidine, the material impregnated in the strip to detect blood. This chemical is oxidized by peroxide, which is produced by the hemoglobin or myoglobin catalase. The reaction turns the strip blue.

Table 44–2 lists the differential diagnosis of hematuria. Further evaluation is indicated if hematuria cannot be readily explained by one of the common benign causes listed. All dipstick-positive urine samples should be examined microscopically to confirm the presence of RBCs.

If no RBCs are seen in the sediment, a tentative diagnosis of myoglobinuria should be considered. Significant hematuria may cause a positive dipstick reaction for protein as well. If the protein reaction is strong, however, true proteinuria is present and glomerular pathology should be suspected.

TABLE 44–2. DIFFERENTIAL DIAGNOSIS FOR HEMATURIA

Exercise	Polycystic disease	Thrombocytopenia purpura
Trauma	Glomerulonephritis	Anticoagulants
Cystitis	Schönlein-Henoch purpura	Thrombotic thrombocytopenic purpura
Calculi	Malignant hypertension	
Genitourinary tumors	Focal embolic glomerulitis	

Glucose

Glucose is spilled into the urine when the tubular threshold for its reabsorption is exceeded. Glycosuria usually indicates a serum level >170 mg%. The dipstick test for glucose is very specific; there is no cross-reaction with other reducing substances, such as lactose, fructose, or pentose.

The dipstick reading is caused by the conversion of glucose to gluconic acid by glucose oxidase that is impregnated on the strip. The reaction releases peroxide, which oxidizes ortho-toluidine, with which this area of the strip is also impregnated. A positive reaction is noted when the color changes from yellow to different shades of blue. The dipstick for glucose is not as reliable as the Clinitest tablets for the quantification of urine glucose concentration.

The urine dipstick for glucose has a sensitivity and specifity of >95%.[8] False-negative results may occur in the presence of large amounts of ascorbic acid.[9] In one study, pH, creatinine, uric acid, and protein had no effects on the glucose dipstick.[10] False-positive results can occur if the urine is contaminated with bleach or hydrogen peroxide.

Ketones

The dipstick test for ketones is based on the reaction of ketone with nitroprusside impregnated on the test strip, which in the presence of glycine produces a color change from lavender to purple. The dipstick is sensitive to acetoacetic acid but is somewhat less sensitive to acetone and does not react with β-hydroxybutyric acid.

Leukocyte Esterase

Urine can be screened by dipstick for significant pyuria (corresponding to a count of >10 WBC/HPF on the spun sediment or >8 WBC/mm^3 on the unspun urine). The dipstick test has been reported in several studies to have a sensitivity and specificity of >88%.[11–13] The sensitivity is lower when there are <10 WBC/HPF. One study reported a sensitivity of only 44% when there were 6 to 12 WBC/HPF.[14] The dipstick is impregnated with indoxyl carboxylic acid ester, which reacts with esterase released by WBCs. The reaction converts the substrate into indoxyl, which is then oxidized in room air to an indigo color.

A positive test does not always indicate urinary tract infection. Noninfectious causes such as renal stones, interstitial nephritis, bladder irritation secondary to pelvic and abdominal pathogy, vaginal discharge, and chronic kidney disorders can produce significant pyuria and not be associated with bacteriuria. In addition, contamination of the urine by vaginal secretions can be a cause of false-positives.[1]

Infectious etiologies other than the usual urinary tract infections that cause pyuria but no bacteriuria should also be mentioned. Of these, prostatitis and genitourinary tuberculosis are the most notable. A negative test result almost always rules out infection; a 100% negative predictive value was noted in one study.[11] Nevertheless, if the clinical suspicion of urinary tract infection is high and the dipstick is negative, the urine should be sent for microscopic examination and possible culture.

NITRITE

The dipstick nitrite reaction depends on the reduction of endogenous nitrates by nitrate-reducing bacteria. Not all bacteria that cause urinary tract infection have the ability to reduce nitrate. False-negative nitrite results can occur with dilute urine, non–nitrate reducing bacteria, bacterial inhibition secondary to antibiotics, and urinary ascorbic acid. Although not very sensitive, the test's specificity approaches 100%.

When the nitrite test is used in conjunction with the leukocyte esterase test, the negative predictive value is >95% if both are negative.[15] In the same study, the positive predictive value for urinary tract infection when both the nitrite and leukocyte esterase were positive was significantly lower than that of the nitrite test alone because of the high sensitivity of the leukocyte esterase test and the low prevalence of urinary tract infection in the study population.[15] The microscopic examination, a clean midstream catch, and culture help the clinician to decide whether infection is present.

Bilirubin

Normal urine contains no bilirubin. The urine dipstick test for bilirubin turns positive when urinary bilirubin is >0.5 mg/dL. A positive bilirubin and a negative urobilinogen are highly suggestive of biliary obstruction. False-positive results can occur with phenazopyridine, and false-negative results can occur with chlorpromazine, selenium,[16] and high urinary ascorbic acid levels.[16]

Urobilinogen

Urobilinogen is a by-product of the bacterial degradation of conjugated bilirubin in the intestine. It has an enterohepatic circulation and is excreted in the urine. Normal adult excretion for a 24-hour period is up to 2.5 mg.[17] Increased urine urobilinogen occurs with hemolysis and intrinsic liver disease and is absent in total biliary obstruction. The urobilinogen dipstick has a range of 0.1 to 1.0 per deciliter. It gives a slight reaction with most urines, however. The test should not be used to determine the absence of urobilinogen. High nitrite concentrations in the urine artifactually decrease color reactivity, and phenazopyridine dyes give false-positive results.[4]

URINE SEDIMENT

The urinary sediment is the most valuable part of the urinalysis examination for the detection of renal disease. As noted previously, WBCs, RBCs, and casts degenerate over several hours.

Ten mL of fresh urine should be spun in a centrifuge for 5 minutes at 2000 rpm. The supernatant is poured off and the sediment button is resuspended in the few drops of urine that remain in the bottom of the tube. A drop is then placed on a slide and a coverslip is applied. The urine is initially examined under low power. Under high power (400×), the number of cells and casts seen per HPF is quantitated. Ten HPFs should be viewed and the cell count per HPF should be averaged over the ten fields. Casts are reported in a similar manner, but counts are done on low-power fields. Several variables may affect cell counts. The method for centrifuging and resuspending the sediment should be consistent. The volume of urine that is spun, amount of urine used to resuspend the sediment, size of the drop used for examination, coverslip size, and field size all affect the cell count.

Cells and casts are not normally found in the urine, except for an occasional tubular epithelial cell, which may be increased with fever and exercise. The presence of WBCs in the urine usually represents infection, as noted earlier. Generally, a finding of >5 to 10 WBC/HPF in a clean catch midstream urine represents significant pyuria. If associated with bacteria noted on microscopic examination, the likeli-

TABLE 44–3. MICROSCOPIC EXAMINATION OF URINARY SEDIMENT AND ITS CLINICAL SIGNIFICANCE

Cells	Clinical Significance
Red blood cells	Urinary tract infection, renal calculi, urinary tract inflammation, genitourinary tumors
White blood cells	Urinary tract infection or inflammation
Squamous epithelial cells	Contamination
Casts	
Red cell	Glomerulonephritis, vasculitis, subacute bacterial endocarditis, renal vein thrombosis
White cell	Pyelonephritis, interstitial nephritis, papillary necrosis
Epithelial	Tubular damage, recovery from acute tubular necrosis
Hyaline	May be normal, dehydration states, fever
Granular	Renal parenchymal disease
Fatty	Nephrotic syndrome, diabetes glomerulosclerosis
Waxy	Advanced renal disease

TABLE 44–4. CRYSTALS FOUND IN ACID AND ALKALINE URINES

Acid	Alkaline
Calcium oxalate	Triple phosphate
Uric acid	Amorphous phosphates
Cystine	Calcium phosphate
Amorphous urate	Calcium carbonate
Sodium urates	Ammonium urate

hood of infection is high. If red blood cells are noted, a cause must be sought. Table 44–2 lists the differential diagnosis of hematuria. Casts in the urine often indicate intrinsic renal disease. Red blood cell casts indicate glomerular involvement and are seen primarily in glomerulonephritis. White blood cell casts imply inflammation of the renal parenchyma. Table 44–3 correlates sediment findings with clinical significance.

The presence of crystals for the most part has no diagnostic value. Calcium oxalate crystals are seen in the urine 30 to 50% of the time in ethylene glycol ingestion. Their presence may support the diagnosis but their absence is of no help. Urinary pH plays an important part in the type of crystal that is seen. Table 44–4 lists the types of crystals in acid and alkaline urines.

REFERENCES

1. McGuckin M, Cohen L, MacGregor RR: Significance of pyuria in urinary sediment. *J Urol.* 1978;120:452.
2. Monzon OT, Ory EM, et al: A comparison of bacterial counts of the urine obtained by needle aspiration of the bladder, catheterization and midstream-voided methods. *N Engl J Med.* 1958;259:764.
3. Brody LH, Salladay JR, Armbruster K: Urinalysis and the urinary sediment. *Med Clin North Am.* 1971;55:243.
4. Sheets C, Lyman JL: Urinalysis. *Emerg Med Clin North Am.* 1986;4:263.
5. Triger DR, Smith WG: Survival of urinary leucocytes. *J Clin Pathol.* 1966;19:443.
6. Frew AJ, McEwan J, Bell G, et al: Estimation of urine specific gravity and osmolality using a simple reagent strip. *Br Med J.* 1982;285:1168.
7. Said R: Contamination of urine with povidone-iodine: Cause of false positive test for occult blood in urine. *JAMA.* 1979;242:748.
8. Dyerberg J, Pedersen L, Aagaard O: Evaluation of a dipstick test for glucose. *Clin Chem.* 1976;22:205.
9. Smith BD, Peake MJ, Fraser CG: Urinalysis by use of multi-test reagent strips: Two dipsticks compared. *Clin Chem.* 1977;23:2337.

10. Nakamura RM, Reilly EB, Fujita K, et al: False negative reactions and sensitivity in the urine glucose oxidase test. *Diabetes.* 1965;14:224.
11. Chernow B, Zaloga GP, Soldano S, et al: Measurement of urinary leukocyte esterase activity: A screening test for urinary tract infection. *Ann Emerg Med.* 1984;13:150.
12. Gillenwater JY: Detection of urinary leukocytes by chemstrip-L. *J Urol.* 1981;125:383.
13. Kusumi RK, Grover PJ, Kunin CM: Rapid detection of pyuria by leukocyte esterase activity. *JAMA.* 1981;245:1653.
14. Propp DA, Weber D, Ciesta ML: Reliability of a urine dipstick in emergency department patients. *Ann Emerg Med.* 1989;18:560.
15. Bartkett RC, O'Neill D, McLaughlin JC: Detection of bacteria by leukocyte esterase, nitrite, and the automicrobic system. *Am J Clin Pathol.* 1984;82:683.
16. Fody EP: Preanalytic variables. *Clin Lab Med.* 1983;3:525.
17. Balikov B: Urobilinogen excretion in normal adults. *Clin Chem.* 1957;3:145.

Chapter

Thoracentesis and Analysis of Pleural Effusions

Joanne Gould Kuntz

Only a few milliliters of pleural fluid is normally present in the pleural space. Visible blunting of the costophrenic angle on the lateral chest radiograph is one of the earliest findings of pleural effusion and represents the accumulation of more than 300 mL of fluid,[1] although effusions as large as 2000 mL have been reported without any blunting of the angle.[2] Chest radiographs may reveal the presence of an unsuspected effusion or may confirm physical findings suggesting its presence.[3] The emergency physician must decide when it is appropriate to aspirate the effusion and which diagnostic tests will be most time- and cost-effective in determining the etiology (Table 45–1). This chapter discusses the indications for diagnostic and therapeutic thoracentesis in the emergency department and the diagnostic tests that may prove useful in certain clinical settings.

TABLE 45–1. DIAGNOSES THAT CAN BE ESTABLISHED DEFINITIVELY BY THORACENTESIS

Etiology	Findings from Thoracentesis
Malignancy	Malignant cells
Empyema	Aspiration of pus[a]
Tubercular pleurisy	Positive AFB smear or culture
Fungal infection	Positive KOA stain or culture
Lupus pleuritis	LE cells
Chylothorax	High triglycerides or presence of chylomicrons
Urinothorax	Pleural fluid/serum creatines, ratio >1.0
Esophageal rupture	Increased pleural fluid amylase and pH of 6.00[b]

[a]Only diagnosis that may be established immediately at the bedside.
[b]Diagnosis at bedside if food particles are present.
Adapted from Sahn SA: The state of the art. The pleura. *Am Rev Resp Dis.* 1988;138:184–234.

PATHOPHYSIOLOGY

Pleural fluid accumulates in the following settings:

1. increased hydrostatic pressure
2. increased vascular permeability
3. decreased oncotic pressure
4. increased negative intrapleural pressure
5. decreased lymphatic drainage
6. movement of fluid from the peritoneal space.

Pleural effusions have traditionally been divided into transudates and exudates. A transudate develops as a consequence of derangements in the formation or absorption of pleural fluid even when the pleural surfaces are not diseased. An exudate results when disease involves the pleural surfaces.

The differential diagnosis of pleural effusion includes a long list of disorders involving almost every major organ system in the body (Table 45–2).

INDICATIONS FOR THORACENTESIS

Therapeutic thoracentesis, according to the recommendations of the American Thoracic Society, ". . . may be indicated for relief of symptoms due to large pleural effusions. When repeated thoracentesis is

TABLE 45–2. COMMON CAUSES OF EFFUSION

Common Causes of Transudates
- Congestive heart failure
- Cirrhosis with ascites
- Nephrotic syndrome
- Hypoproteinemia
- Acute atelectasis
- Acute glomerulonephritis
- Myxedema
- Peritoneal dialysis
- Superior vena caval obstruction

Common Causes of Exudates
- Pulmonary infarction
- Lung abscess
- Bacterial pneumonia (parapneumonic effusion)
- Neoplasm
- Viral illness
- Tuberculosis
- Fungal illness
- Rickettsia
- Certain parasites
- Collagen vascular disease (especially lupus erythematosus or rheumatoid pleuritis)
- Pancreatitis
- Drug reactions (nitrofurantoin, methysergide, practolol)
- Asbestosis
- Meigs' syndrome
- Dressler's syndrome
- Lymphatic disease
- Trapped lung
- Subphrenic and hepatic abscess
- Sarcoidosis
- Chronic atelectasis
- Uremia
- Chylothorax

From Vukich DJ: Diseases of the pleural space. *Emerg Med Clin North Am.* 1989;7:309–324.

required for effusions that re-accumulate, consideration should be given to referral for tube drainage and pleurosclerosis.''[4]

Diagnostic thoracentesis is indicated whenever the etiology of the effusion is unknown. In instances when the cause can be reasonably deduced from clinical circumstances, the procedure may be deferred and the response to therapy observed.[4]

In patients with congestive heart failure (CHF), 50% have pleural effusions.[5] Although the pleural effusions may be simply observed while treatment for CHF proceeds, diagnostic thoracentesis should be performed if any of the following is noted: fever; pleuritic chest pain; unilateral, left-sided, or greatly disparate effusions; or absence of cardiomegaly on the chest radiograph.[1, 4, 6]

CONTRAINDICATIONS TO THORACENTESIS

There are no absolute contraindications to thoracentesis. Relative contraindications relate to the type of patient, the size of the effusion, and the presence of physiologic derangements.

Thoracentesis is contraindicated in patients who are unable to cooperate in the procedure. Appropriate sedation may be employed, however, to overcome this obstacle.

An effusion that measures <10 mm across on chest radiograph is likely to be too small to be aspirated.[6] If a fluid sample is required for diagnostic purposes, one may employ real-time ultrasound guidance, reducing the likelihood of a dry tap as well as other complications. Although the presence of coagulopathy is associated with an increased risk of complications, a small gauge needle in skilled hands and attempted removal of only a small amount of fluid reduce this risk. In performing the procedure, one should also take care to enter the pleural space through skin that is not obviously involved by infection or malignancy.

It has been cautioned that a transudative effusion due to CHF may acquire the biochemical characteristics of an exudate if the fluid is sampled after diuresis, thus subjecting the patient to the morbidity and expense of an unnecessary workup. Shinto and Light demonstrated in a prospective study that this occurrence is uncommon, even after aggressive diuresis over a 24- to 48-hour period, concluding that "If pleural fluid is found to meet exudative criteria in this situation further investigation should be directed toward the pleura."[5]

COMPLICATIONS OF THORACENTESIS

Thoracentesis is a relatively safe procedure with reported complication rates ranging from 0 to 46%.[7] The frequency and severity of complications are dependent on the skill of the clinician and the method of collection.

Thoracentesis techniques fall into three categories: ultrasound guided, needle-through-catheter, and needle only. In a prospective study by

Grogan and coworkers of 52 patients with free-flowing pleural effusions, the only complication associated with real-time ultrasound-guided thoracentesis (in three of 19 patients) was pain that was characterized as self-limited and mild to moderate in severity. In contrast, complications such as pneumothorax, subcutaneous hematoma, dry tap, inadequate yield, and persistent pain were associated with thoracentesis attempted without sonographic guidance.[7]

Pneumothorax is the most common complication following thoracentesis, especially therapeutic thoracentesis in which large volumes of fluid are collected. Review of several series indicates a variable incidence from 3 to 20%; of these, 2 to 10% require tube thoracostomy. Pneumothorax is most commonly caused by the generation of negative pleural pressure, which causes air to move from the atmosphere into the pleural space. Less commonly, pneumothorax follows laceration of lung tissue.

Reported cases of retention of catheter fragments when a catheter-through-needle technique is used appear to have been due to improper use of the instrument. Retention of the foreign body does not appear to have had long-term sequelae, although a retained fragment could clearly serve as a nidus for infection.

Approximately 2% of all pleural space infections are due to contamination during thoracentesis. Strict adherence to aseptic technique is thereby necessary.[6]

Hemothorax results when an intercostal artery is lacerated during needle insertion or removal. Although the risk of this mishap is greatly reduced when one enters just superior to the rib, it may still occur owing to the presence of tortuous vessels, especially in some elderly patients.

Rare but significant complications of liver and splenic laceration occur when thoracentesis is attempted lower in the thoracic wall. This risk is reduced by entering above the eighth intercostal space.

It has been held that removal of more than 1 L of fluid from the pleural space greatly increases the risk of reexpansion pulmonary edema in the rapidly reexpanded lung. This condition may be associated with hypoxia and hypotension, sometimes requiring mechanical ventilation, and it occasionally results in death. The exact mechanism of reexpansion pulmonary edema is unknown. It was initially thought to result from the reduction of pulmonary interstitial pressure that occurs after aspiration, causing a marked increase in pulmonary capillary wedge pressure and resultant transudation of fluid across the capillary endothelium. However, there is some evidence that reexpansion pulmonary edema is actually due to a reperfusion injury associated with free radical formation in areas of hypoxia. This finding is supported by the observation that administration of O_2 during thoracentesis helps to prevent reexpansion pulmonary edema. It is further supported by experiments in rabbits in which premedication with antioxidants minimized the capillary permeability and inflammation.[6]

ANALYSIS OF THE ASPIRATE

The differential diagnosis of pleural effusion includes an array of organ systems and diseases (see Table 45–2), yet analysis of pleural fluid yields a definitive diagnosis in a relatively small number of disease entities. Analysis of the aspirate can, however, narrow the differential diagnosis, and when the history and clinical setting are taken into account a diagnosis may be made in 85% of cases. It is generally accepted that effusions that prove to be transudative require no further evaluation.[8] Exudative processes, however, suggest more serious illness (eg, malignancy, collagen vascular disease) and require further investigation.

Light[12] has proposed the most widely accepted criteria for differentiating transudative from exudative effusions:

- Pleural fluid LDH > 2/3 upper limits of normal for serum LDH
- Pleural fluid LDH/serum LDH > 0.6
- Pleural fluid protein/serum protein > 0.5.

An exudate is characterized by the presence of at least one of these criteria, whereas a transudate is characterized by the absence of all three. A small prospective study by Scheurich and coworkers[8] showed the specificity of Light's criteria for the identification of transudates and exudates to be 87.5 and 88%, respectively. In this study clinical judgment performed as well as Light's criteria. In a larger retrospective study of 320 patients, Peterman and Spiecher found the sensitivity and specificity to be 94 and 87%, respectively.[9]

Visual Inspection

Information from the gross characteristics of the fluid aid in formulating the differential diagnosis and may be used to guide selection of further tests (Table 45–3).

Cell Count and Cytology

Total and differential leukocyte counts are useful only in confirming the presence of infection. Large population-based studies have found

TABLE 45–3. GROSS CHARACTERISTICS OF PLEURAL FLUID

Characteristics	Significance
Most transudates	
Clear, straw-colored	Further pleural fluid analysis usually unnecessary
Most exudates	
Anchovy-paste color	Suggests amebic liver abscess ruptured into pleural space
Turbid, green/yellow	Suggests rheumatoid pleuritis
Reddish tinge to bloody	If not traumatic tap, suggests tumor, pulmonary infarction, or trauma with pleuropulmonary contusion or laceration
Cloudy, white	Suggests chylous effusion and indicates disruption of thoracic duct from trauma, tumor
Yellow, thick, metallic sheen	Suggests longstanding chyliform effusion (pseudochylothorax), eg, tuberculous or rheumatoid pleuritis, trapped lung
Pus (with or without putrid odor)	Empyema; tube thoracostomy indicated
Viscous, hemorrhagic	Suggests malignant mesothelioma

Adapted from Jay SJ: Pleural effusions. I. Preliminary evaluation—Recognition of the transudate. *Postgrad Med.* 1986;80:164–167, 170–177.

cell count to be of no diagnostic value, with the exception of cytology when a neoplasm is suspected.

Cytologic analysis of three serial aspirates carries a sensitivity of 80%. When pleural biopsy is performed as well, the sensitivity is increased to 90%, with a low false-positive rate. In tuberculosis, pleural biopsy has been shown to have a sensitivity and specificity of 77 and 100%, respectively.[13]

pH

Normal pleural fluid has a pH of approximately 7.6. Transudates generally have a pH in the range of 7.4 to 7.55, whereas exudates are in the range of 7.3 to 7.45. Pleural fluid acidosis is believed to result from an increased production of hydrogen ions by pleural cells or bacteria, direct contamination with GI contents (as in esophageal rupture), or decreased escape of fluid from the pleural space that results from fibrosis or tumor involvement.[10]

Glucose

Extremely low levels of glucose are seen in pleural effusions resulting from rheumatoid arthritis.[11]

Amylase

Pleural fluid amylase levels are elevated in pancreatitis. When the levels are twice that of the serum or >160 Somogyi units/dL, the differential diagnosis includes acute pancreatitis, pancreatic pseudocyst, malignancy, and esophageal rupture.[11]

Lipids

A chylous pleural effusion is suggested by the milky white appearance of the aspirate. The presence of lipids may be confirmed microscopically with a Sudan stain and by chemical analysis for lipids and triglycerides. Lipid levels >400 mg/dL, triglyceride levels >110 mg/dL, or levels greater than twice those measured in the serum are consistent with a chylous effusion.

Acid-fast Bacillus Staining and Culture

Staining the pleural fluid for acid-fast bacilli (AFB) has a low sensitivity. In fact, one study reported a 0% sensitivity of AFB staining of pleural fluid from patients with radiographic and culture-proven tuberculosis (TB). Pleural biopsy is dramatically more sensitive and specific in identifying tuberculous effusions.

Acid-fast bacillus cultures of pleural fluid in suspected TB have a 100% specificity but, as with AFB staining, carry an unacceptably low sensitivity. Escudero and colleagues reported on 414 patients with pleural effusions of unknown etiology. Excluded from the study were patients with CHF, hepatic cirrhosis, or purulent effusion as well as those with a bleeding diathesis and those with other known causes of a transudate. Of the 414 patients, 107 had a final diagnosis of tuberculosis. The investigators advocated the use of both anaerobic and aerobic cultures and reported a sensitivity from 28 to 39%.[13]

CONCLUSION

A systematic approach to ordering tests is invaluable in terms of time, cost, and most importantly making the correct diagnosis. More than 90% of pleural effusions are caused by CHF, cirrhosis, pleuropulmonary infection, malignancy, and pulmonary embolism.[14] The history and physical examination play important roles in determining the necessity of thoracentesis as well as in deciding which tests to order.

Testing of transudative pleural fluid beyond what is necessary to differentiate it from an exudate may be associated with false-positive results that confuse the clinical picture and increase costs. Inappropriate analysis of pleural fluid may actually lead to a more prolonged hospital course.[9]

REFERENCES

1. O'Connor RE, Feldstein JS, Bouzoukis JK: Thoracentesis in the emergency department. *J Emerg Med.* 1985;2:433–442.
2. Henschke CI, Davis SD, Romano PM, et al: Pleural effusions: Pathogenesis, radiologic evaluation, and therapy. *J Thorac Imaging*. 1989;4:49–60.
3. Vukich DJ: Diseases of the pleural space. *Emerg Med Clin North Am.* 1989;7:309–324.
4. Sokolowski JW Jr, Burgher LW, Jones FL Jr: Guidelines for thoracentesis and needle biopsy of the pleura. (This position paper of the American Thoracic Society was adopted by the ATS Board of Directors, June 1988.) *Am Rev Respir Dis*. 1989;140:257–258.
5. Shinto RA, Light RW: Effects of diuresis on the characteristics of pleural fluid in patients with congestive heart failure. *Am J Med.* 1990;88:230–234.
6. Light RW: *Pleural Diseases.* Philadelphia: Lea & Febiger; 1983.
7. Grogan DR, Irwin RS, Channick R, et al: Complications associated with thoracentesis. A prospective, randomized study comparing three different methods. *Arch Intern Med.* 1990;150:873–877.
8. Scheurich JW, Keuer SP, Graham DY: Pleural effusion: Comparison of clinical judgment and Light's criteria in determining the cause. *South Med J.* 1989;82:1487–1491.
9. Peterman T, Speicher C: Evaluating pleural effusions: A two-stage laboratory approach. *JAMA.* 1984;252:1051–1053.
10. Sahn SA, Good JT Jr: Pleural fluid pH in malignant effusions. Diagnostic, prognostic, and therapeutic implications. *Ann Intern Med.* 1988;108:345–349.
11. Anonymous: Diagnostic thoracentesis and pleural biopsy in pleural effusions. Health and Public Policy Committee, American College of Physicians (published erratum appears in *Ann Intern Med.* 1986;104:290.) *Ann Intern Med.* 1985;103:799–802.
12. Light RW, MacGregor MI, Luchsinger PC, et al: Pleural effusions: The diagnostic separation of transudates and exudates. *Ann Intern Med.* 1972;77:507.
13. Escudero BC, Garcia CM, Cuesta CB, et al: Cytologic and bacteriologic analysis of fluid and pleural biopsy specimens in Cope's needle. Study of 414 patients. *Arch Intern Med.* 1990;150:1190–1194.
14. Jay SJ: Pleural effusions. I. Preliminary evaluation—Recognition of the transudate. *Postgrad Med.* 1986;80:164–167, 170–177.
15. Sahn SA: The state of the art. The pleura. *Am Rev Resp Dis.* 1988;138:184–234.

Chapter

Cerebrospinal Fluid

Louis Profeta

Since its reference in the "Edwin Smith surgical papyrus" of the 17th century B.C., the cerebrospinal fluid (CSF) has been recognized as a valuable tool for study and interpretation in the understanding of a variety of disease states. This chapter addresses some of the more common tests ordered on CSF and discusses their interpretation and applicability in the emergency department setting. It also explores the limitations of these tests and provides the reader with a better appreciation of the low sensitivity of many of the CSF parameters traditionally used to diagnose disease.

WHITE BLOOD CELL COUNT

The white blood cell (WBC) count is most often used to establish a diagnosis of meningitis and to differentiate between viral and bacterial etiologies. Although a count of 20,000 cells/mm^3 with 100% polymorphonuclear leukocytes (PMNs), in the correct setting, is classic for bacterial meningitis, a count <1000 cells/mm^3 is much less specific, especially when there is a preponderance of lymphocytes.

In the normal healthy child and adult, there should be fewer than 5 WBC/mm^3 in the CSF. In the past, a single PMN was considered pathologic; with newer, more efficient centrifuges, one PMN in the sediment is quite commonly seen in individuals without disease.[1] Parameters for infants are different from those for adults. Term infants are reported to have a mean CSF count of 8.2 WBCs/mm^3, with a range of 0 to 32 WBCs/mm^3 and <57% PMNs. In preterm infants the average count increases to 9.0 WBC/mm^3, with a range of 0 to 22 WBC/mm^3 and <61% PMNs. In infants over 1 month of age, the values tend toward adult levels.[1–3]

Classically, a count of >1000 WBCs/mm^3 with >50% PMNs is highly suggestive of bacterial infection.[4] Strict application of this rule guarantees that the clinician will diagnose some patients with bacterial meningitis as having a viral infection. No single CSF parameter has a perfect 100% positive or negative predictive value, and there is no substitute for a careful history and physical examination in conjuction with analysis of the CSF.[5] In a review of patients with viral meningitis, many were noted to have counts of >1000 WBCs/mm^3, with some values approaching 6000 WBCs/mm^3; the percentage of PMNs ranged from 0 to 66%. Fewer than 4% of patients with viral meningitis had counts >1000 WBCs/mm^3; the percentage of PMNs ranged from 0 to 100% in these patients.[6]

In general, 30 to 60% of patients with viral meningitis have a predominance of PMNs in the CSF, and 10% of patients with bacterial meningitis have a lymphocytic predominance.[4, 6, 7] Individuals with bacterial meningitis and counts <1000 WBCs/mm^3 tended to have lymphocytic predominance, especially in neonates and children without meningismus.[8, 9]

It has been observed that viral meningitis often begins with a PMN pleocytosis and then shifts to lymphocytic predominance. The overlap in CSF WBC count and differential has thus led some investigators to suggest that the lumbar puncture be repeated after a period of observation in patients with PMN pleocytosis who do not appear toxic and who have only marginally abnormal glucose or CSF protein levels and negative Gram stain.[5, 7] This practice could decrease the patient's length of hospital stay or even avoid the unnecessary initiation of intravenous (IV) antibiotic therapy.[5, 7, 10]

The WBC count and differential are even less useful in distinguishing fungal, mycobacterial, and viral etiologies for meningitis. There is roughly a 30 to 40% overlap in each CSF parameter among these agents.[11]

In cryptococcal meningitis, the CSF frequently demonstrates a lymphocytic-predominant pleocytosis of 40 to 400 WBC/mm^3, usually <150 WBC/mm^3, and rarely exceeding 800 WBC/mm^3.[14] Not infrequently, cryptococcosis has been seen with a count of <5 WBC/mm^3.[12]

Cell counts in mycobacterial meningitis are similar to those in fungal and viral meningitis. In one review, the range of CSF WBC counts was 1 to 340/mm^3 for tuberculous meningitis, and 25% of patients had a predominance of PMNs.[13] In another study, 17% of patients had counts >400 WBC/mm^3, and 27% demonstrated a PMN-predominant differential.[15] Some cases have been reported with cell counts >3000 cells/mm^3 and a range of 10 to 100% PMNs.[6]

In summary, the CSF WBC count and differential cannot be used as the sole distinguishing feature of viral, bacterial, fungal, or mycobacterial etiologies of suspected meningitis. The cell count and differential should be utilized in conjunction with other CSF parameters and the overall clinical picture.

GRAM STAIN

The Gram stain can supply valuable information regarding not only the presence of a CSF infection but also the type of organism responsible. Grossly purulent CSF should be examined immediately without centrifugation because cell debris may interfere with staining.[20, 21] Otherwise, the CSF should be centrifuged at 1500 × g for at least 15 minutes prior to the suspension and staining of the remaining pellet.

The sensitivity of Gram stain in identifying organisms in the CSF is reported to range from 80 to 90% in individuals with previously untreated culture-positive bacterial meningitis. The sensitivity falls to about 60 to 70% in patients who have received prior antibiotic therapy.[16, 18] In general, the greater the number of organisms/mL, the greater the sensitivity of the Gram stain.[23] False-negative results are thought to be particularly likely when the number of organisms is <1000/mL.[20, 21] Pneumococcus and *Haemophilus influenzae* are the organisms most often identified on the smear, owing to their higher concentrations in the CSF of patients with these infections.[17]

False-positive CSF Gram stains are most often the result of contaminated stains, alcohol baths, CSF kits, and slides and of occluded needles used for lumbar puncture.[19, 21, 22] In one report, 50 screw-top tubes from lumbar puncture kits were crushed, centrifuged, and resuspended; six of the 50 had positive Gram stains.[19]

Up to 40% of cases of culture-proven bacterial meningitis may be associated with a negative Gram stain. Organisms with cell walls that have been destroyed in the phagocytic process may not be visible by conventional Gram stain, in which case acridine orange staining may improve the yield. Thus, in patients who are suspected of having bacterial meningitis but who have negative Gram stains, acridine orange stain should be considered. In any case, all patients with suspected bacterial meningitis should have treatment initiated promptly regardless of the Gram stain results.

TOTAL PROTEIN

The CSF contains a myriad of protein components that vary in concentration and composition depending on age, gender, disease, and nutritional status. The major components are albumin, prealbumin, immunoglobulin, transferrin, and a variety of other globulins and enzymes. Levels are typically higher in infants and the elderly and are slightly greater in males than females. Although much is made of the observation that CSF protein tends to be higher in bacterial than in nonbacterial meningitis, there is considerable overlap, especially when fungal and mycobacterial infections are included in the differential diagnosis. An elevated CSF protein thus offers little more than an indication of the presence of some pathologic process affecting the CSF.[24]

Traditionally, a total CSF protein level >40 mg/dL has been considered abnormal. Other investigators report values in adults of 38 ± 20 mg/dL, with a normal range of 18 to 58 mg/dL.[25] Normal preterm and term infants have higher CSF protein concentrations, possibly owing to an immature blood brain barrier.[2]

A CSF protein concentration >150 mg/dL in the setting of hypoglycorrhachia and PMN-predominant CSF pleocytosis is suggestive of bacterial meningitis.[25] Some patients with bacterial meningitis may have normal or only slightly elevated protein levels. The CSF protein is also elevated in 90% of patients with cryptococcal and mycobacterial meningitis, with values ranging from 30 to 312 mg/dL in the former and 21 to 1500 mg/dL in the latter.[13, 14] In contrast, one review of 111 cases of viral meningitis found that no patients had CSF protein levels >150 mg/dL. This study excluded cases due to lymphocytic choriomeningitis virus and mumps, which are frequently associated with substantially higher protein levels, approaching 300 to 400 mg/dL.[6] Other investigators have reported CSF protein levels in the 100- to 200-mg/dL range with viral meningitis.[5]

Other causes of elevations of CSF protein include drugs such as ethanol and phenytoin, traumatic tap, and subarachnoid hemorrhage. Cerebrospinal fluid protein typically increases by 1 mg/dL for each 1000 RBCs/mm^3.[1, 21, 24, 25]

In summary, the CSF protein concentration provides little help to the clinician. At best, when used with the cell count and CSF glucose concentration, the CSF protein level may be of some utility in guiding the investigator toward a final diagnosis. This is probably the test that can best be eliminated if only a small amount of CSF is available for analysis.

CEREBROSPINAL GLUCOSE

Cerebrospinal fluid is not an ultrafiltrate of plasma. Its protein, glucose, and electrolyte composition are the result of a variety of active and passive transport mechanisms as well as simple diffusion. The concentration of glucose in the CSF reflects the activity of a carrier-mediated transport mechanism that tends to maintain a plasma-to-CSF glucose ratio of about 0.6. When this pathway is saturated, typically at a serum glucose of 300 mg/dL and CSF glucose of 200 mg/dL, further increases in CSF glucose tend to result in a decrease of this ratio. Moreover, it requires about 2 hours for the CSF glucose to reach peak levels when serum levels rise (eg, when D50 is given in the setting of mental status changes) and 4 hours for it to equilibrate with the plasma.[23] Thus, it is likely to be difficult to determine the significance of relative hypoglycorrhachia in an individual who has received IV glucose because of altered mental status and then has a lumbar puncture performed a short time later. It has been suggested that Dextrostix or similar oxidase-impregnated strips can be utilized as a rapid means of determining CSF glucose in the emergency department setting.

The decrease in CSF glucose levels in pyogenic meningitis may reflect an interference with the carrier-mediated pathway, although some believe that it is a function of increased glycolysis by PMNs and glucose utilization by bacteria.[26, 27] Hypoglycorrhachia has also been reported to occur in about 15 to 20% of patients 1 to 8 days following subarachnoid hemorrhage, but the mechanism is unknown.[27] In term and preterm infants less than 6 months of age, the active transport systems are less developed and the normal CSF-to-plasma ratio ranges from 0.74 to 0.96.[28]

In an excellent review of meningitis by Karandanis and Shulman, a wide range of CSF glucose levels was found in both bacterial and mycobacterial meningitis.[6] More than 50% of patients had CSF glucose concentrations <40 mg/dL. Whereas a CSF glucose level <40 to 50 mg/dL or a CSF-to-plasma ratio <0.60 suggests a pathologic process in the CSF, about 40% of patients with pyogenic meningitis have normal levels. In contrast, only 4% of patients with a final diagnosis of viral (aseptic) meningitis manifested hypoglycorrhachia, a frequency similar to that found in other studies.[6] Studies reporting higher rates of hypoglycorrhachia tend to include infants, to have small sample sizes, and to focus on infections involving a single viral organism (eg, mumps and lymphocytic choriomeningitis virus, which seem to be associated with higher incidence of hypoglycorrhachia).[6]

RED BLOOD CELL COUNT AND XANTHOCHROMIA

One of the more common problems facing the emergency physician is to determine whether the cause of blood found on lumbar puncture is a subarachnoid hemorrhage (SAH) or a traumatic tap. At least 6000 RBC/mL must be present for the fluid to appear grossly bloody.

A progressive decrease in the RBC count from tube 1 to tube 3 is suggestive of a traumatic tap. As the bloody CSF around the lumbar puncture site is collected, it is replaced by normal CSF. With a traumatic tap, when RBC counts exceed 200,000 cells/mL one can expect the CSF to show signs of clotting, whereas in patients with SAH in vivo defibrination hinders clot formation.[23]

In addition, in a traumatic tap the ratio of RBCs to WBCs is comparable to the peripheral blood ratio of 500:1. In SAH, free hemoglobin acts as a chemotactic agent for inflammatory cells and tends to decrease this ratio.[24]

Xanthochromia refers to a pink, orange, or yellow hue of the CSF. In both SAH and encapsulated hemorrhage this color change results from RBC cell lysis, with the resulting formation of oxyhemoglobin, methemoglobin, and bilirubin (the pigments most often responsible for xanthochromia). Whereas methemoglobin is a breakdown product of old encapsulated hemorrhages in the CSF, bilirubin appears in the CSF when RBCs have been in the fluid for more than 12 hours. It peaks at 2 to 4 days and may last for 1 month. Oxyhemoglobin begins to form from RBC lysis within 2 to 4 hours following SAH, peaks at 24 to 36 hours, and may last for 8 days.[24]

False-positive xanthochromia findings can occur. The most common cause is allowing bloody CSF to remain uncentrifuged for more than 1 hour. Red blood cell lysis occurs, with the subsequent formation of oxyhemoglobin. Patients with direct hyperbilirubinemia (usually >10 mg/dL) tend to spill bilirubin into the CSF, thus making it difficult to interpret xanthochromia if seen. Indirect bilirubin often finds its way into the CSF of patients with increased permeability of the blood brain barrier (eg, posttrauma, postcerebrovascular, neonatal).

Less common causes of xanthochromia in the absence of SAH are contamination of the CSF with povidone-iodine, systemic hypercarotenemia in food faddists, CSF protein levels exceeding 150 mg/dL, and melanin in meningeal melanomatosis.[23]

TESTS FOR FUNGI

Although a number of mycoses can be associated with CNS infection, the organism responsible for most CNS fungal infections is *Cryptococcus neoformans.*[30] Fungal infection of the CNS is relatively rare except in the immunosuppressed host, but many clinicians routinely send all CSF samples for fungal cultures and staining. The utility of such a practice is to be questioned. Certainly, patients with risk factors for AIDS or other defects of cell-mediated immunity should be subject to more intensive investigation, but in others only a high level of suspicion should induce the clinician to order these tests.

A common error is to obtain an inadequate volume of fluid when ordering fungal culture and staining. Work by Louria and colleagues suggests that at least 5 mL of fluid should be collected to ensure a positive fungal culture in the setting of disease.[31] The time until a positive culture is noted has been reported to be as long as 10 days.[13, 32]

The India ink stain is a relatively rapid and inexpensive test. Unfortunately, its sensitivity in the setting of a positive CSF culture is only 50 to 60%. Even so, repeated lumbar punctures are often required in patients who eventually prove to be culture-positive before a positive

India ink stain is obtained.[12, 13, 21, 30] Ultimately, the clinician must be cautious in the presence of the high incidence of false-negative results.[30]

False-positive test results, however, are relatively uncommon. The India ink stain can be positive in the presence of negative cultures, especially in individuals who have already begun treatment for cryptococcal meningitis. This occurrence may reflect the presence of organisms that are nonetheless capable of causing a recurrence of CNS infection.[12] False-positive results have also been reported to occur when lymphocytes in the CSF were mistaken for budding yeast or when *Naegleria* was misidentified as *Cryptococcus.*[14, 21]

The latex aggutination (LA) assay for cryptococcal antigen is a rapid and valuable alternative that can facilitate the detection of *Crytococcus.* When properly performed and reported, it is far more sensitive than the India ink stain and has the advantage of providing a quantitative value.

Latex agglutination assay appears to be the most practical and sensitive test for the rapid detection of cryptococcal meningitis. Approximately 90% (reported range: 71 to 100%) of patients with cryptococcal meningitis have detectable antigen levels.[14, 30, 32, 33] The latex agglutination assay can detect as little as 25 ng/mL. In addition, the test is often positive prior to the development of CSF pleocytosis as well as in instances when initial cultures are negative.[14, 34] Moreover, the results are usually available at least 18 hours prior to positive culture results.[21]

False-positive LA assays have been reported to occur when nonspecific factors or rheumatoid factors cause agglutination or in the presence of *Klebsiella* CNS infection.[14, 23, 32, 33] Most of the nonspecific reactions can be identified by the hospital microbiology laboratory. In general, only samples that demonstrate a fourfold greater capacity to agglutinate the immune-coated particles than control particles should be reported as positive. The clinician should ask the hospital laboratory if positive results are determined in this fashion.[14, 32, 33] Even so, 0.4% of samples still yield false-positive results.[34]

In summary, LA is the test of choice for the rapid detection of cryptococcal antigen in the CSF. A positive test result is a clear indicator of *Cryptococcus* in the CSF.[21, 23] In contrast, India ink stain is not sufficiently sensitive to rule out the disease.

STAINING AND CULTURE FOR ACID-FAST BACILLUS

Although it is true that tuberculosis (TB) and atypical mycobacterial infections are lately being found with increasing incidence, routine ordering of acid-fast bacillus (AFB) smears and cultures is not warranted. Only when the clinical or the geographic setting makes it more likely for these organisms to be the cause of CNS disease should the clinician utilize valuable laboratory resources in the pursuit of this diagnosis.

One retrospective study of 1883 CSF samples failed to yield a single positive culture for TB, prompting the suggestion that CSF samples be refrigerated for at least 5 hours and that only specimens from cases with other laboratory findings suggestive of infection be cultured.[35] In another study, of 4816 CSF cultures for TB, all were negative.[36] Both of these studies took place in settings in which the incidence of TB was reported to be 1 in 1000.

In a review of 52 cases of tuberculous meningitis, cultures were positive in only 83% of the cases. In the rest, the diagnosis was made on the basis of a positive AFB smear or CNS manifestations in the presence of disseminated tuberculosis. At least 100,000 organisms/mL must be present to allow for detection of *Mycobacterium tuberculosis* by AFB smear.[13] A successful search for AFB on the slide typically requires patience and diligence by the microbiologist and laboratory personnel.

Although tuberculous meningitis is a lethal and devastating infection, the time to definitive diagnosis by positive culture is typically quite long, and often several cultures are performed before one becomes positive. Moreover, AFB smears are insufficiently sensitive to be relied on to rule out infection. Although findings from cell counts and chemistries may be suggestive, tuberculous meningitis is a diagnosis made by the astute clinician based on emergency department presentation, clinical course, immune status, geography, and patient demographics.

ACRIDINE ORANGE STAIN

Acridine orange is an inexpensive staining compound that has long been recognized for its utility in identifying organisms in the CSF and other body fluids.[21, 37, 38] Unlike the Gram stain, which visualizes cell wall components, acridine orange highlights the nucleic acids found in both bacteria and somatic cells. Bacteria appear bright orange on a yellow to pale-green background.[21] This often allows for easier identification of organisms in the presence of low cell counts.[38] Acridine orange cannot distinguish between gram-positive and gram-negative species. Its utility is most evident in partially treated infections.

In one study, the CSF of patients with culture-proven bacterial meningitis who had received antibiotic therapy for 18 hours or longer was analyzed by both conventional Gram stain and acridine orange stain.[38] Of 47 patients, 45 (96%) had positive staining by acridine orange, whereas none of the patients had identifiable organisms on Gram stain. More surprising was the finding that, of patients who had *not* received antibiotic therapy but then had culture-proven *N. meningitis* infections, seven of seven had a positive acridine orange stain, compared with only two of seven with a positive Gram stain. This improved yield was attributed to the staining of bacteria within phagocytes.

The rapidity, high sensitivity, and low cost of this test make it a promising adjunct in the diagnosis of bacterial meningitis. This stain should be considered when the clinical picture is suggestive for bacterial meningitis but the Gram stain is negative or the patient has previously been treated with antibiotics. Nevertheless, one must keep in mind that the incidence of false-positive staining with acridine orange has yet to be addressed.

REFERENCES

1. Conly JM, Ronald AR: Cerebrospinal fluid as a diagnostic body fluid. *Am J Med.* 1983;75:102–108.
2. Sarff LD, Platt LH, McCrachen GH Jr: CSF evaluation in neonates: Comparison of high risk infants with and without meningitis. *J Pediatr.* 1976;88:473–477.
3. Lane H: *Handbook of Pediatrics.* St. Louis: Mosby Year Book, 1991;57–58.
4. Benson CA, Harris AA: Acute neurologic infections. *Med Clin North Am.* 1986;70:987–1101.
5. Ratzan KR: Viral meningitis in adults. *Med Clin North Am.* 1985;69:399–413.
6. Karandanis D, Shulman J: Recent survey of infectious meningitis in adults. *South Med J.* 1976;69:449–457.
7. Varki AP, Puthuran P: Value of second lumbar puncture in confirming the diagnosis of aseptic meningitis. *Arch Neurol.* 1979;36:581–582.
8. Powers WJ: CSF lymphocytosis in acute bacterial meningitis. *Am J Med.* 1985;79:216.
9. Dagbjartsson A, Ludvigsson P: Bacterial meningitis: Diagnosis and initial antibiotic therapy. *Pediatr Clin North Am.* 1987;34:219–231.
10. Feigin RD, Shackelford PG: Value of repeat lumbar puncture in the differential diagnosis of meningitis. *N Engl J Med.* 1973;289:571–574.
11. McGee ZA, Kaiser AB: *Principles and Practice of Infectious Disease.* New York: John Wiley & Sons, 1985;560–573.
12. Lewis JL, Rabinovich S: The wide spectrum of cryptococcal infections. *Am J Med.* 1972;53:315–322.
13. Stockstill MT, Kauffman CA: Comparisons of cryptococcal and tuberculosis meningitis. *Arch Neurol.* 1983;40:81–85.
14. Sebetta JR, Andriole VI: Cryptococcal infection of the central nervous system. *Med Clin North Am.* 1985;69:333–344.
15. Kennedy KH, Fallon RJ: Tuberculosis meningitis. JAMA. 1979;241:264–268.
16. Roberge R: Meningitis. In Harwood-Nuss A, Linden C, Luten RC, et al (eds):

The Clinical Practice of Emergency Medicine. Philadelphia: JB Lippincott, 1991;1033–1037.
17. Feldman WE: Concentrations of bacteria in CSF of patients with bacterial meningitis. *J Pediatr.* 1976;88:549–552.
18. Bolan G, Barza M: Acute bacterial meningitis in children and adults. *Med Clin North Am.* 1985;69:231–241.
19. Musher D, Schell R: False-positive Gram stains of cerebrospinal fluid. *Ann Intern Med.* 1973;79:603–604.
20. Martin W: Rapid and reliable techniques for the laboratory detection of bacterial meningitis. *Am J Med.* 1983;75:119–123.
21. Dougherty J, Jones J: CSF fluid culture and analysis. *Ann Emerg Med.* 1986;16:317–323.
22. Ericson C, Carmichael M, et al: Erroneous diagnosis of meningitis due to false positive Gram stains. *South Med J.* 1978;71:1524–1525.
23. Herndon R, Brumback R: *The CSF.* Boston: Kluwer Academic, 1989.
24. Ward PCJ: Cerebrospinal fluid data: Interpretation in intracranial hemorrhage and meningitis. *Postgrad Med.* 1989;68:181–188.
25. Tintinelli JE, Krome RL, Ruiz E: *Emergency Medicine, A Comprehensive Study Guide.* New York: McGraw-Hill, 1988.
26. Wyngaarden JB, Smith LH: *Cecil Textbook of Medicine.* 18th ed. Philadelphia: WB Saunders, 1988.
27. Vincent FM: Hypoglycorrhachia after subarachnoid hemorrhage. *Neurosurgery.* 1981;8:7–14.
28. Silver TS, Todd JK: Hypoglycorrhachia in pediatric patients. *Pediatrics.* 1976;58:67–71.
29. Fisher M: Identification of xanthochromia. *JAMA.* 1985;253:39.
30. McGinnis MR: Detection of fungi in cerebrospinal fluid. *Am J Med.* 1983;75:129–138.
31. Louria DB, Feder N, Mitchell W, et al: Influence of fungus strain and lapse on time in experimental histoplasmosis and of volume of inoculum in cryptococcosis upon recovery of the fungi. *J Lab Clin Med.* 1959;53:311–317.
32. Prevost E, Newel R: Commercial cryptococcal latex kit: Clinical evaluation in a medical center. *J Clin Microbiol.* 1978;8:529–533.
33. Kauffman CA, Bergman AG, Severence PJ, et al: Detection of cryptococcal antigen: Comparison of two latex agglutination tests. *Am J Clin Pathol.* 1981;75:106–109.
34. Snow SM, Dismukes WE: Cryptococcal meningitis: Diagnostic value of cryptococcal antigen in CSF. *Arch Intern Med.* 1975;135:1155.
35. Crowson TW, Rich EC, Woolfrey BF, et al: Overutilization of cultures of CSF for mycobacteria. *JAMA.* 1984;251:70–82.
36. Bromberg K: Policy for fungal and mycobacterial culture requests on CSF. *Lancet.* 1980;2:1023.
37. Kronvall G: Differential staining of bacteria in clinical specimens using acridine orange buffered at low pH. *Acta Pathol Microbiol Scand.* 1977;85:249.
38. Kleinman MB, Reynolds JK, Watts NH, et al: Superiority of acridine orange stain versus Gram stain in partially treated bacterial meningitis. *J Pediatr.* 1984;104:401–404.

Chapter

Synovial Fluid Analysis

John M. Lorei

The analysis of the synovial fluid from an affected joint space is frequently necessary for the appropriate management of the patient presenting with acute mono- or pauciarticular arthritis. The differentiation between inflammatory and noninflammatory arthritides can usually be made on the basis of careful history and physical examination. Most important for the emergency department physician is the differentiation between the various inflammatory arthritides. The decision to admit the patient and the aggressiveness of treatment are usually based on the likelihood of infectious arthritis, which can lead rapidly to joint destruction with significant morbidity. The diagnosis of the other inflammatory arthritides is less urgent.

Physical examination cannot reliably distinguish between an infectious and a noninfectious inflammatory arthritis in the evaluation of the patient with acute monoarticular or pauciarticular involvement. Fever, leukocytosis, marked inflammation, and limitation of movement can occur in all inflammatory arthritides.[4, 12] The appropriate use of the clinical laboratory for synovial fluid analysis can assist in making a definitive diagnosis (Table 47–1).

In the emergency department evaluation of the patient with a nontraumatic acute mono- or pauciarticular arthritis, the need to identify and treat a potential bacterial infection is of major importance. Certain historical and physical examination clues can assist in differential diagnosis. In septic arthritis, the rapid onset of joint pain and fever is the most common presentation. Septic arthritis may result from direct penetration of the joint capsule, from a contiguous focus of osteomyelitis, or, most commonly, from hematogenous dissemination from a remote site of infection or intravenous drug abuse. In gonococcal arthritis, patients may have experienced migratory polyarthralgias prior to the onset of monoarticular arthritis.

The most commonly infected joint is the knee in adults and the hip in children, although any joint may be infected. There is a predisposition toward infection of the large joints, although septic arthritis of the sternoclavicular, sternochondral, and sacroiliac joints appears to be more common in the settings of rheumatoid arthritis, diabetes mellitus, and intravenous drug abuse.[14, 15] The first metatarsal phalangeal joint is most commonly affected in acute gouty arthritis. If the history is consistent with gout, it is unlikely to be the initial site of septic arthritis.

TABLE 47–1. SYNOVIAL FLUID ANALYSIS IN ACUTE MONO- OR PAUCIARTICULAR ARTHRITIS

Type of Arthritis	History	Appearance	Cell Count	Gram Stain	Crystals
Hemorrhagic	Trauma Coagulopathy	Bloody	Primarily RBCs	Negative	Negative
Infectious	Underlying infection Osteomyelitis Pneumonia Gonorrhea Urosepsis Endocarditis Penetrating joint injury Arthrocentesis Arthrotomy IV drug abuse Prior arthritis	Opaque, turbid	Often >50,000 WBC/μL	75% positive in nongonococcal arthritis <40% positive in gonococcal arthritis	Negative
Crystal induced	Gout/pseudogout Hyperuricemia Drugs: diuretics, alcohol	Opaque	2000–50,000 WBC/μL	Negative	Gout: monosodium urate crystals[a] Pseudogout: calcium pyrophosphate dihydrate crystals[b]
Inflammatory	Psoriasis Reiter's syndrome (urethritis, conjunctivitis, iritis)	Opaque	2000–50,000 WBC/μL	Negative	Negative

[a]MSU: needle shaped and possess strong negative birefringence, ie, yellow on red background when long axis is parallel to axis of compensator.
[b]CPPD: usually rhomboid shaped or platelike; possess weak positive birefingence, ie, appear blue on red background when parallel to axis of compensator.

SYNOVIAL FLUID TESTS

Total White Blood Cell Count

A total WBC count of >2000/mm^3 has been shown to be at least 80% sensitive and 80% specific in identifying an inflammatory joint effusion.[9] Although there is considerable overlap between the total WBC counts of infectious vs noninfectious inflammatory joint effusions, total WBC counts >50,000/mm^3 are present in 70% of bacterial infections,[7] and counts >100,000mm^3 are present virtually exclusively in bacterial infections.[2, 9]

Immunocompromise may result in an inability to mount a normal synovial fluid leukocytosis.[5, 8] The common underlying medical problems associated with blunting of the leukocyte response are malignant neoplasm, neutropenia of any cause, intravenous drug abuse, AIDS, alcoholism, diabetes, and rheumatoid arthritis. Patients on antibiotics and corticosteroids may also have a diminished leukocyte response to infection of the synovial fluid.[2, 5, 8]

White Blood Cell Differential

A percentage of polymorphonuclear cells (PMNs), over 75%, is about 75% sensitive and >90% specific in defining an inflammatory joint effusion. Percentages of PMNs over 75% do little to assist in the differentiation of infectious arthritis from other inflammatory causes, but PMN percentages less than 75% have a negative predictive value for the presence of bacterial infection of >90%.[5, 9]

Synovial Fluid Gram Stain

Unfortunately, the Gram stain reveals organisms in only 75% of cases with culture-proven gram-positive bacterial infections, 50% of gram-negative infections, and <40% of gonococcal infections in the synovial fluid.[1, 2] Obviously, in the absence of contamination of the synovial fluid, a positive Gram stain is virtually diagnostic of infection. Care must be taken to avoid false-positive readings from synovial fluid mucin, which may take up precipitated Gram stain and appear as gram-positive cocci.[2] Acridine orange stain may provide better visualization of gram-negative organisms than the standard Gram stain.[2]

Gram stain is most reliable when performed on a centrifuged pellet in cloudy or clear fluid or on an unspun droplet in grossly purulent fluid.[2]

Acid-fast bacillus smears are positive in only about 20% of proven cases of tuberculous arthritis and would rarely be of value in the emergency department.[7]

Synovial Fluid Culture

The culture is positive in virtually 100% of nongonococcal bacterial infections in patients who are not on antibiotics.[2, 4] Gonococcal infections are identified on synovial fluid culture in only 25 to 50% of patients, hence the importance of oropharyngeal, urethral, rectal, and cervical cultures in patients suspected of the disease.[2, 4]

The highest culture yields are obtained when fluid is immediately plated on broth and solid media, including chocolate agar. If it is not possible to plate immediately, the fluid can be placed into aerobic and anerobic blood culture bottles.[2]

Blood cultures should be obtained in patients in whom bacterial arthritis is considered because up to 50% of patients with nongonococcal bacterial arthritis have positive cultures.[2, 7, 10] Cultures of any extraarticular site of infection should also be obtained in patients being evaluated for infectious arthritis.

Crystal Analysis

The identification of crystals within the synovial fluid aspirate can greatly assist in the differential diagnosis. As the crystal-induced arthritides predispose patients to bacterial arthritis, the presence of crystals in the synovial fluid does not rule out a coexistent bacterial infection.[2]

There are two major types of crystals implicated in acute arthritis: monosodium urate monohydrate (MSU) and calcium pyrophosphate dihydrate (CPPD). These are associated with gout and "pseudogout," respectively. Monosodium urate monohydrate crystals appear needle shaped and possess strong negative birefringence, ie, they appear yellow on a red background when their long axis is parallel to the axis of the compensator. Monosodium urate monohydrate crystals are said to be seen in the synovial fluid of >95% of patients with gout.[13] The presence of intracellular MSU crystals is pathognomonic for acute gout,[13] whereas the presence of extracellular crystals strongly suggests the presence of gouty arthritis.[13]

Calcium pyrophosphate dihydrate crystals are seen in >75% of patients suffering from acute exacerbations of pseudogout.[3] These crystals can appear needle shaped like MSU crystals but are usually rhomboid or platelike. The rhomboid crystals can usually be identified by ordinary light microscopy and are diagnostic of CPPD crystal deposition. They possess a weak positive birefringence on polarizing microscopy, ie, they appear blue on a red background when parallel to the longitudinal axis of the compensator and yellow when perpendicular (the ''opposite'' of MSU crystals). The crystals are usually intracellular during the acute inflammatory phase of pseudogout and extracellular between acute attacks.[3]

Steroid crystals may persist long after an intraarticular injection. They may be intracellular or extracellular and can resemble those seen in the common crystal-induced arthritides.[1, 7, 11] The evaluation of synovial fluid following previous corticosteroid injection must take into consideration the possibility of steroid crystal–induced arthritis and the presence of steroid crystals.

Cholesterol crystals can be seen in chronic joint effusions, most notably in rheumatoid arthritis.[1]

Synovial Fluid Glucose

The glucose concentration in the synovial fluid is normally slightly less than that in serum.[1] A synovial fluid glucose level <50% of the serum glucose after a 4-hour fast is strongly suggestive of infection, but this finding is insensitive. It is also nonspecific in that extremely low synovial glucose determinations may also be observed in rheumatoid arthritis.[1] The variability of equilibration between serum and synovial fluid makes this an unreliable test in most circumstances.[1]

Synovial Fluid Total Protein

The measurement of synovial fluid total protein is insensitive in detecting an inflammatory arthritis and nonspecific in defining its presence. It is thus not indicated in the evaluation of synovial fluid in acute arthritis.[9]

Synovial Fluid Lactate Dehydrogenase

An elevation of the synovial fluid lactate dehydrogenase (LDH) above 250 U/L has a sensitivity of >80% in detecting inflammatory effusions but a specificity of only 70% in distinguishing inflammatory fluid from noninflammatory fluid.[9] It provides no useful information in distinguishing between infectious and noninfectious inflammatory effusions.

Mucin Clot Test

This test is used to measure the integrity of hyaluronate in synovial fluid. A normal clot reflects a noninflammatory effusion and a poor or friable clot indicates dilution and destruction of hyaluronate protein in an inflammatory effusion. This test, although quick and inexpensive, is less reliable than WBC counts in differentiating inflammatory from noninflammatory effusions.[1] It provides little useful information to distinguish between infectious and noninfectious inflammatory effusions.

RECOMMENDATIONS FOR SYNOVIAL FLUID ANALYSIS IN ACUTE ARTHRITIS

The following tests are recommended for the analysis of most synovial fluid specimens:

- Gram stain
- Crystal analysis
- Aerobic and anaerobic cultures (Thayer-Martin media if gonococcus is suspected)
- Total WBC count and differential.

CLINICAL "PEARLS" IN SYNOVIAL FLUID ANALYSIS

1. Septic arthritis can reliably be ruled out only after synovial fluid analysis.
2. The presence of crystals does not rule out infection.
3. A negative Gram stain does not rule out infection.
4. A total WBC count $<50,000/mm^3$ does not rule out infection, although a count over $100,000/mm^3$ almost certainly indicates infection.
5. Synovial fluid glucose, protein, and LDH offer little useful information in the differential diagnosis of joint effusions.

REFERENCES

1. Schumacher HR: Synovial fluid analysis and synovial biopsy, in Kelley WN, Harris ED, Ruddy S, et al (eds): *Textbook of Rheumatology*. 3rd ed. Philadelphia: WB Saunders; 1989:637–649.
2. Goldenberg DL: Bacterial arthritis, in Kelley WN, Harris ED, Ruddy S, et al (eds): *Textbook of Rheumatology*. 3rd ed. Philadelphia, WB Saunders; 1989:1567–1585.
3. Moskowitz RW: Diseases associated with the deposition of calcium pyrophosphate or hydroxyapatite, in Kelley WN, Harris ED, Ruddy S, et al (eds):

Textbook of Rheumatology. 3rd ed. Philadelphia: WB Saunders; 1989:1449–1467.
4. McCune WJ: Monoarticular arthritis, in Kelley WN, Harris ED, Ruddy S, et al (eds): *Textbook of Rheumatology.* 3rd ed. Philadelphia: WB Saunders; 1989:442–454.
5. Krey PR, Bailen DA: Synovial fluid leukocytosis: a study of extremes. *Am J Med.* 1979;67:436–442.
6. Schumacher HR, Smolyo AP, Tse RL, et al: Arthritis associated with apatite crystals. *Ann Intern Med.* 1977;87:411–416.
7. Ward PCJ: Interpretation of synovial fluid data. *Postgrad Med.* 1980;68:175–184.
8. McCutchan HJ, Fisher RC: Synovial leukocytosis in infectious arthritis. *Clin Orthop.* 1990;257:226–230.
9. Schmerling RH, Delbanco TL, Tosteson ANA, et al: Synovial fluid tests—What should be ordered? *JAMA.* 1990;264:1009–1014.
10. Schlapbach P, Ambord C, Blochlinger AM, et al: Bacterial arthritis: Are fever, rigors, leucocytosis and blood cultures of diagnostic value? *Clin Rheum.* 1990;9:69–72.
11. Wolf AW, Benson DR, Shoji H, et al: Current concepts in synovial fluid analysis. *Clin Orthop.* 1978;134:261–265.
12. Freed JF, Nies KM, Boyer RS, et al: Acute monoarticular arthritis—a diagnostic approach. *JAMA.* 1980;243:2314–2316.
13. Kelley WN, Fox IH, Palella TD: Gout and related disorders of purine metabolism, in Kelley WN, Harris ED, Ruddy S, et al (eds): *Textbook of Rheumatology.* 3rd ed. Philadelphia: WB Saunders; 1989:1395–1448.
14. Gillis S, Friedman B, Caraco Y, et al: Septic arthritis of the sternoclavicular joint in healthy adults. *J Intern Med.* 1990;228:275.
15. Chandrasekar PH, Narula AP: Bone and joint infections in intravenous drug abusers. *Rev Infect Dis.* 1986;8:904.

Chapter

Ascitic Fluid

Dean Johnson

Ascites is the abnormal collection of fluid within the abdomen. It most frequently accompanies cirrhosis and portal hypertension but can accompany severe right heart failure, tuberculosis, or malignancy. In itself, ascites is generally a problem only by virtue of its bulk and discomfort. In up to 25% of patients with ascites, however, the fluid can become infected.[1] These infections are often unrecognized and can lead to sepsis and with associated mortality often greater than 50%.[3] Diagnostic paracentesis is often used to diagnose infections within the ascitic fluid. This chapter addresses which tests are most useful and which culture methods are most reliable for the diagnosis of spontaneous bacterial peritonitis.

It is necessary to define spontaneous bacterial peritonitis (SBP). In most texts, SBP is defined as culture-positive ascitic fluid in the absence of other localized sources of infection.[2] The exact method of bacterial inoculation is uncertain, with theories ranging from the translocation of bacteria through the intestinal walls to transport through the lymphatic fluid. Regardless of the method of inoculation, the morbidity remains high and the diagnosis important.

To determine that cultures are positive, it is necessary to collect the fluid in such a way as to yield the highest rate of true-positive results. In the past fluid was usually collected in syringes, transported to the laboratory, and inoculated on chocolate agar plates. Bedside inoculation of blood culture bottles with ascitic fluid, however, has a higher positive culture rate (81%), indicating that conventional plating methods (52%) may be inadequate for the detection of infection. Another study found that cultures planted after a 4-hour delay also reduced the yield of positive results, with only 75.9% of known positive cultures testing positive.[3] Thus, immediate, bedside inoculation of ascitic fluid into blood culture bottles appears to be the preferred method for culturing. Both of these studies used an inoculum of 10 mL of ascitic fluid; the relative sensitivities with different amounts of fluid inoculation are unknown.

Many tests besides cultures have been proposed to aid in the diagnosis of spontaneous bacterial peritonitis. Among these are LDH, protein, amylase, serum-to-ascites albumin gradient, PMN cell count, Gram stain, glucose, pH, and lactate.

The most commonly ordered test is the cell count and differential. A sample of ascitic fluid with >500 PMN/mm^3 can be considered to be positive for SBP with a sensitivity of 90% and specificity of 98%.[4] The Gram stain may be positive in only 33% of culture-proven SBP.[2] Total LDH in ascitic fluid has been studied as a marker for SBP. It is often elevated in cases attributed to SBP and decreases after successful treatment. In one study, however, it was determined that total LDH values overlap considerably between the SBP and non-SBP groups, making the test insensitive and nonspecific.[5] Total protein ratios of blood to ascitic fluid are nonspecific; one study demonstrated a large overlap between values in SBP, malignancy, and sterile ascitic fluid.[4] In the same study, an ascitic fluid-to-blood glucose ratio <1 had a sensitivity of only 43% and a specificity of 78%.[4] A blood-to-ascites albumin difference of <1.1 g/dL is useful for the detection of malignant ascites but not for the detection of SBP. Ascitic fluid pH of <7.32 had a sensitivity of only 42% and a specificity of 87% in one study; in another series of 41 patients there was no correlation between pH and the presence of SBP.[5, 6] Ascitic fluid lactate and blood-to-ascitic fluid lactate ratios both had a sensitivity of 68% and a specificity of 90%.[4]

On the basis of these figures, therefore, the most useful diagnostic marker for SBP is ascitic fluid PMNs >500/μL. Other tests may be considered supportive, but none has the sensitivity and specificity of the ascitic fluid cell count. If other tests are ordered to confirm the diagnosis of SBP but their results are equivocal or contradictory to the cell count, the additional tests may serve only to confuse the clinical picture.

REFERENCES

1. Montserrat A, Sola R, Sitges-Serra A, et al. Risk factors for spontaneous bacterial peritonitis in cirrhotic patients with ascites. *Gastroenterology.* 1993;104:1133–1138.
2. Sagatelian M, Gallo SH: Spontaneous bacterial peritonitis. *Hospital Physician.* 1993;29:46–50.
3. Runyon BA, Antillon M, Akriviadis EA, et al: Bedside inoculation of blood culture bottles with ascitic fluid is superior to delayed inoculation in the detection of spontaneous bacterial peritonitis. *J Clin Microbiol.* 1990;28:2811–2812.
4. Al A, Cu-Mons V, et al: Ascitic fluid polymorphonuclear cell count and serum to ascites albumin gradient in the diagnosis of bacterial peritonitis. *Gastroenterology.* 1990;98:134–140.
5. El-Touny M, Osman L, Abd-El Hamid T, et al: Re-evaluation of the value of ascitic fluid pH lactate dehydrogenase and total proteins in the value of diagnosing spontaneous bacterial peritonitis. *J Trop Med Hyg.* 1992;92:6–9.
6. Runyon B, Antillon M: Ascitic fluid pH and lactate: Insensitive and nonspecific tests in detecting ascitic fluid infection. *Hepatology.* 1991;13:929–935.

Chapter

Guaiac and Gastroccult

William Jenkins

Effective therapy for the patient with suspected gastrointestinal (GI) bleeding depends first on establishing that the patient is in fact bleeding and then on identification of the site of hemorrhage. Technologically advanced methods (endoscopy, laparoscopy, angiography) have been developed to aid in the identification of bleeding sources in the GI tract. These studies, however, are far too invasive and time consuming for use as screening and diagnostic measures in the emergency department (ED).

Stool guaiac testing and gastric aspiration, however, are valuable screening tools for the identification of GI hemorrhage. The ease with which these tests are performed, low cost, and reliability make them ideal for ED use.

The tests for occult blood in the stool and gastric aspirate depend on the conversion of a colorless substance to a substance with detectable color in the presence of blood.

STOOL GUAIAC

In the detection of occult blood in the stool, substances such as guaiac, benzidine, and amidopyrone are oxidized by a developing agent, usually hydrogen peroxide, to yield a positive result in the presence of hemoglobin.[1]

The sensitivity and specificity of the stool guaiac test have been extensively studied primarily in relation to the detection of colorectal cancer. The sensitivity of Hemoccult (Smith Kline Diagnostics, Sunnyvale, CA) has been reported to be 63 to 89% and its specificity about 93%.[5, 6]

The reaction forming the basis for the guaiac card test is complex and susceptible to many interfering factors. Agents that can adsorb hemoglobin, strong reducing agents, strong dyes, and low pH diminish the test's sensitivity, as does decomposed or contaminated developer.[2]

False-positive guaiac test results may cause significant expense and inconvenience to the patient because of unneeded follow-up diagnostic procedures. Oral iron ingestion has long been accused of causing false-positive guaiac tests, but, although studies over many decades have yielded conflicting results, most findings indicate that oral iron ingestion does not affect the stool guaiac reaction.[7–10, 12]

Because the stool guaiac test is not specific for human hemoglobin, false-positive results can be caused by a variety of foods and commonly prescribed medications. Peroxidase-containing foods such as those listed in Table 49–1 are known to cause false-positive guaiac results. Because large amounts of these foods in the diet may confound test results, appropriate inquiries should be included in the history of the patient with a positive test result. Medications that are blue in color, either in tablet or liquid form, may cause a false-positive result by yielding a blue color on the test card even before the developer is added. Aspirin, even in therapeutic doses, has also been shown to cause a positive guaiac reaction.[13] Long-distance running and contamination from vaginal bleeding or hematuria are other potential causes of a false-positive stool guaiac test.[13]

False-negative results may lead to significant patient morbidity and even mortality if potentially life-threatening conditions remain undetected. A dangerously low hemoglobin is a cause of a false-negative or only weakly positive test result. In one report, a young man with a hemoglobin of 3.7 mg/dL had only a faintly positive result despite a bleeding GI lesion.[1] Vitamin C (ascorbic acid) is a cause of false-negative guaiac test results; ingested ascorbic acid inhibits the oxidation of guaiac, thus inhibiting the guaiac reaction and the blue color production.[14] Other drugs that are known to cause a false-negative guaiac test include *N*-acetylcysteine, rifampin, and hydralazine.[2] Factors such as expired developer and card exposure to excessive heat or moisture can also decrease the test's sensitivity.

In summary, guaiac tests are a safe and inexpensive means of detecting occult blood in the stool and should be a part of all thorough physical examinations. Knowledge of the factors that interfere with the

TABLE 49–1. FOOD THAT CAN AFFECT THE GUAIAC RESULT

Broccoli	Plum	Walnut	Carrot
Banana	Watermelon	Potato	Pear
Beet	Cabbage	Red meat	Grape
Peach	Zucchini	Apple	Blackberry
Celery	Artichoke	Apricot	Pepper
Fig	Parsley	Olive	Mint
Grapefruit	Cucumber	Raspberry	Pineapple
Pumpkin	Radish	Turnip	

From Johnson DA: Fecal occult blood testing: Problems, pitfalls and diagnostic concerns. *Postgrad Med.* 1989;85:287–299. With permission.

test is essential to accurately interpret a positive or negative result and to employ the information gained for maximal patient benefit.

GASTROCCULT

Gastric aspirates that are grossly hemorrhagic pose no diagnostic difficulty, but in other cases the ability to detect occult blood in gastric samples can be more difficult. In the past, clinicians have attempted to use the standard guaiac card intended for use with stool samples to detect blood in gastric aspirates. A low pH, such as that found typically within the stomach, adversely affects the oxidation of guaiac, thus causing a false-negative result. This can be explained by the fact that hemoglobin is denatured in acid and loses the peroxidase activity on which the guaiac reaction depends.[4] Studies with gastric samples have found marked insensitivity of the guaiac reaction in detecting blood in acidic conditions, despite blood concentrations in the samples of up to 4% hematocrit.[16] The reaction is invariably negative when pH is <2. Neutralization of the gastric juice with sodium hydroxide or another buffer restores the guaiac card's sensitivity and ability to detect blood.[3, 16]

More simply, one may use Gastroccult (Smith Kline Diagnostics, Sunnyville, CA), a test card made specifically for the accurate and rapid detection of blood in gastric juice.[2–4] Gastroccult has been shown to be sensitive at low pH in detecting blood within gastric samples. It is able to detect low concentrations of blood (150 μg/dL) even at pH <2.[3] Little has been published regarding substances that adversely affect the results of the Gastroccult card. Substances capable of causing false-positive and false-negative results require further investigation.

In summary, gross upper GI hemorrhage is easily identified, but occult upper GI bleeding can be missed if standard guaiac test cards are used for testing. Gastroccult, a test card made exclusively for use with gastric juice, is an accurate means to detect occult blood in samples withdrawn from the upper GI tract.

REFERENCES

1. Forshaw JWB, Mason GM, et al: Evaluation of occult blood tests on feces. *Lancet.* 1954;ii:470–473.
2. Gogel HK, Tandberg D, Strickland RK: Substances that interfere with guaiac card testing: Implications for gastric aspirate testing. *Am J Emerg Med.* 1989;7:474–479.

3. Rosenthal P, Thompson J, Singh M: Detection of occult blood in gastric juice. *J Clin Gastroenterol.* 1984;6:119–121.
4. Long PC, Wilentz KV, Sudlow G, et al: Modification of the Hemoccult slide test for occult blood in gastric juice. *Crit Care Med.* 1982;10:692–693.
5. Johnson DA: Fecal occult blood testing: Problems, pitfalls, and diagnostic concerns. *Postgrad Med.* 1989;85:287–299.
6. Mandel JS, Bond JH, Bradley M, et al: Sensitivity, specificity, and positive predictivity of the Hemoccult test in screening for colorectal cancers. *Gastroenterology.* 1989;97:597–600.
7. Laine LA, Bentley E, Chandrasoma P: Effect of oral iron therapy on the upper gastrointestinal tract. *Dig Dis Sci.* 1988;33:172–177.
8. McDonnell WM, Ryan JA, Seeger DM, et al: Effect of iron on the guaiac reaction. *Gastroenterology.* 1989;96:74–78.
9. Kulbaski MJ et al: Oral iron and the Hemoccult test: A controversy on the teaching wards. (Letter) *N Engl J Med.* 1989;22:1500.
10. Lifton LJ, Kreiser J: False positive stool occult blood tests caused by iron preparations. *Gastroenterology.* 1982;83:860–863.
11. Morgan TE, Roantree RJ: Evaluation of tests for occult blood in the feces. *JAMA.* 1957;164:1664–1667.
12. Bratshaw JR, Harris F, McCurdy PR: The effect of oral iron therapy on the stool guaiac and orthotolidine reactions. *Ann Intern Med.* 1963;59:172–179.
13. Fleming JL, Ahlquist DA, McGill DB, et al: Influence of aspirin and ethanol on fecal blood levels as determined by using the HemoQuant assay. *Mayo Clin Proc.* 1987;62:159–163.
14. Jaffe RM, Kasken B, Young DS, et al: False negative stool occult blood tests caused by ingestion of ascorbic acid (vitamin C). *Ann Intern Med.* 1975;241:576–578.
15. Luk GD, Bynum TE, Hendrix TR: Gastric aspiration in localization of gastrointestinal hemorrhage. *JAMA.* 1979;241:576–578.
16. Layne EA, Mellow MH, Lipman TO: Insensitivity of guaiac slide test for detection of blood in gastric juice. *Ann Intern Med.* 1981;94:774–776.

MICROBIOLOGY

Chapter

Blood Cultures

J. Stephan Stapczynski

Blood culture has become an important diagnostic test in the evaluation of the patient with potential infection (Table 50–1). In daily clinical practice, however, blood cultures are often either not used to their fullest potential or used inappropriately. Although the extensive literature on the use of blood cultures has been summarized in several reviews,[1–5] this chapter focuses on the use of blood cultures in adult patients presenting to the emergency department (ED).

TEST DEFINITION

The primary purpose of a blood culture is to detect bacteremia. The test is performed when a sample of blood is drawn and incubated in a liquid medium. If bacterial growth is identified, the organism or organisms are isolated and antibiotic susceptibility is determined. The drawing and incubation of one sample constitutes a single blood culture, even if that sample is divided and inoculated into multiple bottles. Optimally, several samples of blood should be drawn and incubated separately, constituting a blood culture series.

Several technical factors affect the performance of blood culturing (Table 50–2),[6–8] and a number of these are relevant to the use of blood cultures in the ED.

TIMING. For patients with episodic symptoms of bacterial infection, bacteremia is most frequently detected before fever and rigor occur.[9] The issue of timing for patients with continuous symptoms (sustained fever) is less understood, with little published literature upon which to base recommendations.[10] In this regard, Crowley[11] found that, in patients admitted to the hospital, the rate of positive blood cultures decreased if they were drawn more than 12 hours after the onset of symptoms, with the exception of bacterial endocarditis.

TABLE 50–1. USES OF BLOOD CULTURES

Identify: primary diagnosis in high-risk population
A. Febrile neutropenic or immunosuppressed patients
B. Febrile adults without localizing symptoms or signs to detect primary bacteremias or clinically occult infections
Establish or confirm: bacterial etiology of a focal infection
A. Culture from focal source easily available: eg, pyelonephritis (urine), dysentery (stool), meningitis (CSF)
B. Culture from focal source subject to contamination: eg, pneumonia (sputum)
C. Culture from focal source has low yield: eg, cellulitis (subcutaneous aspiration)
D. Culture from focal source technically difficult to access: eg, osteomyelitis (bone)
Definitive test: for some disorders
A. Primary bacteremia
B. Intravascular infections: eg, bacterial endocarditis
C. Disseminated phase of bacterial infection: eg, disseminated gonococcal infection
Prognostic information and detection of complications
A. Pneumonia, meningitis
Monitoring therapy
A. Bacterial endocarditis

This list is illustrative of the use of blood cultures and should not be considered as the indications for blood cultures.

SITE PREPARATION. A cardinal principle of blood culturing is that the skin at the venipuncture site must be cleaned and the concentration of commensal flora reduced with disinfectant to minimize the likelihood of contamination.[1–3, 6–8] The necessity for rigorous disinfection has been challenged by Shahar and associates,[12] who found a nearly identical rate of contamination after either strict antiseptic cleaning with alcohol and povidone-iodine (4.4%) or routine preparation with 70% alcohol (3.3%) in their study of patients.

TABLE 50–2. TECHNICAL FACTORS AFFECTING BLOOD CULTURE PERFORMANCE

Timing of phlebotomy	Method of vascular access
Site preparation	Volume of blood
Number of samples	Specimen handling
Number of sample sites	Growth media characteristic
Sampling interval	System to detect bacterial growth

NUMBER OF SAMPLE SITES IN A BLOOD CULTURE SERIES. The concept of drawing each sample from a different site is that this will minimize the chance that contamination will affect the entire series[1] and decrease the clinician's ability to discriminate contamination from significant bacteremia.[3, 13–15]

METHODS OF VASCULAR ACCESS. Blood cultures are obtained most commonly by phlebotomy using a sterile needle through intact skin into a peripheral vein without indwelling devices.[1–3] The rate of contamination when blood is withdrawn from established intravascular lines is reported to be increased by two to 12 times over that observed with simple venipuncture.[16–18] Thus, if the presence of "contaminant" bacteria in blood cultures will affect clinical decision making, sampling from established vascular lines is not recommended. Conversely, if bacteremia from commensal bacteria is not a realistic possibility and their presence on blood cultures will not affect the physician's judgment, sampling from established intravascular lines may yield acceptable results, because the findings can be expected to be the same as those from peripheral venipuncture about 90% of the time.[17, 18] In a small study of children, the rate of contamination from blood sampled from freshly inserted intravenous lines was not increased, approximately 1% with each technique.[19] The applicability of this finding to adults remains unproven.

VOLUME OF BLOOD SAMPLED. The volume of blood sampled directly affects the results—the rate of bacteremia increases with greater sample size, especially with low levels of bacteremia.[3, 13] A significant number of bacteremias are in fact low level, less than 10 colony forming units/mL in 84% of patients with gram-negative bacteremia[20] and 30% in patients with gram-positive bacteremia.[21] It is recommended that individual samples be at least 10 mL in volume, although yields have been observed to be higher when the sample size is increased to 15 or 20 mL.[13] For practical reasons, the sample size cannot be increased without limit; little additional benefit appears to be obtained from samples larger than 20 mL.

SPACING INTERVAL BETWEEN SAMPLES. It has been recommended that "sampling should be spaced at wide intervals, if practical, to detect transient or intermittent bacteremia."[1] This recommendation must be balanced by the need to obtain the necessary cultures urgently before administering intravenous antibiotics to patients with serious or life-threatening infections. Waiting 30 to 60 minutes between samples in stable patients is a common practice,[1–3] although these times are chosen more because of practical considerations than any scientific basis.

SPECIMEN HANDLING AND NEEDLE CHANGES. The necessity of changing needles after phlebotomy and before inoculation into the growth medium has been the focus of four studies (Table 50–3).[22–25]

TABLE 50–3. EFFECT OF NEEDLE CHANGE IN RATE OF CONTAMINATION

Author	Population	No Needle Change	Needle Change
Isaacman and Karasic[22]	Pediatric ED	2/92 (2.2%)	2/211 (0.9%)
Krumholz et al[23]	Inpatient and ED	7/451 (1.6%)	6/462 (1.3%)
Leisure et al[24]	Healthy adults	4/182 (2.2%)	1/182 (0.6%)
Chapnick et al[25]	Inpatient and elderly	4/75 (5.3%)	1/75 (1.3%)

Data from Isaacman and Karasic RB[22]; Krumholz et al[23]; Leisure et al[24]; and Chapnick et al.[25]

Overall, the rate of contamination was low using standard technique (needle changes), but a small trend was noted toward increased contamination without needle changes. The opinion that needle changing is not required because the rate of contamination is not statistically different has been criticized because of the small sample size and low rates of contamination. A study of over 30,000 patients would be required to demonstrate a difference in the rate of contamination.[26] A practical concern is that needle changing exposes the phlebotomist to an increased risk of a needle-stick injury. The decision to continue or discontinue needle changing must take these two issues into account.

DISEASE DEFINITION

Because the primary purpose of blood cultures is to detect bacteremia, the condition must first be defined. Bacteremia is the presence of viable, intact bacteria within the liquid component of blood. Intraerythrocytic infections thus are not commonly considered "bacteremia." Bacteremia can be divided into different categories for a clearer understanding of this condition (Table 50–4).

Transient bacteremia is a common condition and a normal occurrence of daily life,[27] not surprising given the extensive colonization of the oropharynx, gastrointestinal tract, skin, and external genitalia. Fortunately, the pathogenicity of commensal flora is low, the degree of bacteremia is minimal, and the immune system is capable of neutralizing the organisms.

Significant bacteremia is associated with an infectious disease and may be intermittent or continuous.[9, 10]

Contaminant "bacteremia" continues to be a problem.[28] Because a positive blood culture is the diagnostic test for bacteremia and there is

TABLE 50–4. CLASSIFICATION OF BACTEREMIA

Transient
A. Oral bacteria (eg, dental procedures) (10–50%)[a]
B. GU bacteria (eg, urologic procedures) (8–25%)
C. GI bacteria (eg, barium enema) (11%)
D. Cutaneous bacteria (eg, incision and drainage of abscesses) (up to 30%)

Significant
A. Intermittent
   1. Focal infection (eg, undrained abscesses, pyelonephritis)
   2. Short bacteremic phase (eg, disseminated gonococcal infection)
B. Continuous
   1. Intravascular infection (eg, bacterial endocarditis, suppurative thrombophlebitis)
   2. Prolonged bacteremic phase: eg, typhoid fever or brucellosis

Contaminant
A. Cutaneous bacteria

[a]Reported ranges for transient bacteremia.

no alternative standard, any bacteria isolated in the culture bottles must be explained, often leading to increased testing and cost.[28] These false-positive blood cultures are usually distinguished from true-positives, considering both test and clinical characteristics (Table 50–5). A multivariate scoring system has been described to help in this matter (see Table 50–5).[29] Depending on the patient population, the incidence of false-positive (contaminated) blood cultures in outpatient and ED settings may approach the incidence of true-positives (Table 50–6).

TEST PERFORMANCE

There are limited data concerning the pretest probability of bacteremia in patients presenting to the ED or similar settings (see Table 50–6). These rates, especially when associated with infections that produce intermittent bacteremia, are undoubtedly underestimates because of the imperfect timing and techniques of blood culturing characteristic of clinical practice. Therefore, the emergency physician can generally only roughly estimate the pretest probability of bacteremia within a relatively broad range.[1]

Sensitivity

Because there is no alternative standard for bacteremia, the sensitivity of blood culturing cannot be accurately defined.[1–3] Operationally, sensitivity has been defined in the literature by evaluating the sensitivity of

TABLE 50–5. DIFFERENTIATION BETWEEN CONTAMINANT AND SIGNIFICANT BACTEREMIA

Criteria Modeled After Aronson and Bor[2]

Test Characteristics

A. Isolated bacteria, typically normal cutaneous flora
B. Reduced rate of bacteremia with subsequent culturing
C. Slow or delayed growth in culture media

Clinical Characteristics

A. Clinical course inconsistent with bacterial infection
B. Bacteremic isolate not found at site of focal infection
C. Absent predisposing factors for bacteremia
D. Absent leukocytosis or bandemia

Multivariate Clinical Risk Score After Bates and Lee[29]

Components of Clinical Risk Score

VARIABLE	POINTS
Maximum temperature, ≥38.3°C	3
Rapidly fatal disease (<1 mo)	4
Ultimately fatal disease (>1 mo but <5 y)	2
Presence of shaking chills	3
Intravenous drug abuse	4
Examination showing acute abdomen	3
Major comorbidity	3

Performance of the Prediction Rule

	RISK SCORE			
	0–7	8–11	12–14	>15
Derivation set (n = 219), no. (%)				
Contaminant	65 (92)	28 (80)	8 (33)	3 (3)
True bacteremia	6 (8)	7 (20)	16 (67)	86 (97)
Validation set (n = 129), no. (%)				
Contaminant	51 (86)	13 (81)	3 (30)	5 (11)
True bacteremia	8 (14)	3 (19)	7 (70)	39 (89)

Reproduced with permission from Aronson MD, Bor DH: Blood cultures. *Ann Intern Med.* 1987;106:246. From Bates DW, Lee TH: Rapid classification of positive blood cultures. Prospective validation of a multivariate algorithm. *JAMA.* 1992;267:1962–1965. Copyright 1992, American Medical Association.

a series of blood cultures in patients who had clinical features of bacterial infection and at least one positive blood culture with an organism believed to be significant. The "best" studies utilize at least three sets of cultures collected at different sites over an interval of time. Within the limitations of these studies, the initial blood culture is about 80% sensitive, a series of two increases the sensitivity to about 90%, and a third culture increases sensitivity to over 98%.[1–3, 13, 14] In most

TABLE 50–6. APPROXIMATE INCIDENCE OF BACTEREMIA IN DIFFERENT POPULATIONS

Population	Site	No. Patients	True Bacteremia*	Contaminant Bacteremia*
Healthy[30]	Outpt	240[a]	0/240	5/240 (2.1%)
Febrile[31]	ED	565	10/210 (4.8%)	10/210 (4.8%)
Unstated[32]	ED	411	29/411 (7.1%)	20/411 (4.9%)
Febrile IVDU[33]	Inpt	87	16/87 (18.4%)	NS
Febrile IVDU[34]	ED	283	29/276 (10.5%)	NS
AIDS (about ⅔ with fever)[35]	ED/Inpt	About 800	44/800 (5%)	NS
Fever without focal symptom/sign[36]	ED	135	21/135 (16%)	NS
Cellulitis[37]	ED	50	2/50 (4%)	NS
Pyelonephritis[38]	Inpt/ED	194	21/95 (22%)	NS

NS = not stated.
*Number positive/number of patients with blood count drawn. Inpt = inpatients; outpt = outpatients.

circumstances three blood cultures are necessary to maximize the yield; additional cultures produce diminishingly small returns.

Under some conditions, the ability of blood cultures to detect bacteremia is reduced and sensitivity decreases. This has been found to occur in patients with infections due to unusual organisms with atypical growth characteristics. Some of these bacteria are part of the normal flora of the oropharynx or skin. It has also been observed that administration of oral antibiotics (either prescribed or self-administered) reduces the ability of blood cultures to detect bacteremia in patients with bacterial endocarditis. Therefore, in patients with a potential infection due to unusual organisms or to bacteria that are part of normal cutaneous or oropharyngeal flora, or with endocarditis partially treated with oral antibiotics, a minimum of four blood cultures is required for additional sensitivity.[1, 2]

Specificity

As previously noted, the correct determination of false-positive blood cultures remains a problem. The false-positive rate is influenced both by technique and by patient characteristics. The ability of poor technique to cause false-positive results is obvious. Not so obvious is the influence of patient characteristics. Bacteremia is often found in patients with conditions that impair the immune system, alter host defenses, or require indwelling prosthetic devices. Normal bacterial flora of the skin, oropharynx, or perineal area, which are usually considered contaminants when found in blood cultures, may infect these patients and produce true bacteremia. Between 5 and 20% of blood culture isolates of bacteria normally considered contaminants may represent true infection.[1,2] Overall, the incidence of false-positive blood cultures varies between 1 and 5% for individual cultures, depending on the setting (see Tables 50–3 and 50–6). For cultures obtained in the ED, often under difficult circumstances, values tend to be found toward the higher range; a value of 3 to 4% seems consistent with clinical experience.

Ordinarily, the specificity of a test decreases with repeated application in a single patient. In other words, if a healthy patient is repeatedly tested with some technique that has less than 100% specificity, the likelihood increases that one "abnormal" result will be obtained by chance alone, and the specificity decreases. This is true of a series of blood cultures, provided any "positive" is considered significant. Using the criteria previously noted (see Table 50–5) to differentiate true- from false-positives, individual contaminated cultures can be identified and excluded without increasing the specificity of the entire series.[1]

INDICATIONS FOR TESTING

As with all testing, there should be reasonable indications for the appropriate use of blood cultures, not just a suspicion of infection. These indications may be based on clinical characteristics (obtained from the history or physical examination) or from the results of other ancillary tests.

There should be a clinically relevant use for the results of blood cultures. For example, in acute pyelonephritis, blood cultures may be positive in about 22% of cases, but urine cultures are just as easy and available and are more sensitive for this disease. Routine blood cultures in this setting add little to diagnostic or therapeutic decision making.

Because the clinical relevance of bacteremia varies according to patient characteristics, disease, and bacteriology, it is not possible to make blanket recommendations concerning the indications for blood cultures. Instead, the discussion reviews the factors that have been found to be associated with clinically significant bacteremia.

History and Physical Examination

Because fever is a cardinal sign of infection, it is not surprising that fever has been correlated with an increased risk for bacteremia in several patient populations: febrile ED patients, febrile intravenous drug users (IVDU), febrile AIDS patients, febrile adults without focal symptoms or signs, sepsis syndrome patients, and hospitalized patients.[31, 33–36, 39–44] In most clinical settings, fever is the chief indication for blood culturing. In the absence of fever, the incidence of clinically significant bacteremia in most adult patients falls below 1%.

In a study of hospitalized patients, shaking chills, history of intravenous drug use, presence of acute abdomen, major comorbidity, and fatal or ultimately fatal underlying disease were all associated with an increased risk of bacteremia.[40] These factors could be combined into a prediction rule: for patients at the highest risk, the incidence of bacteremia was 15% and, for patients at the lowest risk, the incidence was 1 to 2%.

In another study, hypotension and fever were the best clinical predictors of bacteremia in patients with the sepsis syndrome, although no valid prediction rule could be developed from this population.[39]

For febrile adults without localizing symptoms or signs seen in the ED, Mellors and coworkers[36] first developed a multivariate risk index using the results of the CBC and ESR that was also studied by Liebovici and coworkers[45] on inpatient service. The results of both studies were similar (Table 50–7). Additional conclusions of these studies were

- A significant portion of adults with fever unexplained by history or physical examination had a bacterial infection (about 30%) often with bacteremia (about 15%).
- These "clinically occult" infections were most often due to common bacteria in common locations.
- The incidence of diagnostic abnormalities on the routine urinalysis was 16 and 13% and on chest radiography 4 and 3%, respectively. From the perspective of detecting as many clinically occult infections as possible, routine urinalysis and chest radiography detected approximately half.
- Increasing age, underlying host illness, leukocytosis, or left shift on the white cell differential was associated with an increased risk of bacterial infection.

White Blood Cell Count and Differential

Overall, the total WBC and differential is believed to be insensitive in detecting bacterial infections or bacteremia and lacks specificity to exclude them as well. Abnormal total WBC counts and percent of neutrophilic bands are associated with an increased risk of bacteremia in febrile adults, but the risk is only relative, and bacteremia can be absent with abnormal values or present with normal values.

TABLE 50–7. MULTIVARIATE INDEX FOR CLINICALLY OCCULT BACTERIAL INFECTION (FEBRILE ADULT PATIENTS WITHOUT LOCALIZING SYMPTOMS OR SIGNS)

Score one point for each factor

a. Age ≥50 y
b. Diabetes mellitus
c. WBC ≥15,000
d. Neutrophil band count ≥1500
e. ESR ≥30 mm/h

Emergency Department Patients[a, 36]

Score	*Bacterial Infection*	*Bacteremia*
0	1/21 (5%)	0/21 (0%)
1	15/45 (33%)	3/45 (7%)
2	15/38 (39%)	6/38 (16%)
≥3	17/31 (55%)	12/31 (39%)

Hospitalized Patients[b, 45]

Score	*Bacterial Infection*	*Bacteremia*
0	1/11 (9%)	0/11 (0%)
1	12/44 (27%)	5/44 (11%)
2	13/41 (32%)	7/41 (17%)
≥3	9/17 (53%)	6/17 (35%)

[a]After history and physical examination in ED.
[b]After initial assessment on inpatient unit including ancillary tests.
From Mellors JW, Horwitz RI, Harvey MR, et al: A simple index to identify occult bacterial infection in adults with acute unexplained fever. *Arch Intern Med.* 147:666–671. Copyright 1987, American Medical Association; Leibovici L, Cohen O, Wysenbeek AJ: Occult bacterial infection in adults with unexplained fever. Validation of a diagnostic index. *Arch Intern Med.* 150:1270–1272. Copyright 1990, American Medical Association.

In selected subgroups, however, the WBC count can be used to increase the possibility of bacterial infection and bacteremia. These include adults with fever unexplained by history and physical examination[36, 45] and febrile patients with neutropenia.[46, 47] In the latter group, a neutrophil count <1000/mm^3 is associated with a 20 to 30% incidence of bacteremia.[46, 47]

Is it possible to develop low-risk criteria using a combination of WBC count and differential that would identify some patients at such low risk for bacteremia that blood cultures are not indicated? Using the multivariate analysis of Mellors and coworkers in evaluating the febrile adult without localizing symptoms or signs (and assuming age <50, absence of diabetes, and ESR <30 mm/h), with a total WBC <15,000/mm^3 and an absolute neutrophil band count <1500/mm^3, the incidence of bacteremia was 0 of 32 patients.[36, 45] Although the numbers of patients studied have been small and the conclusions are tentative, a combination of the total WBC count and differential may be useful to assign a low risk for bacteremia to subgroups of febrile adults and obviate the need for some blood cultures.

Erythrocyte Sedimentation Rate

In unselected febrile adults, the ESR does not appear to be a useful test in discriminating between those with serious or bacterial infections and those without.[48] As with leukocytosis, an elevated ESR is associated with an increased incidence of bacteremia. In their study of the febrile adult without localizing symptoms or signs, Mellors and coworkers found that an ESR >30 mm/h had a sensitivity of 85% and a specificity of 39% for detecting bacteremia.[36] The incidence of bacteremia in patients with an ESR >30 mm/h was 30%; the rate with an ESR <30 mm/h was 10%.[36, 45]

RECOMMENDATIONS

The analysis of Aronson and Bor contains the following general recommendations:[2]

- When the probability of bacteremia is low to moderate and the anticipated pathogen is different from the commensal flora, two blood cultures are generally sufficient.
- When the probability of bacteremia is high or continuous bacteremia is suspected (eg, bacterial endocarditis), three blood cultures should be obtained.
- When the probability of bacteremia is high and the anticipated pathogens are part of the indigenous flora, four or more blood cultures should be drawn.
- If a patient with suspected bacterial endocarditis has received antibiotics in the previous 2 weeks, four or more blood cultures should be drawn.

Intravenous drug users have an increased incidence of bacterial infection and bacteremia, and blood cultures are an important tool in the evaluation of these patients. The evaluation of febrile intravenous drug users is complicated because of the possibility of endocarditis and the inability to accurately predict its presence or absence upon ED evaluation.[33, 34] Two studies from municipal hospitals in New York City and Boston found that the most common infection in the febrile IVDU was pneumonia, seen in 38 and 34%, whereas the incidence of bacterial endocarditis was 13 and 6%.[33, 34] Other serious bacterial infections found in these febrile patients were cellulitis, abscess, septic arthritis, and pyelonephritis. Importantly, only a minority, 26 and 32%, of the patients had "minor" illnesses.

Whereas some clinical features or ancillary test results were associated with occult bacterial infection or endocarditis, no single feature or combination was accurate enough to guide the evaluation or disposition decisions. In the study by Marantz and colleagues two of seven (28%) of the patients predicted to have a minor illness upon ED evaluation developed major illness during hospitalization.[33] Three of the 28 (11%) patients predicted *not* to have endocarditis did indeed have endocarditis. In the study by Samet and associates, seven of 79 patients predicted *not* to have bacteremia had positive blood cultures (9%) and six of 140 patients predicted *not* to have endocarditis did indeed have endocarditis (4%).[34]

SUMMARY

Blood cultures are a valuable technique in the diagnosis of bacterial infection. They are not always necessary, especially in patients with focal infections in whom a bacteriologic diagnosis can be made by another means. To maximize the utility of blood cultures, clinicians should pay close attention to the use of adequate number of samples, practice careful technique, and interpret the results with common sense.

REFERENCES

1. Bor DH, Aronson MD: Blood cultures: clinical decisions, in Sox HC (ed): *Common Diagnostic Tests. Use and Interpretation.* 2nd ed. Philadelphia: American College of Physicians; 1990:265–285.
2. Aronson MD, Bor DH: Blood cultures. *Ann Intern Med.* 1987;106:246–253.
3. Washington JA: Blood cultures. Principles and techniques. *Mayo Clin Proc.* 1975;50:91–98.
4. Lyman JL: Use of blood cultures in the emergency department. *Ann Emerg Med.* 1986;15:308–311.
5. Ristuccia PA, Hoeffner RA, Digamon-Beltran M, et al: Detection of bactermia by buffy-coat smears. *Scand J Infect Dis.* 1987;19:215–217.
6. Reller L, Murray P, McLowry J, et al: *Blood Cultures II.* Washington, DC: American Society for Microbiology; 1982:1–11.
7. Isenberg HD, Washington JA, Balows A, et al: Collection, handling and processing of specimens, in Lennette EH, Balows A, Hauser WJ, et al (eds):

Manual of Clinical Microbiology. 4th ed. Washington, DC: American Society for Microbiology; 1985;73–98.

8. Washington JA, Ilstrup DM: Blood cultures: Issues and controversies. *Rev Infect Dis*. 1986;8:792–802.
9. Bennett IL, Beeson PB: Bacteremia: A consideration of some experimental bacteremias. *Yale J Biol Med*. 1954;226:241–262.
10. Beeson PB, Brannon ES, Warren JV: Observations on the sites of removal of bacteria from the blood in patients with bacterial endocarditis. *J Exp Med*. 1945;81:9–23.
11. Crowley N: Some bacteraemias encountered in hospital practice. *J Clin Pathol*. 1970;23:166–171.
12. Shahar E, Wohl-Gottesman BS, Shenkman L: Contamination of blood cultures during venepuncture: Fact or myth? *Postgrad Med J*. 1990;66:1053–1058.
13. Weinstein MP, Reller LB, Murphy JR, et al: The clinical significance of positive blood cultures: A comprehensive analysis of 500 episodes of bacteremia and fungemia in adults. I. Laboratory and epidemiologic observations. *Rev Infect Dis*. 1983;5:35–53.
14. MacGregor RR, Beaty HN: Evaluation of positive blood cultures. Guidelines for early differentiation of contaminated from valid positive cultures. *Arch Intern Med*. 1972;130:84–87.
15. Flournoy DJ, Adkins L, McCaffree RD: Bacteremia in adult men. *J Natl Med Assoc*. 1987;79:816–824.
16. Tonnesen A, Peuler M, Lockwood WR: Cultures of blood drawn by catheters versus venipuncture. *JAMA*. 1976;235:1877.
17. Tafuro P, Colbourn D, Gurevich I, et al: Comparison of blood cultures obtained simultaneously by venipuncture and from vascular lines. *J Hosp Infect*. 1986;7:283–288.
18. Bryant JK, Strand CL: Reliability of blood cultures collected from intravascular catheter versus venipuncture. *Am J Clin Pathol*. 1987;88:113–116.
19. Isaacman DJ, Karasic RB: Utility of collecting blood cultures through newly inserted intravenous catheters. *Pediatr Infect Dis J*. 1990;9:815–818.
20. DuPont HL, Spink WW: Infections due to Gram-negative organisms: An analysis of 860 patients with bacteremia at the University of Minnesota Medical Center, 1958–1966. *Medicine*. 1969;48:307–332.
21. Kluge RM, DuPont HL: Factors affecting mortality of patients with bacteremia. *Surg Gynecol Obstet*. 1973;137:267–269.
22. Isaacman DJ, Karasic RB: Lack of effect of changing needles on contamination of blood cultures. *Pediatr Infect Dis J*. 1990;9:274–278.
23. Krumholz HM, Cummings S, York M: Blood culture phlebotomy: switching needles does not prevent contamination. *Ann Intern Med*. 1990;113:290–292.
24. Leisure MK, Moore DM, Schwartzman JD, et al: Changing the needle when inoculating blood cultures. A no-benefit and high-risk procedure. *JAMA*. 1990;264:2111–2112.
25. Chapnick EK, Schaffer BC, Gradon JD, et al. Technique for drawing blood for cultures: is changing needles truly necessary? *South Med J*. 1991; 84:1197–1198.
26. Elliott WJ: Switching phlebotomy needles. (letter) *Ann Intern Med*. 1991; 114:94.

27. Everett ED, Hirschmann JV: Transient bacteremia and endocarditis prophylaxis. A review. *Medicine*. 1977;56:61–77.
28. Bates DW, Goldman L, Lee TH: Contaminant blood cultures and resource utilization. The true consequences of false-positive results. *JAMA*. 1991; 265:365–369.
29. Bates DW, Lee TH: Rapid classification of positive blood cultures. Prospective validation of a multivariate algorithm. *JAMA*. 1992;267:1962–1965.
30. Wilson WR, Van Scoy RE, Washington JA: Incidence of bacteremia in adults without infection. *J Clin Microbiol*. 1975;2:94–95.
31. Eisenberg JM, Rose JD, Weinstein AJ: Routine blood cultures from febrile outpatients. Use in detecting bacteremia. *JAMA*. 1976;236:2863–2865.
32. Sklar DP, Rusnak R: The value of outpatient blood cultures in the emergency department. *Am J Emerg Med*. 1987;5:95–100.
33. Marantz PR, Linzer M, Feiner CJ, et al. Inability to predict diagnosis in febrile intravenous drug abusers. *Ann Intern Med*. 1987;106:823–828.
34. Samet JH, Shevitz A, Fowle J, et al: Hospitalization decision in febrile intravenous drug users. *Am J Med*. 1990;89:53–57.
35. Krumholz HM, Sande MA, Lo B: Community-acquired bacteremia in patients with acquired immunodeficiency syndrome: Clinical presentation, bacteriology, and outcome. *Am J Med*. 1989;86:776–779.
36. Mellors JW, Horwitz RI, Harvey MR, et al: A simple index to identify occult bacterial infection in adults with acute unexplained fever. *Arch Intern Med*. 1987;147:666–671.
37. Hook EW III, Hooton TM, Horton CA, et al: Microbiologic evaluation of cutaneous cellulitis in adults. *Arch Intern Med*. 1986;146:295–297.
38. Safrin S, Siegel D, Black D: Pyelonephritis in adult women: Inpatient versus outpatient therapy. *Am J Med*. 1988;85:793–798.
39. Peduzzi P, Shatney C, Sheagren J, et al: Predictors of bacteremia and Gram-negative bacteremia in patients with sepsis. *Arch Intern Med*. 1992;152:529–535.
40. Bates DW, Cook EF, Goldman L, et al: Predicting bacteremia in hospitalized patients. A prospectively validated model. *Ann Intern Med*. 1990;113:495–500.
41. Leibovici L, Greenshtain S, Cohen O, et al: Bacteremia in febrile patients. A clinical model for diagnosis. *Arch Intern Med*. 1991;115:1801–1806.
42. VonReyn CF, Levy BS, Arbeit RD, et al: Infective endocarditis: An analysis based on strict case definitions. *Ann Intern Med*. 1981;94:505–518.
43. Werner AS, Cobbs CG, Kaye D, et al: Studies on the bacteremia of bacterial endocarditis. *JAMA*. 1967;202:199–203.
44. Pelletier LL, Petersdorf RG: Infective endocarditis: A review of 125 cases from the University of Washington Hospitals 1963–72. *Medicine*. 1978;56:287–313.
45. Leibovici L, Cohen O, Wysenbeek AJ: Occult bacterial infection in adults with unexplained fever. Validation of a diagnostic index. *Arch Intern Med*. 1990;150:1270–1272.
46. Meunier F: Infections in patients with acute leukemia and lymphoma, in Mandell GL, Douglas RG, Bennett RE (eds): *Principles and Practice of Infectious Diseases*. 3rd ed. New York: Churchill-Livingstone; 1990:2265–2275.

47. Whimbley E, Kiehn TE, Brannon P, et al: Bacteremia and fungemia in patients with neoplastic disease. *Am J Med.* 1987;82:723–730.
48. Sox HC, Liang MH: The erythrocyte sedimentation rate. Guidelines for rational use, in Sox HC (ed): *Common Diagnostic Tests. Use and Interpretations.* 2nd ed. Philadelphia: American College of Physicians; 1990:204–226.

Chapter

Vaginal Wet and KOH Preparations

Elaine B. Josephson

Microscopic examination of the vaginal smear is a rapid and readily available means of evaluating a variety of vaginal disorders in the emergency department. Three basic diagnostic tests are used: the saline or wet mount (''wet prep''), the potassium hydroxide (KOH) preparation (''KOH prep''), and the Gram stain.

The *wet prep* is performed by adding a drop of saline to the smeared vaginal secretions, applying a coverslip, and examining directly by simple light microscopy.

The *KOH prep* is performed in a similar fashion, but a drop of 10% KOH is used rather than saline. The slide may be gently heated to promote the dissolution by KOH of any cellular elements, allowing for direct visualization of fungal hyphae and spores. (The *Gram stain* is discussed elsewhere.)

SPECIFIC CLINICAL ENTITIES

Vaginal smears and microbiologic studies are directed generally at diagnosing one or more of three disorders: trichomonal vaginitis, *Candida* vaginitis, and bacterial vaginosis (formerly termed nonspecific vaginitis).[1, 2]

Trichomonal Vaginitis

Trichomonal vaginitis is caused by *Trichomonas vaginalis*, a motile flagellated protozoan. The infection is sexually transmitted, but its presence may not necessarily be responsible for the symptoms for which the patient has sought medical attention.[3, 4] *Trichomonas,* generally is easily identified on wet prep. The motile trichomonads are somewhat oval or pear-shaped and bear active flagella. Many polymorphonuclear leukocytes are also typically present.[4]

Although Papanicolaou (PAP) smear, culture, and other various staining techniques have been shown in some studies to be more sensitive than the wet prep for diagnosis of trichomonal vaginitis,[3, 6] they offer no immediate advantage, particularly in the ED setting.[4] If done properly and examined shortly after collection of the specimen, the wet prep yields sensitivity values equivalent to those of culture, as well as cytodiagnostic and other special staining methods (in one report as high as 55% sensitivity on wet mount).[4, 7, 8] A negative wet prep does not rule out trichomonal vaginitis, however, because organisms have been reported to be visible in only approximately 70% of cases.[5] Eddie[8] reported an accuracy of >90% in detecting trichomonal infection using the wet mount. A study by Thomason[9] found an 86% sensitivity for both culture and wet mount in detecting *Trichomonas.* The wet mount is clearly preferable because of its rapidity and low cost.[7]

Candida Vaginitis

Candida usually is readily identified on wet prep, KOH prep, or Gram stain. The yeast can be isolated on various culture media as well and can also be detected using the slide latex agglutination (SLA) test.

The wet prep in *Candida* vaginitis reveals leukocytes, epithelial cells, and clumps of budding spores, nongerminating spores, and branched mycelia (hyphae). The KOH prep is, however, more sensitive.[5, 11] The wet prep and KOH prep are very specific in detecting *Candida* but are less sensitive than culture. A Gram stain of a vaginal smear taken from a patient with *Candida* vaginitis can also reveal the presence of germinating and nongerminating spores as well as branching yeast filaments.[7]

Several studies have demonstrated fungal culture to be more sensitive than KOH prep in detecting *Candida* infection. A general recommendation is made to obtain specimens for culture in any woman with vulvovaginal symptoms whose wet mount or KOH smear is negative before a diagnosis of a yeast infection can be definitively excluded.[7, 8, 11, 12] *Candida* can take up to 2 to 3 days to grow on culture, however. Bertholf and Stafford[7] describe the KOH prep as being only 70% sensitive in screening for *Candida,* and 34% of symptomatic culture-positive women in their study were missed by KOH prep. As a screening test, however, the KOH prep appears to be both time- and cost-effective.

McCormack and associates[12] have recommended that patients who are still symptomatic despite having negative slide test results and for whom other causes of vaginitis are ruled out should be further evaluated with cultures. A study by Eddie[8] reported a 52% rate of detecting positive cases of *Candida* by wet smears stained with methylene blue, with 93% of the cases studied being culture positive.

Sobel and colleagues[13] evaluated the use of the slide latex agglutination test for diagnosing *Candida* vaginitis. They found the KOH prep to have a sensitivity of 90% in symptomatic women, and the SLA to have a sensitivity of only 72.7%. Sobel and colleagues[13] concluded that the SLA test offered no advantage over the KOH prep.

Bacterial Vaginosis

Bacterial vaginosis, also known as nonspecific vaginitis, is a common cause of vaginital symptoms in women. It is characterized by a decrease in the normal vaginal flora and an overgrowth of other organisms such as *Gardnerella vaginalis.*[1, 10]

The United States Department of Health and Human Services[14] as well as Amsel and coworkers[2] have formulated specific criteria for the clinical diagnosis of bacterial vaginosis. At least three of the four following features must be present: (1) a typical thin homogeneous vaginal discharge, (2) a vaginal fluid pH of >4.5, (3) a positive amine test (ie, a ''fishy odor'' is emitted when 10% KOH is added to vaginal secretions), and (4) a finding of clue cells on wet prep or a Gram-stained smear. The clue cells are somewhat flat squamous epithelial cells with surfaces that are covered with many adherent bacteria, and they can have a granular appearance; few leukocytes are seen.[1, 2, 5, 7, 9] Larsson and Platz-Christensen,[15] using rehydrated air-dried wet smears, found the presence of clue cells to be 98% specific and 96% sensitive in diagnosing bacterial vaginosis.

Cultures can be obtained to isolate the various bacterial vaginosis organisms, but these are time-consuming and not cost-effective compared with the wet prep and vaginal Gram stain, which have higher levels of specificity and similar sensitivity and correlate with patients' symptoms.[1]

SUMMARY

Examination of the vaginal smear provides a relatively quick and simple method for evaluating vaginal complaints in the ED. Testing the vaginal secretions for pH and examining them using a wet prep, Gram stain, and KOH prep can in most cases rapidly make the diagnosis and allow for prompt and appropriate treatment. Cultures are not necessary except in unusual cases.

REFERENCES

1. Hillier S, Holmes KK: Bacterial vaginosis, in Holmes KK, et al (eds): Sexually Transmitted Diseases. 2nd ed. New York: McGraw-Hill; 1990:547–559.
2. Amsel R, Totten PA, Spiegel CA, et al: Nonspecific vaginitis: Diagnostic criteria and microbial and epidemiologic associations. *Am J Med.* 1983; 74:14–22.
3. McLellan R, Spence MR, Brockman M, et al: The clinical diagnosis of trichomoniasis. *Obstet Gynecol.* 1982;60:30–34.
4. Rein MF, Muller M: Trichomonas vaginalis and trichomoniasis, in Holmes KK, et al (eds): Sexually Transmitted Diseases. 2nd ed. New York: McGraw-Hill; 1990:481–492.
5. Gilly PA: Vaginal discharge: Its causes and cures. *Postgrad Med.* 1986;80:231–237.
6. Krieger JN, Tom MR, Stevens CE, et al: Diagnosis of trichomonas: Comparison of conventional wet-mount examination with cytologic studies, cultures, and monoclonal antibody staining of direct specimens. *JAMA.* 1988; 259:1223–1227.
7. Bertholf ME, Stafford MJ: An office laboratory panel to assess vaginal problems. *Am Fam Physician.* 1985;32:113–125.
8. Eddie DAS: The laboratory diagnosis of vaginal infections caused by *Trichomonas* and *Candida (Monilia)* species. *J Med Microbiol.* 1986;1:153–159.
9. Thomason JL: Comparison of four methods to detect *Trichomonas vaginalis. J Clin Microbiol.* 1988;26:1869–1870.
10. Friedrich EG: Vaginitis. *Am J Obstet Gynecol.* 1985;152:247–251.
11. Siapco BJ, Kaplan BJ, Berstein GS, Moyer DL: Cytodiagnosis of Candida organisms in cervical smears. *Acta Cytol.* 1986;30:477–480.
12. McCormack WM, Starko KM, Zinner SH: Symptoms associated with vaginal colonization with yeast. *Am J Obstet Gynecol.* 1988;158:31–33.
13. Sobel JD, Schmitt H, Meriwether C: A new slide latex agglutination test for the diagnosis of acute candida vaginitis. *Am J Clin Pathol.* 1990;94:323–325.
14. United States Department of Health and Human Services, Public Health Service, Division of Sexually Transmitted Diseases: Bacterial vaginosis in the 1989 sexually transmitted diseases treatment guidelines. *MMWR* 1989;38:36–37.
15. Larsson PG, Platz-Christensen JJ: Enumeration of clue cells in rehydrated air-dried vaginal wet smears for the diagnosis of bacterial vaginosis. *Obstet Gynecol.* 1990;76:727–730.

Chapter

Gonorrheal Culture

Eric Davis

Correctly diagnosing gonorrheal infection is an important aspect of emergency medicine. Gonorrhea (GC) is the most common reportable bacterial infection in the United States and is the best single indicator of unsafe sexual behavior and risk of HIV infection.[7, 11] As a result, it is important that emergency physicians understand proper diagnostic methodology for this disease.

WHO SHOULD BE TESTED

The first step is to determine whom to test. Gonorrheal illness may manifest in many forms, including urethritis, epididymitis, and proctitis in males and urethritis, cervicitis, and salpingitis in females. Other syndromes less commonly associated with a gonorrheal origin are conjunctivitis, pharyngitis, vaginitis, and arthritis. The incidence of genital GC is highest in those who are under 25 years of age, unmarried, of low socioeconomic status, and who have multiple sexual contacts or sexual contacts known to be positive for GC. Urethral gonorrhea in the male manifests as a discharge that is purulent in 75% of cases. Anal GC has a higher incidence in homosexual males, as does pharyngeal GC. Disseminated GC and its sequelae are more common in females, especially those with pharyngeal GC, and has an increased incidence during pregnancy and just after menses. Although only 10 to 15% of infections in males are asymptomatic, 75 to 80% are asymptomatic in females.

If the diagnosis of gonococcal infection is suspected, testing is warranted. In a male with a purulent urethral discharge that stains for gram-negative intracellular diplococci, the diagnosis of gonorrhea may be made without further testing (positive predictive value greater than 95%[32]). A reasonably specific positive diagnosis may be made in females who have a purulent cervical discharge with a pH greater than 4.5 and at least ten polymorphonuclear neutrophils (PMNs) per high power field.[1] Gram stain is characteristically positive in about 50% of this population.[1, 16] These tests, although highly specific, are sensitive in only 40 to 50%.[1] All others must have confirmation by specific testing.

In addition to those clinically suspected of the disease, patients with known positive contacts as well as certain high-risk groups (sexually active teens, pregnant women of lower socioeconomic standing) should be routinely cultured for GC during the pelvic examination.

CULTURE MEDIA

The type of medium chosen to plate the specimen depends on the area of the body from which the culture is taken (Table 52–1). For specimens not likely to be contaminated by other bacteria, standard culture medium is sufficient. Otherwise, special selective media (GC-Lect, Thayer-Martin, Martin-Lewis, NYC media) should be used. These media are impregnated with a variety of antibiotics (vancomycin, colistin, trimethoprim, and nystatin)[1] designed to inhibit normal flora while permitting growth of *Neisseria gonorrhoeae*. Approximately 10% of *N. gonorrhoeae* have been found to be sensitive to vancomycin, however.[2, 4, 15] These aerobic cultures should be enriched with 5 to 10% carbon dioxide, which may increase positive yields by up to 10%. Candle jars, the JEMBEC transportation system (citric acid-bicarbonate tablet), and a bottle chamber containing CO_2 are all effective.[23] Although the culture plates must be kept refrigerated to prevent inactivation of antibiotics, they must be warmed to room temperature at the time of inoculation. The medium must be kept moist but not wet, as excessive fluid will inhibit growth. This is facilitated by storing the media plates upside down. The specimens should then be transported directly to the laboratory for incubation.

WHERE AND HOW TO CULTURE

The single most important element in the laboratory diagnosis of GC is culturing of the appropriate site and collection of the specimen.

TABLE 52–1. SELECTION OF CULTURE MEDIA BY SITE

Selective Media	Nonselective Media
Pharynx	Joint effusion
Urethra	Blood
Endocervix	Conjunctiva
Rectum/anus	Skin vesicles
Nasopharynx	

Improper collection technique is a common cause of false-negative results. The proper technique varies by location.

Endocervical Cultures

In women, regardless of the presentation, cultures should always be obtained from the endocervical canal. Cervical mucus should first be removed with a cotton pledget, followed by insertion of a sterile, cotton-tipped swab 1 cm into the canal. The swab should then be rotated and moved side-to-side for 10 to 30 seconds to promote adherence and absorption,[26] and then immediately plated. For best results, a second swab should be utilized and plated on the opposite side of the original swab.[16] Lubricants should not be used while the culture is being obtained, because they may inhibit growth of the organisms. Under ideal conditions, endocervical cultures are 85 to 95% sensitive in localized infection, and 80% sensitive in disseminated GC.[18] In high-risk women with negative cultures, repeat cultures in 1 week may uncover an additional 5 to 10% of cases.[21] Cultures are obtained from the endocervix only, as the vagina is usually not infected, perhaps owing to the lack of mucus glands and the presence of cornified epithelium. Vaginal cultures may, however, be useful in children as well as in women who have had a hysterectomy.

Urethral Cultures

All males with suspected infections should have urethral cultures. An unmoistened calcium alginate swab is inserted 2 cm into the urethra and rotated for 30 seconds to 2 minutes.[22] The specimen is then immediately plated. Sensitivity is reported to be in the 85 to 95% range and higher, if those determined to be positive by Gram stain are included.[19] As with females, if repeat cultures are done in culture-negative patients after 1 week, the overall yield is improved.[3, 12]

Rectal Cultures

Rectal cultures are obtained by inserting a sterile cotton-tipped swab into the canal to the level of the crypts of Morgagni (2 to 3 cm), the site of infection. As with endocervical cultures, lubricants should not be used. The swab is pressed against the side wall, moved circumferentially for 10 to 30 seconds, and then removed. If fecal material is present, the swab should be discarded and another specimen obtained. The material is then immediately plated onto selective media. The sensitivity of rectal cultures is reported to be 30 to 50%. When obtained in conjunction with cervical culture in females,[21] rectal cultures increase the detection of GC by about 5 to 10%.

Throat Cultures

The pharynx is a common source for disseminated GC, and a difficult area to eradicate the organisms. Throat cultures are obtained by swabbing the posterior pharynx and tonsillar crypts with a sterile cotton-tipped applicator. When a specimen from the crypts is obtained, it is recommended to press the swab into the area and rotate it for 10 to 15 seconds and to repeat this procedure in two or three different areas. The specimen is then plated onto selective media. Best results are obtained when both sides of the pharynx are cultured and plated on opposite sides of the agar. The sensitivity of pharyngeal GC culture has been reported to vary from 15 to 80%.[10, 24] Culturing the throat does not appear to improve the overall detection of infection.

Joint Effusion Cultures

Neisseria gonorrheoeae has been reported to be the most common cause of bacterial arthritis in urban centers.[24] All joint effusions in cases of suspected disseminated GC should be aspirated. The fluid should be Gram-stained (positive for GC in less than 25% of cases) and cultured (positive in less than 50% of cases). Culture should be obtained utilizing standard methods and media. Leukocyte counts are typically lower than in other forms of bacterial arthritis, but the mean count is over 50,000 cells/mm^3.[24] Some sources recommend also sending the fluid for complement fixation, which becomes positive 2 to 6 weeks after the initial infection. When negative, the test should be repeated after 1 week if the diagnosis is still in doubt.

Culture of Vesicular Skin Lesions

Vesicular skin lesions are present in 33 to 50% of patients with disseminated GC; overall, 75% of these patients have positive blood cultures and 15% have positive joint effusion cultures. The technique involves cleansing the vesicle with normal saline, followed by aspiration using a sterile needle. Material is immediately plated onto selective media and is Gram-stained if there is sufficient volume.

Blood Cultures

It is recommended that all patients with suspected disseminated GC have blood cultures drawn. Usual blood culture bottles should be used, but the laboratory should be notified that GC is suspected. The sensitivity of blood culture for disseminated GC infection has been reported to be 20% overall[24] but higher when nonselective media are used.

Choice of Culture Site(s)

The choice of site or sites to culture for GC must be guided by the clinical presentation, exposure history, and risk factors. In general, patients with suspected infections should have urethral cultures if male, and endocervical cultures if female. The yield in females is reported to approach 100% if two endocervical cultures are obtained 24 hours apart[5] and a rectal culture is included. Rectal cultures are also recommended for homosexual males. Cultures of the pharynx add little in the asymptomatic or low-risk patient but should be routinely obtained in high-risk populations, such as homosexual males, prostitutes, sexual abuse victims, and those known with positive oral-genital contacts. In patients with suspected disseminated GC, culture specimens should be obtained from all primary sites (genital, pharyngeal, rectal) as well as from the blood and all disseminated sites (joints, vesicles). Test-of-cure cultures are recommended in 3 to 7 days for all those with positive cultures.

NEWER METHODS

The traditional method of identifying *N. gonorrhoeae* infection has some limitations. As previously mentioned, false-negative cultures are obtained when the organism is susceptible to vancomycin (up to 10% of all infections). The culture may also be falsely negative if proper collection, handling, and storage guidelines are not followed. Cultures take up to 3 days to grow, and more time may be needed for confirmatory testing. Alternative methods have therefore been developed for the direct detection of gonococcal infection.

The *urinary leukocyte esterase* test, in which a first-catch urine sample is tested with an esterase test strip, has been utilized for screening in males. Cases that test positive are then cultured. The sensitivity, specificity, and positive and negative predictive values have been reported to be 72%, 93%, 58% and 96%, respectively, in males presenting to an sexually transmitted disease clinic.[17] The test's ultimate value for screening has yet to be determined.

Tests to detect *gonococcal antigen* directly in urethral and endocervical fluid have also been developed. The specimen is mixed with a reagent in which antigonococcal antibody conjugated to peroxidase produces a color change in the presence of gonococci. The reaction is related to the number of organisms present and, thus, is more sensitive in males than in females. It may be falsely negative in asymptomatic individuals. Moreover, it cannot be used as a test-of-cure, because residual antigen may be present even in the absence of live gonococci, yielding a false-positive result. A similar test that utilizes the spun urine sediment in males is also available. In one study, it was shown to have a sensitivity of 93% and a specificity of 99%.[25] Its utility would seem to be greatest in a high-risk, symptomatic population.

A relatively new technique for the direct detection on *N. gonorrhoeae* uses a *DNA probe* that detects chromosomal sequences in gonococcal organisms. This 2-hour test has been shown to be extremely sensitive and specific and, in some cases, superior to traditional culture methods.[4, 8, 19, 27] Its utility in the acute setting has yet to be determined.

It must be remembered that, unlike culture, these newer tests do not provide information about antibiotic sensitivity. Penicillin resistance has been reported to vary from 0 to 6% in the United States to as high as 10 to 30% in parts of Asia and Africa.[9, 21]

REFERENCES

1. Eschenback D, Dillior S: Advances in diagnostic testing for vaginitis and cervicitis. *J Reprod Med*, 1989;34:555–565.
2. US Preventative Services Task Force: Screening for sexually transmitted diseases. Am *Fam Physicians*. 1990;42:693–396.
3. Young H, Moyes A: Utility of monoclonal antibody coagglutination to identify *Neisseria gonorrhoeae. Genitourin Med.* 1989;65:8–13.
4. Granato P, Franz M: Evaluation of a prototype DNA probe test for the noncultural diagnosis of gonorrhea. *J Clin Microbiol.* 1989;27:632–635.
5. Thomason J, Gelbart S, Sobieski V, et al: Effectiveness of gonozyme for detection of gonorrhea in low-risk pregnant and gynecologic populations. *Sex Transm Dis*. 1989;16:28–31.
6. Gradus S, Clemet N, Silver K: Comparison of the quad term and 2 hour identification system with conventional carbohydrate degradation tests for confirmatory identification of *Neisseria gonorrhoeae. Sex Transm Dis.* 1989;6:57–59.
7. Begley C, McGill L, Smith P: The incremental cost of screening, diagnosis and treatment of gonorrhea and chlamydia in a family planning clinic. *Sex Transm Dis*. 1989;16:63–67.
8. Schoone G, Cornelissen W, Veenhoijsen P, et al: Comparison of dot blot with in-situ hybridization for the detection of *Neisseria gonorrhoeae* in urethral exudate. *J Appl Bacteriol.* 1989;66:401–405.

9. Ingram C: Gonorrhea: An overview for North Carolina physicians. *N C Med J*. 1989;50:129–130.
10. Brown R, Lossick J, Mosure D, et al: Pharyngeal gonorrhea screening in adolescents: Is it necessary? *Pediatrics* 1989;84:623–625.
11. Giacomini G, Bianchi G, Moretti D: Detection of sexually transmitted diseases by urethral cytology, the ignored male counterpart of cervical cytology. *Acta Cytol*. 1989;33:13–15.
12. Rajasekarian G, Edward S, Shapira D, et al: Direct detection of *N. gonorrhoeae* with monoclonal antibodies characterized by serotyping reagent. *J Clin Microbiol*. 1989;27:1700–1703.
13. Shalor M, Schuactor J, Moscecki A, et al: Urinary leukocyte esterase screening test for asymptomatic chlamydial and gonococcal infections in males. *JAMA*. 1989;262:2562–2566.
14. Cavicchini S, Alessi E: Monoclonal antibody direct immunofluorescence for the identification of *Neisseria gonorrhoeae* strains grown on selective culture media. *Sex Transm Dis*. 1989;16:195–197.
15. Rossan R, Duhamel M, Van Dyck E, et al: Evaluation of an rRNA-derived nucleotide probe for culture confirmation of *Neisseria gonorrhoeae*. *J Clin Microbiol*. 1990;28:944–948.
16. Judson F: Gonorrhea. *Sex Transm Dis*. 1990;74:1353–1366.
17. Dealler S, Gough K, Campbell L, et al: Identification of *Neisseria gonorrhoeae* using the Neisstrip rapid enzyme detection test. *J Clin Pathol*. 1991;44:376–379.
18. Korle K, Mascola J, Miller T: Disseminated gonococcal infection. *Am Fam Physician*. 1992;45:209–214.
19. Panke E, Yang L, Leist P, et al: Comparison of Gen-Probe, DNA probe test and culture for the detection of *Neisseria gonorrhoeae* in endocervical specimens. *J Clin Microbiol*. 1991;29:883–888.
20. Boehm D, Bernhardt M, Kurzynski T, et al: Evaluation of two commercial procedures for rapid identification of *Neisseria gonorrhoeae* using a reference panel of antigenically diverse gonococci. *J Clin Microbiol*. 1990;28:2099–2100.
21. Ravel R (ed): *Clinical Laboratory Medicine*. 5th ed. Chicago: Year Book Medical; 1989;196–197.
22. Tietz N (ed): *Clinical Guide to Laboratory Tests*. 2nd ed. Philadelphia; WB Saunders, 1990;773–777.
23. Henry JB: *Clinical Diagnosis and Management by Laboratory Methods*, 18th ed. Philadelphia: WB Saunders; 1991;1045–1048.
24. Goldenberg D, Reed J: Bacterial arthritis. *N Engl J Med*. 1985;312:764–771.
25. Schuchter J, Pang F, Parks R, et al: Use of gonozyme on urine sediment for diagnosis of gonorrhea in males. *J Clin Microbiol*. 1986;23:124–125.
26. Masi A, Eisenstein B: Disseminated gonococcal infection (DGI) and gonococcal arthritis (GCA) II: Clinical manifestations, diagnosis, complications and prevention. *Semin Arthritis Rheum*. 1981;10:173–197.
27. Totten P, Holmes K, Handsfield J, et al: DNA hybridization technique for the detection of *Neisseria gonorrhoeae* in men with urethritis. *J Infect Dis*. 1983;148:462–471.

Chapter

Chlamydial Culture and Immunoassay

Phil B. Fontanarosa

Chlamydial infection is the most common sexually transmitted disease in the United States, and the incidence appears to be increasing.[1, 2] Clinical findings in symptomatic cases are often indistinguishable from those of other genital infections.[3, 4] More important, many chlamydial infections are asymptomatic or cause only mild symptoms and thus remain untreated, often resulting ultimately in more severe disease and providing a reservoir for further spread of infection.[5]

Reliable, practical, cost-effective, and timely methods for diagnosing and screening for chlamydial infections would clearly be of greater use in the emergency department (ED). Cell culture for *Chlamydia trachomatis* is the most reliable diagnostic method, but it is relatively difficult and expensive, requires considerable processing time, and is not universally available in emergency centers.[6] Nonculture techniques for the rapid detection of chlamydial antigens represent a significant advance in the diagnosis of chlamydial infections and are easily adapted for use in the ED setting.

DIAGNOSTIC STUDIES FOR THE DETECTION OF *CHLAMYDIA* INFECTIONS

Available methods[8–12] for establishing the presence of *C. trachomatis* infections include identification of the organism by direct visualization of intracytoplasmic inclusions, isolation of the organism in tissue cell culture, and detection of chlamydial antigen.

Serum antibody assays are of limited value for the diagnosis of chlamydial infections. Although the characteristic increase in antibody titers between acute and convalescent phases is observed commonly in patients with systemic or more invasive chlamydial infections (e.g., psittacosis, lymphogranuloma venereum), a similar serologic response seldom occurs in patients with urethritis or uncomplicated cervicitis and is uncommon even in patients with documented chlamydial pelvic inflammatory disease.[13] In fact, less than one-third of patients with documented chlamydial genital tract infections ever develop evidence of these antibodies.[14, 15]

Specimen Collection

The reliability of tests for chlamydial infection is highly dependent on the collection, quality, and handling of the specimens. Several important factors must be considered, such as the site sampled, type of swab used, the transport medium, and specimen storage prior to testing.

The optimal specimen for evaluation of *C. trachomatis* infection requires sampling of infected epithelial cells rather than collection of urine, seminal secretions, or vaginal discharge.[9] In men, urethral specimens are collected by inserting a special, thin urethral swab 3 to 5 cm into the urethra and gently rotating the swab. Deep urethral swabbing, rather than meatal swabbing, is necessary for optimal recovery of the organism. In women, exocervical discharge must be removed before the specimen is obtained. The collection swab is then placed in the endocervical canal and rotated against the canal wall for 10 to 15 seconds. The swab should be withdrawn carefully, without touching the vaginal mucosa.

Specimens should be collected with rayon- or cotton-tipped swabs with aluminum or plastic shafts.[10] Specially developed collection brushes also have been advocated and are purported to increase the number of infected cells obtained for examination. Clinical investigations, however, have not proven that these devices are superior to standard swabs for culture and suggest that they are not necessary or cost-effective for routine specimen collection.[11, 12] Swabs provided in commerical enzyme immunoassay kits may be toxic to *C. trachomatis* and, if so, should not be used for collecting specimens for culture.[13]

Immediately after specimen collection, the swab should be placed in appropriate transport medium, which serves to maintain the viability of the organism until the diagnostic assay is performed and suppresses the growth of fungi and other bacteria.[11, 14] Proper transport, handling, and storage of the specimen are essential for an accurate assay and are usually specified by the testing laboratory.

Microscopic Evaluation

Although microscopic examination with vital dyes was the first method used to diagnose chlamydial infections, direct microscopy of stained smears is used infrequently today.[3] Microscopy is most likely to reveal the characteristic signs of intracytoplasmic inclusion bodies in stained infected host cells when tissues have a high concentration of infected cells, as occurs with acute chlamydial conjunctivitis in neonates. This method is unreliable for identifying genital chlamydial infections in adults and usually is not available in the emergency setting.

Gram-stained smears of genital secretions may be helpful in selecting patients in whom infections may be confirmed by other studies. Chlamydial infection is suggested by the presence of 10 or more white blood cells (WBCs) per high power field (HPF) and the absence of intracellular gram-negative diplococci (indicative of *Neisseria gonorrhoeae*) on a Gram-stained smear of urethral discharge in men or cervical discharge in nonmenstruating women.[16, 17]

Cell Culture

Chlamydia are obligate intracellular bacterial pathogens and are somewhat like viruses in that they require viable cells in which to replicate.[7] Consequently, specialized cell culture techniques are necessary to isolate the organism. Traditional cell culture is regarded as the method of choice for definitely establishing chlamydial infection.[14] The specificity of cell culture approaches 100% and thereby provides the rationale for regarding culture as the standard against which nonculture methods are compared.[1, 11] False-positive reports are uncommon but can occur occasionally as a result of technical problems such as reading or staining errors.

Cell culture is far from perfect in diagnosing chlamydial infection. Although the sensitivity of cell culture has been estimated at 80 to 90,[1, 4] later studies report the sensitivity of culture using a single cervical swab to range from 33 to 86%.[18, 19] Approximately 10 to 15% of men with nongonoccocal urethritis who have negative chlamydial cultures develop serum IgM antibody to *C. trachomatis.* Although not a sensitive sign, it is indicative of recent infection.[20]

The occurrence of false-negative results from cell cultures has led some investigators to question cell culture as the definitive diagnostic test.[21] Factors that increase the likelihood of false-negative cultures include a duration of symptoms of less than 7 days, infection with small numbers of organisms, elevated serum antibody level to *C. trachomatis,* and previous treatment with antibiotics. Specimen-dependent factors are the presence of inhibitory substances such as seminal fluid or contraceptive foams, contamination with vaginal secretions, and improper sampling. Technical factors contributing to false-negative studies are the use of improper collection swabs, devices, or transport medium, improper storage of specimens prior to analysis, and delays in inoculating the specimen into cell culture.

Chlamydial cell culture has several other disadvantages. First, the technique requires rigorous transport conditions; specimens must be refrigerated at 4°C to maintain the viability of the organism. Second, the culture procedure is time-consuming, technically difficult to perform, and somewhat limited by cytologic interpretation. Third, cell cultures are expensive, costing approximately $30 to $65 per assay. Fourth, and perhaps of most importance in limiting the usefulness of culture in the ED, is that cultures require a 2- to 5-day turnaround time and are not available in all hospitals.

Antigen Detection Methods

The development of tests that detect chlamydial antigen has been a major advance in the diagnosis of chlamydial genital infections. Two types of antigen detection systems have been developed: (1) direct fluorescent antibody (DFA) staining using monoclonal antibodies and (2) enzyme-linked immunoassay (EIA).

Direct fluorescent antibody requires immunofluorescent microscopy and specialized training for accurate interpretation. Enzyme-linked immunoassay lends itself to automation and is more convenient to use when large batches of specimens are tested. The major advantage of both antigen detection methods is rapidity of results, with estimated turnaround times for the DFA of approximately 35 minutes and for EIA of less than 4 hours, compared with at least 40 hours for traditional cell culture.[22] Antigen detection methods generally are less expensive than tissue cell culture but are also less sensitive. They are a reasonable diagnostic alternative when cell culture technology is not available or is not feasible.[23]

The performance of nonculture methods for the detection of *Chlamydia trachomatis* is summarized in Table 53–1.

Direct Fluorescent Antibody Testing

Stamm[24] analyzed 15 studies that evaluated the DFA technique in high-prevalence and intermediate-prevalence populations. In high-risk women (prevalence of chlamydial infection 15 to 26%), the median sensitivity for the DFA was 90% and the median specificity was 95%. In women with disease prevalence rates of 9 to 11%, DFA had a median sensitivity of 77% and a median specificity of 97%. Kellogg[21] pooled data from 25 studies evaluating DFA for detection of *C. trachomatis* from cervical specimens in women. Patients were not grouped according to risk factors or disease prevalence. The overall sensitivity of the DFA ranged from 55.9 to 100%, and the specificity from 91.8 to 100%.

Similar findings were noted in symptomatic men. In Stamm's[24] analysis, DFA had a median sensitivity of 92% and a specificity of 97% for detecting chlamydial infection. Pooled data from nine additional studies conducted in high-risk or symptomatic men demonstrated sensitivities ranging from 47.8 to 92% and specificities from 90 to 100%.[21]

TABLE 53–1. DETECTION OF *Chlamydia trachomatis* BY NONCULTURE METHODS COMPARED WITH CULTURE[a]

Method and Population	Sensitivity (%)[b]	Specificity (%)[b]	Predictive Value[b]	
			Positive	*Negative*
Direct Immunofluorescence				
Women				
High-prevalence (15–26%)	90 (88–99)	95 (89–99)	90 (68–98)	98 (94–100)
Intermediate-prevalence (9–11%)	77 (61–96)	97 (94–99)	79 (65–93)	98 (94–99)
Low-prevalence (4–8%)	80 (59–100)	98 (95–99)	76 (65–95)	99 (97–100)
Men				
Symptomatic	92 (90–100)	97 (72–99)	87 (82–93)	98 (95–100)
Enzyme Immunoassay				
Women				
High-prevalence (15–26%)	89 (70–98)	95 (86–98)	80 (61–94)	98 (94–99)
Intermediate-prevalence (9–11%)	85 (60–96)	97 (93–98)	70 (45–80)	98 (96–99)
Low-prevalence (4–8%)	83 (78–89)	96 (93–98)	61 (44–80)	99 (98–99)
Men				
Symptomatic	79 (62–95)	97 (96–100)	93 (84–100)	90 (89–94)
Asymptomatic	49 (48–50)	95 (90–100)	85 (69–100)	88 (79–98)

[a]Data compiled and reproduced with permission from Stamm WE: Diagnosis of *Chlamydia trachomatis* genitourinary infections. *Ann Intern Med.* 1988;108:710–717, and Kellogg JA: Clinical and laboratory considerations of culture vs antigen assays for detection of *Chlamydia trachomatis* from genital specimens. *Arch Pathol Lab Med.* 1989;113:453–460. Copyright 1989. American Medical Association.

[b]Values given are median, with range shown in parentheses.

Enzyme Immunoassay

Evaluation of EIA has yielded slightly higher sensitivities than DFA in women with intermediate risk of infection, with similar results in women with high-risk and in men with urethritis. Pooled data from 12 studies of EIA in high-prevalence women revealed a median sensitivity of 89% and a median specificity of 95%, whereas among intermediate-prevalence populations, the median sensitivity and specificity were 85% and 97%, respectively.[24] In another analysis of 14 studies with a total of 6744 women, the overall sensitivity of EIA ranged from 44.4 to 100%, and specificity ranged from 93 to 98%.[21]

Review of seven studies of high-risk or symptomatic men revealed sensitivities ranging from 78.8 to 92% and specificities from 93 to 100%.[21] According to Stamm's analysis,[24] EIA had a median sensitivity of 79% and a median specificity of 95% in symptomatic men, whereas in asymptomatic men, the sensitivity was only 49%.

Within the past several years, technically simple, ultra-rapid EIAs have been introduced. These "desktop" assays, which were designed specifically for office processing of genital specimens, require no specialized equipment or training, take less than 30 minutes to perform, and are estimated to cost approximately $15 per test.[25, 26]

In a study of 1694 endocervical specimens obtained from patients in an intermediate-prevalence (11.6%) population, Coleman and coworkers,[25] reported that, compared with cell culture, rapid chlamydial assays had a sensitivity of 76.5% and a specificity of 99.5%. In a group of high-risk pregnant women with a 13.2% prevalence of chlamydial infection, Grossman and colleagues[26] reported that the rapid assay had a sensitivity of 66.7% and a specificity of 95.4%. In an investigation performed in the ED setting, Thrasher and colleagues[27] examined 166 patients at high risk for chlamydial infection and reported a sensitivity of 68% and a specificity of 97%. Arumainayagam and coworkers[28] evaluated 376 patients using a novel rapid solid-phase immunoassay and reported a sensitivity of 93.% and a specificity of 99% compared with cell culture.

The use of monoclonal antibodies to detect *chlamydia* is a promising technique to improve diagnosis.[29–31] Jawad and associates[29] evaluated the use of an amplified enzyme-linked immunoassay for chlamydia using first-catch morning urine samples in 623 sexually active men. Compared with routine urethral cell culture, this test had a sensitivity of 72.6% and a specificity of 98.6%.

DIAGNOSING CHLAMYDIAL INFECTIONS IN THE ED

The decision to order diagnostic tests for chlamydial infections in the ED should be based on the clinical profile and risk factors of the individual patient, the estimated prevalence of chlamydial infection in the ED population, the intended purpose of the test, and the type of diagnostic studies available.

Indications for Diagnostic Testing in Symptomatic Patients (Table 53–2)

Infections in Women

Specific indications[32–35] for diagnostic testing for *Chlamydia* are (1) clinical evidence of mucopurulent cervicitis, salpingitis, pelvic inflammatory disease, or acute urethritis in women, (2) acute urethritis, proctitis, or epididymitis in men, and (3) a history of exposure to *C. trachomatis* or any other sexually transmitted disease. Even though symptomatic women are treated empirically with agents such as doxycycline or azithromycin prior to the availability of culture results, confirmation of *Chlamydia* infection has several advantages, including clarification of the diagnosis, improvement of the patient's understanding of the illness, possible increased likelihood of medication compliance, and facilitation of management of sexual partners.[24]

Infections in Men

Indications[36–40] for laboratory studies for chlamydial infection are (1) history of high-risk exposure, such as a sexual partner with cervicitis,

TABLE 53–2. INDICATIONS FOR DIAGNOSTIC TESTING FOR *Chlamydia trachomatis*

Symptomatic Women
Mucopurulent cervicitis
Salpingitis
Pelvic inflammatory disease
Acute urethritis
Concomitant gonorrhea infection
History of exposure to *C. trachomatis* or any other STD
Symptomatic Men
Urethritis—urethral discharge, dysuria
Gram stain of urethral discharge with >5 WBCs per HPF
Pyuria in first-voided morning urine specimen
Proctitis
Epididymitis
Sexual partner with cervicitis, pelvic inflammatory disease, documented chlamydia infection, or other STD

pelvic inflammatory disease, or documented chlamydial infection, (2) evidence of urethral infection, such as dysuria or urethral discharge, (3) demonstration by Gram stain of urethral discharge of >5 PMNs/HPF, and (4) pyuria in a first-voided morning urine specimen. Although most infected men can be identified presumptively and are treated empirically before culture results are available, confirmation of chlamydial genital infection has several potential benefits. Knowledge of chlamydial infection improves the ability to identify and treat sexual contacts, has educational benefits for the patient, may have prognostic significance, and has public health implications.[24]

Strategies for Chlamydial Screening (Table 53–3)

The majority of men with nongonococcal urethritis are symptomatic. Chlamydial urethritis can be asymptomatic, however, up to 21 days after exposure.[36] One study reported that nearly one-third of men with documented *Chlamydia* urethral infection seen at a sexually transmitted disease (STD) clinic had no signs or symptoms of urethritis.[37]

Because sexually active women with chlamydial infections may be asymptomatic, liberal screening has been advocated as a necessary and cost-effective public health measure.[33, 41] Routine screening is recommended for sexually active women in health care settings with high rates of chlamydial genital infection.[33–35] Prevalence rates of *C. trachomatis* have been documented as 3 to 5% in women seen in private practice,[42, 43] 9% in a family planning clinic,[33] 10% in a university student health center,[34] 8 to 20% in clinics for adolescent patients,[44, 45]

TABLE 53–3. SCREENING CRITERIA FOR *Chlamydia trachomatis* IN SEXUALLY ACTIVE WOMEN

Adolescents
Adults younger than 25 years old
Nonwhite race
New sexual partner within preceding 2 months
More than one sexual partner within 6 months
Unmarried, pregnant
Bleeding induced by swabbing of endocervical mucosa
Inflamed tissue adjacent to the cervical os
Cervical secretions with >20 WBCs per HPF
Use of no contraception or use of nonbarrier method
Lack of use of antibiotics active against *C. trachomatis* within the preceding month
Patient population with prevalence of chlamydia infection >7%

and 17 to 28% in STD clinics.[32, 43] The ED may provide an appropriate setting for chlamydial screening, although problems with patient compliance and follow-up may limit the effectiveness of the screening program. Screening is indicated for women with specific risk factors for chlamydial infection, including adolescent age range, nonwhite race, new sexual partner, multiple sexual partners, clinical evidence of cervicitis, and being unmarried and pregnant.[1, 24]

Universal screening is prohibitively expensive and impractical, primarily because there is no ideal screening test. Rapid assays are less expensive and easier to perform than cell cultures but may result in unacceptable levels of false-positive tests in low-prevalence populations and of false-negative tests in high-prevalence populations. Therefore, selective screening of women based on their risk of infection appears to be a reasonable strategy.

Several investigators have developed models that group women according to their risk for chlamydial infection. Magder and colleagues[32] prospectively evaluated women attending an STD clinic and identified three high-yield criteria for *C. trachomatis* infection: age less than 25, unmarried status, and concomitant gonorrhea infection or contact. Handsfield and coworkers[33] evaluated 1059 patients attending family planning clinics and identified five independent factors associated with *C. trachomatis* infection: (1) age 24 years or less, (2) intercourse with a new partner within the preceding 2 months, (3) purulent or mucopurulent cervical discharge on examination, (4) bleeding induced by swabbing of the endocervical mucosa, and (5) use of no contraception or a nonbarrier method. These investigators estimated that a screening program that tested women with two or more of these risk factors would detect 90% of all chlamydial infections in the population studied.

Johnson and colleagues[34] developed and prospectively validated a clinical diagnostic model for chlamydial infection in 2271 sexually active university students. They identified the following high-yield variables: new sexual partner within 2 months, more than one sexual partner within 6 months, inflamed tissue adjacent to the cervical os, bleeding from the cervix when touched by an endocervical swab, purulent endocervical discharge with at least 20 PMNs/HPF in cervical secretions, PMNs in vaginal secretions, and lack of use of an antibiotic active against *C. trachomatis* within the preceding month.

Several investigators argue that routine screening becomes cost-effective in populations in which the prevalence of chlamydial infections is greater than 7%.[35, 41] In a decision analysis designed to estimate the clinical and economic implications of testing for chlamydial infection in women during routine gynecologic office visits, Phillips and associates[35] compared a no-test strategy with a strategy involving either the routine use of cultures or the routine use of rapid nonculture tests. In their analysis, overall costs from chlamydial infections would be reduced by routine use of a rapid test if the prevalence of infection was greater than 7% and would be reduced by routine use of culture if the prevalence was 14% or greater.

Selection of the Appropriate Diagnostic Study

The choice of cell culture or antigen detection system is dependent on the capabilities and logistic factors of the particular institution, such as availability of personnel and equipment, volume of studies performed, individual or batch analysis, reagent and assay costs, expected turnaround and reporting times, and quality assurance considerations.

Cell Culture

Despite its disadvantages of cost, relatively long turnaround time, and potential for false-negative results, cell culture remains the standard method for detection of chlamydial infections in ED patients. Because of its high specificity (nearly 100%), cell culture is indicated for the evaluation of low-risk women in low-prevalence ED populations and is the preferred study for screening asymptomatic patients from low-risk populations. In these patients, negative antigen testing does not rule out chlamydial infection, and positive antigen results must be confirmed by culture.

Confirmation by culture is essential in cases in which litigation may be an issue, such as in alleged sexual assault.[14] Cell culture also is recommended for analysis of genital specimens from children because of the increased risk of false-positive antigen detection assays, the increased possibility of contamination with fecal flora, and the association of positive culture results with child abuse.[46]

Antigen Detection Methods

Antigen detection assays are a reasonable alternative to culture for the ED evaluation of chlamydial infections in symptomatic or high-risk women, in populations of women in whom the prevalence of infection is moderately high (>10%), and in symptomatic men. In these patients, DFA and EIA are comparable; both have adequate sensitivity and specificity for reliable diagnosis.[21, 24] In suitably equipped laboratories, results can be available as soon as 30 to 40 minutes after specimen collection, thus confirming the diagnosis while the patient is in the ED, thereby facilitating specific treatment.

Some workers argue, however, that establishing a diagnosis on the basis of positive antigen tests alone and unsupported by confirmatory tests is unacceptable. They therefore recommend routine use of cultures in order to avoid false-positive diagnoses.[14] They argue that false-positive findings would result in unnecessary costs related to antibiotic therapy, follow-up cultures, and repeat office visits. These might then provoke unwarranted anxiety when the patient is erroneously informed of the diagnosis of a sexually transmitted infection.[34]

Furthermore, for low-risk groups, the predictive value of a positive screening test may be low even if the test is highly sensitive and highly specific. For example, in a patient population with a 5% prevalence of chlamydial infection, a rapid antigen screening test with 95% sensitivity and specificity has a positive predictive value of only 50%.[1] Thus, positive results on screening tests require confirmation by other methods such as culture.

By virtue of providing rapid results and being relatively simple to perform in the ED without reliance on the microbiology laboratory, the ultra-rapid EIAs are ideally suited to the emergency setting. Unfortunately, the sensitivity of these assays is unacceptably low and defeats the purpose of an effective screening test. Until these assays are evaluated more carefully in clinical trials, preferably in the ED population, their use cannot be advocated for routine testing in the emergency setting.

CONCLUSION

Despite the increasing incidence of chlamydial infections in ED patients and the ready availability of sophisticated microbiologic tests to detect them, the diagnosis of chlamydial genital infections in the ED remains a challenge. Cell culture is the most commonly used laboratory procedure and remains the standard for diagnosis in most laboratories and clinical settings.[13] Antigen detection methods have achieved widespread popularity, largely because of claims of acceptably high diagnostic accuracy compared with cell culture in symptomatic patients. Clinical investigations have demonstrated that the various antigen detection assays have comparable sensitivity and specificity but that they are highly population-dependent and have significantly lower sensitivity than does cell culture in low-prevalence populations and in screening asymptomatic patients.

In current emergency practice, diagnostic testing for *C. trachomatis* in patients with clinical evidence of genital infection generally does not affect immediate patient management, because empiric treatment is usually instituted before the results of the test are available. The cost-benefit ratio of routine testing in symptomatic patients with suspected chlamydial infections and of widespread ED screening in asymptomatic patients remain to be established.

REFERENCES

1. *Chlamydia trachomatis* infections: Policy guidelines for prevention and control. *MMWR.* 1985;34 (suppl 3S):53S–74S.
2. Thompson SE, Washington AE: Epidemiology of sexually transmitted *Chlamydia trachomatis* infections. *Epidemiol Rev.* 1983;5:96–123.
3. Schachter J: Chlamydial infections. *N Engl J Med.* 1978;298:428–435;490–495;540–549.
4. Krasnoff MJ: Diagnosis and treatment of pelvic inflammatory disease. *Medical Rounds* 1990:3;49–62.
5. Heller M: Chlamydial infections. Ann Emerg Med 1984;13:170–174.
6. Amortegui AJ, Meyer MP: Enzyme immunoassay for detection of *Chlamydia trachomatis* from the cervix. Obstet Gynecol 1985;65:523–526.
7. Bowie WR, Holmes KK: *Chlamydia trachomatis,* in Mandell GL, Douglas RG, Bennett JE (eds): *Principles and Practice of Infectious Diseases,* 3rd ed. New York: Churchill Livingstone; 1991:1426–1440.
8. Magnusson AR, Jui J: Rapid microbial detection systems, in Roberts JR, Hedges JR (eds): *Clinical Procedures in Emergency Medicine.* 2nd ed. Philadelphia: WB Saunders; 1991:1086–1091.
9. Smith TF, Weed LA: Comparison of urethral swabs, urine, and urinary sediment for the isolation of *Chlamydia. J Clin Microbiol.* 1975;2:134–135.
10. Mahony JB, Chernesky MA: Effect of swab type and storage temperature on the isolation of *Chlamydia trachomatis* from clinical specimens. *J Clin Microbiol.* 1985;22:865–867.
11. Weiland TL, Noller KL, Smith TF, et al: Comparison of Dacron-tipped applicator and the Cytobrush for detection of chlamydial infections. *J Clin Microbiol.* 1988;26:2437–2438.
12. Lees MI, Newnan DM, Plackett M, et al: A comparison of Cytobrush and cotton swab sampling for the detection of *Chlamydia trachomatis* by cell culture. *Genitourin Med.* 1990;66:267–269.
13. Taylor-Robinson DT, Thomas BJ: Laboratory techniques for the diagnosis of chlamydial infections. *Genitourin Med.* 1991;67:256–266.
14. Ridgway GL, Taylor-Robinson DT: Current problems in microbiology: Chlamydial infections: Which laboratory test? *J Clin Pathol.* 1991;44:1–5.
15. Sierra MF, Clarke LM, Boyle JF: The laboratory diagnosis of chlamydial infections. *Laboratory Medicine.* 1988;19:311–314.
16. Brunham RC, Paavonen J, Stevens CE, et al: Mucopurulent cervicitis—the ignored counterpart in women of urethritis in men. *N Engl J Med.* 1984;311:1–6.
17. Faro S: *Chlamydia trachomatis. Res Staff Phys.* 1990;36:59–66.
18. Dunlop EM, Goh BT, Darouger S, et al: Triple culture tests for diagnosis of chlamydial infection of the female genital tract. *Sex Transm Dis.* 1985;12:68–71.
19. Smith JW, Rogers RE, Katz BP, et al: Diagnosis of chlamydial infections in women attending antenatal and gynecologic clinics. *J Clin Microbiol.* 1987;25:868–872.
20. Bowie WR, Wang SP, Alexander ER, et al: Etiology of nongonococcal urethritis: Evidence for *Chlamydia trachomatis* and *Ureaplasma urealyticum. J Clin Invest.* 1977;59:735–742.
21. Kellog JA: Clinical and laboratory considerations of culture vs antigen assays

for detection of *Chlamydia trachomatis* from genital specimens. *Arch Pathol Lab Med.* 1989;113:453–460.

22. Baselski VS, McNeeley SG, Ryan G, et al: A comparison of nonculture-dependent methods for detection of *Chlamydia trachomatis* infections in pregnant women. *Obstet Gynecol* 1987;70:47–52.
23. Evans DL, Demetriou E, Shalaby H, et al: Detection of *Chlamydia trachomatis* in adolescent females using direct immunofluorescence. *Clinical Pediatr.* 1988;27:223–228.
24. Stamm WE: Diagnosis of *Chlamydia trachomatis* genitourinary infections. *Ann Intern Med.* 1988;108:710–717.
25. Coleman P, Varitek I, Mushahwar K, et al: TestPack Chlamydia, a new rapid assay for the direct detection of *Chlamydia trachomatis. J Clin Microbiol.* 1989;27:2811–2814.
26. Grossman JH, Rivlin ME, Morrison JC: Detection of chlamydia infection in pregnant women using the Testpack Chlamydia diagnostic kit. *Obstet Gynecol.* 1991;77:801–803.
27. Thrasher G, Terpylak M, Fontanarosa PB, Thomson RB: Evaluation of a rapid immunoassay for the detection of *Chlamydia trachomatis* genital infection [abstract]. *Ann Emerg Med.* 1990;19:958.
28. Arumainayagam JT, Matthews RS, Uthayakumar S, et al: Evaluation of a novel solid-phase immunoassay, Clearview Chlamydia, for the rapid detection of *Chlamydia trachomatis. J Clin Microbiol.* 1990;28:2813–2814.
29. Jawad AJ, Manual G, Matthews R, et al: Evaluation of a genus-specific monoclonal antibody in an amplified enzyme-linked immunoassay in the detection of Chlamydia in urine samples from men. *Sex Transm Dis.* 1990;17:87–89.
30. Horn JE, Hammer ML, Falkow S, et al: Detection of *Chlamydia trachomatis* in tissue culture and cervical scrapings by in situ DNA hybridization. *J Infect Dis.* 1986;153:1155–1159.
31. McPherson JR: DNA probe to detect sexually transmitted disease in female sexual assault victims. [abstract]. *Ann Emerg Med.* 1992;21:623.
32. Magder LS, Harrison HR, Ehret JM, et al: Factors related to genital *Chlamydia trachomatis* and its diagnosis by culture in a sexually transmitted disease clinic. *Am J Epidemiol.* 1988;28:298–308.
33. Handsfield HH, Jasman LL, Roberts PL, et al: Criteria for selective screening for *Chlamydia trachomatis* infection in women attending family planning clinics. *JAMA.* 1986;255:1730–1734.
34. Johnson BA, Poses RM, Fortner CA, et al: Derivation and validation of a clinical diagnostic model for chlamydial cervical infection in university women. *JAMA.* 1990;264:3161–3165.
35. Phillips RS, Aronson MD, Taylor WC, et al: Should tests for *Chlamydia trachomatis* cervical infection be done during routine gynecologic visits? *Ann Intern Med.* 1987;107:188–194.
36. Stamm WE, Cole B: Asymptomatic *Chlamydia trachomatis* urethritis in men. *Sex Transm Dis.* 1986;14:21–25.
37. Stamm WE, Koutsky LA, Benedette JK, et al: *Chlamydia trachomatis* urethral infections in men: Prevalence, risk factors, and clinical manifestations. *Ann Intern Med.* 1984;100:47–51.
38. Karam GH, Martin DH, Flotte TR, et al: Asymptomatic *Chlamydia trachomatis* infections among sexually active men. *J Infect Dis.* 1986;154:900–903.

39. Podgore JK, Holmes KK, Alexander ER: Asymptomatic urethral infections due to *Chlamydia trachomatis* in male U.S. military personnel. *J Infect Dis.* 1982;146:828.
40. Adger H, Shafer MA, Sweet RL, et al: Screening for *Chlamydia trachomatis* and *Neisseria gonorrhoeae* in adolescent males: Value of first-catch urine examination. *Lancet* 1984;2:944–945.
41. Schacter J, Grossman M: Chlamydial infections. *Ann Rev Med.* 1981;32:45–61.
42. Phillips RS, Hanff PA, Holmes MD, et al: *Chlamydia trachomatis* cervical infection in women seeking routine gynecologic care: Criteria for selective screening. *Am J Med.* 1989;86:515–520.
43. Chernesky MA, Mahony JB, Castriciano S, et al: Detection of *Chlamydia trachomatis* antigens by enzyme immunoassay and immunofluoresence in genital specimens from symptomatic and asymptomatic men and women. *J Infect Dis.* 1986;154:141–148.
44. Chacko MR, Lovchik JC: *Chlamydia trachomatis* infection in sexually active adolescents: Prevalence and risk factors. *Pediatrics.* 1984;73:836–840.
45. Fraser JJ, Rettig PJ, Kaplan DW: Prevalence of cervical *Chlamydia trachomatis* and *Neisseria gonorrhoeae* in female adolescents. *Pediatrics.* 1983;71:333–336.
46. Alexander ER: Misidentification of sexually transmitted organisms in children: Medicolegal implications. *Pediatr Infect Dis.* 1988;7:1–2.

Chapter

Sputum Gram Stain

Robert W. Neumar and Michael J. Fine

The sputum Gram stain has traditionally played a key role in the initial diagnostic evaluation of patients with suspected pulmonary infections and is one of the few studies available to the emergency physician that is easily performed with immediately available results at little cost or morbidity. The results can provide a presumptive etiologic diagnosis and prognostic information to guide initial antibiotic therapy and emergency department disposition. Proper use of sputum Gram stain results in clinical decision-making requires an understanding of the sequential steps involved in carrying out and interpreting this procedure. Difficulties in obtaining adequate sputum samples; systematic technical errors in slide preparation; and test sensitivity, specificity, and predictive values must all be considered in the interpretation of results.

INDICATIONS

Sputum Gram stain in the emergency department is indicated for patients in whom pneumonia is suspected according to clinical or radiographic criteria. The main purpose of this test is to determine the etiologic agent of the pneumonia in order to guide antimicrobial therapy and provide prognostic information. The results may also influence the decision to hospitalize the patient. Sputum Gram stain is also critical in determining whether a sputum sample will yield reliable culture results.[1] Kalin and Krook[2] demonstrated that sputum culture positivity for *Pneumococcus* decreased from 52% prior to antibiotic therapy to 8% when sputum was obtained after initiation of antibiotics.[2] Thus, if antibiotics are to be started in the emergency department, a sputum Gram stain should be performed first to confirm that an adequate sputum sample has been obtained. Sputum Gram stain to determine sputum purulence in patients with chronic obstructive pulmonary disease (COPD) exacerbation may be useful in the decision to use empiric antibiotic therapy, but determination of an etiologic agent is difficult because of the high degree of respiratory tract colonization in these patients.[3, 4]

METHODS

Sample Acquisition

The first step in performing a sputum Gram stain is obtaining an adequate sputum specimen. The specimen should always be collected in a sterile container, because the same sample is often sent for routine bacteriologic culture. Ideally, an expectorated sputum sample is representative of secretions from deep in the bronchoalveolar tree; frequently, however, patients provide only oral secretions. Several published prospective studies have reported that expectorated sputum could be obtained in only 78 to 81% of hospitalized patients.[5–7] Of expectorated sputum samples obtained, only 58 to 89% are considered "purulent" or adequate for diagnostic purposes.[6, 8, 9] Thus, an adequate sputum sample is likely to be obtained in less than two thirds of patients with suspected pneumonia. There is some evidence to suggest that sputum collection performed by trained personnel (eg, respiratory technicians) may result in a greater yield of purulent specimens, but studies designed to compare the relative efficacy of different collection methods do not exist.[10] Multiple methods of optimizing sputum acquisition have been reported, including patient observation, instructing the patient to cough deeply prior to expectoration, chest physical therapy, postural drainage, aerosolized saline, mouthwash, and rinsing sample with tap water.[10–12]

If an adequate expectorated sputum sample cannot be obtained, more invasive procedures can be used, such as nasotracheal suctioning, transtracheal aspiration, and bronchoscopy with protected brush techniques.[13, 14] Other than nasotracheal suctioning, these techniques are rarely indicated in the emergency department. Although transtracheal aspiration has been shown to be superior to expectorated sputum in isolation of lower respiratory pathogens, anaerobes in particular,[8, 15] the risk of complications must be weighed against any potential benefit to the patient. Reported complications include subcutaneous emphysema and mediastinal emphysema in less than 5% of patients, hemoptysis, vagal stimulation with associated bradycardia, paroxysmal cough, and hypoxia.[16] This procedure is contraindicated in patients with known coagulopathy, and the risk of subcutaneous and mediastinal emphysema is increased in patients with uncontrolled cough.

Initial Evaluation of Sputum Samples

The purpose of initial evaluation of the sputum sample is to identify the portion of the specimen that is purulent, because this portion is most likely to represent uncontaminated lower airway secretions. Even a sample collected under ideal conditions, however, may be contaminated with upper airway secretions or saliva. The purulent portion of the sample should be identified macroscopically and separated from the remainder of the specimen using a sterile wire loop or wooden spatula. This portion of the specimen is then applied to a glass microscope slide and spread to achieve a uniform application of the sputum sample. After air drying, the sample is heat-fixed by passing the slide through a flame several times. The slide should not become too hot to touch, because overheating may cause staining artifact. The eventual quality of a Gram stain slide is highly dependent on the successful completion of this initial identification and application process. Errors in the application of the sputum sample to the glass slide may actually prevent a meaningful Gram stain interpretation. A 1991 study showed that up to half of Gram stain smears improperly prepared by house staff were so classified because the specimen application was either too thick or too thin.[6]

The Gram Staining Technique and Interpretation

Figure 54–1 summarizes a commonly used and easily applied Gram stain method.[17] The stained specimen should first be reviewed under low-power magnification to confirm the quality of the actual stain. In an appropriately stained specimen, granulocyte nuclei and gram-negative organisms such as *Haemophilus influenzae* stain red, and gram-positive

THE GRAM STAIN METHOD

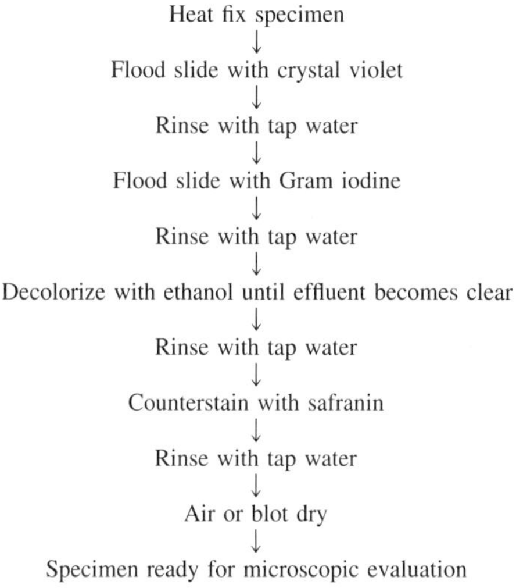

FIGURE 54–1. The heat-fixed specimen is first stained with crystal violet for 10 seconds. After rinsing with tap water, the slide is flooded with Gram iodine for a similar period of time. During the critical decolorizing step, the slide is rinsed with ethanol only until the effluent becomes colorless. Following application of the safranin counterstain for 10 seconds, the slide is rinsed for a final time and then dried in preparation for microscopic evaluation. The entire staining process requires less than 5 minutes to complete. Adapted from Donowitz GR, Mandell GL. Acute pneumonia. In: Mandell DG, Douglas RG, Bennett JE (eds), *Principles and Practices of Infectious Diseases.* New York: Churchill Livingstone, 1990, pp. 541–554.

organisms such as staphylococci stain purple. The most common staining error is under- or over-decolorizing, which can be avoided by decolorizing only until the effluent is colorless.[17]

Once the adequacy of the stain has been established, the specimen should be evaluated to determine whether it is purulent or representative of lower respiratory tract secretions on a microscopic level. Microscopic characteristics of lower respiratory tract specimens are the presence of alveolar macrophages, ciliated bronchial epithelial cells, neutrophils, and elastin fibrils and the relative absence of squamous epithelial cells (which originate from the oropharyngeal cavity and signify contamination by upper airway secretions).[18, 19] Numerous studies have been performed to establish what criteria should be used to determine whether the specific etiologic agent found on Gram stain is indeed the cause of the respiratory infection. These studies are difficult to compare, because no true standards exist and various methods for diagnosing the etiologic agent of pneumonia are used. The various criteria employed to determine purulence include number of buccal epithelial cells, number of polymorphonuclear leukocytes (PMNs), ratio of PMNs to buccal epithelial cells, and location of bacteria on the slide (inside PMNs, associated with PMNs, associated with epithelial cells).[1, 7, 20] In general, if more than 10 to 25 PMNs are present per 100× field and fewer than 10 to 25 buccal epithelial cells per 100× field, or if the ratio of PMNs to buccal epithelial cells is greater than 5:1, the sample can be considered purulent. When these criteria are met, an etiologic diagnosis can be made most accurately if a predominant organism (greater than 50%) is present in a region of the slide not associated with buccal epithelial cells. On the basis of these data, many microbiologists reject sputum specimens that fail to meet these criteria for further Gram stain interpretation or bacteriologic culture because of the high likelihood of contamination by oropharyngeal flora.

An evaluation of the Gram stain appearance and bacterial morphology is initiated after establishing the adequacy of the Gram stain and sputum sample. Several areas of the microscope slide should be scanned under high power (oil immersion lens) to search for areas near leukocytes, because these areas often provide the best opportunity to identify bacterial pathogens from the lower respiratory tract. In contrast, bacteria surrounding epithelial cells almost always represent upper respiratory tract flora.[17] The assessment of the Gram stain appearance includes identification of both gram-positive and gram-negative organisms, if present. When identifying gram-positive organisms, remember that aged or antibiotic-treated gram-positive bacteria may appear gram-negative because their walls are often more permeable to the decolorizing agent.[21]

Once the staining characteristics of the bacteria are established, the next step is to determine the morphology of the potential pathogens. The two basic morphologic forms are the coccus and bacillus. Some bacteria may have a morphology that is intermediate between these forms. If irregularly shaped gram-positive forms are seen, they usually represent precipitated crystal violet, rather than gram-positive cocci or bacilli.

The common bacterial agents in community-acquired pneumonia and their Gram stain and microscopic appearances are summarized in Table 54–1.[17, 22] Although a single pathogen is often identified in a stained sputum specimen, it is not uncommon to have a mixed bacterial pneumonia etiology (eg, *H. influenzae* and *Streptococcus pneumoniae*).[22] The presence of mixed organisms is often overlooked on a Gram stain slide because of an inadequate review of the background of the stained sample. In a sputum specimen from a patient with a mixed infection,

TABLE 54–1. MICROSCOPIC GRAM STAIN AND MORPHOLOGIC APPEARANCE OF COMMON PATHOGENS IN COMMUNITY-ACQUIRED PNEUMONIA

Organism	Gram Stain Appearance	Morphologic Appearance
Streptococcus pneumoniae	Positive	Lancet-shaped diplococci or cocci in pairs or short chains
Haemophilus influenzae	Negative	Coccobacilli
Staphylococcus aureus	Positive	Cocci in clusters
Other streptococcal species	Positive	Cocci in pairs or chains of variable length
Moraxella (Branhamella) catarrhalis	Negative	Intracellular cocci or coccobacilli
Gram-negative rods	Negative	Bacilli or slender rods
''Atypical'' organisms[a]	None	No organisms (predominance of leukocytes)

[a]Atypical organisms in community-acquired pneumonia include *Chlamydia* species *(C. pneumoniae, C. psittaci), Mycoplasma pneumoniae, Legionella* species, *Coxiella burnetii*, and a wide spectrum of viral etiologies.

Data from Donowitz GR, Mandell GL: Acute pneumoniae, in Mandell DG, Douglas RG, Bennett JE (eds): *Principles and Practices of Infectious Diseases.* New York: Churchill Livingstone; 1990:541–544, and Fang GD, Fine MJ, Orloff JJ, et al: New and emerging etiologies for community-acquired pneumonia with implications for therapy: A prospective multicenter study of 359 cases. *Medicine.* 1990;69:307–316.

faintly staining gram-negative organisms such as *H. influenzae* may be rendered nearly invisible by the prominent gram-positive organisms on the smear.[6]

Although it is often assumed that it is possible to define an exact microbiologic etiology on the basis of a sputum Gram stain study, assignment of a microbiologic etiology from the Gram stain alone may result in diagnostic errors. Common bacterial pathogens have characteristic Gram stain appearances, but variations in morphology and appearance frequently exist. For example, *Staphylococcus* may form pairs and short chains mimicking *Streptococcus* rather than the more typical clusters of cocci.[21] As a result, Gram stain findings should be interpreted in conjunction with diagnostic sputum and blood culture results prior to assignment of a definitive or final microbiologic diagnosis.

DIAGNOSTIC PERFORMANCE

Beyond recognition of the appropriate methods of collection, staining, and interpretation, effective use of the sputum Gram stain for clinical decision-making requires an understanding of the diagnostic performance and clinical significance of this test in patients with community-acquired pneumonia. Few studies have attempted to determine the sensitivity and specificity of sputum Gram stain. Results depend on the screening criteria chosen for adequacy of samples, who performs the staining and interprets the slide, and the method used to diagnose the etiologic organism. The methods for determining etiologic agents include quantitative sputum cultures, Gram stain or culture of transtracheal aspirate, blood culture, immunologic techniques, and mouse peritoneal cultures. When bacteriologic sputum culture results are used as the reference standard, the overall sensitivity of the sputum Gram stain has ranged from 48 to 100%.[6, 7, 9, 23] Utilizing blood culture as the reference standard, Gleckman and associates[23] found that the sputum Gram stain had an overall diagnostic sensitivity of 85%. Table 54–2 shows the sensitivity, specificity, and predictive values determined in two prospective studies. With sensitivities ranging from 62 to 86% and specificities ranging from 72 to 88%, it is obvious that the predictive value of the test is extremely dependent on the prevalence of pneumonia in the population studied. In a review of the literature on community-acquired pneumonia, Fang and colleagues[22] found the reported incidence of *Pneumococcus* to range from 9 to 76% and that of *H. influenzae* from 3 to 46%, with no etiologic diagnosis in 30% of cases. Because of this wide variability, it is extremely difficult to determine the predictive value of a sputum Gram stain unless the patient population is well defined.

IMPACT ON PATIENT CARE

Sputum Gram stain has classically been considered an essential part of the standard workup for patients with suspected pulmonary infection. This test is inexpensive, noninvasive, and rapidly performed, and it can provide immediate diagnostic information in patients with community-acquired pneumonia. Difficulties in obtaining adequate sputum samples limit the number of patients who can be studied in this manner. Errors in preparation and interpretation significantly alter the sensitivity and specificity of the tests. Unless the incidence of a particular etiologic agent in the population is known, the predictive value of a positive or negative result cannot be accurately determined. With these limitations in mind, what is the impact of sputum Gram stain on patient care?

Gleckman and associates[23] suggest that in theory, appropriate antibiotic monotherapy could be selected in up to 94% of pneumonia cases when selective, defined criteria for the microbiology of valid sputum are met. Clinicians appear to be more reluctant, however, to prescribe a single antibiotic on the basis of Gram stain results alone. Fine and coworkers[6] reported that only 50% of hospitalized patients with commu-

TABLE 54–2. SENSITIVITY, SPECIFICITY AND PREDICTIVE VALUE OF SPUTUM GRAM STAIN

				Predictive Value (%)		
Study	**Etiologic Agent**	**Sensitivity (%)**	**Specificity (%)**	*Positive*	*Negative*	**Prevalence (%)**
Fine et al (1991)[6]	*Pneumococcus*	86	72	43	95	10
	Haemophilus influenzae	80	88	73	92	7
Rein et al (1978)[7]	*Pneumococcus*	62	85	90	50	69

nity-acquired pneumonia were treated with single-antibiotic therapy when a predominant organism was identified on Gram stain, versus 30% when no predominant organism was identified ($P < 0.05$). Although early identification of a specific bacterial pathogen has been shown to predict a rapid clinical improvement with directed antibiotic therapy, the marked difference between the theoretic and actual selection of monotherapy in patients with a predominant etiologic agent identified reflects clinicians' lack of confidence in the diagnostic performance of sputum Gram stains. The use of narrow-spectrum or single antibiotic agents certainly has the potential for reducing the cost of caring for patients with pneumonia. The cost of not initially covering the etiologic agent, however, in terms of hospital days and possible ICU time, must also be considered.

Sputum Gram stain can provide information to aid the emergency physician in deciding the disposition of patients with community-acquired pneumonia. Fine and coworkers[24] studied the impact of the etiology of pneumonia on the risk of a complicated course in patients without indication for admission. Patients with a confirmed diagnosis of staphylococcal, gram-negative rod, aspiration, or postobstructive pneumonia had a relative risk of 23.1 (95% confidence interval 2.7–200.7) for complications. Fourteen percent (6/44) of the patients in this study without clinical criteria for admission (based on modified Appropriateness Evaluation Protocol) had either confirmed staphylococcal or gram-negative pneumonia. Thus, demonstration of predominantly gram-negative rods or *Staphylococcus* on Gram stain should be considered an indication for hospital admission in a patient who may otherwise have been discharged.

It is well documented that COPD patients with a documented bacterial cause of exacerbation benefit from antibiotic therapy. The determination of bacterial bronchitis may be aided by a sputum Gram stain more by showing purulence than by confidently identifying the etiologic agent. Focused antibiotic therapy is difficult, however, because of the colonization of the upper respiratory tract in these patients.

REFERENCES

1. Murray PR, Washington JA II: Microscopic and bacteriologic analysis of expectorated sputum. *Mayo Clin Proc.* 1975;50:339–344.
2. Kalin M, Krook A: Comparison of three methods for detection of pneumococcal antigen in sputum of patients with community-acquired pneumonia. *Eur J Clin Microbiol Infect Dis.* 1989;8:956–961.
3. Chodosh S: Sputum cytology in chronic bronchial disease. *Adv Asthma Allergy.* 1977;4:8–27.
4. Baigelman W, Chodosh S, Pizzuto D: Quantitative sputum Gram stains in chronic bronchial disease. *Lung.* 1979;156:265–270.

5. Levy M, Dromer F, Brion N, et al: Community-acquired pneumonia; importance of initial noninvasive bacteriologic and radiographic investigations. *Chest.* 1988;92:43–48.
6. Fine MJ, Orloff JJ, Rihs JD, et al: Evaluation of housestaff physician's preparation and interpretation of sputum Gram stains for community acquired pneumonia. *J Gen Intern Med.* 1991;6:189–198.
7. Rein MF, Gwaltney JM, O'Brien WM, et al: Accuracy of Gram's stain in identifying pneumococci in sputum. *JAMA.* 1978;239:2671–2673.
8. Glecker RW, Gremillion DH, McCallister CK, Ellenbogen C: Microscopic and bacteriological comparison of paired sputa and transtracheal aspirates. *J Clin Microbiol.* 1977;6:396–399.
9. Kalin M, Lindberg AA, Tunevall G: Etiological diagnosis of bacterial pneumonia by Gram stain and quantitative culture of expectorates. *Scand J Infect Dis.* 1983;15:153–160.
10. Chodosh S: Sputum examination, in Fishman AP (ed): *Pulmonary Diseases and Disorders.* New York: McGraw-Hill; 1988:411–426.
11. Spada EL, Tinivella A, Carli S, et al: Proposal of an easy method to improve routine sputum bacteriology. *Respiration.* 1989;56:137–146.
12. Bartlet JG, Finegold SM: Bacteriology of expectorated sputum with quantitative culture and wash technique compared to transtracheal aspirates. *Am Rev Respir Dis.* 1978;117:1019.
13. Winterbauer RH, Hutchinson JF, Reinhardt GN, et al: The use of quantitative cultures and antibody coating of bacteria to diagnose bacterial pneumonia by fiberoptic bronchoscopy. *Am Rev Respir Dis.* 1983;128:98–103.
14. Kalinske RW, Parker RH, Brandt D, et al: Diagnostic usefulness and safety of transtracheal aspiration. *N Engl J Med.* 1967;276:604–608.
15. Bartlett JG, Rosenblatt JE, Finegold SM: Percutaneous transtracheal aspiration in the diagnosis of anaerobic pulmonary infection. *Ann Intern Med.* 1973;79:535–540.
16. Spencer DC, Beaty HN: Complications of transtracheal aspiration. *N Engl J Med.* 1972;6:304–306.
17. Donowitz GR, Mandell GL: Acute pneumonia, in Mandell DG, Douglas RG, Bennett JE (eds): *Principles and Practices of Infectious Diseases.* New York: Churchill Livingstone; 1990:541–554.
18. Shlaes DM, Lederman MM, Chmielewski R, et al: Sputum elastin fibers and the diagnosis of necrotizing pneumonia. *Chest.* 1984;85:763–766.
19. Epstein RL: Constituents of sputum: A simple method. *Ann Intern Med.* 1972;77:259–265.
20. Heineman HS, Chawla JK, Lofton WM: Misinformation from sputum cultures without microscopic examination. *J Clin Microbiol.* 1977;6:518–527.
21. Gardner P, Provine HT: Lower respiratory tract infections, in *Manual of Acute Bacterial Infections.* Boston: Little, Brown; 1984:37–66.
22. Fang GD, Fine MJ, Orloff JJ, et al: New and emerging etiologies for community-acquired pneumonia with implications for therapy: A prospective multicenter study of 359 cases. *Medicine.* 1990;69:307–316.
23. Gleckman R, DeVita J, Hibert D, Pelletier MR: Sputum Gram stain assessment in community-acquired pneumonia. *J Clin Microbiol.* 1988;26:846–849.
24. Fine MJ, Smith DN, Singer DE: Hospitalization decision in patients with community-acquired pneumonia: A prospective cohort study. *Am J Med.* 1990;89:713–721.

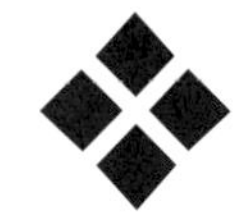

Chapter 55 Chest Radiography

W. Scott Morse

Even in this day of ultrasound, computed tomography, and magnetic resonance imaging, the chest radiograph remains the most frequently ordered radiologic examination. The chest radiograph (CXR) can provide the emergency physician with a wealth of information in a short time with little risk to the patient and at relatively low cost. As with any test, the effective use of the CXR is determined by several factors. What are the indications for the test? What is the likelihood that it will yield useful information? What are the costs and risks involved?

INDICATIONS

Patients for whom a chest radiograph is performed in the emergency department fall into two categories: those in whom the radiograph is obtained to detect disease and those in whom it is obtained for other reasons, such as to provide a baseline, for medicolegal indications, or for patient reassurance.[1] Radiographs done to detect disease can be divided into two further categories—diagnostic chest radiographs (DCXRs) (ie, studies directed by physical signs or symptoms related to diseases of the thorax, such as chest pain, hemoptysis, and cough) and screening chest radiographs (SCXRs) performed to detect occult disease.

It was hoped at one time that the SCXR would be an effective means of identifying patients with occult disease. In particular, it was thought that early detection of lung carcinoma and tuberculosis would result in an improvement in the cure rate of the former and prevent the spread of the latter. In neither case, however, has this hope been borne out.

Feingold[2] reviewed the admission radiographs of over 39,000 patients from the Grady Memorial Hospital in 1972. Of the six previously unsuspected cases of tuberculosis that were discovered, all would have

TABLE 55–1. FINDINGS IN THE PATIENT'S HISTORY ASSOCIATED WITH POSITIVE FINDINGS ON CHEST RADIOGRAPHY

Fever	COPD
Shortness of breath	Chills
Occupational exposure	Cough
Cancer anywhere	Smoking
Asthma	Myocardial infarction
Weight loss	AIDS
Hemoptysis	Chest pain
Age > 40??	Angina
Stroke	

required DCXRs because of associated signs or symptoms. No patients without signs or symptoms were found to have TB.

Boucot and Weiss[3] found that patients whose cancer was discovered early by mass screening had no improvement in 5-year survival. In a Mayo Clinic study of 12,000 women who had prenatal SCXRs, 48 patients were found to have appreciable abnormalities on radiography. Abnormal findings from the history or physical examination, however, would have led to the performance of a DCXR in all 48. No abnormalities were found in patients with normal histories and physical findings.[4]

Screening CXRs have also proved to be unrewarding in children. In an analysis of SCXRs done on 1000 children from high-prevalence tuberculosis areas in New York, 6% had radiographic abnormalities, 66% of which were minor skeletal abnormalities and none of which required medical or surgical treatment.[5] Similar studies have corroborated these findings.[6, 7]

When does screening radiography become diagnostic radiography? What are the history and physical findings that indicate the possibility of abnormal CXR findings? Tables 55–1 and 55–2 present symptoms and signs found by various groups to be associated with a higher incidence of abnormal radiographic findings.[1, 7, 8, 9, 10]

Sagel and associates[7] found that of 5975 SCXRs reviewed, only 4%

TABLE 55–2. FINDINGS ON PHYSICAL EXAMINATION ASSOCIATED WITH SIGNIFICANT CHEST RADIOGRAPHY FINDINGS

Altered mental status	Severe murmurs
Fever	Abdominal tenderness
Tachypnea	Organomegaly
Abnormal breath sounds or dullness	Ascites
Tachycardia	

showed abnormalities and only 7 (0.12%) of the patients had radiographic abnormalities that changed therapeutic management. In contrast, CXRs that were done because of signs or symptoms detected serious abnormalities 54% of the time. Rucker and colleagues[8] noted a similar absence of radiographic findings on the screening chest radiographs of 504 patients.

Benacerraf and coworkers[9] concluded, from their study of 1102 patients with complaints related to the chest, that any patient who has signs or symptoms of thoracic disease and is over the age of 40 years should receive a DCXR. The frequency of abnormal radiographic findings in these patients continued to increase with age. In patients under the age of 40, positive physical findings or hemoptysis was an especially good predictor of abnormal radiographic findings.

White and associates[10] found that patients who did not have signs and symptoms directly related to the thorax but who were members of ''high-risk'' groups (65 years or older, cigarette smokers, HIV positive, with altered mental status) had a significant number of abnormal findings on radiography that subsequently altered treatment. Of patients who were not in the high-risk groups, some had abnormalities detected on SCXR but for none was treatment altered by the finding.

Although studies to date overwhelmingly indicate that the absence of pertinent findings from the history or physical examination makes it unlikely that the CXR will contribute to the patient's management, it must be emphasized that whether it is to safer eliminate the CXR from the workup depends on the accuracy with which the history and physical examination are performed. Hubbell and coworkers[1] found that of 20 patients classified by house staff as candidates for SCXR and found to have new abnormalities on chest radiography, eight actually had findings on history and physical examination that, if detected, would have indicated a greater likelihood of chest disease. Seemingly unrelated signs and symptoms may be associated with CXR abnormalities (eg, the intoxicated patient who may have aspirated, the patient with an altered level of consciousness who has pneumonia). Berk and colleagues[11] noted that among elderly patients with *Escherichia coli* pneumonia, lethargy was the earliest symptom, preceding cough and fever by 1 to 2 days. Likewise, the CXR is an integral part of the workup in a child with an unexplained source of fever or in the neonate who presents with a history of lethargy, poor feeding, or irritability.[12]

If the patient's signs and symptoms are not indicative of thoracic pathology, the emergency physician may still find it valuable to obtain a CXR. For instance, the examination may be of use as a baseline study in the patient about to undergo emergency surgery or an invasive procedure (eg, central line placement). Mendelson and coworkers'[13] study of postoperative patients' chest radiographs showed that the preoperative radiographs were essential to accurate interpretation of the postoperative CXRs 51% of the time. In 9% of 369 patients undergoing general surgery, the quality of postoperative care was improved by the availability of a baseline study.

The physician ordering the CXR must decide whether there is value to be gained from a medicolegal standpoint or from the reassurance that a normal radiograph provides the concerned patient. As to the former issue, certain clinical situations (motor vehicle accidents, assaults) may require radiographic documentation for legal or insurance purposes. In addition, performing a chest radiograph on a patient who unreasonably demands one may in fact be extremely cost-effective in preventing complaints or litigation. In any event, it may also keep the patient from seeking the same test at another emergency department.[14] The value of the CXR in providing reassurance should also not be underestimated.

RISKS

In the realm of imaging studies, the radiograph is relatively risk-free, the main concern being that of patient exposure to radiation. The radiation exposure from chest radiography is minimal, however. Dosage received from a PA view of the chest is about 10 millirems (mrem), whereas that from a lateral view is in the range of 50 to 100 mrem.[15] These doses do not significantly increase the risk of cancer.[16]

Certainly, no activity is without risk. It is estimated that a chest radiograph may increase the risk of death by .000001. This makes the risk of undergoing chest radiography equivalent to that of flying 1000 miles by jet, smoking 1.4 cigarettes, living 2 days in New York, or traveling 6 minutes by canoe.[17]

With respect to the pregnant patient, radiation exposure should at all times be minimized. If there are indications for the study, however, it should not be postponed or omitted. With shielding, the exposure of the fetus to radiation from chest radiography is about 1 mrem. Fetal risk from radiation exposure is not considered problematic unless the exposure has been greater than 5 rads (approximately equivalent to 5 rem).[18]

COST

The charge to the patient for a chest radiograph in most hospitals remains under $100.[19] Little has been written about the actual cost of providing the service. It is difficult to estimate the actual savings to society that would come about as a result of reducing the number of CXRs. Hubbell and coworkers[1] have estimated that 30 million screening chest radiographs were performed in 1980. At an average charge of $50, simple arithmetic would imply a cost savings to society of $1.5 billion. Whether this savings would truly be realized or whether the revenue lost to providers by the elimination of this test would simply be made up by increasing the charges for other examinations is unknown.

Other variables that are more difficult to quantitate must also be considered. What are the consequences of a finding that was missed because a CXR was omitted? What harm might befall the patient? How much time might the patient miss from work if the diagnosis is not made as soon as possible? What are the additional costs of a delay in diagnosis to the health care system and to the patient? Given the large number of variables that must be addressed and the relatively inexpensive nature of the examination, it seems advisable to obtain the study whenever signs or symptoms indicative of chest disease are present.

TECHNICAL FACTORS

When considering the CXR, the reviewing physician must first determine whether the technique used in obtaining the film provides adequate visualization of the areas of concern. Second, one must decide whether the position of the patient and the phase of respiration during which the film was taken were appropriate, given the clinical concerns. Some simple guidelines allow the emergency physician to ensure that the radiograph being reviewed is technically reasonable.

First, the entire thorax must be on the film. Second, the patient should be properly centered on the film and should not be rotated. If one side of the thorax is closer to the x-ray beam, that side will appear more lucent than the other. This appearance may lead the reviewer to mistake the abnormal lucency for a pneumothorax or, conversely, to assume that there is a large effusion on the less lucent side. Third, the film should be free of motion, and tissue edges such as those of the ribs and pulmonary vasculature should be sharp. Fourth, for most patients, maximum information is obtained when the film is taken at full inspiration. Fifth, the reviewer should be able to just see the vertebrae and disk spaces of the thoracic spine, and the lung markings behind the heart should be clearly visible. An overexposed film can sometimes be compensated for by increasing the illumination used in reviewing (ie, "bright-lighting"), but an underexposed film is never acceptable.[20]

The density of tissues in the thorax varies widely. The technique generally used is a compromise that allows all the components of the thorax to be seen well but none to be seen optimally. Occasionally, varying the standard technique can improve visualization of a particular area of interest.

Most studies of the chest consist of a posteroanterior (PA) projection and a lateral projection. Although the usefulness of the lateral projection is occasionally questioned, it should be considered an essential part of the examination in the symptomatic or high-risk emergency patient. In Sagel and colleagues'[7] study of 4500 patients with signs or symptoms, the lateral projection was confirmatory or clarifying in 1047 (23%); in 83 patients (2%), an abnormality was detected only on the lateral projection.

In many cases, the patient is unable to be brought to the radiology unit. An examination can be done with a portable machine at the bedside using an anteroposterior projection. Such examinations may be technically inferior to the standard PA projection, because of the need for longer exposure times and patient positioning problems. Care must be taken in interpreting a bedside or portable film, which has a shorter focus-to-film distance, resulting in magnification of the cardiac silhouette by 15 to 20%. Many bedside films are taken with the patient in the supine position; blood flow to the upper lobes is 30% greater in supine patients. Prominent pulmonary vasculature on a supine film should not be mistaken for pulmonary venous hypertension.[20] An erect film may help to differentiate between the two. Despite such limitations, the portable film can be invaluable in the patient's management. Moreover, the technical limitations inherent in the portable film need not preclude accurate interpretation of the study. Humphreys and associates[21] found that the ability of physicians to recognize changes of CHF, cardiomegaly, infiltrate, or pleural effusion on portable films compared favorably with that on PA and lateral projections.

Films normally are taken in full inspiration. The addition of a film taken in expiration may be helpful in two situations. Children with retained bronchial foreign bodies may demonstrate air trapping on expiration. The CXR shows increased lucency of the affected lung, shift of the mediastinum to the opposite side, and failure of the ipsilateral diaphragm to elevate. The expiratory film may also be of use in the patient with a suspected pneumothorax (PTX). Because the amount of air trapped inside the pleural space is proportionately greater relative to the lung on expiration, the separation of the pleural surfaces may be better seen on a view taken during this phase of respiration.

Another projection that may be of help is the lordotic view. Taken with the patient leaning backward against the cassette or with the tube angled 15° cephalad, it can eliminate the overlying clavicular and first rib shadows that can obscure the apices of the lung.

When AP or PA views are questionable for determining the presence of air or fluid in the pleural space, lateral decubitus films may provide the answer. Radiographs taken in this position can reveal as little as 100 mL of fluid.[20] In the patient in whom PTX is suspected but who is unable to control respiration, a decubitus film taken with the affected side up causes the air to rise and makes the PTX visible. The decubitus film may also be of help in the child suspected of having a bronchial foreign body. Because the dependent side of the thorax is effectively splinted against the x-ray table, inflation should be less on that side than on the nondependent side; with air trapping, the affected lobe remains hyperlucent.

Oblique views can be used when the question of retrocardiac or retrohilar pathology arises. Computed tomographic (CT) scanning or standard tomography generally provide better visualization of these areas, however.

CLINICAL APPLICATIONS OF CHEST RADIOGRAPHY

As noted previously, there are very few reasons *not* to order a chest radiograph in a symptomatic patient. The relative sensitivity and specificity of this test vary widely, however, for various medical and surgical problems, as described in this section.

The Trauma Patient

The presence of chest trauma is indication enough to obtain a chest radiograph. Indeed, severe trauma to other areas of the body should be considered an indication for chest radiography, because certain extrathoracic injuries, such as severe head injury, long bone fracture, pelvic fracture, and abdominal injury requiring surgery, have been associated with a higher risk of thoracic injury.[22]

The CXR has proved to be far more accurate than the physical examination in detecting thoracic injuries. A normal CXR, however, should not dissuade the physician from obtaining additional studies if clinical indications warrant. McGonigal and associates[22] found that a number of injuries detected on CT were initially missed on CXR.

Pneumothorax

Most pneumothoraces are readily apparent on CXR, but the diagnosis may be difficult to make when the film is of the patient in the supine position, because the lung tends to collapse posteriorly rather than medially as in the erect patient, making interpretation difficult. The only radiographic evidence of a PTX may be a deep lateral costophrenic angle on the involved side, termed the ‘‘deep sulcus sign’’ by Gordon.[23] A lateral decubitus or cross-table lateral film may be of help in revealing occult air. Computed tomography has been shown to be superior to

CXR in detecting occult pneumothorax.[24] In another series, when compared with CT, the sensitivity of the CXR was only 42% for these small pneumothoraces.[22]

Hemothorax

Although as little as 100 mL of blood in the pleural cavity can be detected when special views are used, a large amount of blood can produce only a minor change on the CXR, especially if the film is taken with the patient supine. Schmidgall and Jui[25] estimate that almost 1000 mL of blood can accumulate in the thorax with very little change in radiographic findings. Decubitus films or CT scans may aid in the diagnosis of hemothorax.

Pulmonary Contusion

Pulmonary contusion usually manifests on CXR as fluffy white opacities suggesting air space consolidation. Absence of CXR findings does not indicate absence of pulmonary contusion, and CT scanning can demonstrate significant lung injury that escapes detection on CXR.[23] Johnson and associates[26] found that the extent of pulmonary contusion as assessed on the admission CXR was not predictive of mortality or of the need for intubation. The extent of pulmonary compromise was better assessed by a combination of CT and the PO_2/FIO_2 ratio.[26]

Traumatic Aortic Rupture or Great Vessel Injury

Various findings on the CXR have been reported in patients with thoracic aortic tears[27, 28] and are listed in Table 55–3. Unfortunately,

TABLE 55–3. CHEST RADIOGRAPH FINDINGS REPORTED IN PATIENTS WITH TRAUMATIC RUPTURE OF THE THORACIC AORTA

Mediastinal widening
Loss of the aortic arch contour
Focal bulge in the aorta
Deviation of the trachea to the right
Presence of a pleural cap
Fractures of the first and second ribs
Elevation and rightward shift of the right mainstem bronchus
Depression of the left mainstem bronchus
Obliteration of the space between the pulmonary artery and the aorta
Deviation of the NG tube to the right
Displaced right paraspinous stripe

none of these has been shown to be reliably accurate in detecting aortic injury.

Much attention has been directed toward mediastinal widening in particular. Mediastinal widening can be seen on the CXRs of normal patients taken in the supine position, and the widening reverts to normal when the radiographs are repeated in the upright position. Woodring and King[29] found that only 5% of normal subjects had a mediastinal width greater than 7.5 cm. Of 32 patients with known aortic injury, however, 41% had normal mediastinal width. These researchers noted that if a cutoff width small enough to detect all of the abnormal cases was used, the false-positive rate among patients without injury rose to 74%. Interestingly, however, Woodring and King[29] found evidence of one of the other radiographic signs of injury listed in Table 55–3 in 94% of their injured patients.

Building on this work, Huang and coworkers[30] performed a regression analysis of various CXR findings in an attempt to determine whether a combination of plain film findings might allow for accurate prediction of aortic injury. They found that a formula using a combination of loss of aortic contour, tracheal deviation, and abnormal mediastinum-to-chest width ratio allowed them to detect all patients with rupture and to exclude patients without aortic injury. These investigators cautioned that a prospective study needed to be done to confirm the validity of their approach. Computed tomography may have a role in excluding patients from angiography,[31] but until additional work is done with this modality, the indications for angiography remain subjective, and it should not be postponed on the basis of normal CXR findings.

Diaphragmatic Injury

The chest radiograph is notoriously insensitive in detecting diaphragmatic injuries.[31, 32] A lateral view can be of help in detecting a ruptured diaphragm, as can a small amount of barium instilled into the gastrointestinal tract. If questions persist, a CT scan may provide the answer.[23]

Medical Emergencies

The CXR can be invaluable in discriminating among the large number of medical problems that can cause the signs and symptoms listed in Tables 55–1 and 55–2. Radiographic changes representing effusions, infiltrates, collapse, vascular overload, and other pulmonary and mediastinal pathology can be readily detected. As in the trauma patient, however, a normal chest radiograph should not provide a sense of security about patients who present with signs and symptoms of thoracic disease.

The chest radiograph remains a valuable part of the diagnostic process. Although not worthwhile as a screening examination, the CXR can provide critical clinical information in the symptomatic patient. Care must be taken, however, not to overemphasize the significance of a normal study in the symptomatic patient.

Pulmonary Embolism

Patients with pulmonary emboli are notable for presenting with dyspnea or chest pain and having a normal chest radiograph. Various radiographic signs have been associated with the presence of pulmonary embolism (eg, triangular pleural-based mass with the apex toward the hilum, abrupt cutoff of a pulmonary artery, unilateral hypolucent lung). The CXR, however, has proved to be unreliable in the detection of pulmonary embolism,[33] and pulmonary angiography remains the standard. Still, omission of the chest radiograph in the patient with signs and symptoms of pulmonary emboli is ill-advised, because any of a number of other problems can cause these symptoms. Moreover, accurate interpretation of the ventilation/perfusion scan requires correlation with a chest radiograph. Thus, the CXR remains a necessary part of the workup.

Tuberculosis

Tuberculosis is found commonly in patients who are infected with HIV or who are otherwise relatively immunocompromised (eg, diabetics, transplant patients, elderly patients). Although upper lobe infiltrates or cavitary lesions should suggest the possibility of TB, the proportion of patients with extrapulmonary TB is increasing, especially HIV-infected patients.

Pneumocystis carinii *Pneumonia (PCP)*

The CXR signs of PCP can be very subtle, consisting of fine reticular perihilar changes that progress to air space consolidation.[34] These findings, however, are often not present. In one study, seven of 20 patients (35%) with proven PCP had a normal CXR on admission.[35] Doppman and associates[36] found characteristic radiographic findings in only 43% of their patients with PCP.

Pneumonia

Physicians have been known to underestimate and overestimate the presence of pneumonia in patients presenting with respiratory symptoms.[37] In an attempt to more clearly identify patients who would benefit from radiography, several researchers have proposed decision rules that would decrease the number of radiographs ordered.[38–40] Comparison of these methodologies with the clinician's judgment was made by Emerman and colleagues.[37] Clinical judgment was found to be more sensitive, but the presence of certain clinical features was more specific and more accurate overall. These features were the presence of at least one abnormal vital sign, decreased breath sounds or rales, absence of asthma, temperature greater than 37.8°C, or pulse greater than 100.

In patients with positive radiographs, the findings may vary from a focal area of increased opacification, small diffuse areas of increased density, or increased interstitial markings, to a combination of the three. The presence of a particular radiographic pattern is not specific for a particular organism, and attempting to identify an organism from the patient's chest radiograph is not worthwhile. As with other conditions discussed, a normal radiograph in the patient with clinical indications of pneumonia may be misleading. The leukopenic or dehydrated patient with pneumonia may not initially have CXR findings. As with other patients, the overall clinical impression should guide therapy.

Sickle Cell Crisis

Patients with known sickle cell disease often present with painful vaso-occlusive crisis. The sickle chest pain syndrome in and of itself does not produce radiographic findings (unless there is primary pulmonary infarction). There has been some question as to whether the CXR is worthwhile in these patients. In a 1991 study, however, 12% of children and 6% of adults presenting with painful sickle cell crisis were found to have underlying pneumonia, indicating that the CXR may remain a worthwhile evaluation in these patients.[41]

Asthma

Patients with asthma usually present with dyspnea, cough, wheezing, or tachycardia, any one of which is a reasonable indication for obtaining a CXR. Some investigators have argued, however, that the low incidence of positive radiographic findings in adults and children with asthma should preclude obtaining a CXR unless the patient shows no response to initial bronchodilator therapy or, in children, if rales or rhonchi were present.[42] White and colleagues[43] confirmed that patients with asthma unresponsive to an initial course of bronchodilators had a high incidence (34%) of CXR abnormalities. Aronson and coworkers[44] built on these findings, noting that no abnormal CXRs were found in their group of 81 patients with uncomplicated asthma (no fever, chills, or underlying disease), whereas in 13 of the 44 patients with complications, the initial CXR had an impact on admission.

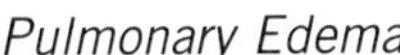

Pulmonary Edema

Pulmonary edema is most practically diagnosed using chest radiography, and it can be detected earlier by CXR than by physical examination.[45] Engorgement of pulmonary vessels, increased interstitial markings, and alveolar infiltrates are the radiographic findings traditionally used to make the diagnosis. Milne and associates,[45] employing these findings along with vascular pedicle size, distribution of edema, and heart size, were able not only to diagnose the presence of edema but also to differentiate between types of edema 89% of the time.

Aortic Dissection

The sensitivity and specificity of the CXR for detecting dissection of the thoracic aorta are poor.[46] Aortography, magnetic resonance imaging (MRI), or transesophageal echocardiography should be employed if aortic dissection is suspected.

Exacerbation of COPD

The initial diagnosis of chronic obstructive pulmonary disease is usually made on the basis of a patient's history, physical examination, and pulmonary function testing. Radiographic findings such as an increased anteroposterior diameter, flattened diaphragms, increased lung volumes, and loss of pulmonary vascular and interstitial markings have a secondary role in diagnosis. Patients who present with a history of COPD or comorbid underlying conditions[44] were found to have a treatment-altering radiographic abnormality 21% of the time.[47] Other researchers have similarly recommended that CXR should be routine in patients experiencing acute exacerbations of COPD.[48]

REFERENCES

1. Hubbell FA, Greenfield S, Tyler JL, et al: The impact of routine admission chest X-ray films on patient care. *N Engl J Med.* 1985;312:209–213.
2. Feingold AO: Routine chest roentgenograms on hospital admission do not discover tuberculosis. *South Med J.* 1977;70:579–580.
3. Boucot RB, Weiss W: Is curable lung cancer detected by semiannual screening? *JAMA.* 1973;224:1361–1365.
4. Bonebrake CR, Noller KL, Loehnen CP, et al: Routine chest roentgenography in pregnancy. *JAMA.* 1978;240:2747–2748.
5. Brill PW, Ewing ML, Dunn AA: The value (?) of routine chest radiography in infants and adolescents. *Pediatrics.* 1973;52:156–158.
6. Farnsworth PB, Steiner E, Klein RM, et al: The value of preoperative chest roentgenograms in infants and children. *JAMA.* 1980;244:582–583.

7. Sagel SS, Evens RG, Forrest JV, et al: Efficacy of routine screening and lateral chest radiographs in a hospital based population. *N Engl J Med.* 1974;291:1001–1004.
8. Rucker L, Frye EB, Staten MA: Usefulness of screening chest roentgenograms in preoperative patients. *JAMA.* 1983;250:3209–3211.
9. Benacerraf BR, McCloud TC, Rhea JT, et al: An assessment of the contribution of chest radiography in outpatients with acute chest complaints: A prospective study. *Radiology.* 1981;138:293–299.
10. White CS, Austin JHM, Lubetsky HW, et al: The impact of chest radiography on the management of patients admitted from an emergency service. *Invest Radiol.* 1990;25:720–723.
11. Berk SL, Neumann P, Holtsclaw S, et al: *Escherichia coli* pneumonia in the elderly: With reference to the role of *E. coli* capsular polysaccharide antigen. *Am J Med.* 1982;72:899–902.
12. Berkowitz C: The febrile child, in Tintinalli JE, Rothstein RJ, Krome RL (eds): *Emergency Medicine.* New York: McGraw-Hill; 1985:550–553.
13. Mendelson DS, Khilnani N, Wagner LD, et al: Preoperative chest radiography: Value as a baseline examination for comparison. *Radiology.* 1987;165:341–343.
14. McNamara RM, O'Brien MC, Davidheiser S: Post-traumatic neck pain: A prospective and follow-up study. *Ann Emerg Med.* 1988;17:906–911.
15. Sprawls P: *Physical Principles of Medical Imaging.* Rockville: Aspen Pub; 1987:485.
16. Ritenour RE: Health effects of low level radiation: carcinogenesis, teratogenesis, and mutagenesis. *Semin Nucl Med.* 1986;16:106–117.
17. Sorenson JA: Perception of radiation hazards. *Semin Nucl Med.* 1986;16:158–170.
18. Swartz HM, Reichling BA: Hazards of radiation exposure to pregnant women. *JAMA.* 1978;239:1907.
19. Straub WH: Cost benefit considerations: Dollars, rads and utils, in *Manual of Diagnostic Imaging.* Boston: Little, Brown; 1989:4.
20. Fraser RG, Pare JAP: *Synopsis of Diseases of the Chest.* Philadelphia: WB Saunders; 1983:101–123.
21. Humphreys T, Goldman JM, Stemhagen M, et al: Chest radiography in the emergency department: Lack of superiority of PA/lateral films over single view portable AP films. *Ann Emerg Med.* 1990;19:448.
22. McGonigal MD, Schwab CW, Kauder DR, et al: Supplemental emergent chest computed tomography in the management of blunt torso trauma. *J Trauma.* 1990;330:1431–1434.
23. Gordon R: The deep sulcus sign. *Radiology.* 1980;136:25–27.
24. Toombs BD, Sandler CM, Lester RG: Computed tomography of chest trauma. *Radiology.* 1981;140:733–738.
25. Schmidgall JR, Jui J: Diagnostic techniques in the evaluation of chest injury. *Top Emerg Med.* 1988;10:19–59.
26. Johnson JA, Cogbill TH, Winga ER: Determinants of outcome after pulmonary contusion. *J Trauma.* 1986;26:695–697.
27. Advanced Trauma Life Support Program: *Instructors Manual.* Chicago: American College of Surgeons; 1989.
28. Barcia TC, Livoni JP: Indications for angiography in blunt thoracic trauma. *Radiology.* 1983;147:15–19.

29. Woodring JH, King JC: Determination of normal transverse mediastinal width and mediastinal-width to chest-width ratio in control subjects with aortic or brachiocephalic arterial injury. *J Trauma.* 1989;29:1268–1272.
30. Huang P, Fong C, Rademaker A: Prediction of traumatic aortic rupture from plain chest film findings using stepwise logistic regression. *Ann Emerg Med.* 1987;16:1330–1333.
31. Richardson P, Mirvis SE, Scorpio R, et al: Value of CT in determining the need for angiography when findings of mediastinal hemorrhage on chest radiographs are equivocal. *AJR.* 1991;156:275–279.
32. Gelman R, Mirvis SE, Gens D: Diaphragmatic rupture due to blunt trauma: Sensitivity of plain chest radiographs. *AJR.* 1990;156:52–57.
33. Greenspan RH, Ravin CE, Polansky SM, et al: Accuracy of the chest radiograph in the diagnosis of pulmonary embolism. *Invest Radiol.* 1982;17:539–543.
34. Walzer PD: *Pneumocystis carinii* pneumonia, in Kelley WN (ed): *Textbook of Internal Medicine.* Philadelphia: JB Lippincott; 1989:1694–1696.
35. Barron TF, Birbaum BA, Shane LB, et al: *Pneumocystis carinii* pneumonia studied by gallium-67 scanning. *Radiology.* 1985;154:791–793.
36. Doppman JL, Geelhoed GW, DeVita VT: Atypical radiographic features in *Pneumocystis carinii* pneumonia. *Radiology.* 1975;114:39–44.
37. Emerman CL, Dawson N, Speroff T, et al: Comparison of physician judgment and decision aids for ordering chest radiographs for pneumonia in outpatients. *Ann Emerg Med.* 1991;20:1215–1219.
38. Singal BM, Hedges MJR, Radack KL: Decision rules and clinical prediction of pneumonia: Evaluation of low yield criteria. *Ann Emerg Med.* 1989;18:13–20.
39. Diehr PH, Wood RW, Bushyhead JB, et al: Prediction of pneumonia in outpatients with acute cough—a statistical approach. *J Chronic Dis.* 1984;37:215–225.
40. Heckerling PS, Tape TG, Wigton RS, et al: Clinical rule for pulmonary infiltrates. *Ann Intern Med.* 1990;113:664–670.
41. Pollack CV, Jorden RC, Kolb JC: Usefulness of chest radiography and urinalysis testing in adults with acute sickle cell pain crisis. *Ann Emerg Med.* 1991;20:1210–1214.
42. Zieverink SE, Harper PA, Holden RW, et al: Emergency room radiography of asthma: An efficacy study. *Radiology.* 1982;145:27–29.
43. White CS, Randolph P, Lubetsky HW, et al: Acute asthma: Admission chest radiography in hospitalized adult patients. *Chest.* 1991;100:14–16.
44. Aronson S, Gennis P, Kelly D, et al: The value of routine admission chest radiographs in adult asthmatics. *Ann Emerg Med.* 1989;11:1206–1208.
45. Milne E, Pistolesi M, Miniati M, Giuntini C: The radiologic distinction of cardiogenic and noncardiogenic edema. *AJR.* 1985;144:879–894.
46. Petasnick JP: Radiologic evaluation of aortic dissection. *Radiology.* 1991;180:297–305.
47. Tsai T, Gallagher E, Lombardi G, et al: Guidelines for selective ordering of admission chest radiography in adult obstructive airway disease. *Ann Emerg Med.* 1993;22:1854–1858.
48. Emerman C, Cydulka R: Evaluation of high-yield criteria for chest radiography in acute exacerbation of chronic obstructive pulmonary disease. *Ann Emerg Med.* 1993;22:680–684.

Chapter

Rib Radiographs

Thomas Russell Jones and Robert W. Lasek

The detection of injuries to vital structures should be the primary concern when one is evaluating injuries to the thorax. Rib fractures can provide clues to serious chest injuries, yet major intrathoracic injuries can occur in the presence of an intact rib cage. Rib fractures are frequently overlooked on a routine chest radiograph, because technique places emphasis on the soft tissues. Freed and Shields[1] report that rib fractures were the most frequently missed fractures in a university teaching hospital.

The upright posteroanterior (PA) chest radiograph is the most clinically useful and cost-effective study for detecting major thoracic trauma.[2] Hemothorax, pneumothorax, and mediastinal injuries are most readily screened on this view. From a radiologic viewpoint, the optimal views for the detection of rib fractures are (1) an upright PA chest film, (2) a well-penetrated AP view of the lower ribs, (3) oblique views, and (4) a ''coned-down'' view of the suspected area.[3]

The sensitivity of rib radiographs is difficult to study, because they are considered the standard for the radiographic diagnosis of rib fracture. Hence, the incidence of false-negative studies is unknown unless they are correlated with serial radiographic examinations or radionucleotide bone scans, which are seldom warranted. The sensitivity of rib radiographs can be expected to vary with the appropriateness of radiographic technique for body habitus, mineral bone density, and experience of the individual interpreting the films. When a lesion is identified, specificity is high.

Even when a ''rib series'' is obtained, a fracture may not be apparent initially. Fractures are recognized when the fracture line is perpendicular to the x-ray beam. Fracture lines that are parallel to the x-ray beam are not seen unless there is displacement of fragments. Extrapleural soft tissue swelling from hemorrhage may be the only sign of rib fracture but, when correlated with the history of trauma or physical examination, is sufficient evidence of rib fracture. Follow-up clinical and radiologic examination at 24 to 48 hours ensures that no significant complications have developed and that the therapeutic goal of adequate pain relief has been achieved. Fracture lines not seen at the time of initial examination commonly become visible on radiographs after several days as bony fragments become slightly displaced. Bavendam and Nedelman[4] describe a trauma patient admitted with pleuritic pain in whom one rib fracture was identified initially. Serial examination demonstrated four rib fractures on the second day, six fractures at 1 week, and callus formation suggesting fracture of eight ribs at 1 month. Fractures through the costal cartilage are very difficult to detect and are often more painful than osseous fractures.[5]

Injuries to the rib cage most commonly involve the fourth through ninth ribs. The bones and muscles of the shoulder girdle form a protective buffer for the first three ribs. The lower three ribs are more mobile and yielding, and thus are less likely to be fractured.

Despite the widely held belief that fractures of the first rib are associated with vascular injuries, Poole and Meyers[6] found no correlation in a retrospective review of 168 patients. The need for vascular imaging procedures such as transesophageal echocardiography and contrast aortography should be dictated by clinical judgment, which is based on the radiologic appearance of the mediastinal structures and suspicion of injury, not on the presence of rib fractures. Fractures of the lower three ribs may raise suspicion of intraabdominal solid organ injury and warrant further evaluation with diagnostic peritoneal lavage, computed tomography, or ultrasound evaluation as the clinical setting dictates.

With the increasing concern over health care costs, serious thought should be given to the utility of rib films. In the evaluation of the victim of thoracic trauma, the highest priority should be placed on the identification of serious intrathoracic injuries. The presence or absence of isolated rib fractures usually does not significantly influence either patient management or outcome.[2, 7, 8] Rib radiographs may be useful and important when there are medicolegal concerns, such as in assault or suspected child abuse. The presence of multiple rib fractures in elderly patients, individuals with significant cardiopulmonary compromise, or patients in whom there is question of their ability to provide self-care may require hospital admission. In these cases, the selective application of rib radiographic imaging is probably indicated.[9] The presence of multiple old rib fractures has been correlated with alcoholism. In this instance, rib radiographs are not indicated to establish a diagnosis of alcoholism; rather, their presence noted on routine chest radiographs can help confirm a clinical suspicion.[10, 11] In addition, the documentation of rib fractures may have physician reimbursement implications, eg, billing for closed treatment of rib fracture.

REFERENCES

1. Freed HA, Shields NN: Most frequently overlooked radiographically apparent fractures in a teaching emergency department. *Ann Emerg Med.* 1984;13:900–904.

2. Thompson BM, Finger W, Tonsfeldt D, et al: Rib radiographs for trauma: Useful or wasteful? *Ann Emerg Med.* 1986;15:261–265.
3. Merril V: *Atlas of Roentgenographic Positions and Standard Radiologic Procedures.* St Louis: CV Mosby; 1991:382–391.
4. Bavendam FA, Nedelman SH: Some considerations in the roentgenology of fractures and dislocations. *Semin Roentgenol.* 1966;1:407–463.
5. Kattan KR: Trauma of the bony thorax. *Semin Roentgenol.* 1978;8:69–77.
6. Poole GV, Meyers RT: Morbidity and mortality rate in major blunt trauma to the upper chest. *Ann Surg.* 1981;193:70–75.
7. Kattan KR: What to look for in rib fractures and how. *JAMA.* 1980;143:262–264.
8. deLuca SA, Rhea JT, O'Malley TO: Radiographic evaluation of rib fractures. *Am J Roentgenol.* 1982;138:91–92.
9. Cantrill SV: The appropriate utilization of rib radiographs, in Cantrill SV, Karas S (eds): Cost-effective diagnostic testing in emergency medicine. Dallas: American College of Emergency Physicians; 1994:163–166.
10. Lindsell DR, Wilson AG, Maxwell JD: Fractures on the chest radiograph in detection of alcoholic liver disease. *Br Med J.* 1982;285:597–599.
11. Keso L, Kivisaari A, Salaspuro M: Fractures on chest radiographs in detection of alcoholism. *Alcohol Alcohol.* 1988;23:53–56.

Chapter

Cervical Spine Radiography

Jay M. Goldman

The development of standardized trauma treatment protocols (Basic Trauma Life Support and Prehospital Trauma Life Support for prehospital care, and Advanced Trauma Life Support for emergency department resuscitation) has led to widespread use of aggressive spinal immobilization techniques for victims of blunt trauma. Similarly, very liberal, almost indiscriminate, use of cervical spine radiography in the emergency department evaluation of blunt trauma patients has been recommended in order to avoid the potentially catastrophic consequences of missing an "occult" spinal cord injury.[1–3]

The routine use of cervical spine radiography for all victims of blunt trauma has resulted in vast numbers of radiographic examinations yielding normal findings. Attempts to reduce the number of studies have focused on defining a subgroup of trauma patients who are indeed at risk of cervical spine injury and limiting cervical spine radiography to this subgroup. The benefits of such an approach would be multiple: It would eliminate the cost of personnel and materials for unnecessary films, reduce potential risks of unnecessary radiation to patients and clinicians, and minimize the direct risk to the patient of delaying the evaluation and treatment of other, more immediately threatening injuries. In addition, unnecessary radiographs prolong the evaluation of the trauma patient and thus lengthen the time during which resources may be unavailable to other critically ill emergency department patients.

The selective application of cervical spine radiography to a high-risk group is an unusually difficult challenge, however. Because the potential consequences of missing a cervical spine injury (and thus producing a permanent, functionally significant cervical spinal cord injury) are so catastrophic, criteria used to define a high-risk subgroup must identify every patient with a cervical spine injury, ie, the prediction rule's sensitivity must be 100%.

This chapter focuses on the development of a rational approach to the use of cervical spine radiography in the evaluation of patients with multiple trauma.

TECHNICAL FACTORS IN CERVICAL SPINE IMAGING

The primary goal of examining the cervical spine in a patient with blunt trauma is the identification of potentially unstable cervical spine injuries, thus minimizing the risk of further injury to the spinal cord as well as optimizing the patient's comfort level and functional status. A critical fact is that significant morbidity from spinal cord injury may occur in the absence of cervical spine injury. Cervical spine radiographs are commonly normal, for example, in the central cord syndrome in adults and in the spinal cord injury without radiographic abnormality syndrome in children.[4] This observation reinforces the importance of the physical examination in "clearing the C-spine" and emphasizes the limitations of plain cervical spine radiography in predicting spinal cord injury.

Within this framework, then, the contribution of cervical spine radiography is a series of images, in at least two planes, of the entire cervical spine from the atlanto-occipital junction to and including the superior portion of T1. At one time, a single supine cross-table lateral view served as the standard radiologic means of evaluating the trauma patient with potential cervical spine injury. During this same period, however, the diagnosis of cervical spine injury was delayed or missed in up to one third of patients.[1] The supine cross-table lateral view provides an image in only one plane and is further limited at both ends of the cervical spine (at C1–2 and at C7–T1). Although applying downward traction to the arms while maintaining cervical spine immobilization is believed to improve the likelihood of imaging C7–T1, the overall sensitivity of this view alone for unstable cervical spine injury is only about 85%.[5–7] The "swimmer's" view (ie, taken by directing the x-ray beam through the axilla after externally rotating and fully extending the arm on the side of the x-ray source) may improve visualization of C7–T1 to allow the identification of subluxations and dislocations, but multiple overlying shadows on this view make identification of fractures in this area difficult.

Addition of the odontoid (atlantoaxial) and supine anteroposterior (AP) views increases the sensitivity of plain radiography for unstable cervical spine injury to 92 to 94%.[5, 6, 8, 9] Addition of bilateral supine oblique views to complete a five-view series has been advocated by some,[10–12] but the value of these additional views is open to debate.[13] Flexion-extension views may be useful in a subset of alert, cooperative patients who have subtle (2-mm) "antero-" or "retro-listhesis" on static views or in patients who have complaints strongly suggesting ligamentous injury despite a normal cervical spine series. In these two patient subsets, active flexion and extension views (with all movement performed by an alert, cooperative patient who is instructed to stop when he or she feels discomfort) may increase sensitivity to 99%.[12–14]

Some workers have advocated routine use of computed tomography (CT) scanning of C1–2 in all blunt trauma patients undergoing CT of the head (especially patients with intracranial hemorrhage or skull fracture) and of C7–T1 whenever the initial cross-table lateral view is inadequate.[5, 6, 10, 15–17] Computed tomography is also useful in delineating the extent of injuries first identified on plain cervical spine radiography. Computed tomography may carry some risk, however, if it requires removing the multiply-injured patient from the resuscitation area.

Adequate initial cervical spine imaging (cross-table lateral, odontoid, and AP views) can usually be obtained rapidly and efficiently in the trauma resuscitation unit. Jewelry, identification tags, hair clips, and other nonessential paraphernalia are removed, but cervical spine immobilization devices and backboards are left in place. If the patient is cooperative enough to hold still, the anterior portion of the cervical collar may be removed to allow the patient's mandible to drop further, improving the quality of the odontoid view. If C1–2 or C7–T1 is not adequately imaged initially, the next imaging attempt should be with CT scanning, because repetitive attempts to image this area with plain films are rarely fruitful. Perhaps most important, the resuscitation team must keep the effort to clear the cervical spine in perspective and address other immediately life-threatening problems first. When necessary, cervical spine radiography may be delayed and cervical immobilization maintained until more urgent needs are addressed in the operating room and the patient is sufficiently stable to undergo more complete radiographic imaging.

INDICATIONS FOR CERVICAL SPINE RADIOGRAPHY

Identifying those victims of blunt trauma who require cervical spine radiography has been an issue of considerable debate. Standard trauma treatment guidelines currently teach prehospital personnel to apply complete spinal immobilization to any patient (1) has been subjected to sudden deceleration forces, (2) has had a seizure or been found unconscious, or (3) has suffered any injury above the clavicle.[18] Similarly, Advanced Trauma Life Support guidelines recommend liberal use of cervical spine radiography for any patient with multisystem trauma and particularly one with blunt trauma above the clavicle.[3] The liberal application of cervical spine radiography to all patients who arrive with spinal immobilization has resulted in a negative examination rate of well over 98%.[19–21] A number of investigators have attempted to reduce the unnecessary use of cervical spine radiography by defining clinical subgroups of blunt trauma patients who are at essentially no risk of cervical spine injury and thus do not require radiography.

Mechanism of Injury

Although motor vehicle crashes are virtually always reported as the most common mechanism of cervical spine injury, motor vehicle crashes alone have not been shown to be an independent predictor of cervical spine injury. Similarly, falls have been shown to correlate with cervical spine injury, but the relationship is not strong enough to mandate cervical spine radiography in every patient brought to the emergency department after a fall.[22, 23] One large prospective study found that none of 283 patients with "whiplash" had cervical spine injury[24]; nevertheless, fractures have previously been described in these patients.[25]

Concurrent Injuries

The presence of facial or mandibular fractures has been commonly thought to indicate a high risk for cervical spine injury. Two retrospective studies and one prospective study have failed, however, to show any increased incidence of cervical spine injury in patients with facial fractures.[26–28]

Head injury is also frequently considered to be associated with higher risk of cervical spine injury, perhaps because of the association of these two injuries in fatal motor vehicle crashes.[29] In patients surviving motor vehicle crashes long enough to undergo trauma center evaluation, however, no statistically significant relationship has been shown in retrospective or prospective studies. The same is true for patients who have sustained traumatic loss of consciousness.[20, 22, 24, 28]

In contrast to these findings in patients with isolated head or facial injuries, alert patients with multiple other blunt injuries may be sufficiently distracted by the pain of their other injuries that they fail to notice neck pain or tenderness. Reports of patients with supposedly ''asymptomatic'' or ''occult'' cervical spine injuries commonly note the presence of concurrent severe ''distracting'' injuries. Although the definition of ''distracting'' is unspecified, injuries so classified in published reports include long bone and pelvic fractures, multiple lacerations and contusions, liver lacerations, and genital injuries.[30–34] In one large study, the examining physicians were prospectively asked to identify patients who, in the physicians' judgment, had ''other severely painful injuries.'' These judgments were made prior to completion of cervical spine radiography and so were unbiased by knowledge of the presence or absence of cervical spine injury. Prospective identification of ''other severely painful injuries'' was independently and statistically significantly associated with the finding of cervical spine injury in blunt trauma patients.[24]

Clinical Findings

Most of the studies attempting to define high-risk and no-risk subgroups for cervical spine injury have focused on clinical features: neck pain, neck tenderness, and neurologic deficits. There is no controversy over the need for cervical spine radiography in patients with neurologic deficits, and prospective studies have confirmed this need.[22, 32] The majority of cervical spine injuries, however, are *not* associated with neurologic deficits. Similarly, as previously mentioned, significant spinal cord injury may occur in the absence of spine injuries.

The signs and symptoms most commonly associated with cervical spine injuries are neck pain and neck tenderness. Numerous studies have consistently established the association between these findings and cervical spine injury. *Neck tenderness* is generally defined as anterior or posterior central neck tenderness; the presence of tenderness over posterolateral neck muscles only was not associated with cervical spine injury in the two reports in which it was studied.[24, 28] Thus, cervical spine radiography is recommended for injured patients who complain of midline neck pain or tenderness.[20, 22, 24, 27, 30, 31, 34]

Injured patients with impaired consciousness are also thought to

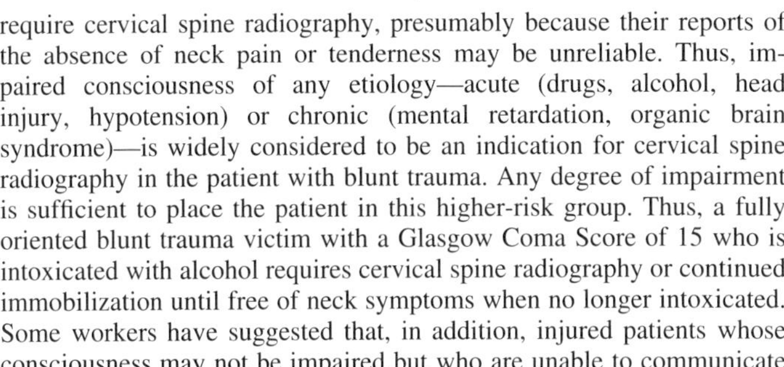

require cervical spine radiography, presumably because their reports of the absence of neck pain or tenderness may be unreliable. Thus, impaired consciousness of any etiology—acute (drugs, alcohol, head injury, hypotension) or chronic (mental retardation, organic brain syndrome)—is widely considered to be an indication for cervical spine radiography in the patient with blunt trauma. Any degree of impairment is sufficient to place the patient in this higher-risk group. Thus, a fully oriented blunt trauma victim with a Glasgow Coma Score of 15 who is intoxicated with alcohol requires cervical spine radiography or continued immobilization until free of neck symptoms when no longer intoxicated. Some workers have suggested that, in addition, injured patients whose consciousness may not be impaired but who are unable to communicate well with the examining physician (language difficulty, endotracheal tube, aphasia) should also undergo cervical spine radiography.

An Algorithmic Approach

In light of the foregoing considerations, a rational approach to cervical spine radiography is thus to order the examination for patients with complaints referable to neck injury, such as central neck pain or tenderness or neurologic deficit. Films are indicated in patients who are unable to communicate or unable to appreciate these symptoms because of impaired consciousness or the distraction of other severely painful injuries. It appears that injured patients without any of these features can be managed without cervical spine radiography, and that the cervical spine may be safely "cleared" clinically.

This approach raises two questions, however. First, is this approach sufficiently sensitive to identify every patient with a cervical spine injury? Second, what are the risks and costs of this approach compared with its benefits and savings?

There is striking consensus in the literature on indications for cervical spine radiography. Analysis of the retrospective studies reveals that, if radiography were performed only in patients with neck signs or symptoms (central neck pain or tenderness, neurologic deficits), impaired consciousness, or other severely painful injuries, every patient with cervical spine injury reported in these studies would have been identified.[19, 20, 31, 35, 36] Still, these findings may be questioned because of the small number of cervical spine injuries identified in the aggregate (fewer than 200 in published studies) and because each study has the limitations of retrospective analysis (missing data and charts, questionable interpretation of findings, and unproven applicability to a prospective population).

To date, there have been only four careful prospective studies designed to evaluate the ability of clinical features to identify patients with cervical spine injury.[23, 24, 32, 37] The findings in these studies entirely support those of the retrospective studies. No cervical spine injury has been found in any patient without symptoms of neck injury, impairment of consciousness, or other concurrent severe ("distracting") injuries. That is, the sensitivity of these clinical indicators has been 100% in all of the prospective studies published to date. In light of the complete concurrence of all published studies, the only realistic reservation one might have is that only about 300 patients with cervical spine injury have been reported in these studies. A large, multicenter prospective study entering an estimated 10,000 to 30,000 patients would be needed to establish, at the 95% confidence level, that this decision rule is at least 99% sensitive in detecting cervical spine injury. Until such a study is completed and widely accepted, the identification of even one patient with cervical spine injury not predicted by the algorithm could invalidate this approach, given the potentially catastrophic consequences of missing even one injury. For this reason, reports of "occult" or "asymptomatic" cervical spine injuries merit close consideration and scrutiny.

"Occult" or "Asymptomatic" Cervical Spine Injuries

Careful examination of all reports of occult or asymptomatic cervical spine injuries reveals that, in every case providing sufficient information to evaluate, the "occult" injury was associated with either mental impairment or other severely painful injuries. In fact, a review of all of these reports, compiled by an advocate of the concept of the "occult, asymptomatic" cervical spine injury, actually confirms this conclusion.[30] Of the 35 patients reported in this review, 25 had one of the identified clinical indicators (neck pain or tenderness, impaired consciousness, other painful distracting injuries). Inadequate information was supplied for nine of the other ten patients, and the tenth denied any trauma whatsoever, his fracture being incidentally discovered on soft tissue films for epiglottitis.

Clinical indicators of central neck pain or tenderness, impaired consciousness, and concurrent severely painful injuries identify a subset of multiply injured patients that appears to include every patient with cervical spine injury. These indicators, defined in retrospective studies, have been confirmed in prospective studies. To date, no convincing case of a truly occult or asymptomatic cervical spine injury has been published.

COST-BENEFIT ANALYSIS

The ultimate judgment about whether to limit cervical spine radiography to a high-risk subgroup of patients that will include virtually all who have cervical spine injury depends on a cost-benefit analysis.

Application of the decision rule to guide selective use of cervical spine radiography in injured patients would reduce the ordering of cervical spine radiographs by 13 to 50%.[12, 19–21, 24, 33, 35] The estimated cost savings of such an approach (approximately 100,000 to 300,000 fewer cervical spine radiographic studies annually) has been estimated at $25 to $75 million per year. In addition, this reduction in cervical spine radiography would decrease radiation exposure of patients and staff, expedite patient care, and decrease the time required for emergency department personnel to care for the acutely injured patient.

The cost savings from selective use of cervical spine radiography must, however, be weighed against the cost potentially incurred if any unstable cervical spine injuries are undetected. If the decision rule indeed performs with a sensitivity of 100% (as it has in all studies to date), there would be no excess costs. Unfortunately, missing an unstable cervical spine injury may result in permanent neurologic disability, with all the attendant costs of additional acute and long-term care, suffering, income loss, and litigation. As stated in the largest prospective study of cervical spine radiography, if even a handful of these injuries is missed, "the fairly large monetary gain (from selective use of cervical spine radiography) would be greatly offset by the costs (human and economic) associated with these . . . cases."[24]

CONCLUSION

Cervical spine radiography is an invaluable adjunct to the history and physical examination in the patient with blunt trauma. With the addition of CT when needed (to visualize C1–2 and C7–T1 if poorly seen on plain radiographs or to visualize C1–2 in the setting of severe head injury), all significant bony injuries may be identified. Current studies suggest that cervical spine radiography is not necessary in every patient with blunt trauma or even in every patient with blunt trauma above the clavicle. Both retrospective and prospective studies provide strong support for the view that cervical spine radiography should be ordered only for the subgroup of patients with blunt trauma who have symptoms or signs referable to the neck (central pain or tenderness, neurologic deficits), impaired consciousness, or other severely painful, distracting injuries. Such an approach could reduce the number of cervical spine radiographic studies by 13 to 50% and result in significant savings in costs, personnel, and time. There is no reliable published report of any patient who has suffered an injury to the cervical spine in the absence of any of these clinical findings. Confirmation of this decision rule at a confidence level acceptable to virtually all clinicians would require completion of a large, multicenter study involving tens of thousands of patients.

REFERENCES

1. Bohlman HH: Acute fractures and dislocations of the cervical spine. *J Bone Joint Surg*. 1979;61A:1119–1142.
2. Wales LR, Knopp RK, Morishima MS: Recommendations for evaluation of the acutely injured cervical spine: A clinical radiologic algorithm. *Ann Emerg Med*. 1980;9:422–428.
3. American College of Surgeons: *Advanced Trauma Life Support*. Chicago: American College of Surgeons; 1989.
4. Pang D, Pollack IF: Spinal cord injury without radiographic abnormality in children—the SCIOWARA syndrome. *J Trauma*. 1989;29:654–664.
5. Ehara S, el-Khoury GY, Clark CR: Radiologic evaluation of dens fracture. *Spine*. 1992;17:475–479.
6. Ross SE, Schwab CW, David ET, et al: Clearing the cervical spine: Initial radiographic evaluation. *J Trauma*. 1987;27:1055–1060.
7. Shaffer MA, Doris PA: Limitation of the cross table lateral view in detecting cervical spine injuries: A retrospective analysis. *Ann Emerg Med*. 1981;10:508–513.
8. Streitweiser DR, Knopp R, Wales LR, et al: Accuracy of standard radiographic views in detecting cervical spine fractures. *Ann Emerg Med*. 1983;12:538–542.
9. Pathria MN, Petersige CA: Spinal trauma. *Radiol Clin North Am*. 1991;29:847–865.
10. Daffner RH: Evaluation of cervical vertebral injuries. *Semin Roentgenol*. 1992;27:239–253.
11. Holliman CJ, Mayer JS, Cook RT, et al: Is the anteroposterior radiograph of the cervical spine necessary in the evaluation of the trauma patient? *Am J Emerg Med*. 1991;9:421–425.
12. Vandemark RM: Radiology of the cervical spine in trauma patients: Practice pitfalls and recommendations for improving efficiency and communication. *AJR*. 1990;155:465–472.
13. Freemyer B, Knopp R, Piche J, et al: Comparison of five-view and three-view cervical spine series in the evaluation of patients with cervical trauma. *Ann Emerg Med*. 1989;18:818–821.
14. Lewis LM, Docherty M, Ruoff BE: Flexion-extension views in the evaluation of cervical-spine injuries. *Ann Emerg Med*. 1991;20:117–121.
15. Roberge RJ: Facilitating cervical spine radiography in blunt trauma. *Emerg Med Clin North Am* 1991;9:733–742.
16. Woodring JH, Lee C: The role and limitations of computed tomographic scanning in the evaluation of cervical trauma. *J Trauma*. 1992;33:698–708.
17. Kirshenbaum KJ, Nadimpalli SR, Fantus R, et al: Unsuspected upper cervical spine fractures associated with significant head trauma: Role of CT. *J Emerg Med*. 1990;8:183–198.

18. Campbell JE (ed): *Basic Trauma Life Support: Advanced Prehospital Care.* Englewood Cliffs, NJ: Prentice-Hall; 1988.
19. Cadoux CG, White JD, Hedberg MC: High-yield roentgenographic criteria for cervical spine injuries. *Ann Emerg Med.* 1987;16:738–742.
20. Fischer RP: Cervical radiographic evaluation of alert patients following blunt trauma. *Ann Emerg Med.* 1984;13:905–907.
21. McNamara RM, Heine E, Esposito B: Cervical spine injury and radiography in alert, high-risk patients. *J Emerg Med.* 1990;8:177–182.
22. Jacobs LM, Schwartz R: Prospective analysis of acute cervical spine injury: A methodology to predict injury. *Ann Emerg Med.* 1986;15:44–49.
23. Roberge RJ, Wears RC, Kelly M, et al: Selective application of cervical spine radiography in alert victims of blunt trauma: A prospective study. *J Trauma.* 1988;28:784–787.
24. Hoffman JR, Schriger DL, Mower W, et al: Low-risk criteria for cervical-spine radiography in blunt trauma: A prospective study. *Ann Emerg Med.* 1992;21:1454–1460.
25. Huelke DF, Mendelsohn RA, States JD, et al: Cervical fractures and fractures-dislocations sustained without head impact. *J Trauma.* 1978;18:533–538.
26. Andrew CT, Gallucci JG, Brown AS, et al: Is routine cervical spine radiographic evaluation indicated in patients with mandibular fractures? *Am Surg.* 1992;58:369–372.
27. Sinclair D, Schwartz M, Gross J, et al: A retrospective review of the relationship between facial fractures, head injuries, and cervical spine injuries. *J Emerg Med.* 1988;6:109–112.
28. Williams J, Jehle D, Cottington E, et al: Head, facial, and clavicular trauma as a predictor of cervical-spine injury. *Ann Emerg Med.* 1992;21:719–722.
29. Bucholz RW, Burkhead WZ, Graham W, et al: Occult cervical spine injuries in fatal traffic accidents. *J Trauma.* 1979;19:768–771.
30. Mace S: The unstable occult cervical spine fracture: A review. *Am J Emerg Med.* 1992;10:136–142.
31. Ringenberg BJ, Fisher AK, Urdaneta LF, et al: Rational ordering of cervical spine radiographs following trauma. *Ann Emerg Med.* 1988;17:792–796.
32. Roberge RJ, Wears RC: Evaluation of neck discomfort, neck tenderness, and neurologic deficits as indicators for radiography in blunt trauma victims. *J Emerg Med.* 1992;10:539–544.
33. Saddison D, Vanek VW, Racanelli JL: Clinical indications for cervical spine radiographs in alert trauma patients. *Am Surg.* 1991;57:366–369.
34. Walter J, Doris PE, Shaffer MA: Clinical presentation of patients with acute cervical spine injury. *Ann Emerg Med.* 1984;13:512–515.
35. Bachulis BL, Long WB, Hynes GD, et al: Clinical indications for cervical spine radiographs in the traumatized patient. *Am J Surg.* 1987;153:473–477.
36. Kreipke DL, Gillespie KR, McCarthy MC, et al: Reliability of indications for cervical spine films in trauma patients. *J Trauma.* 1989;29:1438–1439.
37. Neifeld GL, Keene JG, Hevesy G, et al: Cervical injury in head trauma. *J Emerg Med.* 1988;6:203–207.

Chapter

Spine Radiography for Low Back Pain

Linda G. Allison and John G. Benitez

There is a prevailing notion that a "complete" back examination is not complete without spinal radiographs. "Such notions of completeness are supported by the current system of professional standards review in medicine and by medical malpractice lawsuits, both of which provide ready punishment for 'leaving out' some portion of 'complete medical care' while often ignoring considerations of the marginal gain of information due to, or the marginal cost-effectiveness of, specific diagnostic tests."[1] Therefore, emergency physicians often feel compelled to use lumbosacral (LS) radiography more frequently than may be necessary. What is the best approach in the emergency department (ED) to evaluate back pain? Are radiographs always needed for diagnosis and treatment?

One radiologist in New Zealand had read an average of 48 LS radiographs per year; for 2 years after an accident compensation program was established, he averaged 218 LS radiographs per year. This change represented a 450% increase in the number of radiographs, but the number of accidents did not rise by this amount.[2] In contrast, in occupational medicine settings, the lack of back radiographs has no effect on compensation case proceedings, and radiographs do not play a role in deciding the amount of a judgment.[1]

In order to understand the need for LS spine radiography in the ED, it is necessary to understand the pain syndromes associated with the lower back (Table 58–1), the differential diagnosis of low back pain (LBP), and the history and physical examination (PE) findings. It is also necessary to know exactly what radiographs will and will not show. In addition, the cost-effectiveness and the risk-benefit ratio should be considered. Ultimately, the questions to be answered are as follows: How will radiography affect the management of the patient in the ED? Would other studies be more appropriate?

There are several proposed mechanisms for back pain, most of which focus on the degeneration of the intervertebral disk and abnormalities of the vertebral joints. Early surgical investigations mapped painful areas in the body resulting from nerve root stimulation. They concluded that the nerve root needed only to be touched to cause sciatica, that repeated stimulation caused a root to become hypersensitive, and that gross disk protrusion was not necessary to cause sciatica.[3]

Later studies identified nerve endings in fascia, ligaments, annular

TABLE 58–1. CLINICAL FACTORS PREDICTING PATHOLOGY

1. Age over 50
2. Fever
3. Weight loss, adenopathy, other systemic signs
4. Corticosteroid use
5. Findings suggestive of ankylosing spondylitis
6. Alcohol or drug abuse
7. Prior malignancy
8. Seeking compensation
9. Motor neurologic deficit

From Deyo RA: Early diagnostic evaluation of low back pain. *J Gen Intern Med.* 1986;1:328–338.

ligaments, intervertebral joint capsules, and vertebral periosteum (but none in the vertebral bodies themselves). Injection of hypertonic saline into these areas reproduced root and referred pain syndromes.[4]

Radiographically demonstrable degeneration of the LS spine is a normal process that progresses with age.[5] These changes may or may not be associated with pain, however.[6–8] Congenital lesions have been found with equal frequency in symptomatic and asymptomatic patients.[7, 9, 10–12]

PLAIN RADIOGRAPHY OF THE LS SPINE

Standard views of the LS spine are AP, lateral, and oblique views as well as a ''coned-down'' view of the LS junction. The question has been asked whether it would be cost-effective to limit the use of certain views, thereby reducing cost and radiation exposure but still obtaining the clinical information needed. Oblique views are the best to demonstrate the facet joints and the pars interarticularis, but they add little clinically significant information in most cases; this is especially true in pediatric cases.[13, 14] Omission of the coned lateral view, however, may result in inadequate visualization of the LS joint up to 21% of the time; this has been reported to result in missed diagnoses in up to 4.5% of cases in a high-risk population.[15, 16]

Many studies show no correlation between radiographic findings and back pain.[7, 10–12, 17–21] In the occupational medicine setting, abnormalities on LS films do not help to predict which employees will develop LBP.[9, 17, 20, 22] Although there is a higher incidence of degenerative disk changes in patients with back pain, these changes may not cause the pain but may merely be associated with it.[17, 19–21, 23]

In some syndromes, radiographic changes are not apparent early. Plain films often miss early neoplastic changes, because at least 50% of the cancellous bone must be lost before changes can be seen on the lateral view, and loss of 75% or more is needed for detection on the AP view.[24] Disk prolapse cannot usually be seen in radiographs, because it occurs early in the degenerative process, before disk space narrowing is seen. In other root syndromes (e.g., lateral recess syndrome, spinal stenosis) plain films may show an abnormality, but additional studies are needed to make the diagnosis.[6] Moreover, radiographic findings are not necessarily related to the back pain and do not alter the type of therapy given initially.[25]

Other syndromes *are* manifested by radiographic changes, but their value in subsequent management is minimal. Spondylolysis and facet abnormalities can be seen, but treatment is not based on radiographic findings.[6] Spondylolisthesis has a characteristic wedging of the fifth lumbar vertebra and the slip of one vertebra over another.[26] Vertebral osteomyelitis produces characteristic changes on plain radiography, but in most cases, other historical or physical examination findings point to the diagnosis and the need for imaging studies or other diagnostic maneuvers.[27, 28]

Lumbar spine radiographs may identify degenerative changes with or without osteophytes, osteoarthritis of the apophyseal joints, spina bifida occulta, transitional vertebrae, or asymmetric vertebrae, but the frequency of these findings is the same in symptomatic and asymptomatic patients. Thus, radiography does not help identify the cause of pain and does not aid in patient management. Indeed, most patients become asymptomatic with conservative treatment regardless of the cause and regardless of radiographic findings. Radiographs are not predictive of either the final outcome or the duration of disability.[6, 29, 30] Plain film radiography may be used to exclude conditions such as spondylolysis, ankylosing spondylitis, and metastases, which may mimic mechanical or diskogenic pain. The clinical significance of spondylolysis is disputed, however, and the other diagnoses should be suspected on the basis of historical and physical examination findings.[16, 30]

It is generally accepted that radiography is appropriate in patients sustaining substantial trauma to the spine. For trauma, first a cross-table lateral should be done, and then a standard AP. Oblique films may be ordered to demonstrate spondylolysis associated with spondylolisthesis, but they occasionally fail to do so.[31] Flexion and extension views may be needed to demonstrate ligamentous injury or spinal canal compromise.

The sensitivity of plain radiography in patients with acute uncomplicated low back pain is estimated at 74%, and the specificity is estimated at 64 to 74%. Splithoff[10] compared 100 patients with low back pain and 100 controls without back pain; there was no significant difference in incidence of vertebral abnormalities between the two groups. LaRocca and Macnab[12] compared symptomatic with asymptomatic patients and found no difference in structural abnormalities on radiographs. Rowe[17] followed 500 men with low back pain and 100 men without low back pain who were matched for age and activity for 10 years. There was no significant difference in structural findings, including spondylolisthesis, transitional LS vertebrae, sagittal or asymmetric LS facet joints, and spina bifida occulta. There was an increased incidence of degenerative disk changes by radiography in 54% of patients in the pain group aged 30 to 50 years, compared with 22% in the control group of the same age range.

Torgerson and Dotter[21] confirmed the findings of Rowe[17] in 217 asymptomatic and 387 symptomatic patients between the ages of 40 and 70 years. Radiologic disk degeneration may be more common in those with back pain than in those without. A Swedish study evaluated 68,000 LS radiographs over a 10-year period and found unsuspected and clinically significant radiographic findings in 1/2500 (0.04%) examinations of patients 25 to 50 years old.[6] A British study showed that 0.2% of patients were ultimately diagnosed with a clinically significant disease requiring specific treatment.[32] The predictive value of plain film radiography is low because of the low prevalence of significant pathology.[6–8, 10–12, 17, 20, 21, 33]

There are certain patients in whom the sensitivity is higher. They are usually identified by means of a thorough history and physical examination. Certain characteristics should trigger the physician's suspicions and prompt the use of radiography (see Table 58–1).

Liang and Komaroff[32] analyzed the risk-benefit ratio (as millirads vs days of suffering averted through earlier diagnosis) and cost-effectiveness (as dollars spent vs days of suffering averted through earlier diagnosis) of the initial use of LS radiography in a patient population aged 18 to 60 years. They compared the use of radiographs at the initial visit with no use of radiographs at the initial visit for low back pain. Radiographs were done in both groups 4 or 8 weeks after initial presentation. The researchers assumed that no patient would change from having a curable lesion to having an incurable lesion in 8 weeks without worsening of symptoms. Radiography did not change the length of patient suffering; it increased patient exposure to radiation over 10-fold; and it increased costs of care more than 10-fold.[32] These results suggest that plain films should be obtained only when there is a high probability of finding an abnormality on the radiograph based on history and physical examination data.

The probability of finding specific pathologic conditions on radiography can be estimated (Table 58–2). In most cases in which a specific disease is suspected, the probability of a positive radiographic finding is less than 25% at the time of the initial visit. In cases with suspected mechanical back pain, however, the probability of positive findings

TABLE 58–2. ESTIMATED PROBABILITY OF AN ABNORMAL RADIOGRAPH IN PATIENTS WITH LOW BACK PAIN FROM SELECTED DISEASES

Disease	Initial Visit	4 Weeks	8 Weeks
Chronic epidural infection	0.24	0.38	1.0
Diskitis	0.25	0.85	1.0
Osteomyelitis	0.90	0.99	1.0
Metastatic tumor	0.66	0.76	0.86
Primary bone tumor	0.7	0.8	0.9
Myeloma	0.66	0.76	0.86
Spondylolisthesis	0.99	0.99	0.99
Fracture	0.9	0.98	0.99
Sacroiliitis-spondylitis	0.1	0.1	0.1
Epiphysitis	0.3	0.3	0.3

From Liang M, Komaroff AL: Roentgenograms in primary care patients with acute low back pain: a cost-effectiveness analysis. *Arch Intern Med.* 1982;142:1108–1112.

indicating a serious disease is less than 0.1%. Persistent symptoms (4 to 8 weeks) are associated with a high probability of radiographic findings. History and physical examination (osteomyelitis, primary or metastatic tumor, spondylolisthesis, fractures) usually suggest when radiography may be helpful.[32]

APPROACH TO ED EVALUATION OF LOW BACK PAIN

In the ED, what is important in managing a patient with low back pain? The patient wants the pain alleviated, a diagnosis made, and a prognosis about the worsening or recurrence of pain. In comparison, the emergency physician needs to answer several questions: Is there a serious systemic disease causing the pain? Is there neurologic compromise that might require surgical intervention? Can any of these be demonstrated with radiography? Is there social or psychologic distress that may amplify or prolong pain?[34]

The emergency physician needs to recognize clinical presentations that may indicate the presence of a serious or life-threatening illness or disease. A patient who is writhing in pain may have intraabdominal or vascular pathology, and appropriate investigations should be pursued. When unrelenting pain at rest is the main complaint, one needs to consider cancer or an infectious process, such as acute diskitis, epidural abscess, or spinal osteomyelitis. These infectious processes need to be considered in a patient with a history of diabetes mellitus, intravenous drug use, other immunosuppressive disease, recent spinal surgery, recent urinary tract surgery or procedure, or recent pyelonephritis. Fever, unfortunately, is not always present. An evolving neurologic deficit, caudal anesthesia, or urinary incontinence or retention suggests epidural abscess, epidural hemorrhage, intradural or extradural tumor, or massive central disk herniation. Sudden acute pain in patients with osteoporosis or cancer suggests pathologic fracture.[35]

Back pain secondary to malignancy represents a medical emergency. Tumors account for fewer than 1% of all episodes of low back pain but are the most common systemic disease affecting the spine. About 80% of these patients with back pain secondary to malignancy are over the age of 50. A history of cancer, unexplained weight loss, failure of conservative therapy, or pain lasting longer than 1 month suggests a neoplastic cause. Physical examination is nonspecific except in advanced stages, when the primary tumor source is obvious.[34, 36]

What do plain films add to the management of patients with low back pain? Plain radiography may suggest degenerative conditions and, possibly, abnormal displacements on flexion and extension views. Plain radiographs may be helpful if any of the previous high-risk criteria are

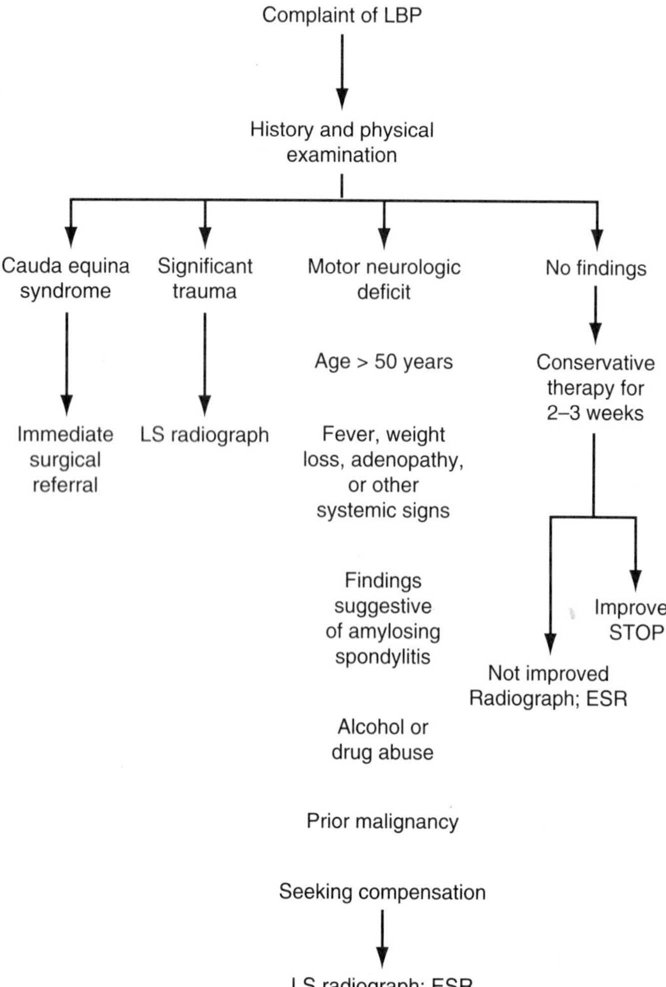

FIGURE 58–1. Proposed algorithm for the initial approach to patients with low back pain. Modified from Deyo RA: Early diagnostic evaluation of low back pain. *J Gen Intern Med.* 1986;1:328–338.

TABLE 58–3. SENSITIVITY AND SPECIFICITY OF DIFFERENT DIAGNOSTIC TESTS FOR HERNIATED LUMBAR DISK[a]

Diagnostic Test	Sensitivity	Specificity
CT scan	0.92	0.88
Metrizamide myelography	0.90	0.87
Iophendylate myelography	0.80	0.90
Diskography	0.83	0.78
Epidural venography	0.87	0.70
Electromyography	0.92	0.38

[a]A diagnosis of herniated disk does not necessarily mean a change in therapy.
From Hudgins WR: Computer-aided diagnosis of lumbar disc herniation. *Spine.* 1983;8:604–615.

present. Oblique projections add information of importance in only 4 to 8% of cases and more than double the patient's radiation exposure.[35] Repeat films are not beneficial; they waste time and money and expose the patient to more radiation. No serious diagnoses are missed, and symptom resolution, functional improvement, and satisfaction are the same whether a patient receives a radiograph or not.[37] Explaining to a patient the problem and the medical care needed help in reducing the number of radiographs ordered, and the patient remains satisfied.[38] A proposed algorithm for the initial approach to the patient with low back pain is presented in Figure 58–1.

What other studies can help in managing patients with low back pain? Imaging techniques such as MRI, CT, myelography, and diskography are useful for diagnosis and for surgical planning in disk disease, spinal stenosis, tumor, and abscesses. Few studies have addressed the sensitivity and specificity of radiography for all lumbar pathology. For herniated lumbar disk, each technique has a different sensitivity and specificity, as shown in Table 58–3. Caution should be used in interpreting these figures, because asymptomatic patients can have visible herniation or other clinically insignificant pathology. In fact, 25 to 30% of these imaging procedures show surgically correctable abnormalities that have no bearing on the patient's clinical status.[16] Magnetic resonance imaging may prove superior to CT because it can show earlier vertebral involvement by tumor or infection.[39]

SUMMARY

The presence of any of several high-risk indicators should make one consider ordering radiographs in patients with low back pain: age greater than 50 or less than 20 years, serious trauma, known cancer, pain at rest, unexplained weight loss, drug or alcohol abuse, and treatment with corticosteroids. Demonstration on physical examination of a fever above 38°C or a neuromotor deficit should also be evaluated carefully.[35, 40]

Lumbar spine radiography is seldom helpful in assessing nontraumatic mechanical low back pain in the emergency department. Patients presenting with high-risk historical or physical examination findings frequently have abnormal radiographs that will help in decision making regarding their management. Missing a diagnosis through failure to obtain plain radiographs of the lumbosacral spine is not common and usually of limited consequence. In most cases, repeat films do not add more information but do increase cost and radiation exposure.

REFERENCES

1. Gift DA, Harris GI, Gard JW, et al: Employment-related administrative roentgenograms: Characteristics of policy formulation and current practice. *J Occup Med.* 1983;25:34–42.
2. MacFarlane RK: The lumbosacral spine and accident compensation. *N Z Med J.* 1976;83:338.
3. Smyth MJ, Wright V: Sciatica and the intervertebral disc. *J Bone Joint Surg.* 1958;40A:1401–1418.
4. Hirsch C, Ingelmark BE, Miller M: The anatomical basis for low back pain. *Acta Orthop Scand.* 1963;33:1–17.
5. Coventry MB: Anatomy of the intervertebral disk. *Clin Orthop.* 1969;47:9–15.
6. Brolin I: Produktkontroll av rontgenundersokningar av londryggraden. *Lakartidningen.* 1975;72:1793–1795.
7. Witt I, Vestergaard A, Rosenklint A: A comparative analysis of x-ray findings of the lumbar spine in patients with and without lumbar pain. *Spine.* 1984;9:298–300.
8. Hirsch C: Studies on the pathology of low back pain. *J Bone Joint Surg.* 1959;41B:237–243.
9. Runge CR: Pre-existing structural defects and severity of compensation back injuries. *Industrial Medicine and Surgery.* 1958;May:249–252.
10. Splithoff CA: Lumbosacral junction: Roentgenographic comparison of patients with and without backaches. *JAMA.* 1953;152:1610–1613.
11. Fullenlove TM, Williams AJ: Comparative roentgen findings in symptomatic and asymptomatic backs. *Radiology.* 1957;68:572–574.
12. LaRocca H, Macnab I: Value of pre-employment radiographic assessment of the lumbar spine. *Indust Med.* 1970;39:31–36.
13. Rhea JT, Salvatore AD, Llewellyn HJ, Boyd RJ: The oblique view: An unnecessary component of the initial adult lumbar spine examination. *Diagn Radiol.* 1980;134:45–47.
14. Roberts FF, Kishore PRS, Cunningham ME: Routine oblique radiography of

the pediatric lumbar spine: Is it necessary? *Am J Roentgenol.* 1978;131:297–298.

15. Lipton ME, Pellegrini V, Harris I: Is the coned lateral lumbosacral junction radiograph necessary for radiological diagnosis? *Br J Radiol.* 1991;64:420–421.
16. Butt WP: Radiology for back pain. *Clin Radiol.* 1989;40:6–10.
17. Rowe ML: Low back pain in industry: A position paper. *J Occup Med.* 1969;11:161–169.
18. Leboeuf C, Kimber D, White K: Prevalence of spondylolisthesis, transitional anomalies and low intercrestal line in a chiropractic patient population. *J Manip Physiol Ther.* 1989;12:200–204.
19. Symmons DPM, van Hemert AM, Vandenbroucke JP, et al: A longitudinal study of back pain and radiological changes in the lumbar spines of middle aged women. II: Radiographic findings. *Ann Rheum Dis.* 1991;50:162–166.
20. Rockey PH, Fantel J, Omenn GS: Discriminatory aspects of pre-employment screening: Low-back x-ray examinations in the railroad industry. *Am J Law Med.* 1979;5:197–214.
21. Torgerson WR, Dotter WE: Comparative roentgenographic study of the asymptomatic and symptomatic lumbar spine. *J Bone Joint Surg.* 1976;58A:850–853.
22. Gibson ES, Martin RH, Terry CW: Incidence of low back pain and pre-placement x-ray screening. *J Occup Med.* 1980;22:515–519.
23. Quinnell RC, Stockdale HR: The significance of osteophytes on lumbar vertebral bodies in relation to discographic findings. *Clin Radiol.* 1982;33:197–203.
24. Edelstyn GA, Gillespie PJ, Grebbell FS: The radiological demonstration of osseous metastases: Experimental observations. *Clin Radiol.* 1967;18:158–162.
25. Deyo RA: Early diagnostic evaluation of low back pain. *J Gen Intern Med.* 1986;1:328–338.
26. Sim GPG: Vertebral contour in spondylolisthesis. *Br J Radiol.* 1973;46:250–254.
27. Komar NN, Gabrielsen TO, Holt JF: Roentgenographic appearance of lumbosacral spine and pelvis in tuberous sclerosis. *Radiology.* 1967;89:701–705.
28. Schweitzer G, Hoosen GM, Dunbar JM, et al: *Salmonella typhi* spondylitis: An unusual presentation. *South African Med J.* 1971;45:126–128.
29. Quinet RJ, Hadler NM: Diagnosis and treatment of backache. *Semin Arthritis Rheum.* 1979;8:261–287.
30. Currey HLF, Greenwood RM, Lloyd GG, Murray RS: A prospective study of low back pain. *Rheumatol Rehab.* 1979;18:94–104.
31. Pope TL, Riddervold HA: Spine, in Keats TE (ed): *Emergency Radiology.* Chicago: Year Book Medical Publishers; 1984:81–114.
32. Liang M, Komaroff AL: Roentgenograms in primary care patients with acute low back pain: A cost-effectiveness analysis. *Arch Intern Med.* 1982;142:1108–1112.
33. Vecchio TJ: Predictive value of a single diagnostic test in unselected populations. *N Engl J Med.* 1966;274:1171–1173.
34. Deyo RA, Rainville J, Kent DL: What can the history and physical examination tell us about low back pain? *JAMA.* 1992;268:760–765.
35. Frymoyer JW: Back pain and sciatica. *N Engl J Med.* 1988;318:291–300.

36. Deyo RA, Diehl AK: Cancer as a cause of back pain: Frequency, clinical presentation, and diagnostic strategies. *J Gen Intern Med.* 1988;3:230–238.
37. Deyo RA, Diehl AK, Rosenthal M: Reducing roentgenography use: Can patient expectations be altered? *Arch Intern Med.* 1987;147:141–145.
38. Deyo RA, Diehl AK: Patient satisfaction with medical care for low-back pain. *Spine.* 1986;11:28–30.
39. Deyo RA, Bigos SJ, Maravilla KR: Diagnostic imaging procedures for the lumbar spine. *Ann Intern Med.* 1989;111:865–867.
40. Deyo RA, Diehl AK: Lumbar spine films in primary care: Current use and effects of selective ordering criteria. *J Gen Intern Med.* 1986;1:20–25.
41. Hudgins WR: Computer-aided diagnosis of lumbar disc herniation. *Spine.* 1983;8:604–615.

Chapter

Imaging After Head Trauma

Donald M. Yealy

Approximately 500,000 to 600,000 patients annually require evaluation and treatment for acute head injuries in the United States. Care ranges from observation to medical and surgical interventions. The history and the physical examination are the most important means of identifying those at risk for significant head injury.[1, 2] Imaging of the skull and brain parenchyma, however, can offer detailed information about the anatomic site of injury and prognosis. Prompt recognition of certain intracranial lesions, such as subdural and epidural hematomas, can help guide treatment and decrease morbidity and mortality.[3]

Until the early 1970s, imaging after head trauma consisted primarily of plain skull radiographs. Pneumocephalography (instillation of air into the midline ventricle) was an adjunct to help diagnose and localize intracranial lesions, although this technique was helpful only in the presence of large mass lesions. With the advent of computed tomography in the 1970s, the utility of plain skull radiography has lessened. Magnetic resonance imaging has now become more widely available and useful for imaging the central nervous system in select cases. The goal of this chapter is to review the major techniques of and indications for radiographic imaging after head trauma. The ED utility of each method is explored; long-term management is not a focus of this review.

PLAIN SKULL RADIOGRAPHY

Plain skull radiography (PSR) is widely available and relatively inexpensive, and it displays good sensitivity and specificity in detecting bony fracture.[2, 4–7] Plain skull radiography can be done quickly in most patients and rarely interferes with monitoring or clinical care. The technique has poor sensitivity and specificity, however, for intracranial lesions. As a result, PSR has a limited value in detecting serious intracranial injury after acute head trauma and offers little information to aid in the management of such cases.

The major usefulness of PSR after head trauma is identification of bony fracture. Depressed or open skull fractures are well defined by PSR, although these are usually evident on physical examination and better defined by computed tomography. Aside from fractures of the basilar areas, most linear nondisplaced fractures are detected by PSR when the films are interpreted by an experienced radiologist or emergency physician. Plain skull radiography can identify and localize penetrating skull injuries containing metallic or glass objects (if 0.5 mm or greater in size).

The presence of a fracture on PSR increases the risk of an intracranial injury, but the magnitude varies from 2 to 200 times according to the clinical scenario and comparison made.[4, 5] For example, a skull fracture in a patient with a depressed sensorium is associated with a 25% risk of developing an intracerebral hematoma. Conversely, the risk of the same lesion is less than 0.2% in a patient with no fracture who has a history of an altered sensorium but is normal throughout the ED evaluation. Although positive PSR (identification of fracture primarily) can help identify those at a higher risk for an intracranial injury, it cannot provide detailed information about the injury. Certain fractures are associated with specific intracranial lesions (eg, a temporoparietal fracture with an epidural hematoma), but PSR will not provide anatomic data to guide surgical therapy. Furthermore, the clinical assessment usually points toward the presence of an intracranial injury and the need for more detailed imaging, so the contribution of plain films to the management of each patient is limited.

In patients with no change in sensorium, a normal physical examination, and a normal skull series, the risk of an intracranial injury is <0.001%.[4] These data have been used to justify routine skull films in all patients with head trauma in order to help identify which patients can be safely discharged. Normal skull radiographs add little to a carefully elicited benign history and normal physical examination, which are associated with a similar low risk (<0.02 to 0.001%) of significant intracranial injury.[2, 5] More simply, the negative predictive value of the clinical data is minimally enhanced by a normal PSR.

In 1971, Bell and Loop[5] developed clinical criteria intended to eliminate the perceived unnecessary routine use of PSR in head trauma patients. Masters and associates[2] have refined these criteria on the basis of data from a Food and Drug Administration (FDA)–sponsored multicenter trial of imaging after head trauma. These guidelines define the role of PSR and other imaging techniques, including computed tomography, in acute head trauma.

Three groups of patients with acute head trauma can be identified according to the history and physical examination (Table 59–1; Fig. 59–1). Patients in the *high-risk group* for significant intracranial pathol-

TABLE 59–1. CLINICAL FEATURES FOR CLASSIFYING PATIENT RISK OF SIGNIFICANT INJURY AFTER HEAD TRAUMA

Low Risk
Asymptomatic
Dizziness
Headache (mild)
Scalp hematoma, laceration, contusion or abrasion
No moderate- or high-risk findings
Moderate Risk
Any history of change in level of consciousness at any time
Progressive or severe headache
Drug or alcohol intoxication
Unreliable or inadequate history
Posttraumatic seizure
Vomiting
Multiple trauma
Serious facial injury
Signs of basilar skull fracture (hemotympanum, otorrhea, rhinorrhea, raccoon eyes, or Battle sign)
Suspected skull penetration or depressed fracture
Suspected child abuse
Bleeding disorder—congenital or acquired (liver disease, drug-induced)
Age less than 2 years (unless trivial injury)
Significant forces by history (even in absence of abnormal exam)
No high-risk findings
High Risk
Depressed level of consciousness (unrelated to drugs, alcohol, other CNS depressants, metabolic derangements, or postictal state)[a]
Glasgow Coma Score (GCS) 8 or less
Focal neurologic findings
Decreasing level of consciousness, or decrease in GCS of 3 or more
Definite skull penetration or depression

[a]Imaging may be needed if these conditions interfere with clinical assessment.

Adapted from Masters SJ, et al: Skull X-ray examinations after head trauma: Recommendations by a multidisciplinary panel and validation study. *N Engl J Med.* 1987;316:84.

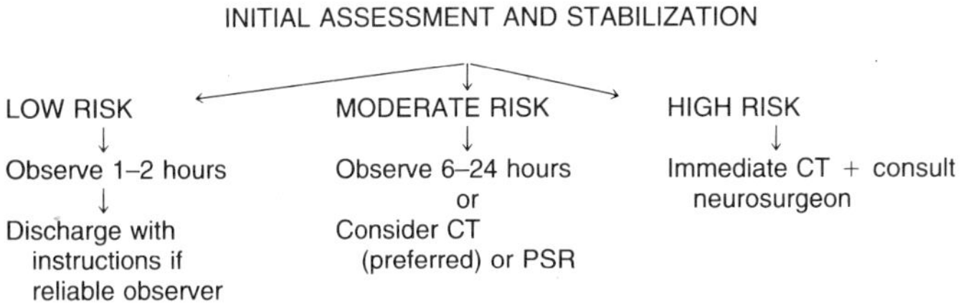

INITIAL ASSESSMENT AND STABILIZATION

LOW RISK	MODERATE RISK	HIGH RISK
↓	↓	↓
Observe 1–2 hours	Observe 6–24 hours or Consider CT (preferred) or PSR	Immediate CT + consult neurosurgeon
↓		
Discharge with instructions if reliable observer		

FIGURE 59–1. Management guidelines for head trauma. The appearance of any moderate- or high-risk criterion automatically places the patient into the higher category. PSR = plain skull radiography; CT = computed tomography (usually unenhanced image is sufficient).

ogy are not candidates for routine PSR, because the examination alone indicates a need for more advanced imaging. These patients are best managed with immediate neurosurgical consultation and computed tomography.

Patients in the *low-risk group* for a significant intracranial injury require no imaging studies. With these clinical criteria, no significant intracranial injuries have been missed in over 7300 patients with low-risk features, and the maximal calculated risk is no greater than 0.02%.[2] Thus, PSR is of no benefit in the practical management of low-risk patients. Although the charge to an individual patient may not seem excessive, the overall cost of routine PSR in low-risk patients is high. It is estimated that up to $100 million could be saved each year in the United States by the elimination of PSR in 80 to 90% of low-risk patients. In spite of these data, PSR continues to be employed frequently in trauma protocols.[8]

Patients with one or more *moderate-risk criteria* should receive either an imaging study or a prolonged observation. Computed tomography is often a more appropriate study, due to its increased sensitivity and specificity for intracranial injury.[9–12] A period of prolonged observation may help further identify patients at varying degrees of risk for serious injury. If PSR is performed in these patients, identification of a fracture should prompt an imaging of the intracranial contents, to search for a concomitant intracranial injury, and a neurosurgical consultation.

Pediatric patients represent one group in whom identification of a linear nondisplaced skull fracture by PSR may have greater significance.[2, 4–7] In children less than 2 years of age, clinical hypovolemia can occasionally result from the extracranial bleeding associated with linear skull fracture. Identifying a skull fracture may also be the initial means of diagnosing child abuse. Leptomeningeal cyst formation is a long-term sequela that must also be observed for after a skull fracture is identified.[7] For these reasons, PSR after head trauma in children under the age of 2 years is recommended unless the history is of a trivial injury. Other imaging modalities more sensitive in detecting intracranial injuries, especially computed tomography, should be used in this age group if significant trauma is reported, because neurologic deficits may be difficult to appreciate in these patients.[1, 13]

COMPUTED TOMOGRAPHY

Computed tomography (CT) currently is the study of choice after head trauma.[3, 9, 10, 12, 15–19] Computed tomography is highly sensitive and specific for both acute bony and intracranial lesions. Its value in identifying which lesions will need immediate operative intervention is unsurpassed, and it offers prognostic information about many injuries. A normal CT scan in a patient with normal neurologic examination findings and normal sensorium has an excellent negative predictive value for delayed neurologic complications.[11, 12, 18, 20] Poor prognostic findings obtained from CT are listed in Table 59–2.

The cost of head CT is approximately twice that of PSR, and it is only slightly less available in the United States (Table 59–3). In order to obtain good images, the patient must remain still to prevent motion artifact. These studies can be obtained in less than 30 minutes in most patients, and invasive monitoring can continue during the procedure.

With the exception of small linear nondisplaced skull fractures, CT can identify bony abnormalities better than PSR.[2, 6, 10, 14] This identification can be done without subjecting the patient to further radiologic exposure simply by manipulating the computer-generated views obtained during the evaluation of the intracranial contents. If CT imaging is indicated after acute head injury, routine PSR to evaluate the bony structures is not recommended, although it may be of benefit in selected cases in which CT findings are equivocal.

TABLE 59–2. POOR PROGNOSTIC FINDINGS ON CT/MRI AFTER HEAD TRAUMA

Bilateral intracerebral hemorrhages
Combined intra- and extraaxial hemorrhages
Shift of midline structures
Delayed intracerebral hematomas
Severe anatomic disruption from penetrating injuries
Hemorrhage within the brain stem, corpus callosum, or basal ganglion
Shear injury findings

TABLE 59–3. COMPARISON OF IMAGING STUDIES FOR PATIENTS WITH ACUTE HEAD TRAUMA

Study	Relative Cost[a]	Relative Availability[a]	Relative Ease[a]	Sensitivity to Detect Injuries		
				Bone	*Blood*	*Edema*
Plain skull radiography (PSR)	1	1	1	Very good	None	None
CT	2	2[b]	2	Excellent	Excellent	Good
MRI	3	3	3	Poor	Good[c]	Excellent

[a]1 = cheapest, most available, and least technical restrictions in trauma patient, and 3 = most expensive, least available, and most restrictions in trauma patient.
[b]Very closely rivals availability of PSR in the U.S.
[c]Equivalent to CT in detecting acute subdural and epidural blood, and better in detecting subacute bleeding and small parenchymal contusions or edema, but less sensitive than CT in detecting acute subarachnoid blood.

Previous limitations of CT in head trauma included basilar skull fractures, posterior fossa lesions, and artifacts from penetrating objects. Newer scanners and thinner slices (5 mm) have improved the ability of CT to detect significant acute injuries in these areas. A normal CT scan still cannot be used to exclude the diagnosis of basilar skull fracture if the physical examination suggests such an injury. A blood-fluid level within the sphenoid sinus or mastoid air cells can provide indirect evidence of a basilar skull fracture.

Extravascular blood is the most common manifestation of an intracranial injury and is well visualized on CT as a hyperdense collection of fluid in the first few days after an injury. Therefore, an unenhanced scan of the head is usually adequate in acute trauma. Contrast enhancement should be used only after evaluation of the unenhanced image, and only if specific injuries are sought. Contrast enhancement may help better characterize isodense intracranial hemorrhages, such those noted with acute bleeding into an old hematoma, or when 7 to 21 days have passed from the time of the initial injury. Computed tomography is often used to evaluate subjective complaints such as headache or mild depression of sensorium in an alcoholic patient or an elderly patient with frequent falls. Isodense hematomas are often seen in these groups, and contrast enhancement may be helpful if the unenhanced image is not diagnostic.

Like PSR, CT is not indicated in the management of low-risk patients. (see Table 59–1 and Fig. 59–1).[2] Patients in the high-risk category for intracranial injury should have immediate neurosurgical consultation and CT after appropriate stabilization to define injuries. Focal neurologic findings or a Glasgow Coma Score (GCS) of 8 or less correlates with a 50 to 75% incidence of CT-proven intracranial injury.[3, 9, 11] In general, of a population of comatose patients imaged with CT after head trauma, approximately 60% have intracranial hemorrhage, 30% are normal, and 10% have edema or infarction.[9, 15, 16]

Computed tomography is also a prudent choice in patients with any head or neurologic complaints after multiple trauma if prolonged anesthesia is imminent for surgical repair of noncranial injuries. If any uncertainty exists, the emergency physician should confer with a neurosurgeon to assist in patient management.

Patients at moderate risk for intracranial injury represent a challenge (see Table 59–1). As noted previously, extended observation (6 to 24 hours) may help identify physical findings that enable reclassification into the high-risk group. Even in those patients who remain stable, the risk of significant intracranial lesion varies depending on the individual case. No generalized recommendation can be made, but it is prudent to employ a low threshold of suspicion to image those with deterioration or in whom neurologic improvement is not noted. Subtle changes, such as increasing headache or mild depression of sensorium, should be sought and should prompt an immediate evaluation of the intracranial contents if found. Patients with one or two moderate-risk criteria who clinically improve during an extended period of observation (6 hours or more) may not require CT imaging.

The use of CT in patients with an inherited or acquired bleeding disorder is controversial; if the history of trauma is trivial and no other complaints or abnormalities are noted, CT may be withheld in lieu of close observation. If any other moderate risk criteria co-exist, however, imaging is best performed promptly because of the risk of seemingly occult intracranial hemorrhage.

Pneumocephalus can be easily seen on CT, with as little as 0.5 cc of air detected. It is a result of fracture through air-containing structures (the petrous bone and mastoid cells or the paranasal sinuses) or from penetrating skull injuries. Computed tomography is also valuable in imaging upper cervical spine, orbit, temporal bone, and facial bone injuries. These can be obtained during the initial scanning period by additional focused views of the desired area.

Head CT Controversies

The cost effectiveness of prolonged observation vs early imaging with CT in moderate-risk patients is debated. A normal CT scan in a patient with a normal neurologic examination (including no altered sensorium) is associated with an extremely low risk of adverse sequelae, allowing for discharge to home if the clinical setting permits. In this case, early imaging by CT scan may cost less and may be equally safe compared with inpatient observation.[18, 20] A normal CT scan in the presence of an abnormal examination, even if nonfocal, requires further observation or testing.[18, 21]

Controversy about "who needs head CT" centers on two issues: How much risk of undiagnosed head injury is acceptable? and What defines "low" risk? Aside from imaging and admitting all patients for extended observation (a costly proposition with indirect risks that are poorly defined), no technique of clinical stratification or management is foolproof. Nonetheless, the data collected prospectively by Masters and associates[2] offer the best information on clinical criteria associated with the patient at risk of intracranial injury in need of treatment. In spite of this information, the terms *low-risk for intracranial injury* and *minimal intracranial injury* are often confused or used imprecisely. Those researchers who advocate CT scans for all "minimally head-injured" patients usually have data limited by retrospective collection techniques and selection biases in the population.[12, 13, 18, 22] More importantly, these studies often place patients with nonfocal neurologic findings into a perceived "low-risk" category, only to prove that some have significant injuries. The Masters criteria are specific, citing a GCS of 13 to 14 or amnesia as abnormal; thus, these patients are not truly at low risk, supporting consideration of CT or extended observation based on resources and clinical judgment.

MAGNETIC RESONANCE IMAGING

Magnetic resonance imaging (MRI) is a relative newcomer to the field of diagnostic imaging and has become more widely available in the United States in the past 10 years. Magnetic resonance images are obtained through the use of magnetic fields instead of exposure to ionizing radiation. Tissues are detailed based on differences in water (proton) density. Those tissues containing higher water content appear darker on MRI. The images obtained by this technique provide a high degree of anatomic and physiologic detail in nonbony tissues.[15, 17, 19, 23–26] In general, the detail offered by MRI is unsurpassed. Magnetic resonance images can be easily obtained in both axial and sagittal planes. This ability is an advantage over CT, which can produce relatively crude sagittal images only after reconstruction of axial views. Although not often required, contrast enhancement of MRI studies with gadolinium-DPTA can better define vascular and selected chronic lesions. Bony structures are not well imaged owing to the poor signal generated.

There are practical limits to MRI in head-injured patients in the emergency department (see Table 59–3). Magnetic resonance imaging is more expensive and less available than CT. Because of the magnetic fluxes, there must be a total absence of ferrous materials in or about the scanning area. Patients with metallic sutures, clips, pacemakers, or other prostheses should not be imaged with MR technology. All monitoring equipment must be suited to this environment. Magnetic resonance imaging studies are quite sensitive to motion artifact and require a relatively long time to complete compared with CT. Because of the need for prolonged immobilization, pharmacologic assistance is usually needed in the absence of exceptional levels of patient cooperation. The physical structure of the MRI scanner limits access to the patient. Collectively, these problems currently make MRI impractical in the seriously ill or acutely traumatized patient in the ED.

MRI is quite sensitive in detecting nonhemorrhagic brain parenchymal injuries (edema)[15–17, 19, 23–30] and is superior to CT in this area. The clinical significance of those asymptomatic nonhemorrhagic lesions undetected by CT is questionable, however, in the initial (ie, first 24 hours) management. In general, MRI and CT offer similar albeit not identical capabilities in detecting hemorrhagic lesions.

The lack of a significant osseous signal creates another advantage over

CT. Magnetic resonance imaging is not affected by bony encasement. In particular, MRI is quite sensitive in detecting lesions in the posterior fossa. The newer CT technologies, however, have dramatically narrowed the gap in this area. Magnetic resonance imaging can detect nonmetallic foreign bodies with the cranium or facial structures and is especially useful in identifying wood or plastic objects.[31]

SPECIFIC INJURIES DETECTED BY IMAGING

Two types of injuries occur after head trauma: hemorrhagic and nonhemorrhagic. Often, both types of injuries coexist after severe head trauma. In the ED evaluation of head-injured patients, CT is clearly the method of choice initially, because of its excellent hemorrhagic and bony lesion detection, good nonhemorrhagic lesion detection, and ease of use.

Patients with hemorrhagic lesions can be categorized into three groups of roughly the same size: those with isolated intraaxial hematomas, those with isolated extraaxial hematomas, and those with both lesions.

Extraaxial Hematomas

Extraaxial (nonparenchymal) hematomas are the most common post-traumatic lesions. The CT scan helps determine the need and approach for surgical intervention. Extraaxial blood appears as an area of increased density outside the brain parenchyma. An exception to this appearance occurs with acute bleeding into the area of an old hematoma, or when 5 to 7 days or more have passed since the initial injury. In these cases, the lesions may be isodense and contrast enhancement often aids diagnosis. Approximately 40% of all extraaxial hematomas are associated with a concomitant intraaxial (parenchymal) lesion. Large hematomas can cause increased intracranial pressure and a shift of the midline structures; these findings are associated with a worsened prognosis.

Acute Subdural Hematomas

Acute subdural hematoma (SDH) is usually the result of venous bleeding. An acute SDH appears as a diffuse hyperdense pattern conforming to the margins of the cortex or, occasionally, as a convex collection of blood if larger. Care in scanning the top of the head helps avoid failure to diagnose a high SDH. A bilateral crescentic SDH can be difficult to appreciate, especially if isodense. Subdural hematomas are commonly associated with an underlying parenchymal contusion. If acute SDH is surgically decompressed within 4 hours of the initial injury, the mortality is 30%. If decompression is achieved after 4 hours, the mortality increases to 90%.[9]

Epidural Hematomas

Epidural hematoma (EDH) is another extraaxial hemorrhage commonly seen after head trauma. A bony fracture is seen in 75 to 90% of patients with EDHs. Classically, EDH results from a fracture of the temporoparietal skull and disruption of the middle meningeal artery. Others sources for an EDH are disruptions of the dural sinuses, venous tributaries, or diploic veins. A history of immediate loss of consciousness (LOC) followed by a ''lucid interval'' and then a decreasing LOC is a classic sign, although not universal. The usual CT appearance of an EDH is a convex blood collection, often in the temporoparietal area. Epidural hematomas usually do not cross suture lines and are contained within the dura and the inner table of the skull. Because they are less commonly associated with an underlying parenchymal contusion and usually symptomatic within minutes to hours (and hence, diagnosed early), the prognosis for EDH is better than for acute SDH.

Subarachnoid Hemorrhage

Subarachnoid hemorrhage (SAH) is the most common hemorrhagic lesion after head trauma. Small amounts of SAH after trauma do not have the serious prognostic findings that nontraumatic SAH has. Increased density within the basal cisterns, interhemispheric fissures, and sulci is pathognomonic for this type of bleeding. Calcification of the falx in elderly adults can mimic acute bleeding; increased density in this region alone must be interpreted with caution.

Intraventricular Hemorrhage

Intraventricular hemorrhage occurs in 5% of head trauma patients and appears as an increased density within the ventricular system.

Parenchymal Hematoma or Contusion

Intraaxial hemorrhage after head trauma is usually in the form of parenchymal hematoma or contusion. The posterior portion of the frontal lobes and the anterior portion of the temporal lobes are common sites for these injuries. Hematomas are usually found within the white matter and can be evacuated surgically, whereas contusions are usually treated medically unless significant intracranial hypertension coexists. Contusions can occur at the site of the trauma (coup injury), opposite the site of the injury (contracoup), or at both sites. The CT appearance of hematoma with contusion is that of a high-density intraparenchymal area, sometimes surrounded by a low-density ring of edema. A small contusion may be difficult to detect by CT, but lesions requiring immediate aggressive surgical management are rarely missed. Contrast enhancement may be of benefit in equivocal cases.

Shearing-Type Injuries

Shearing-type injuries to the cerebral axons can result from significant head trauma and produce multiple small hemorrhages deep in the brain parenchyma at the junction of the gray and white matter. These injuries occur at the corticomedullary junction, corpus callosum, internal capsule, and upper brain stem. Computed tomography often fails to detect shear injuries in the first 24 to 48 hours. The functional prognosis of this type of injury is poor. The shaken-baby syndrome, which is pathognomonic for child abuse, manifests as shear injuries, coup-contracoup contusions, and retinal hemorrhages on CT or MRI, with MRI a more sensitive modality for detection of such lesions.[24–26, 30, 32]

Edema

Edema is the major nonhemorrhagic parenchymal injury after head trauma. Cerebral edema appears as a low-density area on CT and can be distinguished from infarction by serial scanning and contrast enhancement. As with small contusions, some cases of mild cerebral edema may be difficult to detect on CT and are easier to detect on MRI, but these cases rarely require immediate aggressive treatment. Impingement on the cistern or third ventricle may be an early radiographic sign of increased intracranial pressure (ICP). Other areas of ventricular compression are less reliable for predicting ICP.

Delayed intraaxial hemorrhage after an initial severe head injury is a well-recognized phenomenon, occurring 48 hours to 1 week after the injury. Serial imaging can detect these and is indicated when clinical deterioration is noted. These delayed bleeds usually occur in a patient with an abnormal initial physical examination or an abnormal initial CT scan. Those in whom both the neurologic examination and the initial CT scan are normal rarely suffer delayed bleeding. Other sequelae of head trauma, such as recurrent bleeding, abscess formation, and hydrocephalus, can also be assessed by serial CT imaging. Approximately one third of all seriously injured patients have cortical atrophy on a follow-up CT scan or MRI obtained within months of injury.

Although CT and MRI are comparable in detecting acute extraaxial hemorrhagic lesions, CT is superior to MRI in the detection of acute SAH.[16, 17, 19] Conversely, subacute hemorrhagic lesions are better defined by MRI, and chronic hemorrhagic lesions are well visualized by both methods.

Currently, MRI is used as a complementary test to identify injuries that are suspected on clinical examination but not well defined by CT. Most data concerning MRI in acute head trauma have been generated after the initial assessment, stabilization, and imaging with CT, often after 24 to 72 hours. There are no data supporting the routine use of MRI in the first hours after head injury, although this situation may change as the technique evolves and the logistic difficulties are resolved. Patients presenting with ongoing neurologic complaints after previous nondiagnostic CT evaluation for head injury are a group that should receive MRI.

SUMMARY

Decisions about the optimal imaging strategy in patients after acute head trauma can be based on clinical observations (see Tables 59–1 and 59–3; Fig. 59–1) Low-risk patients do not require radiographic imaging. CT is the procedure of choice for imaging moderate- and high-risk patients with head trauma. Because of its limited ability to guide therapy, plain skull radiography should be used sparingly. It may be useful in equivocal cases of bony injury not detected by CT or in selected moderate-risk patients (especially children under the age of 2 years). MRI rivals CT in the detection of intracranial injuries but is more expensive and cumbersome in seriously ill subjects and does not image bony structures.

REFERENCES

1. Davis RL, Mullen N, Makela M, et al: Cranial computed tomography scans in children after minimal head injury with loss of consciousness. *Ann Emerg Med.* 1994;24:640.
2. Masters SJ, McClean PM, Arcarese JS, et al: Skull X-ray examinations after

head trauma: Recommendations by a multidisciplinary panel and validation study. *N Engl J Med.* 1987;316:84.
3. Soloniuk D, Pitts LH, Lovely M, Bartkowski H: Traumatic intracerebral hematomas: Timing of appearance and indication for operative removal. *J Trauma.* 1986;26:787.
4. Balla JI, Elstein AS: Skull X-ray assessment of head injuries: A decision analytic approach. *Methods Inform Med.* 1984;23:135.
5. Bell RS, Loop JW: The utility and futility of radiographic skull examination for trauma. *N Engl J Med.* 1971;284:236.
6. Macpherson P, Teasdale E: Can computed tomography be relied upon to detect skull fractures? *Clin Radiol.* 1989;40:22.
7. Pietrzak M, Jagoda A, Brown L: Evaluation of minor head trauma in children younger than two years. *Am J Emerg Med.* 1991;9:153.
8. Hackney DB: Skull radiography in the evaluation of acute head trauma: A survey of current practice. *Radiology.* 1991;181:711.
9. Clifton GL, Grossman RG, Makela ME, et al: Neurological course and correlated computerized tomography findings after severe closed head injury. *J Neurosurg.* 1980;52:611.
10. Cole HM: Enhanced computed tomography in head trauma. *JAMA.* 1985;254:3370.
11. Livingston DH, Loder PA, Koziol J, Hunt CD: The use of CT scanning to triage patients requiring admission following minimal head injury. *J Trauma.* 1991;31:483.
12. Stein SC, Ross SE: Mild head injury: A plea for routine early CT scanning. *J Trauma.* 1992;33:11.
13. Dietrich AM, Bowman MJ, Ginn-Pease ME, et al: Pediatric head injuries: Can clinical features reliably predict an abnormality on computed tomography? *Ann Emerg Med.* 1994;22:1535.
14. Cohen RA, Kaufman RA, Myers PA, Towbin RB: Cranial computed tomography in the abused child with head injury. *AJR.* 1986;146:97.
15. Gentry LR, Godersky JC, Thompson B, Dunn VD: Prospective comparative study of intermediate-field MR and CT in the evaluation of closed head trauma. *Am J Radiol.* 1988;150:673.
16. Kelly AB, Zimmerman RD, Snow RB, et al: Head trauma: Comparison of MR and CT—experience in 100 patients. *Am J Neuroradiol.* 1988;9:699.
17. Orrison WW, Gentry LR, Stimac GK, et al: Blinded comparison of cranial CT and MRI in closed head injury evaluation. *Am J Neuroradiol.* 1994;15:351.
18. Stein SC, O'Malley KF, Ross SE: Is routine computed tomography scanning too expensive for mild head injury? *Ann Emerg Med.* 1991;20:1286.
19. Zimmerman RA, Bilaniuk LT, Hackney DB, et al: Head injury: Early results of comparing CT and high-field MR. *Am J Radiol.* 1986;147:1215.
20. Livingston DH, Loder PA, Hunt CD: Minimal head injury: Is admission necessary? *Am Surg.* 1991;57:14.
21. Dacey RG, Alves WM, Rimel RW, et al: Neurosurgical complaints after apparently minor head injury. *J Neurosurg.* 1986;65:203.
22. Harad FT, Kerstein MD: Inadequacy of bedside clinical indicators in identifying significant intracranial injury in trauma patients. *J Trauma.* 1992;32:359.
23. Gentry LR, Godersky JC, Thompson B: MR imaging of head trauma: Review

of the distribution and radiopathologic features of traumatic lesions. *Am J Radiol.* 1988;150:633.
24. Levin AV, Magnusson MR, Rafto SE, Zimmerman RA: Shaken baby syndrome diagnosed by magnetic resonance imaging. *Pediatr Emerg Care.* 1989;5:181.
25. Levin HS, Amparo EG, Eisenberg HM, et al: Magnetic resonance imaging after closed head injury in children. *Neurosurgery* 1989;24:223.
26. Yokota H, Kurokawa A, Otsuka T, et al: Significance of magnetic resonance imaging in acute head injury. *J Trauma.* 1991;31:351.
27. Hadley DM, Teasdale GM, Jenkins A, et al: Magnetic resonance imaging in acute head injury. *Clin Radiol.* 1988;39:131.
28. Hesselink JR, Dowd CF, Healy ME, et al: MR imaging of brain contusions: A comparative study with CT. *Am J Roentgenol.* 1988;150:1133.
29. Jenkins A, Hadley MDM, Teasdale G, et al: Brain lesions detected by magnetic resonance imaging in mild and severe head injuries. *Lancet* 1986;2(8504):445.
30. Sato Y, Yuh WTC, Smith W, et al: Head injury in child abuse: Evaluation with MR imaging. *Radiology.* 1989;173:653.
31. Green BF, Kraft SP, Carter KD, et al: Intraorbital wood: Detection by magnetic resonance imaging. *Ophthalmology.* 1990;97:608.
32. Alexander R, Sato Y, Smith W, Bennett T: Incidence of impact trauma with cranial injuries ascribed to shaking. *Am J Dis Child.* 1990;144:724.

Chapter

Cranial Computed Tomography for Nontraumatic Conditions

Phil B. Fontanarosa

Although once regarded as "a paradigm of high-cost technology and unproven value,"[1] computed tomography (CT) of the brain now is considered the diagnostic imaging study of choice in the initial evaluation of acute central nervous system (CNS) disorders. By virtue of being rapid, noninvasive, and highly accurate, cranial CT scanning has revolutionized the evaluation of patients with neurologic emergencies and has become a well-established and indispensable diagnostic tool for the emergency physician.[2, 3]

Yet, despite its widespread availability, extensive use, and increasingly liberal applications, relatively few published reports have evaluated the clinical utility of cranial CT scanning for acute nontraumatic disorders. This chapter reviews the available data regarding emergency department CT scanning for nontraumatic neurologic conditions, focusing on clinical applications, indications, and diagnostic accuracy.

EMERGENCY CT SCANNING: CLINICAL CONSIDERATIONS

Unenhanced CT imaging (ie, without intravenous radiographic contrast agents) is the standard method for evaluating many acute nontraumatic neurologic emergencies (Table 60–1). Routine cranial CT scanning consists of approximately ten scanning images and requires approximately 20 to 30 minutes to complete, depending on the generation of scanner, the expertise of the technician, and the degree of patient cooperation. Head CT without contrast medium clearly reveals acute intracranial hemorrhage, mass effect with midline shift, ventricular enlargement, and cerebral edema.

Enhanced CT imaging, using intravenous (IV) radiologic contrast, is not performed routinely in ED patients but is useful for establishing the diagnosis of certain acute neurologic processes, particularly masses (eg, tumors), inflammatory conditions (eg, abscesses), or vascular le-

TABLE 60–1. RECOMMENDATIONS FOR EMERGENCY CRANIAL CT SCANNING

- Acute altered level of consciousness (not readily explainable by a metabolic etiology)
- New onset of focal neurologic symptoms or deficit
- Headache
  - Abrupt "thunderclap" onset
  - New headache in patient not prone to headache
  - Headache associated with neurologic symptoms or signs
  - Change in chronic headache pattern
- Seizures
  - New-onset seizures
  - Focal seizures
  - Change in chronic seizure pattern
  - Status epilepticus
  - Abnormal postictal neurologic findings
- Evidence of elevated intracranial pressure
- Any neurologic symptoms or signs in high-risk patients
  - Patient with HIV infection
  - Previously diagnosed malignancy
  - Blood dyscrasias (anticoagulant therapy; hemophilia)

sions (eg, arteriovenous malformations) (Table 60–2). Unenhanced cranial CT scanning should be completed before contrast agent is given.

After reviewing the unenhanced CT scan, the emergency physician and neuroradiologist should determine the likelihood, based on the patient's clinical status, that a contrast scan may provide additional useful diagnostic information. If contrast is administered before unenhanced scanning is completed, areas of acute intracranial hemorrhage may be obscured and the identification of intracranial calcifications becomes more difficult. Contrast agent administration may lead to acute neurologic complications in patients with increased cerebral capillary permeability. Contrast material may extravasate through the disrupted blood brain barrier and into the brain parenchyma. Evidence of neurotoxicity typically manifests immediately and consists of sudden seizure, abrupt change in level of consciousness, or acute appearance of focal motor or sensory deficits.[4, 5]

TABLE 60–2. INDICATIONS FOR IV CONTRAST ENHANCEMENT FOR CRANIAL CT SCANNING

Abnormality on unenhanced CT scan
- Mass effect
- Ventricular dilatation or asymmetry
- Focal tissue density abnormalities
- Unexplained intracranial calcification
- Loss of distinction at gray matter/white matter junction
- Localized edema

Suspected vascular lesions
- Aneurysm
- Arteriovenous malformation

Suspected neoplastic disease
- Primary CNS tumor
- Metastatic lesions

Suspected infectious/inflammatory processes
- Brain abscess
- Encephalitis
- AIDS-related infections
- Cerebritis
- Vasculitis

Miscellaneous conditions
- New-onset seizures
- Isodense chronic subdural hematoma
- Ischemic infarction (after acute phase)
- Suspected posterior fossa lesions

HIGH-YIELD CRITERIA FOR CRANIAL CT SCANNING

Although high-yield criteria have been developed for cranial CT scanning following acute head trauma,[6–8] relatively few studies have evaluated cranial CT scanning for nontraumatic conditions. On the basis of limited data, however, several findings have emerged.[9–11] First, the overall yield of cranial CT for acute nontraumatic conditions appears to be relatively high, ranging from 15 to 30%, depending on the indication for obtaining the scan. Second, the frequency of a positive CT scan correlates directly with the patient's presenting complaint and neurologic status. Third, information obtained from emergency CT scanning significantly affects immediate patient management.

In a prospective investigation of high-yield criteria for cranial CT scanning, Mills and coworkers[10] correlated CT findings with clinical findings in 407 ED patients with acute neurologic complaints or conditions. All patients met at least one of the following preselected criteria: (1) clinical suspicion of intracranial hemorrhage, stroke in evolution, mass lesion, or elevated intracranial pressure; (2) blunt head trauma with decreased level of consciousness, focal deficit, seizure, or Glasgow Coma Scale score less than 10; and (3) suspected depressed or open skull fracture or penetrating head injury. Among 304 patients scanned for nontraumatic conditions, 81 (27%) had acutely abnormal CT scans. The yield for a positive CT scan based on presenting condition was 54% for coma, 29% for hemiparesis, 29% for acute headache, 28% for seizures, and 15% for acute alteration of mental status. Based on neurologic condition, the proportion of CT scans that changed immediate management and frequently necessitated acute intervention were coma, 46%; seizures, 23%; hemiparesis, 22%; headache, 21%; and altered mental status, 8%.

Sexton and Caples[11] retrospectively analyzed high-yield criteria in 100 consecutive emergency cranial CT scans, including 23 obtained for head trauma and 71 for nontraumatic conditions. In the absence of head trauma, ten patients (15%) had acute and significant findings on CT scan. Of 35 patients with acute focal neurologic deficits, nine (26%) had positive CT findings. In contrast, the yield for positive CT was only 2.8% among the remaining 36 patients with headache, seizures, or altered mental status without focal neurologic deficits.

In another retrospective study involving 133 consecutive emergency cranial CT scans, ElMallakh[12] reported that 35 patients (26%) had positive scans, and that 47 scans (35%) yielded information that directly altered the patient's immediate management or ultimate disposition.

Reinus and Zwemer[13] evaluated the ability of clinicians to predict the results of emergency cranial CT scans in 536 consecutive patients. Clinical predictions correlated with acute abnormalities on CT scans for 66.7% of patients. However, 36 of the 123 patients with acute CT abnormalities had been predicted to have low probability of abnormal scan results, suggesting that clinical impression alone is not adequate to allow for patient selection for CT scanning.

CRANIAL CT SCANNING FOR NEUROLOGIC CONDITIONS

The clinical utility of cranial CT scans for acute neurologic emergencies has been examined on a limited basis. Studies have evaluated emergency CT scanning for two common neurologic conditions—acute nontraumatic headache and new-onset seizures.

Nontraumatic Headache

Urgent CT scanning is the diagnostic procedure of choice in the evaluation of patients with acute, severe, nontraumatic headache, particularly when acute subarachnoid hemorrhage (SAH) is suspected.[14–19] Because published studies examining emergency CT scanning for acute headache are few, however, indications and high-yield criteria for performing the test are poorly defined, and data regarding sensitivity and specificity are limited.

A prospective investigation[20] examined urgent cranial CT scanning in 160 ED patients with acute onset of nontraumatic headache. Patients with stable chronic headache patterns, such as recurrent migraine headache syndrome, were excluded. Overall, 43 patients (27%) had positive CT scans, including 16 patients with acute cerebral infarction, 14 with subarachnoid or intracerebral hemorrhage, nine with CNS tumor or metastatic lesions, and four with pansinusitis. Neurologic findings significantly associated with positive CT findings included altered mental status, focal motor weakness or sensory deficit, asymmetric reflexes, and abnormal plantar reflexes. Factors that failed to predict positive CT findings were hypertension, a headache described as the ''worst ever,'' neck pain, speech or visual disturbance, and syncope.

These findings are consistent with proposed recommendations for cost-effective use of CT in nontraumatic headache. According to Rothfus,[21] cranial CT scanning is most cost-effective for patients with abrupt onset of severe headache, headache with associated neurologic findings, or recurrent headaches that have an unusual pattern or are progressively worsening. In the absence of these abnormalities, routine use of cranial CT scanning usually is unrewarding.

Seizures

Suggested high-yield criteria for CT scanning in patients with seizures include new-onset seizures in adults, focal seizures, suspected intracranial structural lesions, and persistent abnormal neurologic findings during the postictal period. In a prospective study of 163 patients undergoing a standard seizure workup in an inner city ED, Eisner and colleagues[22] noted that CT was a high-yield test, detecting significant abnormalities in 25% of patients and leading to a change in diagnosis in 44%.

Clinically significant CNS lesions have been documented in as many as 37% of adults presenting with new-onset seizures. The highest rates of positive CT scan were in patients with focal seizures and in those with abnormal postictal neurologic findings.[23–25] Among patients with new-onset alcohol-related seizures, the rate of positive CT findings is even higher. In a retrospective study of 259 such patients, Earnest and coworkers[26] reported that 138 (53%) had abnormal CT scans, including 16 with significant intracranial lesions, the majority of which were unsuspected from clinical examination.

Intracranial Hemorrhage

Intracerebral Hemorrhage (ICH)

Cranial CT scanning is highly sensitive for detecting acute ICH and provides information critical for determining immediate management.[27] According to Weisberg and Nice,[28] there have been no published reports of clinically symptomatic acute ICH that have not been detected by cranial CT.

Computed tomography findings in ICH include hyperdense lesions, usually with smooth, rounded margins and surrounded by hypodense areas of vasogenic edema. Large hemorrhages commonly produce secondary mass effects, such as ventricular compression and midline shift.

Cerebellar Hemorrhage

Acute cerebellar hemorrhage accounts for 10 to 15% of spontaneous intracranial hemorrhages.[28] Immediate diagnosis is imperative, because without prompt surgical intervention, there may be rapid enlargement and acute brain stem compression. Cranial CT is virtually 100% sensitive for detecting acute cerebellar hemorrhage. CT findings include evidence of a posterior fossa hematoma, frequently accompanied by obstructive hydrocephalus, and effacement of the basilar cisterns and fourth ventricle.

Subdural Hematoma (SDH)

Chronic subdural hematoma is virtually always detectable by CT scan.[29] It typically spreads over the entire cerebral hemisphere and conforms to the brain surface and inner aspect of the cranium. As blood denatures and undergoes proteinolysis, the SDH becomes isodense relative to normal brain tissue. A small SDH can easily be missed at this point in its evolution, especially on an unenhanced study.

Unilateral SDH may produce evidence of mass effect, with decreased ipsilateral ventricular size and midline shift. Some patients with bilateral isodense SDH may have no evidence of midline shifts, however. In these cases, decreased ventricular size and loss of the cortical sulci may be the only clues to the presence of SDH. Intravenous contrast medium administration enhances the subdural membrane adjacent to the brain, but there is no contrast medium uptake within the subdural hematoma itself.

Subarachnoid Hemorrhage (SAH)

Emergency CT scanning is the diagnostic modality of choice for spontaneous subarachnoid hemorrhage.[17–19] If performed on the day of hemorrhage, CT demonstrates blood in the subarachnoid space in 90 to 95% of cases.[30–33] Normal scans are more common 2 or more days after SAH occurs. Among 1412 patients with aneurysmal SAH in the Cooperative Aneurysm Study,[31] CT revealed evidence of SAH in 95% of patients who were scanned on the day of bleeding, compared with positive CT findings in only 74% of patients in whom CT scans were performed 3 days after SAH.

In addition to establishing the diagnosis safely and reliably in the majority of cases of acute SAH, CT provides important information. It often helps to localize the probable site of aneurysmal rupture and may demonstrate unruptured aneurysms or arteriovenous malformations (AVMs). CT demonstrates acute complications that may require urgent intervention, particularly acute hydrocephalus and significant intraparenchymal hematoma, and establishes a baseline for the subsequent diagnosis of complications. The modality can also reveal nonaneurysmal bleeding sources, such as hypertensive hemorrhages and AVMs.

Studies also suggest that CT findings are important prognostic indicators that may even be superior to clinical findings in predicting neurologic outcome.[32–34] Gurusinghe and Richardson[33] evaluated the correlation of the quantity of blood in the subarachnoid cisterns and cerebral fissures as visualized on the initial CT scan with the final neurologic outcome in patients with aneurysmal SAH. Ninety percent of patients with extensive bleeding on initial CT scan had poor neurologic outcomes, whereas 90% of patients with no blood on the initial CT had good neurologic outcomes. Likewise, Auer and colleagues[34] reported that prognosis in SAH was less dependent on preoperative clinical grade than on preoperative CT findings. Ninety-three percent of patients in whom CT demonstrated blood only in the subarachnoid space had good neurologic outcomes, whereas only 50% of patients who had associated intracerebral hemorrhage ultimately achieved good outcomes.

Several studies have stressed the significance of a premonitory minor leak prior to major aneurysmal SAH.[35–39] These warning symptoms usually included the sudden onset of a new or unusual headache and are thought to represent a minor initial hemorrhage (''sentinel hemorrhage''). Alternatively, they may be due to an ischemic event, stretching of the aneurysmal wall, or pressure exerted by an unruptured aneurysm. Warning symptoms have been reported in up to 50% of patients with SAH, with a typical interval of 1 to 3 weeks from warning symptoms to major SAH.[40–42] Because CT is unreliable for diagnosing this event, however, patients with suspected warning symptoms Of SAH and negative CT scans should undergo lumbar puncture.[17, 41]

CEREBRAL INFARCTION

Computed tomography is the initial study of choice in patients with suspected acute cerebral infarction. Emergency CT provides important information that may have immediate therapeutic implications, including the presence or absence of hemorrhage, evidence of mass effect, and identification of surgically treatable lesions. The CT scan is typically normal, however, for up to 12 hours after an acute nonhemorrhagic stroke. When performed early in the course of cerebral infarction, cranial CT scanning may occasionally reveal subtle manifestations of localized hypoperfusion, evidenced by minor reductions in tissue density and mild effacement of adjacent cortical sulci.

One to 4 days after cerebral infarction, the CT scan reveals decreased density of the involved parenchyma in the distribution of the affected artery. Five to 6 days after a stroke, CT shows decreased attenuation, often with localized mass effect.[27, 28] In the chronic stages of cerebral infarction, there is cerebral volume loss, as evidenced by ipsilateral dilatation of the ventricular system and widening of the cortical sulci.

CNS TUMORS AND METASTASES

Contrast-enhanced CT has been the conventional first-line study in the evaluation of suspected intracranial neoplasms.[43] In the early stages, the majority of low-grade tumors appear as low-density lesions and usually do not produce mass effect. Higher-grade, larger, and more malignant lesions typically demonstrate patchy, homogeneous, or ring-like patterns with contrast enhancement. Associated mass effect is noted frequently, and extensive white matter edema may occur. Most large tumors (eg, gliomas) are readily visible on CT, especially when they contain cysts, necrotic areas, or neovascular regions capable of contrast enhancement. Meningiomas commonly produce characteristic findings on unenhanced CT, typically appearing as homogeneous, sharply marginated, hyperdense lesions.

Intracranial metastases occur in approximately 20 to 30% of patients with systemic carcinoma.[44] The sensitivity of CT for detecting cerebral metastases depends on tumor size, location, vascularity, surrounding edema, and associated mass effect. Metastatic lesions larger than 10 mm are visualized reliably by CT, although smaller lesions also are commonly detected.[44] Contrast enhancement is essential for delineating cerebral metastases, because many such lesions are isodense on the nonenhanced scan.

CENTRAL NERVOUS SYSTEM INFECTIONS

Brain Abscess

Cranial CT is the diagnostic procedure of choice to confirm the clinical diagnosis of brain abscess. Contrast-enhanced CT is 95 to 99% sensitive for detecting brain abscess and provides important supplemental information, including the presence of midline shift, hydrocephalus, and imminent ventricular rupture.[45–48]

The characteristic appearance of a cerebral abscess is that of a hypodense center (due to leukocytes and necrotic tissue); an outlying smooth, uniformly enhancing ring; and an extensive surrounding hypodense area of white matter edema. Unfortunately, the specificity of CT for brain abscess does not approach its high sensitivity. False-positive study results are most common in patients with necrotic tumors but also may occur with resolving hematomas, cerebral infarction, and granulomas.[47] False-negative scans may occur in immunocompromised patients and patients receiving long-term steroid therapy.

Encephalitis and Meningitis

Findings on contrast-enhanced CT in patients with encephalitis and meningitis depend on the nature and severity of the underlying infectious process. Encephalitis may be suspected from the presence of low-density changes confined to a specific portion of the brain and accompanied by localized mass effect or edema. Herpes simplex infection may produce low-density changes affecting both white matter and adjacent cortical tissue, most commonly in the frontal lobe and medial temporal region; local mass effect if edema is significant; and nonhomogeneous contrast enhancement.[38] Patients with acute bacterial meningitis usually have normal cranial CT scans. Those with chronic meningitis, however, particularly that due to tuberculosis, may display leptomeningeal enhancement in the basal cisterns near the skull base.

AIDS-Related CNS Infections

Emergency CT scanning is indicated for HIV-positive patients who present with neurologic symptoms or signs. Of patients with advanced HIV disease, up to 40% develop significant neurologic symptoms during the course of illness. At autopsy, 80% of cases demonstrate pathologic CNS findings due to HIV or opportunistic infection.[50–51]

According to Hirsch,[50] CT abnormalities in AIDS patients generally can be divided into four categories: (1) enlargement of sulci and ventricles, which results from the direct effects of chronic HIV encephalitis; (2) focal white matter abnormalities, which usually indicate concurrent infection with cytomegalovirus, papovavirus, or herpes simplex; (3) mass lesions, which usually represent primary CNS lymphoma or infection with *Toxoplasma* or *Cryptococcus;* and (4) leptomeningeal thickening and enhancement, which usually suggest meningitis due to fungi, opportunistic bacteria, mycobacteria, or invasive viruses.

CONCLUSIONS

Cranial CT scanning has revolutionized the emergency evaluation and management of patients with acute nontraumatic neurologic disorders. It is readily available, rapid, noninvasive, and highly sensitive. CT is unsurpassed in identifying intracranial lesions that require immediate operative intervention and offers prognostic information about many acute neurologic disease processes.

Despite these advantages, the indiscriminate use of CT scanning cannot be advocated for a variety of reasons, such as logistics, radiation exposure, and cost. Unfortunately, well-designed studies establishing indications, clinical utility, high-yield criteria, and diagnostic accuracy for emergency cranial CT scanning are lacking. Prospective research is necessary to determine criteria for appropriate, cost-effective utilization of this imaging modality in nontraumatic emergency conditions.

REFERENCES

1. United States Congress, Office of Technology Assessment: Policy implications of the computed tomography (CT) scanner. Washington, DC: Government Printing Office; 1978.
2. Wittenberg J: Computed tomography of the body. *N Engl J Med.* 1983;309:1160–1165.
3. Hollerman JJ: Computed tomography, in Tintinalli JE, Krome RL, Ruiz E (eds): *Emergency Medicine—A Comprehensive Study Guide.* 3rd ed. New York: McGraw-Hill; 1991:1126–1136.
4. Whye D, Young J, Barish RA: Altered consciousness and syncope, in Rosen P, Barkin R (eds): *Emergency Radiology.* St Louis: CV Mosby; 1992:388–417.
5. Deck M: Radiologic imaging techniques in the diagnosis and care of the neurologic patient, in Wyngaarden JB, Smith LH (eds): *Cecil Textbook of Medicine.* 18th ed. Philadelphia: WB Saunders; 1995:2058–2060.
6. Melartin E, Taohimac PJ, Dabb R: Neurotoxicity of iodothalamates and diatrizoates: Significance of concentration and reactions. *Invest Radiol.* 1970;5:22–27.
7. Stein SC, Ross SE: The value of computed tomographic scans in patients with low-risk head injuries. *Neurosurgery.* 1990;26:638–640.
8. Rosenthal BW, Bergman I: Intracranial injury after moderate head trauma in children. *J Pediatr.* 1989;115:346–350.
9. Stein SC, O'Malley KF, Ross SE: Is routine computed tomography scanning too expensive for mild head injury? *Ann Emerg Med.* 1991;20:1286–1289.
10. Mills ML, Russo LS, Vines FS, et al: High yield criteria for urgent cranial computed tomography scans. *Ann Emerg Med.* 1986;15:1167–1172.
11. Sexton CC, Caples JM: Emergency CT of the head: Indications and utilization. *Md Med J.* 1987;36:493–495.
12. ElMallakh RS: Utility of emergent computed tomograms of the head in diagnosis and patient management. *Conn Med.* 1987;51:634–637.
13. Reinus WR, Zwemer FL: Clinical prediction of emergency cranial computed tomography results. *Ann Emerg Med.* 1994;23:1271–1278.
14. Linet M, Stewart W, Celentano D, et al: An epidemiologic study of headache among adolescents and young adults. *JAMA.* 1989;261:2211–2214.
15. Leight MJ: Nontraumatic headache in the emergency department. *Ann Emerg Med.* 1980;9:404–407.
16. Diamond ML: Emergency department treatment of the headache patient. *Headache Quarterly* (Suppl). 1992;3:28–33.
17. Fontanarosa PB: Recognition of subarachnoid hemorrhage. *Ann Emerg Med.* 1989;18:1199–1205.
18. Solomon RA, Fink ME: Current strategies for the management of aneurysmal subarachnoid hemorrhage. *Arch Neurol.* 1987;44:769–773.
19. Hillman J: Should computed tomography scanning replace lumbar puncture

in the diagnostic process in suspected subarachnoid hemorrhage? *Surg Neurol.* 1986;26:247–250.
20. Fontanarosa PB, Sargeant L: High-yield criteria to predict intracranial CT findings in patients with acute nontraumatic headache. Presented at the Midwestern Emergency Medicine Research Symposium, Dayton, OH, March 1992.
21. Rothfus WE: Headache, in Straub WH: *Manual of Diagnostic Imaging.* Boston: Little, Brown and Company; 1989:37–42.
22. Eisner RF, Turnbull TL, Howes DS: Efficacy of a "standard" seizure workup in the emergency department. *Ann Emerg Med.* 1986;15:33–39.
23. Ramirez-Lassepas M, Cipolle RJ, Morilo LR: Value of computed tomographic scan in the evaluation of adult patients after their first seizure. *Ann Neurol.* 1984;15:536–543.
24. Russo LS, Goldstein KH: The diagnostic assessment of single seizures: Is cranial computed tomography necessary? *Arch Neurol.* 1983;40:744–746.
25. Hopkins A, Garman A, Clarke C: The first seizure in adult life: Value of clinical features, electroencephalography and computerized tomographic scanning in predicting seizure recurrence. *Lancet.* 1988;1:721–726.
26. Earnest MP, Feldman H, Mark JA, et al: Intracranial lesions shown by CT scans in 259 cases of first alcohol related seizures. *Neurology.* 1988;38:1561–1565.
27. Davis KR, Kistler JP, Buonanno FS: Clinical neuroimaging approaches to cerebrovascular diseases. *Neurol Clin North Am.* 1984;2:655–665.
28. Weisberg L, Nice C: *Cerebral Computed Tomography—A Text Atlas.* 3rd ed. Philadelphia: WB Saunders; 1989:133–162.
29. McMicken DB: Emergency CT head scans in traumatic and atraumatic conditions. *Ann Emerg Med.* 1986;15:274–279.
30. Whiting DM, Barnett GH, Little JR: Management of subarachnoid hemorrhage in the critical care unit. *Cleve Clin J Med.* 1989;56:775–785.
31. Adams HP, Kassell NF, Torner JC, et al: CT and clinical correlations in recent aneurysmal subarachnoid hemorrhage: A preliminary report of the Cooperative Aneurysm Study. *Neurology.* 1983;33:981–988.
32. Weisberg LA: Computed tomography in aneurysmal subarachnoid hemorrhage. *Neurology.* 1979;29:802–808.
33. Gurusinghe NH, Richardson AE: The value of computerized tomography in aneurysmal subarachnoid hemorrhage. *J Neurosurg.* 1984;60:763–770.
34. Auer LM, Schneider GH, Auer T: Computerized tomography and prognosis in early aneurysm surgery. *J Neurosurg.* 1986;65:217–221.
35. Okawara S: Warning signs prior to rupture of an intracranial aneurysm. *J Neurosurg.* 1973;38:575–580.
36. Duffy GP: The "warning leak" in spontaneous subarachnoid hemorrhage. *Med J Aust.* 1983;1:514–516.
37. King RB, Saba MI: Forewarnings of major subarachnoid hemorrhage. *N Y State J Med.* 1974;74:638–639.
38. Ostergaard JR: Headache as a warning symptom of impending aneurysmal subarachnoid hemorrhage. *Cephalgia.* 1991;11:53–55.
39. Verweij RD, Wijdicks EF, van Gijn J: Warning headache in aneurysmal subarachnoid hemorrhage—a case control study. *Arch Neurol.* 1988; 45:1019–1020.

40. Adams HP: Clinical manifestations and diagnosis of subarachnoid hemorrhage. *Semin Neurol.* 1984;4:304–314.
41. Juvela S: Minor leak before rupture of an intracranial aneurysm and subarachnoid hemorrhage of unknown etiology. *Neurosurgery.* 1992;30:7–11.
42. LeBlanc R: The minor leak preceding subarachnoid hemorrhage. *J Neurosurg.* 1987;66:35–39.
43. Council on Scientific Affairs: Magnetic resonance imaging of the central nervous system. *JAMA.* 1988;259:1211–1222.
44. Weisberg LA: Intracranial neoplasms. *Neurol Clin North Am.* 1984;2:695–719.
45. Bleck TP: Increased intracranial pressure, in Schwartz GR, Cayten CG, Mayer TA, et al (eds): *Principles and Practice of Emergency Medicine.* 3rd ed. Philadelphia: Lea & Febiger; 1992:1573–1587.
46. Greenberg JO: Neuroimaging in brain swelling. *Neurol Clin North Am.* 1984;2:677–694.
47. Chun CK, Johnson JD, Hofstetter M, et al: Brain abscess—a study of 45 consecutive cases. *Medicine.* 1986;65:415–431.
48. Wispelwey B, Scheld WM: Brain abscess. *Clin Neuropharmacol.* 1987;10:483–510.
49. McCabe JB, Hochhauser L: Seizures, in Rosen P, Barkin R (eds): *Emergency Radiology.* St Louis: CV Mosby; 1992:418–448.
50. Hirsch WL: AIDS: CNS involvement, in Straub WH: *Manual of Diagnostic Imaging.* Boston: Little, Brown and Company; 1989:64–69.
51. Levy RM, Rosenbloom S, Perrett LV: Neuroradiologic findings in AIDS: A review of 200 cases. *Am J Nucl Radiol.* 1986;7:833–839.

Chapter

61 Extremity Radiography

Alison J. McDonald and Michael P. Bellino

The diagnosis and assessment of extremity injuries by physical examination alone are imperfect. Radiologic imaging helps to determine both the nature and the severity of the injury. Discussions of the overutilization of radiography have focused on several aspects, including an overdependence on radiographs instead of relying on clinical examination; the physician's need for diagnostic certainty; patient demand; and defensive medicine.[1] A study of 500 patients showed that requests for radiographs in the emergency department were made for suspected abnormality in 30% of cases, for patient reassurance in 30%, and for purely medicolegal reasons in 10%.[2]

In an attempt to limit overutilization of radiographs, Brand and associates[3] devised a protocol using clinical indicators in conjunction with physical examination to determine the necessity for upper or lower extremity radiography. Use of this protocol resulted in missing only one fracture in the 848 patients who were examined. Clinical management and outcome for the one patient would not have been affected had radiograph been obtained.

This chapter outlines the diagnostic ED roentgenographic procedures of choice for evaluation of lower extremity injuries and addresses their sensitivity, specificity, and predictive values, when these figures are available.

RADIOLOGY BASICS

Plain film radiography is the most important initial method of evaluating acute extremity injuries in the emergency department. In general, the injured area should be radiographed in two planes that are at right angles to each other. Anteroposterior (AP) and lateral views are sufficient in most simple extremity injuries, but oblique views may be necessary, especially in areas of bone overlap or close to a joint. Stress views may be helpful to document the presence and extent of joint instability and pain. They may be helpful in the first metacarpal joint and in the knees and ankles. Special views of particularly difficult areas, such as the wrist, shoulder, and hip, are needed in certain cases. Magnification views can be helpful if the initial film does not show a fracture (eg, detection of occult scaphoid fractures).

Conventional tomography may help delineate fractures that are not seen well on plain films.[4] Computed tomography (CT) can help define the complex anatomy in shoulder, pelvis, and hip injuries and can be of use in the evaluation of the sternoclavicular joint, distal radioulnar joint, and extremity soft tissue masses. Magnetic resonance imaging (MRI) is being used more commonly in shoulder and knee injuries, obviating arthrography.[4]

UPPER EXTREMITY

The Wrist

Wrist fracture is one of the most commonly seen injuries in emergency department practice. Carpal bone fractures have been reported to be missed initially up to 60% of the time in some series.[5]

The scaphoid, or navicular, is the most commonly fractured carpal bone, accounting for 70 to 80% of all carpal injuries.[5, 6] Scaphoid fractures are, however, the most commonly undiagnosed fracture. Symptoms are frequently minimal, a fracture line may not be immediately visible, and fractures are frequently nondisplaced. The majority of scaphoid fractures occur at the waist (70%); fractures at the proximal pole (20%) and distal pole (10%) constitute the remainder.[7] Initial radiographic views of suspected scaphoid fracture should consist of (1) a posteroanterior view with the wrist in neutral position and gentle ulnar deviation, (2) a lateral view in neutral position, and (3) radial and ulnar oblique views. If a longstanding fracture is suspected, one should include a PA with radial deviation, an AP with a clenched-fist view, and lateral radiographs taken with the wrist in maximal dorsiflexion and volar flexion.[8]

The false-negative rate for initial films of the scaphoid is reported to be between 2 and 16%.[9] A prospective study of 85 emergency department patients with suspected wrist injury revealed an 80% sensitivity for initial standard radiographs, or a 20% false-negative rate. The presence of physical signs of scaphoid fractures, including anatomic snuffbox tenderness, pain with supination against resistance, and pain with axial loading, were found to have sensitivities of 100%, 100%, and 97.5%, respectively. The specificities were also high, although this finding may be misleading because distal forearm injuries were excluded from the analysis.[9]

Another study examined 38 patients seen within 3 days of injury who had mild-to-moderate swelling of the radial aspect of the wrist and anatomic snuffbox tenderness. Initial radiographs, including scaphoid views, were judged to be negative. Repeat radiographic examinations 2 weeks later revealed that 16% of the patients had sustained an occult fracture that had not been seen initially.[7]

An emergency department study of 90 patients with suspected scaphoid fractures added two additional views, 25° wrist pronation and supination, to the standard four views. In this study, anatomic snuffbox tenderness had a sensitivity of 100%, a specificity of 76%, and a positive predictive value of 92%. The four standard views had a sensitivity of 83%, a specificity of 70%, and a positive predictive value of 83%. When all six views were used, the sensitivity, specificity, and positive predictive values were all 100%.[10]

In light of the high incidence of initially negative films in scaphoid fractures, radiographic soft tissue signs have been investigated to see whether they can be used to improve on the initial diagnosis. The scaphoid fat stripe is a radiolucent line parallel to, and slightly convex toward, the radial surface of the scaphoid and is best seen on the PA and oblique views. If the convexity is reversed, obliterated, or indistinct, the fat stripe sign is abnormal and suggests bony injury. The scaphoid fat stripe has been described as present in 90% of normal wrists, but as abnormal in 95% of scaphoid fractures.[7] In one study of 888 patients with wrist injuries, 70% of scaphoid fractures had a positive scaphoid fat stripe and 8% had indistinct fat lines because of obesity; the false-positive rate was 3.4%.[11] In another series of 127 patients, 68.2% of patients with an abnormal scaphoid fat stripe had a scaphoid fracture.[12] A retrospective study concluded that an abnormal fat stripe is a poor predictor of scaphoid injury, whereas a straight or normal fat stripe is a good predictor of the absence of scaphoid injury; if the fat stripe was straight, the probability of a fracture was 9%, whereas the probability of no fracture was 91%.[13] Other injuries that can obliterate the scaphoid fat stripe are fractures of the radial styloid process, first metacarpal bone, and triquetrum.[4]

Dorsal soft tissue swelling has also been described as a sign that may aid in the diagnosis of scaphoid fractures. The dorsal soft tissue is normal if it is concave toward the carpal bones and abnormal if it is convex to them. In one series of 27 patients, 68% of patients with positive dorsal soft tissue swelling had a scaphoid fracture, and 73% patients who had both an abnormal scaphoid fat stripe and a dorsal soft tissue swelling had a fracture.[12] The false-negative rate of dorsal wrist swelling in this series was 27%. In another series, dorsal wrist swelling was seen in only 35% of scaphoid fractures.[11] Thus, the false-positive rate of soft tissue signs in scaphoid fracture varies from 12% to 18%, and the absence of soft tissue signs does not exclude a scaphoid fracture.[11, 12]

Soft tissue signs have also been examined in distal forearm fractures. The pronator quadratus muscle is covered by a thin layer of fatty tissue that is best seen on the true lateral film. Normally, it is gently convex just dorsal to the distal radius and ulna. In one series, 63% of radial and ulnar shaft fractures and 45% of distal radial fractures showed an abnormal pronator stripe. In the same series, 80% of distal radial and ulnar shaft fractures had dorsal radial soft tissue swelling.[11] These numbers are judged to be too low to be of clinical value in excluding fracture.

A negative bone scan 3 days after injury is said to be 100% sensitive in excluding a scaphoid fracture, although soft tissue swelling and tendon inflammation may lead to false-positive readings, reducing the scan's specificity.[8] In view of the difficulty of diagnosing all scaphoid fractures on initial films, the standard of care is to put the patient in a thumb spica cast or splint. The wrist is then radiographed in 2 weeks, when bone resorption at the fracture site will make it more visible. If film findings are negative at this point, a scaphoid fracture has been excluded.[7, 14]

Other wrist injuries have been studied much less extensively than scaphoid injury, and most are visualized on the standard wrist radiographs. Only the more difficult to diagnose are discussed here.

Fracture of the Hook of the Hamate

Rare in the general population but common in athletes, fracture of the hook of the hamate is often difficult to see on routine films. Nonunion is a common sequela, and early identification is important to help prevent this complication.[15] Notably, in one study of 25 patients with a fracture of the hook of hamate, six fractures were not identified initially.

The normal hook, when seen on end in the PA projection, looks like a cortical ring; in 90% of hook fractures, the ring is absent, indistinct, or sclerotic. Special views may be needed. A carpal tunnel view with the wrist prone and in 90° dorsiflexion puts the hook on the ulnar aspect of the carpal tunnel. A nonunited ossification center appears in the same location but has smooth margins; moreover, ossification centers are often bilateral. Computed tomography can also be used to diagnose fractures of the hook of the hamate.[7]

Scapholunate Dislocation

The scapholunate ligaments can be stretched or torn, leading to a widened scapholunate distance. The normal space, taken in the midportion of each bone, usually measures less than 2 mm. A study of 100 patients sent for wrist radiographs added a clenched-fist view in order to increase the scapholunate separation if the ligaments were unstable.[17] Nineteen percent had an abnormal space, but in 15% the abnormality was bilateral. Five percent of patients were believed to have scapholunate dislocation. Jones[17] recommended ordering a clenched-first view when there is concern about scapholunate ligament injury or in patients with chronic wrist pain. If the scapholunate distance is greater than 2 mm, comparison views of the other side should be obtained. Patients with unilateral abnormalities are considered to have scapholunate ligamentous injury.[17]

The Hand

Hand injuries are usually diagnosed on routine radiographs, which should consist of a PA view, a lateral view with flexed fingers, and a 45° pronation oblique view. In order to be properly seen, the thumb requires an AP view with the hand pronated and the dorsal surface of the thumb against the cassette. The lateral view of the thumb requires the hand to be pronated 15°.

Radiographic abnormalities associated with tendon injuries are not uncommon. An avulsed bony fragment can be seen in 25% of cases of ''mallet'' finger. In contrast, avulsion of the profundus flexor tendon owing to forced extension of the distal interphalangeal joint usually shows only soft tissue swelling. Volar plate rupture at the proximal interphalangeal (PIP) joint may show an avulsion fracture at the base of the middle phalanx or dorsal dislocation of the proximal interphalangeal. The lateral view is most helpful, but in 35% of cases of volar plate rupture, the oblique view is needed for the injury to be seen, and 20% are missed initially.[7] Injury to the ulnar collateral ligament of the thumb may show an avulsion fracture at the base of the proximal phalanx, where the ligament inserts, but radiographic findings are often negative. Stress radiographs can be used if the initial film findings are negative; a difference of 10° of abduction between the injured thumb and the normal is considered positive.

The Elbow

The ''fat pad signs'' of elbow injury are well known. The anterior fat pad lies in front of the distal humeral cortex and normally has a teardrop appearance, which becomes a ''ship's sail'' when displaced anteriorly by a joint effusion. This latter appearance is pathognomonic of intraarticular disease. A false-negative anterior fat pad sign may occur with poor positioning, extracapsular fracture, or capsular rupture. The posterior fat pad normally is recessed in the olecranon fossa and is almost never visible normally.[19, 20] Thus, a visible posterior fat pad is generally believed to be pathognomonic of intraarticular disease. A false-positive fat pad sign, however, may occur with elbow extension, an unusually large fat pad in obesity, or elevation of the periosteum by hemorrhage or neoplasm.[19] The fat pad signs are important indicators of trauma but do not necessarily indicate a fracture or ligamentous rupture.[20] Hemarthrosis secondary to a fracture is the most common cause, but other causes of hemarthrosis are hemophilia, transudative joint effusions, crystal arthropathy, and inflammatory arthropathies such as rheumatoid arthritis.[19, 20]

The Shoulder

Radiographic imaging of the shoulder is difficult because of the multiple overlying structures in the area. Standard views include the AP, internal rotation, and external rotation views. In addition, the axillary projection can be used to visualize the glenoid and the coracoid processes; the apical oblique (Neer) view is good for the coracoid or humeral head; and the Y view (scapular projection) is helpful in detecting dislocations and scapular fractures.[20, 21]

Glenohumeral dislocations constitute 85% of all dislocations about the shoulder, and 95% of these are anterior. Associated with the dislocation may be a compression fracture of the posterolateral aspect of the humeral head (Hill-Sachs lesion) or a fracture of the anterorinferior glenoid rim (Bankaert lesion).[20] In the apical oblique (AO) view (Fig. 61–1) the patient faces the tube, and the injured side is rotated 45° dorsally. The beam is directed 45° caudad and centered on the glenohumeral joint, giving a tangential view through the glenohumeral joint with the glenoid rim and scapular neck visible free of other structures. Structures dislocated posterior project cephalad, and those dislocated anteriorly project caudad.[22]

The Y scapular view is obtained by placing the anterolateral aspect of the injured shoulder against the cassette and angling the patient 45 to 60° toward the cassette (Fig. 61–2). The beam is oriented parallel to

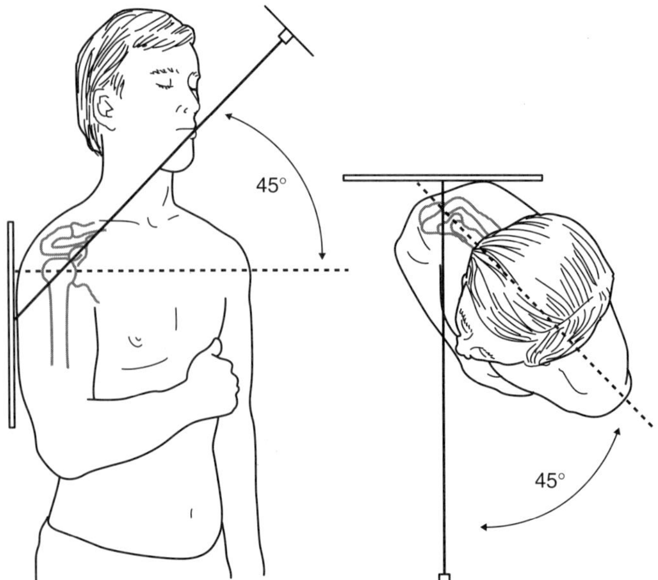

FIGURE 61–1. The apical oblique projection. The injured side is rotated posteriorly, while the central beam is directed 45° caudally, centered on the glenohumeral joint. From Sloth C, Lundgren Just S: The apical oblique radiograph in examination of acute shoulder trauma. *Europ J Radiol.* 1989;9:147–151. Georg Thieme Verlag, Stuttgart.

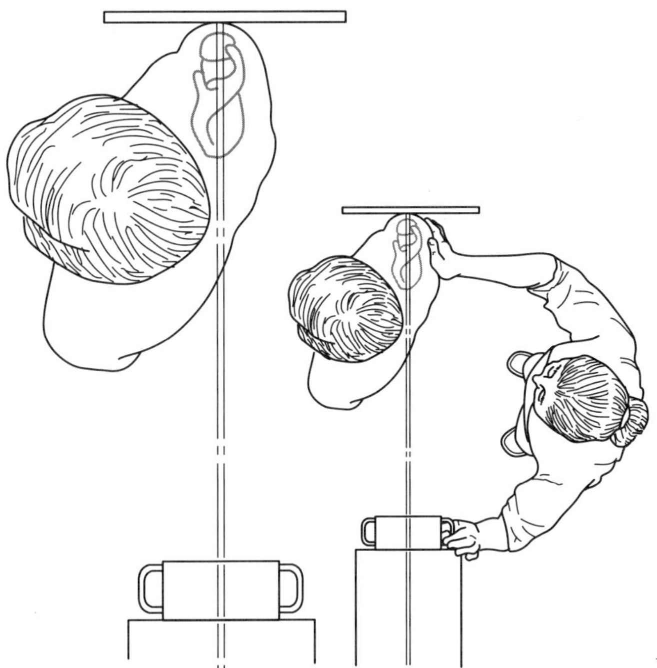

FIGURE 61–2. The scapular Y view, when the patient is able to stand. The patient is placed at an angle of approximately 45° to the cassette. The technician then places a hand on the scapula and orients the x-ray beam parallel to the hand and perpendicular to the cassette. From Silfverskiold JP, Straehley DJ, Jones WW: Roentgenographic evaluation of suspected shoulder dislocation: A prospective study comparing the axillary view and scapular Y view. *Orthopedics.* January 1990;13:64.

the body of the scapula. On the radiograph, the vertical body of the scapula forms the lower limb of the Y, the coracoid forms the anterior arm, and the acromion the posterior arm. The glenoid cavity, seen as the oval between the two arms, is at the junction of the three parts of the Y. The dislocated humerus is then anterior, posterior, or inferior to the center of the Y.

The axillary view is helpful in showing the relationship of the humeral head to the glenoid, as well as in revealing abnormalities of the glenoid rim and humeral head (Fig. 61–3). It is taken with the supine arm abducted approximately 20° or more and with the beam directed from inferior to superior with the cassette above the shoulder. The humeral

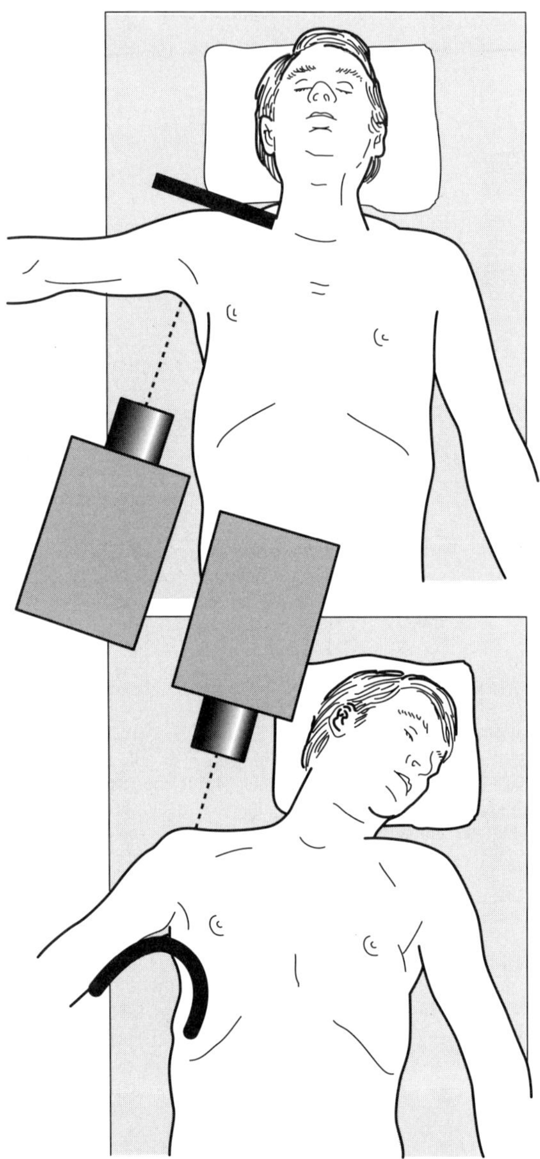

FIGURE 61–3. Illustration depicting the technique for obtaining the axillary view. From Silfverskiold JP, Straehley DJ, Jones WW: Roentgenographic evaluation of suspected shoulder dislocation: A prospective study comparing the axillary view and scapular Y view. *Orthopedics.* January 1990;13:67.

head is seen in the glenoid fossa between the acromion and the anteriorly located coracoid. The dislocated humeral head is outside the glenoid rim in the direction of the dislocation.[5]

In one study, 15% of pathologic shoulder lesions were seen only on the AO view; they included fractures of the glenoid, tubercle, coracoid, and clavicle. Moreover, the AO film provided additional diagnostic information in 23% of patients. The Hill-Sachs lesion was well seen in this projection. This view was not difficult to obtain and allowed less patient discomfort.[23] Another study that compared the AO view with the AP view and the scapular Y view concluded that the apical oblique view was superior in demonstrating the Hill-Sachs lesion and glenoid rim fractures. The apical oblique view also most consistently showed posterior dislocations.[23]

A study of 75 patients with acute shoulder injuries revealed that 92% of the time, the Y view and the axillary view gave the same results. In 8% of cases, the Y view gave an accurate diagnosis that was not seen on the axillary view. The Hill-Sachs lesion, however, was not well seen on the Y view. Eighty-one percent of patients preferred the Y view positioning, because it was less painful, and the technicians judged that the Y view was technically easier to perform. This study did not compare the apical oblique view with the other two special views.[5]

LOWER EXTREMITY

The Hip

The early detection of hip fractures is important both for patient management and for medical, legal, and economic issues. Nondisplaced hip fractures, especially in elderly, osteoporotic women, are often difficult to diagnose. Radionucliotide bone imaging has been useful in diagnosis when the plain film findings are negative. In a study examining the sensitivity and specificity of bone scan in hip fractures, Holder and colleagues[18] found that for patients with normal or equivocal radiographs, the bone scan had a 98% sensitivity and a 95% specificity in excluding a fracture. The positive predictive value was 90% and the negative predictive value was 99%. In addition, these researchers found that it is unnecessary to wait 72 hours to perform the scan. The only cohort of patients in whom bone scan sensitivity dropped if done in the first 72 hours were patients over the age of 70 years. For these patients, the sensitivity was 86% during the first 72 hours after the injury.[18]

The Knee

Knee radiographs are commonly ordered in the ED, with the incidence of clinically significant findings estimated to be 15%.[24] The assessment of knee injuries often involves several radiographic views, including the anteroposterior, lateral, and oblique. Additional views to visualize the intercondyloid fossa (the tunnel view) and the patella (the sunrise view) are often ordered.

Clinical decision rules in ordering knee radiographs can be of value; however, a decision rule must have the standard of being 100% sensitive in order not to miss any clinically significant fractures. One study examined the utility of a clinical decision rule in evaluating patients with knee trauma. Patients involved in a fall or blunt trauma who either were unable to ambulate or were younger than 12 or older than 50 years of age were radiographed. In this series, the sensitivity of the decision rule to predict a fracture was 100%, with the specificity 79%. Using this rule resulted in no false-negative results. The study was limited by its small sample size and a small proportion of fractures.[24]

Another area of controversy is in knee dislocation. Traditionally, any patient with a dislocated knee from blunt trauma undergoes arteriography to exclude a popliteal artery injury. This view was examined in a study recommending selective use of arteriography for knee dislocation. In this study, if the pedal pulse was abnormal, there was a 79% incidence of popliteal artery injury. Of patients in whom the pedal pulse was normal, 90% had a normal arteriogram, 6% demonstrated spasm, and 5% revealed a small nonocclusive arterial injury. The sensitivity for predicting the need for repair was 100% with the pedal pulse examination. No patient with normal pedal pulses required arterial repair.[25]

The Ankle and Foot

The practice of performing ankle radiographs on all patients with ankle injuries has been questioned by several investigators. It is estimated that only 15% of ankle radiographs taken are positive for fractures.[26] Because the majority of ankle injuries in the ED are due to ligamentous injury alone, several investigators have attempted to identify clinical criteria that would allow for the selective use of radiography in the acutely traumatized ankle. An early retrospective study employing strict physical examination criteria found that 50% of ankle radiographs ordered were not indicated.[27] One study prospectively studied 150 patients presenting with ankle injuries and evaluated 24 independent subjective and objective variables. There was a 97.5% probability that the injury was limited to the soft tissue if the patient was able to bear weight and had tenderness over the ankle below the lateral malleolus.[28]

The most publicized decision rules concerning ankle radiography are the Ottawa clinical decision rules. These rules were developed, refined, and validated in an attempt to reduce the number of radiographs taken in the ED. An ankle radiograph was judged to be needed only if the patient had pain near either malleoli and either (a) an inability to bear weight immediately after the injury and to take four steps in the emergency department or (b) a bony tenderness at the posterior edge of the tip of either malleolus.[26, 29] Radiography of the foot was judged necessary if the patient was unable to bear weight initially and to take four steps in the ED or if midfoot pain with tenderness over the navicular bone or at the base of the fifth metatarsal occurred.[26, 29] The refined decision rules were 100% sensitive in detecting ankle and midfoot fractures. In order to achieve this high sensitivity, the specificity was 49% for ankle fractures and 79% for foot fractures. The negative predictive value for both was 100%.[26] The same investigators implemented the Ottawa rules in another study to examine 2342 adults, again finding 100% sensitivity. There was a 28% decrease in ankle radiographs using the rules and a 14% decrease in foot radiographs. Those discharged without radiography spent less time in the ED. Phone follow-up was available for all patients sent home.[30]

Studies have attempted to validate the Ottawa clinical decision rules for ankle radiography in different settings. A New Zealand study found the sensitivity to be only 93%, the specificity 11%, and the positive predictive value 22%. The clinical decision rules would have missed one unstable fracture.[31] This study concluded that the Ottawa clinical decision rule was not adequate to exclude fractures in their setting.

Two investigators have taken this approach a step further by concluding that if there is no swelling adjacent to a malleolus, a radiograph is not necessary.[28, 32] They report that with use of this approach, the only missed fractures have been avulsion fractures of the lateral malleolus. Both studies concluded that because these fractures are safely and adequately managed in a manner identical to that for ligamentous injury, this strategy is reasonable for the evaluation and treatment of patients with ankle injuries.[28, 32]

The issue of selective radiography for ankle injuries continues to be a controversial one. Some investigators believe that the majority of ankle injuries will continue to be radiographed. It might be safe in patients who have sustained minimal trauma and who have very reliable follow-up to forgo radiographs on the initial visit and manage with conservative therapy in the interim. In addition, the clinical decision rules for selective radiography need to be validated in large multicenter trials using examiners at all levels of training and experience.

FUTURE RESEARCH

The major areas that have been studied for radiographic indications are primarily the wrist (specifically the scaphoid bone),[10, 12–14] the shoulder (for suspected dislocation),[5, 6] and the ankle.[26, 29, 30] Many of the published studies have been performed on patients who were referred for orthopedic consultation rather than patients presenting to an emergency department. The indications for ankle radiography are the most recent to have been studied and validated, but prospective studies in different emergency settings are needed. The yield for emergency radiographs in knee injuries has not yet been well studied. Likewise, the indications and yield of radiographs of the injured foot or toes are excellent areas for future investigations.

Decreasing unnecessary radiographs has great cost-saving potential. Despite many recommendations to reduce the ordering of radiographs, it has been noted that physicians are hesitant to comply, especially in the ED setting, for which patient follow-up is not simple or readily ensured.

REFERENCES

1. Abrams HL: The ''overutilization'' of x-rays. *N Engl J Med.* 1979;300:1213–1216.
2. DeLacey GJ, Barker A, Wignall B, et al: Reasons for requesting radiographs in an accident department. *Br Med J.* 1979;1:1595–1597.
3. Brand DA, Frazier WH, Kohlhepp WC, et al: A protocol for selecting patients with injured extremities who need x-rays. *N Engl J Med.* 1982;306:333–339.
4. Becker E, Griffiths HJL: Radiologic diagnosis of pain in the athlete. *Clin Sports Med.* 1987;6:669–711.
5. Silfverskiold JP, Straehley DJ, Jones WW: Roentgenographic evaluation of suspected shoulder dislocation: A prospective study comparing the axillary view and the scapular ''Y'' view. *Orthopedics.* 1990;13:63–69.
6. Richardson JB, Ramsay A, Davidson JK, et al: Radiographs in shoulder trauma. *J Bone Joint Surg.* 1988;70B:457–460.
7. Recht MP, Burk L, Dalinka MK: Radiology of wrist and hand injuries in athletes. *Clin Sports Med.* 1987;6:811–828.
8. Calandra JJ, Goldner RD, Hardaker WT: Scaphoid fractures: Assessment and treatment. *Orthopedics.* 1992;15:931–937.
9. Vargish T, Clarke WR, Young RA, et al: The ankle injury—indications for the selective use of x-ray. *Injury.* 1983;14:507–512.
10. Mehta M, Brautigan MW: Fracture of the carpal navicular: Efficacy of clinical findings and improved diagnosis with six-view radiography. *Ann Emerg Med.* 1990;19:255–257.
11. Wallis MG: Are three views necessary to examine acute ankle injuries? *Clin Radiol.* 1989;40:424–425.
12. Dias JJ, Finlay DBL, Brenkel IF, et al: Radiographic assessment of soft tissue signs in clinically suspected scaphoid fractures: The incidence of false negative and false positive results. *J Orthop Trauma.* 1987;1:205–208.
13. Kirk M, Orlinsky M, Goldberg R, et al: The validity and reliability of the

navicular fat stripe as a screening test for detection of navicular fracture. Ann Emerg Med 1990;19:1371–1376.
14. Mittal RL, Dargan SK: Occult scaphoid fracture: A diagnostic enigma. *J Orthop Trauma.* 1989;3:306–308.
15. Carroll RE, Lakiin JF: Fracture of the hook of the hamate: Acute treatment. *J Trauma.* 1993;34:803–805.
16. Lloyd S: Selective radiographic assessment of acute ankle injuries in the emergency department: Barriers to implementation. *Can Med Assoc J.* 1986;135:973–974.
17. Jones WA: Beware the sprained wrist: The incidence and diagnosis of scapholunate instability. *J Bone Joint Surg.* 1988;7:293–296.
18. Holder LE, Schwarz C, Wernicke PG, et al: Radionuclide bone imaging in the early detection of hip fractures of the proximal femur (hip): Multifactorial analysis. *Radiology.* 1990;174:509–515.
19. Murphy WA, Siegel MJ: Elbow fat pad with new signs and extended differential diagnosis. *Radiology.* 1977;124:659–665.
20. Newberg AH: The radiographic evaluation of shoulder and elbow pain in the athlete. *Clin Sports Med.* 1987;6:785–809.
21. Rozing PM, de Bakker HM, Obermann WR: Radiographic views in recurrent anterior shoulder dislocation. *Acta Orthop Scand.* 1986;57:328–330.
22. Sloth C, Just SL: The apical oblique radiograph in examination of acute shoulder trauma. *Eur J Radiol.* 1989;9:147–151.
23. Kornguth PA, Salazar AM: The apical oblique view of the shoulder: Its usefulness in acute trauma. *Am J Radiol.* 1987;179:113–116.
24. Seaberg DC, Jackson R: Clinical decision rule for knee radiographs. *Am J Emerg Med.* 1994;12:541–543.
25. Trieman GS, Yellin AE, Waver FA, et al: Examination of the patient with a knee dislocation: The case for selective arteriography. *Arch Surg.* 1992;127:1056–1063.
26. Stiell IG, Greenberg GH, McKnight RD, et al: Decision rules for the use of radiology in acute ankle injuries: Refinement and prospective validation. *JAMA.* 1993;269:1127–1132.
27. Auletta AG, Conway WF, Hayes CW, et al: Indications for radiography for patients with acute ankle injuries. *Am J Roentgenol.* 1991;157:789–791.
28. Waeckerle JR: A prospective study identifying the sensitivity of radiographic findings and the efficacy of clinical findings in carpal navicular fractures. *Ann Emerg Med.* 1987;16:733–737.
29. Stiell IG, Greenberg GH, McKnight RD, et al: A study to develop clinical decision rules for the use of radiography in acute ankle injuries. *Ann Emerg Med.* 1992;21:384–390.
30. Stiell IG, McKnight RD, Greenberg GH, et al: Implementation of the Ottawa ankle rules. *JAMA.* 1994;16:271:827–832.
31. Kerr L, Kelly AM, Grant J, et al: Failed validation of clinical decision rule for the use of radiography in acute ankle injury. *N Z Med J.* 1994;107:294–295.
32. Garfield JS: Is radiological examination of the twisted ankle necessary? *Lancet.* 1960;1:1167–1169.

Chapter

Imaging of the Sinuses

Kaveh Ilkhanipour

Clinical diagnosis based on a thorough history and a detailed physical examination is the cornerstone of emergency department evaluation of patients presenting with paranasal sinus pathology. Diagnostic evaluation may also be aided by other modalities, of which sinus radiography is the most helpful.

BASIC RADIOGRAPHIC SIGNS

A working knowledge of common radiographic findings and their clinical significance is also fundamental to effective use of sinus imaging. Sinus disease may be identified radiographically as alterations of the intraluminal sinus air content, the mucous membrane lining of the sinus, and the bony architecture of the sinus.[1]

Opacification of a sinus may be due to mucous membrane thickening, fluid, soft tissue mass, or underdevelopment. It may also reflect improper radiographic technique or the selection of an improper view for visualization of a given sinus. Hypoplastic or opacified maxillary and ethmoid sinuses were found to be common in a study of 100 infants less than 1 year of age who underwent cranial CT scanning for problems other than those related to paranasal sinus disease.[2] In older children and adults, a completely opaque sinus is abnormal, especially if unilateral.

Mucosal thickening is commonly seen on sinus radiographs. It is usually defined as ≥4 mm mucous membrane depth as measured from sinus lumen to bony sinus border. This finding is nonspecific, because it may represent active, inactive, recent, or remote sinus disease. In a study of plain facial film series in 100 patients who had no sinus complaints or known previous history of sinus disease, mucosal thickening was present in 46%.[3] The extent of mucous membrane thickening was not defined, however, and no breakdown of specific sinus involvement was given.

Cysts are quite commonly identified during sinus imaging and may be differentiated from an air-fluid meniscus by their dome-shaped appearance on plain film studies. The most important distinction to be made is between bone-destructive and non–bone destructive cysts. Mucocele is the most common bone-destructive cyst. It results from an obstruction of a major sinus ostium, occurs most commonly in the frontal sinus, and is commonly symptomatic. Advanced radiologic studies (CT scan or MRI) are required to rule out an expansile tumor.

An *air-fluid level* in a sinus may be due to blood, pus, or cerebrospinal fluid. As noted, an air-fluid level can usually be differentiated from a cystic structure by the meniscal appearance of the air-fluid interface. A common error is to misinterpret an unerupted permanent tooth lying at the base of the maxillary sinus as an air-fluid level. This situation can be clarified with a lateral view radiograph of the sinus.

Soft tissue emphysema may be seen in the orbit or cranial cavity. It represents presumptive evidence of fracture of an adjacent sinus cavity, which is the source of air. Air within the orbit indicates possible orbital floor or ethmoid sinus involvement. Pneumocephalus requires mandatory CT examination to look for basilar skull fracture or disruption of the posterior frontal sinus wall.

Calcification and *ossification* are uncommonly seen on conventional sinus films but are most usually secondary to fibrous dysplasia in children and teenagers or to postsurgical thickening of a bony wall or tumor. Bone scans usually lead to a definitive diagnosis.

In almost all instances, *fractures* are secondary to head trauma. Plain film examination provides primarily screening information as to the presence or absence of paranasal sinus involvement. Computed tomography scanning is the standard of care for the evaluation of any facial fracture complex enough to involve a sinus, although a possible exception to this rule is an isolated and uncomplicated orbital blow-out fracture with no extraocular muscle entrapment or enophthalmos.

IMAGING MODALITIES

Conventional Radiography

Conventional plain film radiography is the imaging technique most commonly used in the initial evaluation of the paranasal sinuses. Four views compose the standard plain film sinus series, as follows.

The Waters posteroanterior view is obtained by placing the patient's chin and nose against the film cassette with the mouth open. The x-ray tube is then directed perpendicular to the film. This is the best view for visualizing the maxillary sinuses. The orbit, nasal cavities, nasal septum, and zygomatic arches are also clearly delineated. The other paranasal sinuses are visualized as well but not with optimal detail.

The Caldwell posteroanterior view is obtained by placing the patient's face against the film cassette so that the canthomedial line is perpendicular to the film. The x-ray beam is directed with 15° of caudal tilt from the plane perpendicular to the cassette. This is the primary view for visualizing the frontal and ethmoid sinuses. The orbits, nasal cavities, and nasal septum are well depicted. The maxillary sinuses are also visualized.

The submental–vertex base view, obtained by directing the x-ray beam tangentially to the facial bones, is valuable for visualizing the posterior ethmoidal and sphenoid sinus air cells. The skull base, with its numerous anatomic landmarks, may also be clearly seen.

The lateral view illustrates the sella turcica and posterior nasopharyngeal wall in great detail. The sphenoid and ethmoid sinuses can be visualized with reasonable clarity as well. The maxillary sinuses and nasal bones may also be identified with the use of bright light source.

Use in Children

Radiographic examination of the sinuses is of limited or no benefit in infants less than 1 year of age because of the small size of the sinuses and the high incidence of nonpathologic sinus opacification.[2] In children over 1 year of age, abnormal findings are uncommon in the absence of upper respiratory infection or frank sinusitis.[4] In one study in which clinical signs and symptoms suggestive of acute sinusitis were accompanied by abnormal sinus films (opacification, air-fluid level, mucous membrane thickening ≥4 mm), a sinus aspirate positive for bacteria was present in 75% of cases.[5] Conversely, evidence of clear sinuses on plain film imaging in children makes significant sinus disease unlikely. Mucosal thickening is a common nonspecific finding in children, given the relatively small sinus size and prevalence of redundant mucosa in this age group; fewer than 50% with an isolated finding of sinus mucosal thickening have active sinus disease.[3] A completely opaque sinus is abnormal in older children and indicates sinus disease in a high percentage, especially if it is unilateral.[6]

Sinus films should not be routinely performed in children with obvious clinical findings consistent with a diagnosis of uncomplicated sinusitis. Such a child should be treated on clinical grounds and reevaluated for response to therapy. Plain film imaging should be reserved for the child with an equivocal diagnosis by clinical parameters, the child for whom an initial treatment regimen based on a clinical diagnosis has failed, and the child who is severely ill and is suspected of suffering from a suppurative complication of sinus infection.[7, 8] Plain film imaging of the paranasal sinuses has no utility in children less than 1 year of age; CT scanning is the initial radiographic modality of choice in this age group.

Plain Radiography in Adults

The interpretation of sinus films in adults follows the same general guidelines as those applied to older children. Complete unilateral opacification of an adult sinus represents sinus disease in approximately 75% of cases; an air-fluid level also correlates with infection in 75% of cases.[9] In contrast, mucosal thickening of ≥4 mm correlates with acute sinus pathology in fewer than 50% of cases.[3] Thus, the otherwise healthy adult with clinical signs and symptoms of acute sinus infection should be treated empirically without plain film evaluation. If treatment failure occurs, or if the patient is having recurrent episodes of clinical sinus infection, plain film imaging is indicated. The initial diagnostic impression can be confirmed or cast into doubt, and other abnormalities that could predispose the patient to persistence or recurrence of sinus disease, such as mucocele or polyps, may be identified.

There are two exceptions to the general recommendations of empiric treatment before obtaining sinus films. The first is in the setting of a suspected frontal sinus infection. Because the frontal sinus lies in close proximity to the intracranial cavity, infection may spread anteriorly or posteriorly, either having devastating results. Zimmerman[10] reported that 40% of his patients with subdural empyema had a history of antecedent frontal sinusitis. The potential morbidity and mortality from these complications warrant early identification of frontal sinus disease on initial presentation. Positive findings prompt many clinicians to admit affected patients for intravenous antibiotics or more closely follow their clinical response to outpatient empiric treatment.

Radiographic studies are also indicated in patients who present with signs and symptoms of central nervous system (CNS) involvement secondary to sinus pathology.[11] Computed tomography scanning takes precedence over plain film imaging in this scenario, given CT's ability to visualize the entire intracranial vault and its contained structures in detail.

Complex Motion Tomography

This technique has considerable advantage when one is attempting to identify bony changes in obscure regions of the paranasal sinuses. It permits clear visualization of tissue at a predetermined depth. Since the advent of CT technology, however, conventional tomography is rarely utilized unless CT scanning is unavailable.

Computed Tomography (CT) Scanning

Computed tomography scanning has been an important addition to our ability to evaluate the paranasal sinuses. It has the advantage of showing both bony destruction and soft tissue involvement in great detail, and its high resolution allows excellent visualization of the complex anatomy of the paranasal sinuses. Both axial and coronal plane views may be obtained, depending on the area of interest.

Emergency department use of this diagnostic modality is well delineated. Any paranasal sinus infection that is accompanied by suspicion of intracranial involvement should be evaluated by CT.[11] A suspicion of an extracranial complication of sinus infection, such as frontal osteomyelitis or postseptal periorbital cellulitis, also requires CT, as does evidence of bony destruction or an expansile lesion identified initially on plain films. All complex maxillofacial trauma merits CT examination for proper injury assessment and management.

Magnetic Resonance Imaging (MRI)

Magnetic resonance imaging has largely replaced CT scanning as the imaging modality of choice for evaluating malignant disease in the sinuses. It is also able to differentiate soft tissue inflammation and retained sinus secretions from tumor. Because of its limited availability and high cost, however, MRI has a very small role in the initial emergency department evaluation of paranasal sinus disease.

Ultrasound

Ultrasonography has been used extensively in a variety of clinical settings. It has a number of advantages over the other diagnostic modalities, including safety, simplicity, noninvasiveness, affordability, and relative patient comfort. Over the past decade, interest in its applicability to paranasal sinus imaging has mounted. Because only the anterior wall of the maxilla and floor of the frontal sinus are thin enough to allow for the passage of sound from the ultrasound transducer, only the maxillary and frontal sinuses can be imaged using this technique.

Studies evaluating the utility of ultrasound in the evaluation of paranasal sinus disease have yielded conflicting results. Revonta and Suonpaa[12] found A-mode ultrasound to be 88% sensitive and 98% specific when correlated with sinus puncture and aspiration in the assessment of paranasal sinus infection. Gail and associates[13] compared maxillary sinus radiography with A-mode ultrasound in the diagnosis of sinusitis in 75 patients with a median age of 10 years. Ultrasound had an overall sensitivity of 58% and a specificity of 55%. When patients were stratified by age, ultrasound was slightly better in those older than 21 years. Jenson and von Sydow[14] compared ultrasound with plain film radiography of the maxillary and frontal sinuses in 138 patients with clinical signs and symptoms of acute sinusitis. Maxillary sinus fluid confirmed by antral puncture was detected equally by ultrasound and plain film imaging (80%). Ultrasonography was poor at demonstrating various degrees of mucosal thickening or polyposis. Frontal sinus ultrasound detected only one of 13 abnormal frontal sinuses in the study. The varying results in these studies may be due to differences in equipment and operator experience or technique.

At present, ultrasound examination of the sinuses appears to have little direct application in the emergency department. It might be used as an initial screening tool, however, for the detection of maxillary or frontal sinus fluid in the occasional patient who requires sinus puncture and aspiration. Further applications of ultrasound require improvement and standardization of imaging equipment, combined with growing operator experience.

RADIOGRAPHY OF PARANASAL SINUS TRAUMA

Orbital Blow-Out Fracture

The Waters and modified Caldwell plain film views almost always demonstrate orbital blow-out fractures radiographically.[15] If there is a clinical suspicion of extraocular muscle entrapment, CT scanning is indicated. Computed tomography imaging is useful in differentiating between true herniation of muscle and "pseudoherniation" of submucosal and subperiosteal hematomas of the maxillary sinus roof.[16] Identification of true extraocular muscle entrapment is important, because its treatment is acute surgical decompression of the entrapped muscle.[17]

Ethmoid Sinus Fracture

The Caldwell view is the optimal plain film study for the detection of an ethmoid sinus fracture. If muscle entrapment is suspected on clinical examination, either axial or coronal CT imaging should be obtained. Computed tomography radiography of this region provides excellent visualization of important anatomic landmarks.[18]

Frontal Sinus Fracture

The Caldwell view and lateral projection offer the best plain film radiographic detail of the frontal sinus. A significant limitation of these plain film studies is the relative lack of information regarding the integrity of the posterior frontal sinus wall, which separates the frontal sinus from the cranial cavity. Computed tomography scanning should be employed if there is any clinical suspicion or plain film evidence of frontal sinus injury. Computed tomography can also define any secondary intracranial complications associated with frontal sinus fracture.

Sphenoid Sinus Fracture

The initial suspicion of a sphenoid sinus injury is usually aroused because an air-fluid level or complete sinus opacification is visualized on a lateral film of the face. The standard of care requires further evaluation with high-resolution CT scanning of the sphenoid sinus.[16] In most cases, CT evaluation identifies a sphenoid sinus contusion or submucosal hemorrhage rather than true sinus fracture.

REFERENCES

1. Kuhn JP: Imaging of the paranasal sinuses: current status. *J Allergy Clin Immunol.* 1986;77:6–8.
2. Glacier CM, Mallory GB, Steele RW, et al: Significance of opacification of the maxillary and ethmoid sinus in infants. *J Pediatr.* 1989;114:45–50.
3. Wilson PS, Grocett M: Mucosal thickening on sinus x-ray and its significance. *J Laryngol Otol.* 1990;104:694–695.
4. Kovatch AL, Wald ER, Ledesma-Medina J, et al: Maxillary sinus radiographs in children with nonrespiratory complaints. *Pediatrics.* 1984;73:306–308.
5. Wald ER: Sinusitis and complications in the pediatric patient. *Pediatr Clin North Am.* 1981;28:777–796.
6. Kuhn JP: Imaging of the paranasal sinuses: Current status. *J Allergy Clin Immunol.* 1986;77:6–8.
7. Bluestone CD: Medical and surgical management of sinusitis. *Pediatr Infect Dis.* 1984;3(suppl):513–518.
8. Bluestone CD: Consensus: Medical and surgical management. *Pediatr Infect Dis.* 1985;4(suppl):564.
9. Harmony B: Etiology and antimicrobial therapy of acute maxillary sinusitis. *J Infect Dis.* 1979;139:197–202.
10. Zimmerman C: Radiography and ultrasonography in paranasal sinusitis. *Acta Radiol.* 1987;28:31–34.
11. Carter BL, Bankoff MS, Fisk JD: Computed tomographic detection of sinusitis responsible for intracranial and extracranial infections. *Radiology.* 1984;147:739–742.
12. Revonta M, Suonpaa J: Diagnosis of subacute maxillary sinusitis in children. *J Laryngol Otol.* 1981;95:133.
13. Gail G, Shapiro GG, Furukawa CT, Pierson WE, et al: Blinded comparison of maxillary sinus radiography and ultrasound for diagnosis of sinusitis. *J Allergy Clin Immunol.* 1986;77:59–64.
14. Jenson C, von Sydow C: Radiography and ultrasonography in paranasal sinusitis. *Acta Radiol.* 1987;28:31–34.

15. Zizmor J, Noyek AM: Fractures of the paranasal sinuses. *Otolaryngol Clin North Am.* 1973;6:473–485.
16. Kassel EE: Traumatic injuries of the paranasal sinuses. *Otolaryngol Clin North Am.* 1988;21:455–493.
17. Emery JM, et al: Orbital floor fractures: Long-term follow-up of cases with and without surgical repair. *Trans Am Acad Ophthalmol Otolaryngol.* 1976;75:477–487.
18. Hammerschlag SB, Hughes S, O'Reilly GV, et al: Blow-out fractures of the orbit: A comparison of computed tomography and conventional radiography with anatomic correlation. *Radiology.* 1982;143;487–492.

Chapter

Abdominal Plain Films

Andrew Sucov

Abdominal pain is a common presenting complaint in the emergency department. Abdominal radiographs are frequently ordered to help make the diagnosis—sometimes to rule diseases in, sometimes to rule diseases out.

RADIOLOGIC OPTIONS

Supine View

The supine view is the standard initial view, often referred to as a "flat plate" or "KUB" (ie, kidney, ureter, bladder). These terms refer to a radiographic view of the abdomen in the supine position, from the pubis to the diaphragms. This option allows the lung bases to be evaluated first for pneumonia or effusion; next, the extraabdominal soft tissues for evidence of hernia or masses; and then the skeleton for fractures. When one is evaluating the skeleton, it is important to also look for evidence of scoliosis, which may be seen in up to 14% of cases of appendicitis.[1] The fat-muscle planes should be evaluated for symmetry and contour. These planes consist of the psoas margins medially and the flank stripes laterally. They can be lost when obscured by pus or blood in the peritoneal cavity or in the retroperitoneum. Although classically the fat-muscle planes are expected to be equal bilaterally, the presence of stool or air overlying these areas may impede evaluation, so that loss of distinct shadows is suggestive, but not diagnostic, of a disease process in that region. There are also cases of true peritonitis with intact shadows.

Next, one should evaluate the solid organs, looking for liver, spleen, and kidney shadows. The right kidney is usually located 1 to 2 cm below the left kidney. These organs should be evaluated for size, contour, position, and homogeneity. Loss of these shadows may be reflective of pus or blood obscuring the fat-water density interface.

In evaluating the gas patterns, it is important to note whether anything is displaced or distended. It is normal to see air in the stomach and colon in all individuals, and patients who are currently hospitalized commonly have gas within the small bowel. It is also important to evaluate the size of the small bowel lumen; if the small bowel is not distended, it is probably not pathologic.[2] Any single loop of small bowel can be considered to be abnormal, however, if it is greater than 10 cm in length.[3]

One should then look for any evidence of calcifications, and finally, evaluate the film for any evidence of intraperitoneal air or fluid.

Erect View

In the evaluation of an erect view of the abdomen, all of the preceding steps should be followed. In addition, free air may be seen under either diaphragm as a faint dark region, and air-fluid levels may be noted in the dilated segments.

The better decubitus view is the left lateral, on which free air will be seen contrasting against the density of the liver. This view is used for patients who are too ill to stand for the erect view.

Erect Chest View

Evaluation of the chest is important, as any thoracic pathology can simulate abdominal pain. In addition, the erect chest view (CXR) is the best radiograph to search for small amounts of free air below the diaphragm.[4] Five to 10 cc of free air can reliably be visualized this way.

Most recommend placing the patient in either the decubitus or upright position for a period of 5 to 10 minutes, to allow the air to rise so as to be well visualized, before taking the radiograph.

Which Views to Order

Radiology and surgery texts usually recommend obtaining three views in all patients receiving abdominal radiographs: supine, erect or decubitus, and erect chest. Although there may be some merit to this approach, radiographs should be ordered in the same fashion as other tests, ie, they should be focused toward a predetermined differential diagnosis.[5]

If the concern is free air in the abdomen, the erect abdominal view is unlikely to add to the evaluation. The erect chest or decubitus view allows much smaller amounts of air to be well visualized. The chest radiograph itself enables visualization of the thoracic cavity.

Although radiologists are able to make the diagnosis of obstruction just as easily on the supine view as on the erect view,[6] an erect view usually is necessary if nonradiologists are evaluating the films initially. A potential solution is to order the erect abdominal view instead of the supine view as the initial radiograph, along with a chest view, so that abnormal air-fluid levels (erect abdomen), free air, and intrapleural pathology (CXR) can be visualized.

SPECIFIC CLINICAL ENTITIES

Appendicitis

The diagnosis of appendicitis is mostly a clinical one, with laboratory and radiographic data merely helping to make the diagnosis more or less likely. *Suggestive* findings on radiography may be seen in up to 50% of patients—appendicolith, appendiceal abscess, local ileus, psoas shadow obliteration, lumbar scoliosis, and haziness over the sacroiliac joint.[7]

There are no findings specific for appendicitis, however. The presence of an appendicolith has been mistakenly called pathognomonic for appendicitis, but appendicoliths have been noted in between 3%[8] and 21%[9] of patients with normal appendices at surgery.

Another oft-cited finding, which is thought to rule out appendicitis, is right lower quadrant air in a linear pattern, suggesting that air is filling the appendix. A long appendix, however, may be obstructed distally but appears to be one of normal length that is patent in its entirety.

Obstruction

The "obstructive pattern" can be caused by two very different types of diseases, mechanical obstruction and "paralytic" ileus. Differentiating these two conditions radiographically is often problematic.

If obstruction has been present for more than a few hours, the distal bowel and colon should be empty of gas, helping to define the point of obstruction. With partial small bowel obstruction, however, some gas is allowed to pass beyond the site of obstruction, simulating ileus.

Classically, mechanical obstruction produces air-fluid levels arranged in a "stepladder" fashion. These are seen on the erect film as loops of bowel beginning and ending at different levels, whereas in ileus, the air-fluid levels are more likely to be at the same level. Nevertheless, it takes between 3 and 6 hours for the radiographic picture consistent with obstruction to develop.[10, 11] Early obstruction, therefore, may not show significant air-fluid levels. Similarly, some proximal obstructions do not show air-fluid levels, because the bowel is mostly filled with fluid; in this case, one may be able to see air trapped in the valvulae conniventes (septations), producing the string-of-pearls sign. In addition, as the bowel becomes more atonic with longer periods of obstruction, the air-fluid levels more closely resemble those seen in ileus. Table 63–1 lists other conditions that can simulate obstruction.

Gallstone ileus shows air in the gallbladder or biliary tree in addition to an obstructive pattern. Air in the biliary tree is seen only if the cystic

TABLE 63–1. CONDITIONS MIMICKING INTESTINAL OBSTRUCTION

Metabolic
- Hypokalemia
- Hyponatremia
- Hypoproteinemia
- Anemia
- DKA
- Uremia

Drugs
- Opiates
- Anticholinergics
- Antidiarrheal agents

Irritative
- Any inflammatory process within the peritoneal cavity
- Retroperitoneal hemorrhage
- Renal calculus
- Pneumonia
- Acute MI
- Sickle cell crisis

Air Trapping
- Anxiety or aerophagia
- Pain
- Laxatives or enemas

duct is patent, and it can be differentiated from air in the portal vein by the location: Biliary air is noted to be branching linear lucencies in and below the center of the liver, whereas portal vein air is transversely and peripherally located.[11] The gallstone itself is rarely seen, because it usually does not contain enough calcium to appear on a radiograph.

Several radiographic findings help differentiate between large and small bowel obstructions. Small bowel should show complete septations across the dilated areas, but in the colon, the haustral markings do not completely cross the lumen. The caliber of the colon is usually significantly larger than that of the small bowel. If the ileocecal valve is incompetent, there may be signs of small and large bowel distention. This disorder is due to gas and fluid refluxing back into the ileum and decompressing the colon.

Evaluation of the caliber of the cecum is critical, because this is the portion of the colon most likely to rupture from distention. If cecal diameter is greater than 8 to 10 cm, many investigators would suggest immediate decompression, with either tube cecostomy or operative intervention.[3]

Perforation

Perforation of a viscus other than the stomach or duodenum is rarely accompanied by truly free air, because the intense inflammation walls off the air in an abscess cavity.

Renal Calculi

Although 85% of renal calculi are radiopaque, they are commonly not visualized on the initial abdominal films; a 45% visualization rate is more realistic.[13]

Mesenteric Ischemia

The classic findings in acute mesenteric ischemia are "thumbprinting," gas in the bowel wall and gas in the portal system. These are all considered late findings, however.[2] Early on, the only findings may be a "nonspecific" gas pattern, an obstructive (mechanical or ileus) pattern, or a completely normal radiographic appearance.

Abdominal Aortic Aneurysm

A lateral view of the abdomen enables an estimate of thickness of the aorta, and the supine view shows the width. These views should be utilized to make a diagnosis only if other imaging modalities (eg, bedside ultrasonography) are not available. Nonvisualization of the aorta does not mean that no aneurysm exists, because the degree of calcification may not reflect the size of the aneurysm.

WHEN TO ORDER FILMS

Prospective studies on the use of radiography in the evaluation of abdominal pain have concluded that radiography demonstrates positive findings 10 to 15% of the time but that only under certain circumstances is it actually helpful.[14–17] In the largest and most complete of these studies, Eisenberg and colleagues[17] determined 13 different variables that were significantly associated with positive radiographs, and three variables that were significantly associated with normal radiographs (Table 63–2). These investigators recommended limiting radiographs to patients judged to be *highly likely* to have any of the following: bowel obstruction, perforated viscus, ischemic bowel, renal calculi, and gall-

TABLE 63–2. LIKELIHOOD RATIOS OF HISTORICAL AND PHYSICAL FINDINGS IN PATIENTS WITH ABDOMINAL PAIN

	Ratio[a]
Likelihood Predictive of Abnormality (>1)	
Increased, high-pitched bowel sounds	57.5
Penetrating trauma	38.0
Distention	9.5
Hx of abdominal surgery	7.4
Blood in urine	6.3
Hx of renal-ureteral calculi	5.8
Flank pain/tenderness	5.0
Hx of abdominal tumor	4.7
Hx of gallbladder disease	4.2
Severe abdominal pain and tenderness	3.0
Abdominal pain for less than 1 day	1.8*
Vomiting	1.8*
Likelihood Predictive of Normality (<1)	
Hx of ulcer disease	0.3
Mild abdominal pain	0.3
Abdominal pain for more than 1 week	0.5*

[a]Asterisk [*] denotes $P < 0.05$; all others, $P < 0.01$. (Hx = history.)

From Eisenberg RL, Heineken P, Hedgcock MW, et al: Evaluation of plain abdominal radiographs in the diagnosis of abdominal pain. *Ann Intern Med.* 1982;97:257–261.

stones. The use of radiographs to screen patients who are not at high risk for these diseases should be discouraged, because even in these patients, plain films are not 100% sensitive. Lee[1] found that only 50 to 60% of patients with proven disease had positive radiographs. In populations with a lower incidence, the false-negative rate would be higher.

Perhaps of equal importance is the variability of radiograph readings by different and well-qualified observers. Markus and coworkers[18] found that only certain diagnoses could reproducibly be made when assessed by different attending radiologists (Table 63–3). Other diagnoses could not be made with confidence. These researchers concluded that patients should undergo abdominal radiography only if they have a high likelihood of perforated viscus, ischemic bowel, small bowel obstruction, renal calculi, or gallstones. In this respect, the recommendations derived from clinical and radiographic studies are very similar.

There is poor agreement among radiologists about the diagnosis of

TABLE 63–3. AGREEMENT OF RADIOLOGISTS ON SPECIFIC DIAGNOSES

	Kappa Values[a]		
Diagnosis/Sign	***Range***	***SE***	***Mean***
Pneumobilia	1.000–1.000	0.039	1.000
Renal calculi	0.745–1.000	0.047	0.882
Pneumoperitoneum	0.580–0.908	0.059	0.786
Gallstones	0.646–0.829	0.050	0.740
Colitis	0.476–0.870	0.064	0.679
Small bowel obstruction	0.581–0.817	0.049	0.668
Thumbprinting	0.477–0.853	0.066	0.664
Nonspecific or normal pattern	0.574–0.724	0.040	0.643
Dilated loops of bowel	0.590–0.687	0.036	0.640
Abnormal air-fluid levels	0.595–0.728	0.039	0.638
Normal gas pattern	0.352–0.609	0.053	0.427
Soft tissue mass	0.205–0.646	0.075	0.422
Complete vs incomplete SBO	−0.019–0.428	0.102	0.222
Generalized ileus	−0.012–0.343	0.065	0.153
Nonspecific pattern	−0.009–0.222	0.048	0.134
Ascites	0.000–0.500	0.107	0.083
Localized ileus	−0.026–0.333	0.063	0.068
Ureteric calculi	−0.024–0.234	0.055	0.063
Large bowel obstruction	−0.029–0.419	0.080	0.061
Location of SBO	−0.165–0.416	0.115	0.044

[a]Kappa greater than 0.75 represents excellent agreement; 0.40–0.74, fair–good agreement; less than 0.40, poor agreement. (SBO = small bowel obstruction.)

Adapted from Markus JB, Somers S, Franic SE, et al: Intraobserver variation in the interpretation of abdominal radiographs. *Radiology*. 1989:171:69–71.

ureteric calculi by plain films, however. Roth and associates[13] studied the incremental benefit of ordering plain films in addition to intravenous pyelography (IVP). Prospectively, plain films did not affect the ability to make the diagnosis. Clinical scoring systems and radiographs have been shown to have comparable positive predictive value (82 to 88% vs 86 to 91%, respectively) and sensitivity (73 to 82% vs 58 to 62%, respectively), but at lower cost.[13, 19] In addition, when an IVP is performed, an initial scout film is often obtained. It is also not recommended to obtain a plain radiograph in order to diagnose gallstones.

Thus, radiographs should be obtained only in patients who are likely to have perforated viscus, ischemic bowel, or obstruction. Clinically, these are patients with moderate-to-severe pain, high pitched bowel sounds, distention, prior abdominal surgery, or some combination of these features.

The conclusions of Troupin[2] thus appear to be as applicable in the emergency department as in other settings: "There are clinical settings in which plain films are predictably useless (ie, GI bleeding) and simply distract, dilute, and delay the progress of problem solving. There are other instances in which they offer suspicions that 'are compatible with . . . ' but clearly are just a brief pause along the way to definite imaging. There are, however, some initial situations where plain films may be distinctive and diagnostic: suspected perforation and bowel obstructions."

In patients who are very young, very old, intoxicated, or receiving corticosteroids, the physical examination may be unreliable, and there should be a lower threshold for obtaining films. Patients with inflammatory bowel disease should also undergo radiography early, because toxic megacolon may not be symptomatic until late in its course.

REFERENCES

1. Lee PWR: The plain x-ray in the acute abdomen: A surgeon's evaluation. *Br J Sur.* 1976;63:763–66.
2. Troupin RH. *Diagnostic Imaging in Clinical Medicine.* Chicago: Year Book Medical Publishers; 1985:69–87.
3. Harris JH Jr, Harris WH (eds): *The Radiology of Emergency Medicine.* 2nd ed. Baltimore: Williams & Wilkins; 1981:390–456.
4. Miller RE, Nelson SW. Xray demonstration of tiny amounts of free intraperitoneal gas. *Am J Roentgenol.* 1971;112:574–585.
5. Amberg JR: Acute abdominal pain, in Eisenberg RL, Amberg JR (eds): *Critical Diagnostic Pathways in Radiology: An Algorithmic Approach.* Philadelphia: JB Lippincott Co; 1981:107–114.
6. Mirvis SE, Young JWR, Keramati B, et al: Plain film evaluation of patients

with abdominal pain: Are three radiographs necessary? *Am J Roentgenol.* 1986;147:501–503.

7. Huff JS: Nontraumatic abdomen disorders, in Levy R, Hawkins H, Barsan W (eds): *Radiology Emergency Medicine.* St Louis: CV Mosby Co; 1986:210–63.
8. Lewis FR, Holcroft JW, Boey J, Dunphy JE: Appendicitis: A critical review of diagnosis and treatment in 1000 cases. *Arch Surg.* 1975;110:677–684.
9. Teicher I, Lada B, Cohen M, et al: Scoring system to aid in the diagnosis of appendicitis. *Ann Surg.* 1983;6:753–759.
10. Davis M, Cautman J: The abdomen, in Juhl JH, Crummy AB (eds): *Essentials of Radiologic Imaging.* 6th ed. Philadelphia: JB Lippincott; 1993:501–522.
11. Samuel E, Laws JW: The acute abdomen, in Sutton D (ed): *A Textbook of Radiology and Imaging.* 3rd ed. vol II. Edinburgh: Churchill Livingstone; 1980:759–776.
12. Harris JH Jr, Harris WH (eds): *The Radiology of Emergency Medicine.* 2nd ed. Baltimore: Williams & Wilkins; 1981:390–456.
13. Roth CS, Bowyer RA, Berquist TH: Utility of the Plain Abdominal Radiograph for Diagnosing Ureteral Calculi. *Ann Emerg Med.* 1985;14:311–315.
14. McCook TA, Ravin CE, Rice RP: Abdominal radiography in the emergency department: A prospective analysis. *Ann Emerg Med.* 1982;11:7–8.
15. deLacey GJ, Wignall BK, Bradbrooke S, et al: Rationalizing abdominal radiography in the accident and emergency ward. *Clin Radiol.* 1980;31:453–455.
16. Brewer RJ, Golden GT, Hitch DC, et al: Abdominal pain: An analysis of 1000 consecutive cases in a university hospital emergency room. *Am J Surg.* 1976;131:219–224.
17. Eisenberg RL, Heineken P, Hedgcock MW, et al: Evaluation of plain abdominal radiographs in the diagnosis of abdominal pain. *Ann Intern Med.* 1982;97:257–261.
18. Markus JB, Somers S, Franic SE, et al: Interobserver variation in the interpretation of abdominal radiographs. *Radiology.* 1989;171:69–71.
19. Mugti A, Williams JW, Nettleman M: Renal colic: Utility of the plain abdominal radiograph. *Arch Intern Med.* 1991;151:1589–1592.

Intravenous Pyelography

Kevin O'Toole

The intravenous pyelogram (IVP)[1] in emergency medicine has been largely limited to two specific indications, renal colic and urologic trauma. Ultrasound, radionuclide scanning, and CT scanning have all reduced the need for IVP in some situations.[2–4] Despite these trends, the IVP remains a valuable and frequently employed test in the emergency department setting.

INDICATIONS

The reason for performing an IVP in the emergency department is generally to answer one or both of the following questions: Is there an obstruction? and is the kidney functioning?

Renal function and evidence for an obstruction can almost always be evaluated in a "suboptimal" study. If the study can be delayed until the patient is properly prepared, however, the ability to identify the exact level of obstruction and other more subtle findings is improved.

TECHNIQUE

The initial film usually obtained is the plain abdominal scout film, which is used as a reference point for comparison with subsequent films. The scout film should not be relied on as the sole radiographic study for the evaluation of possible renal calculus. Roth and associates[5] and Zangerle and associates[6] have both shown the plain abdominal film to have poor sensitivity and specificity in the diagnosis of ureteral calculi.

The scout film may, however, show certain suggestive findings that may be helpful in guiding further investigation.[7, 8] These are as follows:

1. Signs of retroperitoneal hemorrhage, such as loss of renal outline, soft tissue mass, loss of psoas shadow, and displacement of the renal shadow
2. Spinal curvature with the concavity toward the side of injury or inflammation caused by spasm of the psoas muscle

3. Enlargement of the renal shadow
4. Pelvic fractures
5. Lumbar transverse process fractures and lower rib fractures, which may indirectly indicate renal injury
6. Elevation of the hemidiaphragm secondary to retroperitoneal bleeding
7. Possible kidney, ureteral, or bladder calculi

The actual performance of the IVP is straightforward.[9] The patient is asked to void the bladder immediately prior to the study. A contrast agent such as Renografin 60 (or, if indicated, a nonionic agent) is given intravenously over 1 minute, and films are obtained at 1, 5, 15, and 30 minutes after the injection. Delayed films at 1, 2, or 4 hours may be necessary in patients with ureteral obstructions. In trauma patients, a one-shot IVP may be obtained to evaluate for renal trauma. This is best obtained at 10 minutes after injection of contrast material.

CONTRAINDICATIONS

There are relatively few contraindications to the performance of an IVP.[9–11] The only *absolute* contraindication is profound hypotension. In the severely hypotensive patient, blood flow to the kidneys is severely restricted, resulting in an inadequate study and potentially contributing to the development of acute renal failure.

There are several *relative* contraindications to doing an IVP, however. In general, one must balance the risk of a possible complication from the procedure with the potential value of the information obtained.

When an IVP is to be performed on an emergency department patient, the patient should first be questioned about any known allergies to iodinated contrast agents. Patients may state that they are allergic to ''IVP dye,'' but when further questioned, they describe normal side effects of its administration, such as nausea, vomiting, and flushing. If the patient describes a true allergic response, with symptoms such as wheezing, urticaria, and hypotension, it is advisable to consider using a nonionic agent or ordering an alternative diagnostic study such as ultrasound.

A history of diabetes mellitus, multiple myeloma, or preexisting renal failure is another relative contraindication to IVP. In addition, evidence of significant dehydration on physical examination should make one cautious about proceeding with the IVP before the fluid deficit has been corrected.

Allergic Reactions

The risk of a severe allergic reaction to contrast media is always a concern, although fatalities from contrast material injection are relatively rare. Hartman and associates[12] reported on 300,000 consecutive patients who underwent IVP over an 18-year period. Four deaths occurred, for a mortality rate of 1:75,000. All the patients who died were older than 50 years and had a history of a hypersensitivity reaction with a respiratory component. Most interestingly, none of the four had ever been given a prior injection of contrast medium. Moreover, all four had received a test dose of contrast agent before the study and had experienced no adverse effects. Other studies have reported mortality rates ranging from 1:117,000 to 1:14,000.[13–17]

Much more common are less severe reactions, which range from mild flushing and urticaria to angioedema, bronchospasm, laryngeal edema, and hypotension. In the largest series to date, Shehadi and Toniolo[18] reported on adverse reactions to contrast media in more than 300,000 patients. The overall incidence of reactions was 4.73%; the incidence of reactions for urography was twice that for arterial procedures. The majority of reactions (approximately 70%) were considered so minor that no treatment was required. An additional 30% were moderate reactions, for which patients received treatment in the radiology suite and were then discharged. Only 1.5% of patients experiencing reactions required hospitalization, and there were only 18 fatalities (~0.006%).

Which patients are more likely to have an adverse reaction to contrast media? Patients with a history of a previous reaction would appear to be at risk for another reaction. Shehadi[17] and Witten and associates[16] found that 16%, and 35%, respectively, of patients who had previous reactions to IVP contrast developed another reaction on repeat contrast injection, but subsequent reactions were no more severe than the first one, and this pattern held true for any number of subsequent examinations. A history of reactive airways disease, conditions such as hay fever and eczema, or a history of previous allergies to other materials increased the risk of developing a contrast reaction to a level estimated to be five times greater than the risk in the general population.[19]

It has been standard procedure in the past to administer a test dose of contrast material in an attempt to determine which patients would develop a reaction, but this practice has been found to be unreliable and has now been abandoned. Currently, if a patient is known to be allergic to contrast media and the IVP is judged to be necessary, the physician has two available options: pretreatment with steroids or proceeding with low-osmolarity contrast medium. Pretreatment with steroids has been shown to significantly decrease reactions to contrast media. Treatment should begin at least 12 hours prior to the study, however, thereby making this alternative unrealistic for most emergency departments. The second option is to use a low-osmolarity contrast medium. Standard contrast media have been shown to cause subclinical, as well as clinical, bronchospasm in a number of patients who have received it, whereas this effect is reported to be quite uncommon with either the nonionic or the ionic dimeric low-osmolarity media.[20] One drawback to the use of the newer low-osmolarity agents is that they cost 10 to 15 times more than conventional agents. At present, their utilization should be limited to patients with known reactions to conventional contrast media, asthma, hay fever, or other allergies.

Contrast-Induced Nephropathy

The majority of patients suffer no renal damage from an IVP. There is a subset of patients, however, who have a significant risk of developing contrast-induced renal failure. This subset includes those with diabetes mellitus, preexisting renal failure, age greater than 60 years, volume depletion, or multiple myeloma, and those receiving large doses of contrast medium.[21] Some evidence indicates, however, that the number of cases of contrast-induced renal failure may have been overestimated.[22] Moreover, the decrement in renal function is, as a rule, transient and of only modest degree.

The risk of contrast-induced nephropathy may be minimized in a number of ways.[21] The BUN and creatinine levels should be checked prior to performing an IVP in patients in a high-risk category. A history of previous contrast-induced renal failure should prompt consideration of an imaging modality other than IVP. The patient should be well hydrated prior to and during the study. One should use the minimum amount of contrast material needed for an acceptable study and should avoid the use of additional contrast studies during the subsequent 3 days. The newer nonionic contrast agents may also decrease the risk of renal damage. In any event, one should attempt to estimate the relative risks and benefits of performing the IVP in individuals with any of the preceding medical conditions, and alternative imaging procedures should be considered.

RENAL COLIC AND THE IVP

What are we looking for on the IVP that is evidence for a renal calculus? In normal patients, the first film taken after contrast injection shows symmetric bilateral nephrograms. By the 5-minute film, the ureters contain contrast material. Because of ureteral peristalsis, contrast material is generally not seen over the entire length of the ureter in any one film. By 15 minutes, there should be enough contrast material in the bladder to give a good cystogram. There should be no evidence of dilation of the collecting system, and both kidneys should show prompt excretion of contrast, with equal degrees of opacification at all times.

The following radiographic findings indicate or suggest renal colic:[7, 9, 11]

1. A dense nephrogram with delay in excretion of contrast on the affected side.
2. Hydronephrosis and hydroureter, or a column of dye along the length of the ureter.
3. A cutoff of the dye column at the level of the obstruction, or a relative filling defect representing the calculus with contrast material surrounding it.
4 Nonvisualization of the kidney on the affected side. This is evidence of high-grade obstruction. Delayed films taken up to 24 hours after contrast injection may be needed to show a nephrogram.
5. Urinary extravasation. This is rare but usually indicates high-grade obstruction that has been present for many hours. Extravasation usually occurs at the fornices and is associated with significantly elevated intrarenal hydrostatic pressures. Although extravasation is generally a benign finding per se, prompt urologic consultation is indicated when this finding is present.
6. Occasionally, there is evidence of hydroureter and hydronephrosis, but no calculus is seen. One explanation for this combination of findings is that there may be a very small calculus that cannot be visualized. The second possibility is that a calculus has just been passed and there is some residual ureteral edema and spasm.

THE IVP IN RENAL TRAUMA

The indications for IVP in the trauma patient are not as straightforward as in the patient with renal colic. With the wide availability of CT scanning, the IVP is less commonly used in the trauma patient. Recommendations range from performing an IVP in all trauma patients, to ordering it only if there is gross hematuria. Between these two extremes is an approach suggested by Uehara and Eisner,[4] in which patients should have immediate IVP if there is (a) gross hematuria, (b) pain or tenderness that is referable to the genitourinary (GU) tract, even in the absence of hematuria, (c) flank hematoma or ecchymosis, or (d) penetrating injury in the vicinity of the GU tract. Fortune and colleagues[23] believe that for trauma patients without gross hematuria, a one-shot IVP is adequate initially to rule out occult renal arterial injury.

IVP findings suggestive of urinary tract injury are as follows:

- Nonvisualization of a kidney
- Enlargement or disruption of the kidney outline
- Caliceal distortion
- Delayed excretion or decreased concentration of contrast material
- Extravasation of contrast material
- Collecting system filling defects.

Any trauma patient who has a solitary kidney on IVP should immediately undergo arteriography to evaluate for a renal vascular injury. Both IVP and arteriography should be done before the urethrogram and cystogram, so that extravasated contrast material from those procedures does not block visualization of the ureters.

ALTERNATIVE STUDIES

A number of alternative imaging studies have been compared with the IVP for evaluation of both renal colic and renal trauma. For suspected renal colic, it has generally been reported that ultrasound is not as sensitive as IVP, and the latter remains the examination of choice.[2, 24–29] Ultrasound may be useful as an initial screening test, however.[2] If the ultrasound shows hydronephrosis, the patient can be treated for renal colic, and the IVP delayed unless the patient's symptoms persist. If the ultrasound findings are negative but renal colic is still suspected clinically, an IVP could then be done. Ultrasound is also valuable for pregnant patients and for patients with a history of allergy to contrast material.

For the evaluation of renal trauma, radionuclide scans have been found to be as accurate as the IVP, but they are not generally as readily available.[3, 4, 30, 31] In a stable patient with suspected renal trauma who may have a contrast allergy, a radionuclide scan is a reasonable alternative to IVP.

Computed tomography (CT) has gained wider acceptance in the evaluation of renal trauma. Federle and associates[31] found that CT was superior to IVP in diagnosing renal trauma and in differentiating minor injuries from major injuries. Uehara and Eisner[4] concur with this view in proposing the following approach to the evaluation of suspected renal trauma. If an isolated renal injury is suspected, an emergent IVP is performed. If the IVP is normal and the patient is stable clinically, the patient is observed, and no specific treatment is initiated. If the IVP is abnormal or the patient's symptoms persist, a CT scan is done emergently. An emergency CT scan should be the *initial* diagnosic test, however, for any stable multiple-trauma patient or any patient who appears likely on clinical evaluation to have sustained a severe renal injury.

SUMMARY

The IVP is the diagnostic study of choice in the patient with suspected renal colic. It is an appropriate screening test for renal trauma in selected patients and in areas where CT scanning is not readily available. When used in a rational manner and with due consideration of its possible side effects, the IVP is a valuable tool for the emergency physician.

REFERENCES

1. Swick M: The discovery of intravenous urography: Historical and developmental aspects of the urographic media and their role in other diagnostic and therapeutic areas. *Bull N Y Acad Med.* 1966;42:128–51.
2. Sinclair D, Wilson S, Toi A, Greenspan L: The evaluation of suspected renal colic: Ultrasound versus excretory urography. *Ann Emerg Med.* 1989;18:556–559.
3. Flax S, McLorie G, Churchill BM, Gilday DL: A comparative study of intravenous urograms and radionuclide renal scans in diagnosis of renal trauma. *Urology.* 1989;34:62–64.
4. Uehara DT, Eisner RF: Indications for intravenous pyelography in trauma. *Ann Emerg Med.* 1986;15:266–269.
5. Roth CS, Bowyer BA, Berquist TH: Utility of the plain radiograph for diagnosing ureteral calculi. *Ann Emerg Med.* 1985;14:311–315.
6. Zangerle KF, Iserson KV, Bjelland JC, Criss E: Usefulness of abdominal flat plate radiographs in patients with suspected ureteral calculi. *Ann Emerg Med.* 1985;14:316–319.
7. Harris JH Jr, Harris WH: *The Radiology of Emergency Medicine.* 2nd ed. Baltimore: Williams & Wilkins; 1981:458.
8. Roberts JR, Hedges JR: *Clinical Procedures in Emergency Medicine.* Philadelphia: WB Saunders;1985:827.
9. Stine RJ, Avila JA, Lemons MF, Sickorez GJ: Diagnostic and therapeutic urologic procedures. *Emerg Med Clin North Am.* 1988;6:555–558.
10. Freeman S, Chapman J: Urologic procedures. *Emerg Med Clin North Am.* 1986;4:543–560.
11. Stewart C: Nephrolithiasis. *Emerg Med Clin North Am.* 1988;6:617–630.
12. Hartman GW, Hattery RR, Witten DM, Williamson B Jr: Mortality during excretory urography: Mayo Clinic experience. *Am J Roentgenol.* 1982;139:919–922.
13. Pendergrass HP, Tondreau RL, Pendergrass EP, et al: Reactions associated with intravenous urography: Historical and statistical review. *Radiology.* 1958;71:1–12.

14. Wolfromm R, Dehouve A, Degand F, et al: Les accidents graves par injection intraveineuse de substances iodées pour urographie. *J Radiol Electrol.* 1966;47:346–357.
15. Ansell G: Adverse reactions to contrast agents: Scope of problem. *Invest Radiol.* 1970;5:374–384.
16. Witten DM, Hirsh FD, Hartman GW: Acute reactions to urographic contrast medium: Incidence, clinical characteristics and relationship to history of hypersensitivity states. *AJR.* 1973;119:832–840.
17. Shehadi WH: Adverse reactions to intravascularly administered contrast media: A comprehensive study based on a prospective survey. *AJR.* 1975;124:145–152.
18. Shehadi WH, Toniolo G: Adverse reactions to contrast media: A report from the Committee on Safety of Contrast Media of the International Society of Radiology. *Radiology.* 1980;137:299–302.
19. Ansell G, Tweedie MC, West CR, et al: The current status of reactions to intravenous contrast media. *Invest Radiol.* 1980;15(6 Suppl):32–39.
20. Longstaff AJ, Henson JH: Bronchospasm following intravenous injection of ionic and non-ionic low-osmolality contrast media. *Clin Radiol.* 1985;36:651–653.
21. Fontanarosa PB: Radiologic contrast-induced renal failure. *Emerg Med Clin North Am.* 1988;6:601–615.
22. Benvon CC, Patrick PS, Hutchinson TA, et al: Renal function following infusion of radiologic contrast material: A prospective controlled study. *Arch Intern Med.* 1985;145:87–89.
23. Fortune JB, Brahme J, Milligan M, et al: Emergency intravenous pyelography in the trauma patient. *Arch Surg.* 1985;120:1056–1059.
24. Erwin BC, Carroll BA, Sommer PG: Renal colic: The role of ultrasound in initial evaluation. *Radiology.* 1984;152:147–150.
25. Pollack HM, Anger PM, Goldberg BB, et al: Ultrasonic detection of non-opaque renal calculi. *Radiology.* 1978;127:233–237.
26. Edell S, Zegel H: Ultrasonic detection of renal calculi. *AJR.* 1978;130:261–263.
27. Svedstrom E, Alanen A, Nurmi M: Radiologic diagnosis of renal colic: The role of plain films, excretory urography, and sonography. *Eur J Rad.* 1990;11:180–183.
28. Lang FC, Jeffery RB, Wing VA: Ultrasound vs. excretory urography in evaluating acute flank pain. *Radiology.* 1985;154:613–616.
29. Hill MC, Rich JI, Mardiat JG, et al: Sonongraphy vs. excretory urography in acute flank pain. *AJR.* 1985;144:1235–1238.
30. Lang EK, Sullivan J, Frentz G: Renal trauma: Radiological studies: Comparison of urography, computed tomography, angiography, and radionuclide studies. *Radiology.* 1985;154:1–6.
31. Federle M, Kaiser J, McAninck J, et al: The role of computed tomography in renal trauma. *Radiology.* 1981;141:455–460.

Chapter

Ultrasonography

Vincent P. Verdile and Michael B. Heller

Ultrasound was first used as a diagnostic modality in the 1940s. Few imaging modalities have achieved such broad application in such a relatively short time. In addition to its use in a variety of clinical conditions, ultrasound has also been adopted as a diagnostic tool by many different medical specialists in a myriad of settings. Both the Society of Academic Emergency Medicine[1] and the American College of Emergency Physicians[2] have published position papers on ultrasonography, and a model curriculum has been developed for training emergency physicians.[3] This chapter outlines the current role of diagnostic ultrasound for the emergency department patient and discusses the ability of emergency physicians to function as ultrasonographers.

TECHNICAL ASPECTS

The parlance of ultrasound can be confusing. First of all, the terms *ultrasound, ultrasonography,* and *sonography* are synonymous. Echocardiography has essentially the same equipment as regular ultrasound but is adapted for imaging the heart and its structures. Transesophageal echocardiography (TEE) serves the same diagnostic role as transthoracic (traditional) echocardiography but offers a different vantage point for viewing the heart and mediastinal structures.[4] TEE has been suggested as an alternative method for evaluating the thoracic aorta in patients with blunt chest trauma.[5, 6] Doppler ultrasound is used to study flow information, primarily in the evaluation of blood vessels.[7]

Ultrasound equipment has evolved tremendously over the past 20 years. Modern-day ultrasound employs a real-time scanning mode that is two-dimensional (2-D) and can assess both anatomic structures and motion, in a manner analogous to fluoroscopy. M-mode ultrasound is single-dimensional scanning that displays changes in position of anatomic structures over time. M-mode was first utilized for visualizing cardiac anatomy but has since been surpassed by 2-D echocardiography, which is essentially real-time scanning. B-mode ultrasound, once the most commonly selected for diagnostic purposes, is also 2-D, but the images are static. Hence, B-mode has generally been replaced by real-time scanning.[7–9]

For the majority of ultrasound units, the transducer serves to both generate and receive the ultrasound beam or sound wave. The returning sound wave is called the *echo,* because it is reflected off the tissue being studied. Within each transducer, there is a crystal that vibrates in cycles per second to create the ultrasonic beam, which is described in terms of megahertz (MHz). After the beam is sent, the transducer pauses to receive the returning echo. The time that elapses between sending and receiving an ultrasound beam provides information about the depth of the tissue being studied, and the quality of the returning echo provides some information about the tissue characteristics.[7, 9, 10] Ultrasound images are displayed as electrical signals on a monitor.

Different transducers are chosen for examining different tissues, according to the depth of the tissue and the resolution desired. For example, a 3.5-MHz transducer has great tissue penetration but inferior resolution compared with a 7.5-MHz transducer. The 3.5-MHz transducer might be used to scan kidneys or the abdominal aorta, whereas a 7.5-MHz transducer may be best used to localize a foreign body under the skin. As a rule, the higher the transducer frequency, the greater the resolution, but the more superficial the examination has to be (Table 65–1).

The cost of the actual ultrasound machine can vary greatly, depending on the size, applications, and resolution needed. Small portable units that would be most adaptable to the ED can cost as little as $20,000 to $50,000 (Fig. 65–1). The larger units, which are found in the ultrasound department, can cost as much as several hundred thousand dollars. Although the transducers are fundamentally important to image reproduction, the ultrasound machine is responsible for generating the images. The larger, more sophisticated units do this the best. Additional transducers increase costs substantially for any size ultrasound machine.

Each specific organ or type of tissue yields a reproducible visual echo pattern, determined by its structure and composition. The visual recognition of tissue types is an essential skill and one that emergency physicians must acquire in order to perform ultrasound on their own.[10]

Air and bone reflect the entire ultrasound beam and do not allow the

TABLE 65–1. TRANSDUCER FREQUENCIES AND APPLICATIONS

3.5 MHz	5.0 MHz	7.5 MHz
Adults	Pediatrics	Small parts
Abdomen	Abdomen	Breast
Pelvis	Pelvis	Testis
Cardiac	Cardiac	Foreign body

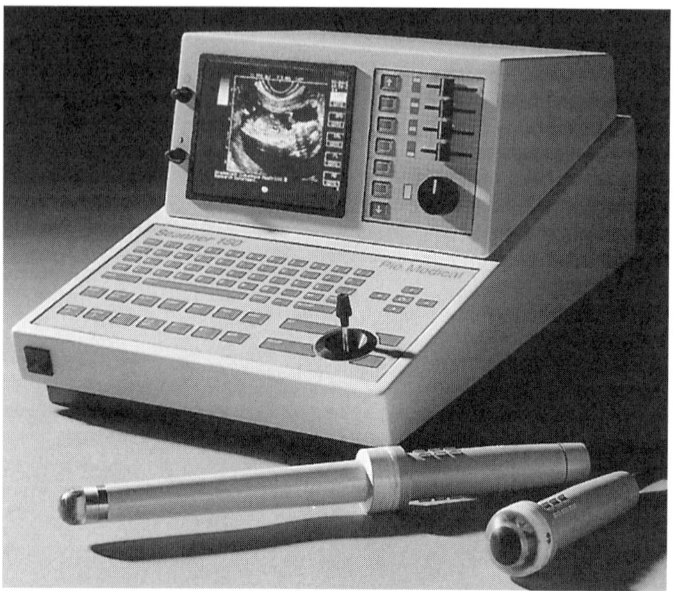

FIGURE 65–1. An example of a tabletop portable ultrasound machine. (Courtesy of Leisegang Medical, Boca Raton, Florida.)

structures beyond them to be visualized. Fluids and fluid-filled structures by comparison facilitate the ultrasonic evaluation of structures near them; hence the importance of a full bladder to image pelvic structures in the female patient. In general, fluid-filled structures, such as a gallbladder or an ovarian cyst, are easily studied by ultrasound.[9, 10]

The image produced by the real-time scanners is displayed as a pie-shaped image. This is referred to as *sector scanning,* with the apex of the pie shape representing the skin-transducer interface. *Linear array* scanning, most often used for obstetric purposes, creates a rectangular image. Sector scanning, by virtue of the smaller transducer size, is much more versatile and maneuverable and so more adaptable to the emergency applications of ultrasound.

Ultrasonography (because it is noninvasive, not dependent on organ function, and for the newer models quite portable) is an ideal imaging modality for the emergency department. Many clinical conditions seen in the emergency department are amenable to evaluation by sonography.

ABDOMINAL APPLICATIONS

The most common emergency application for ultrasound is probably in the evaluation of abdominal pathology.

Cholelithiasis

Gallbladder disease is a common reason for patients to seek medical attention.[11] Although plain radiographs are often taken of the patient who complains of abdominal pain, they are of only limited use for detecting gallstones, because fewer than 20% of these stones contain enough calcium to be visualized. Oral or intravenous cholecystography and radionuclide imaging studies are not always available through the emergency department and are usually not cost- and time-efficient for emergency patients. Ultrasound has demonstrated its superiority as a right upper quadrant imaging modality, with 95 to 99% accuracy in the detection of gallstones.[12–14]

Gallstones, even when visualized, may or may not be the etiology of abdominal pain. Asymptomatic gallstones are quite common, particularly in the elderly.[15–18] There are, however, well-accepted criteria for the ultrasonic diagnosis of acute cholecystitis. An enlarged, tender gallbladder (sonographic Murphy sign) with intraluminal stones is an exceptionally specific finding for the diagnosis of acute cholecystitis in patients with abdominal pain.[13, 14, 19] Ultrasound is 90 to 95% sensitive and 94 to 98% specific for the detection of acute cholecystitis in patients with acute right upper quadrant abdominal pain.[13, 14, 19] What makes ultrasonography even more valuable in the evaluation of abdominal pain is its ability to essentially rule out gallbladder disease, in the patient with a normal-appearing, nontender gallbladder, with greater than 95% certainty.[13]

Emergency physicians have demonstrated some success in using ultrasound in the detection of gallbladder pathology in emergency department patients.[20, 21] Gussow and colleagues[21] compared the emergency physician's interpretation of a right upper quadrant ultrasound scan for the presence or absence of gallstones with that of a formal ultrasound scan performed by a technologist and interpreted by a radiologist. Of 44 patients suspected of having acute cholecystitis, 57% had gallstones. Two of 35 emergency department ultrasounds (one false-positive and one false-negative) disagreed with the formal ultrasound interpretation. Nine scans were interpreted by the ED physicians as indeterminate, 3 of which were formally read as positive and 6 as negative. Gussow and colleagues[21] concluded that emergency physicians can perform ultrasound with some degree of accuracy, thereby facilitating diagnosis and management in patients presumed to have cholecystitis.[21]

Abdominal Aortic Aneurysm

Ultrasound is commonly used in nonemergency situations to evaluate patients suspected of having abdominal aortic aneurysm (AAA). The limitations of the physical examination and of plain film radiography in the detection of AAA are well described.[22–25] Sonographic evaluation of the aorta is safe, rapid, and accurate and can be performed at the bedside in the hemodynamically unstable patient.

Shuman and associates[26] described what is perhaps the first use of ultrasound for the initial evaluation of patients who present to an emergency department and have signs and symptoms suggestive of a leaking AAA. In their study, prehospital health care providers notified the emergency department of the patients being transported who were suspected have symptomatic AAA. An ultrasound technologist was called to the emergency department, where a portable ultrasound machine was stationed. Abdominal ultrasonography was performed during the initial evaluation and resuscitation to determine the presence or absence of an AAA or periaortic extraluminal blood. Sonographic findings were correlated with surgical results and clinical outcome. Ultrasound was accurate in demonstrating the presence or absence of an AAA in 98% of the 60 patients studied, but extraluminal blood was detected in only 4%. The sonographic confirmation of an AAA in the setting of abdominal pain and hemodynamic instability resulted in the correct decision to take 21 of 22 patients immediately to surgery. The negative predictive value of a normal-appearing aorta was 96% (26).

Patients who present with the classic AAA findings, namely, abdominal or back pain, shock, and pulsatile abdominal mass, generally pose little problem in diagnosis. The clinical picture is not always so clear, however, and there can be significant delays in the diagnosis. Bedside ultrasound can be a very useful tool in these circumstances. Most aneurysms appear as fusiform dilatations, and 95% lie below the renal arteries.[25] Ultrasound equipment permits the measurement of the aneurysm during real-time scanning. The presence or absence of thrombus, although discussed in the ultrasound literature, is not clinically relevant to the diagnosis and initial management of AAA.[23, 25]

Ultrasound has been demonstrated to be quite accurate in the diagnosis of AAA and is often suggested as the primary imaging modality.[23, 25, 27] The experience of emergency physicians with ultrasound for the detection of AAA is limited. Jehle and coworkers[20] discovered AAAs in five patients who presented with unexplained abdominal pain or pulsatile mass. Three patients were found to have AAAs that were greater than 5 cm in diameter, which were later confirmed by surgery or other imaging techniques.

Although the use of ultrasound for the detection of acute AAA in the ED seems very reasonable, there is not a wealth of clinical research to support its use in this setting. Clinical research directed at the population of ED patients with the atypical presentation, in whom an AAA must be expeditiously diagnosed, is still needed. Nevertheless, it appears likely that ultrasound will play a significant role in the early evaluation of acute AAA. A brief ED ultrasound examination demonstrating a dissecting AAA may be all that is necessary to convince a surgeon to take a patient directly to the operating room.

Acute Appendicitis

Ultrasound has also been used in the evaluation of patients suspected of having acute appendicitis and has proved to be quite helpful.[28–30]

Jeffrey and associates[28] evaluated 90 patients with clinically suspected acute appendicitis, using high-resolution real-time sonography. The ultrasonic diagnosis was made when the appendix was visualized and noncompressible. (A normal appendix cannot usually be visualized.)

Ultrasonography had a sensitivity of 89% and a specificity of 95%, with an overall accuracy of 93%, in detecting acute appendicitis, comparable with a previous report on the use of ultrasound to make this diagnosis.[29] If female patients were analyzed separately, the sensitivity was 86%, the specificity was 98%, and the overall accuracy was 96%. It was proposed that ultrasound may actually decrease the incidence of unnecessary laparotomy for presumed acute appendicitis, particularly in young female patients, when it is used in conjunction with the other relevant clinical indicators.[28]

GENITOURINARY SYSTEM

Renal Ultrasound

Excretory urography (ie, intravenous pyelography) remains the standard for the evaluation of patient with suspected nephrolithiasis.[31–34] Ultrasound does have a role in the evaluation of these patients, however, particularly to address specifically the presence or absence of hydronephrosis.[32, 34–36] In addition, ultrasound may be the preferred diagnostic study in the patient with compromised renal function or an allergy to intravenous contrast material and in the pregnant patient.[31, 33, 36]

Ultrasound has been reported to have a sensitivity of 98 to 100% for the detection of moderate-to-severe urinary tract obstruction (hydronephrosis).[36–37] It can detect the presence of both opaque and nonopaque renal calculi, especially those located in the proximal collecting system or the bladder.[34, 38, 39] Bowel gas and stool make the evaluation of the midportion of the ureter more difficult.[33, 35]

One report described a sensitivity of 100% and a specificity of 95% for ultrasonic evaluation of patients with presumed renal calculus.[35] The sonographic criterion was the presence of unilateral hydronephrosis or the presence of a renal calculus, or both. The number of patients was small, however, thus limiting the significance of the study. Sinclair and associates[34] prospectively evaluated 98 patients, also comparing the diagnostic accuracy of ultrasound with IVP. Overall, these investigators judged that the diagnostic abilities of these procedures were equal in the detection of renal calculi or hydronephrosis.

Sonography has not been uniformly successful, however, in the evaluation of patients with acute flank pain. Several studies have suggested that ultrasound alone is not particularly useful.[31–33, 35] Hill and coworkers[33] prospectively studied 61 patients with acute flank pain and compared ultrasound with urography. Urography had a diagnostic accuracy of 85%. Ultrasound was correct only 66% of the time. Lang and colleagues[32] also reported that urography is superior to ultrasound for the evaluation of patients with acute flank pain. Both the Hill[33] and Sinclair[34] studies, however, concluded that ultrasound was superior to IVP in the detection of calculi at the ureterovesical junction.

Perhaps the most appropriate role for ultrasound in the evaluation of the emergency department patient suspected of having nephrolithiasis is as an initial screen for the detection of hydronephrosis or renal calculi.[36] Svestrom and associates[31] have demonstrated that ultrasound, combined with plain radiographs of the abdomen, has a sensitivity of 80% and a specificity of 58%. Other investigators have proposed the same role for ultrasound and plain films as initial screening tools or as the preferred studies in the patient in whom urography is contraindicated.[33, 35] To date, no controlled, prospective clinical trial has been undertaken to critically evaluate this position.

Pelvic Ultrasound

Ultrasound is commonly used in the emergency department to determine the presence or absence of an ectopic pregnancy in the female patient of reproductive age with lower abdominal pain.[40–43] The transabdominal approach of ultrasound scanning, however, is rapidly being replaced by the transvaginal approach with specially designed transducers.[42, 43–45] The transvaginal approach can detect an intrauterine gestational sac almost 1 week younger than with the transabdominal approach.[41] Most reports describe identification of an intrauterine gestational sac between 23 and 35 days' menstrual age using the endovaginal transducer,[41–43] a stage that coincides with a positive urine pregnancy test. More significant, however, is the superiority of the transvaginal approach for the detection of ectopic pregnancies.[43–46]

Thorsen and colleagues[44] prospectively evaluated 193 patients with a clinical diagnosis of suspected ectopic pregnancy and compared the transvaginal approach with the transabdominal approach. Patients underwent both procedures. Transvaginal sonography was able to detect ectopic pregnancy in 38% of the 60 women with surgically proven ectopic pregnancy, compared with 22% detected by the transabdominal approach. All 83 intrauterine pregnancies were detected by transvaginal ultrasound, versus only 34 detected by the transabdominal transducer. Thorsen and colleagues[44] concluded that transvaginal ultrasound is superior to transabdominal ultrasound for the evaluation of patients with suspected ectopic pregnancies. Other investigators have confirmed these results.[43, 45]

Cacciatore[46] compared transvaginal ultrasound findings with surgical findings in 120 women in an attempt to determine the ability of transvaginal ultrasound to evaluate the status of a tubal pregnancy. The size of the tubal mass was predicted accurately with transvaginal ultrasound, as well as the determination of an intact or ruptured ectopic pregnancy. Furthermore, the presence of hemoperitoneum was detected with a sensitivity of 91%, a figure supported by other studies.[45, 47, 48]

Gussow and Alberto[49] have reported that emergency physicians can reliably perform transabdominal ultrasound to determine the presence or absence of an intrauterine pregnancy in patients suspected of having ectopic pregnancies. These two emergency physicians evaluated 17 patients suspected of having ectopic pregnancy and compared their ultrasound results with those of formal ultrasound. Of the seven scans interpreted as demonstrating an intrauterine pregnancy, all were confirmed by formal ultrasonography. Ten patients were judged by emergency ultrasound not to have intrauterine pregnancy, and these findings were again confirmed by formal ultrasound examination in all ten. Although extremely limited in scope and based on only a small number of patients, these results suggest that emergency physicians may be able to utilize transabdominal ultrasonography successfully to facilitate the ED evaluation of this group of patients.

In a later study, Mateer and associates[50] demonstrated that emergency physicians were capable of performing transvaginal ultrasound to exclude the presence of ectopic pregnancy. Their prospective study of 152 patients found that emergency physicians had a 100% sensitivity and a 95% specificity for the presence or absence of an ectopic pregnancy. The role of ED ultrasonography for the diagnosis of ectopic pregnancy is clearly an exciting area for clinical research.

Transvaginal ultrasound, then, is more sensitive than transabdominal ultrasound in the detection of either intrauterine or ectopic pregnancy. In addition, the transvaginal approach has emerged as a useful tool for the evaluation of other pelvic pathology and may supersede transabdominal ultrasound in this regard as well.[48, 51, 52] The application of this relatively new diagnostic modality to the ED setting promises to become widespread in the not too distant future.

TRAUMA SONOGRAPHY

Some experience has been reported with the use of sonography for the detection of hemoperitoneum in the trauma patient.[53–56] One study found ultrasound to be 87% sensitive and 100% specific, with an accuracy of 97%, in determining the presence of blood in the peritoneal cavity of patients suffering from blunt abdominal trauma.[54] There were no negative laparotomies in patients who had ultrasound findings of hemoperitoneum. Bode and colleagues[55] have reported similar results in a study of 353 patients undergoing sonography in the ED after blunt abdominal trauma.

The ability of nonradiologists to perform ultrasound on patients with blunt abdominal trauma was examined by Forster and coworkers.[57] These investigators demonstrated that proficiency with ultrasonography increased with years of experience with the device. Positive predictive values for ultrasonographic findings were 60% for surgeons with less than 1 year, 76% for those with less than 3 years, and 92% for those with more than 3 years of experience. Forster and coworkers[57] concluded that ultrasound is highly sensitive and specific for detecting injuries after blunt abdominal trauma and that, for the 17 surgeons in their study, it was an easy diagnostic test to master.

In the pregnant trauma patient, ultrasound is very useful in identifying abruptio placentae and in evaluating the status of the fetus.[58] For the unstable patient, of course, this examination can be performed at the bedside with a portable scanner.

Ultrasound is beginning to demonstrate its utility as an imaging modality for the evaluation of solid organs that are subjected to blunt force trauma. The kidney,[59] the liver and spleen,[60–63] and the testes[64] have all been evaluated by ultrasound for the presence or absence of parenchymal injury after trauma. The role of ultrasound in the evaluation of trauma patients has been limited thus far because of the ready availability and the reliability of computed tomography in the detection of traumatic injuries in solid organs.[65]

OTHER EMERGENCY APPLICATIONS

A few other applications of ultrasound may be of interest or use to the emergency physician. Sonography has been shown to be a superior imaging modality for the detection of soft tissue foreign bodies.[66–69] Ultrasound can identify both radiopaque and nonradiopaque foreign bodies and can, in addition, facilitate localization and extraction of a foreign body.[67–69] In an experimental model of beef cubes, emergency physicians were able to detect 59 of 60 foreign bodies, which included gravel, cactus spine, plastic, metal, and wood.[68] High-frequency transducers, 7.5 MHz or greater, are best for the purpose of detecting foreign bodies.

Some preliminary work suggests that real-time ultrasound may be an effective screening tool to identify proximal deep venous thrombosis of the lower extremity.[70, 71] A prospective study was conducted comparing ultrasound with contrast venography in the detection of proximal deep vein thrombosis.[70] Negative ultrasound readings were consistent with venogram interpretations in all 56 patients studied, giving a negative predictive value of 100%. Eighteen patients had positive ultrasound scans for deep venous thromboses, only 14 of which were verified by venography, giving a positive predictive value of 78%. Because of the preliminary nature of this information, coupled with the serious morbidity and mortality associated with missed deep vein thrombosis, it is not likely that emergency physicians will be performing bedside ultrasound to diagnose this clinical entity.

Sonography has also been utilized to guide central venous catheter placement, an application that may be of some utility to the emergency physician.[72, 73] Ultrasound has demonstrated its utility for guiding suprapubic needle aspiration of the bladder in pediatric patients.[74] A successful suprapubic aspiration was accomplished in 79% of the attempts in the ultrasound-guided group, compared with 52% in the blind aspiration group. Ultrasound was able to significantly improve the success rates for suprapubic aspiration in the hands of pediatric residents and pediatric emergency medicine fellows.[74]

SUMMARY

Ultrasound has broad application as a diagnostic modality for many different clinical conditions. There are many conditions for which ultrasound could provide the emergency physician with valuable clinical information. Clinical research to demonstrate the efficacy of ultrasound by emergency physicians is needed. It is likely that ultrasound will assume a role in emergency medicine analogous to that of a stethoscope, serving as an extension of the physical examination. For appropriately selected ED patients, ultrasound can be a very valuable asset in emergency department evaluation, clinical decision making, and patient management.

REFERENCES

1. Society of Academic Emergency Medicine: Ultrasound position statement. *SAEM Newsletter.* 1991;3:3.
2. American College of Emergency Physicians: Council resolution on ultrasound. *ACEP News.* April 1991:(insert).
3. Mateer J, Plummer D, Heller M, et al: Model curriculum for physicians training in emergency ultrasonography. *Ann Emerg Med.* 1994;23:95–102.
4. Khandheria BK, Seward JB, Tajik AJ: Transesophageal echocardiography. *Mayo Clin Proc.* 1994;69:856–863.
5. Shapiro MJ, Yanofsky SD, Trapp J, et al: Cardiovascular evaluation in blunt thoracic trauma using transesophageal echocardiography. *J Trauma.* 1991;31:835–839.
6. Kearney PA, Smith DW, Johnson SB, et al: Use of transesophageal echocardiography in the evaluation of traumatic aortic injury. *J Trauma.* 1993;34:696–703.
7. Council on Scientific Affairs, American Medical Association: Medical diagnostic ultrasound instrumentation and clinical interpretation: Report of the Ultrasonography Task Force. *JAMA.* 1991;265:1155–1159.
8. James AE, Goddard J, Price RR, et al: Advances in instrument design in image recording. *Radiol Clin North Am.* 1980;18:3–20.
9. Walter JP: Physics of high-resolution ultrasound—practical aspects. *Radiol Clin North Am.* 1985;23:3–12.
10. Price RR, Jones TB, Goddard J, et al: Basic concepts of ultrasonic tissue characterization. *Radiol Clin North Am.* 1980;18:21–30.
11. Diehl AK, Sugarek NJ, Todd KH: Clinical evaluation for gallstone disease: Usefulness of symptoms and signs in diagnosis. *Am J Med.* 1990;89:29–33.
12. Ferrucci JT: Radiologic and ultrasonographic diagnosis of gallstones. *J Clin Gastroenterol.* 1988;10(suppl 2):S22–S24.
13. Laing FC: Diagnostic evaluation of patients with suspected acute cholecystitis. *Radiol Clin North Am.* 1983;21:477–492.
14. Martin KI, Doubilet P: How to image the gallbladder in suspected cholecystitis. *Ann Intern Med.* 1988;109:722–729.
15. Ratner J, Lisbona A, Rosenbloom M, et al: The prevalence of gallstone disease in very old institutionalized persons. *JAMA.* 1991;265:902–903.
16. McSherry CK, Ferstenberg H, Calhoun FW, et al: The natural history of diagnosed gallstone disease in symptomatic and asymptomatic patients. *Ann Surg.* 1985;202:59–63.
17. Friedman GD, Raviola CA, Fireman B: Prognosis of gallstones with mild or no symptoms: Twenty-five years of follow-up in a health maintenance organization. *J Clin Epidemiol.* 1989;42:127–136.
18. Thistle JL, Clearly PA, Lachin JM, et al: The natural history of cholelithiasis: the National Cooperative Gallstone Study. *Ann Intern Med.* 1984;101:171–175.
19. Laing FC, Federle MP, Jeffrey RB, et al: Ultrasonic evaluation of patients with acute right upper quadrant pain. *Radiology.* 1981;140:449–455.
20. Jehle D, Davis E, Evans T, et al: Emergency department sonography by emergency physicians. *Am J Emerg Med.* 1989;7:605–611.
21. Gussow L, Himmelman R, Zalenski R: Portable ultrasound in patients with

suspected cholecystitis: Performance and interpretation by emergency physicians [abstract]. *Ann Emerg Med.* 1989;18:441.
22. Quill DS, Colgan MP, Sumner BS: Ultrasonic screening for the detection of abdominal aortic aneurysms. *Surg Clin North Am.* 1989;69:713–720.
23. Paivansalo M, Lahde S, Myllyla V, et al: Ultrasonography in the diagnosis of abdominal aortic aneurysms. *Fortschr Röntgenstr.* 1984;140:683–685.
24. Hardy BC, Lee JKT, Weyman PJ, et al: Measurement of the abdominal aortic aneurysm. *Radiology.* 1981;141:821–823.
25. Godwin JD, Korobkin M: Acute disease of the aorta. *Radiol Clin North Am.* 1983;21:551–565.
26. Shuman WP, Hastrup W, Kohler PR, et al: Suspected leaking abdominal aortic aneurysm: Use of sonography in the emergency room. *Radiology.* 1989;168:117–119.
27. Leopold GR, Goldberger LE, Bernstein EF: Ultrasonic detection in evaluation of abdominal aortic aneurysms. *Surgery.* 1982;72:939–945.
28. Jeffrey RB, Laing FC, Lewis FR: Acute appendicitis: High resolution real-time US findings. *Radiology.* 1987;163:11–14.
29. Puylaert JBCM: Acute appendicitis: US evaluation using graded compression. *Radiology.* 1986;158:355–360.
30. Puylaert JBCM, Rutgers PH, Lalisang RI, et al: Prospective study of ultrasonography in the diagnosis of appendicitis. *N Engl J Med.* 1987;317:666–669.
31. Svestrom E, Alanen A, Nurmi M: Radiologic diagnosis of renal colic: The role of plain films, excretory urography and sonography. *Eur J Radiol.* 1990;11:180–183.
32. Laing FC, Jeffrey RB, Wing VW: Ultrasound versus excretory urography in evaluating acute flank pain. *Radiology.* 1985;154:613–616.
33. Hill MC, Rich JI, Mardiat JG, et al: Sonography versus excretory urography in acute flank pain. *AJR.* 1985;145:1235–1238.
34. Sinclair D, Wilson S, Toi A, et al: The evaluation of suspected renal colic: Ultrasound scan versus excretory urography. *Ann Emerg Med.* 1989;18:556–559.
35. Erwin BC, Carroll BA, Sommer FG: Renal colic: The role of ultrasound in initial evaluation. *Radiology.* 1984;152:147–150.
36. Ellenbogen PH, Scheible W, Talner LB, et al: Sensitivity of gray scale ultrasound in detecting urinary tract obstruction. *Am J Roentgenol.* 1978;130:731–733.
37. Lee JKT, Baron RL, Melson GL, et al: Can real-time ultrasonography replace static B-scanning in the diagnosis of renal obstruction? *Radiology.* 1981;139:161–165.
38. Pollack HM, Arger PH, Goldberg BB, et al: Ultrasonic detection of non-opaque renal calculi. *Radiology.* 1978;127:233–237.
39. Edell S, Zegel H: Ultrasonic evaluation of renal calculi. *Am J Roentgenol.* 1978;130:261–263.
40. Lawson TL: Ectopic pregnancy: Criteria and accuracy of ultrasonic diagnosis. *Am J Roentgenol.* 1978;131:153–156.
41. Council on Scientific Affairs, American Medical Association: Report of the Ultrasonography Task Force: Gynecologic sonography. *JAMA.* 1981;265:2851–2855.
42. Marn CS, Bree RL: Advances in pelvic ultrasound: Endovaginal scanning

for ectopic gestation and graded compression sonography for appendicitis. *Ann Emerg Med.* 1989;18:1304–1309.
43. Dashefsky SM, Lyons EA, Levi CS, et al: Suspected ectopic pregnancy: Endovaginal and transvesical US. *Radiology.* 1988;169:181–184.
44. Thorsen MK, Lawson TL, Amin EJ, et al: Diagnoses of ectopic pregnancy: Endovaginal versus transabdominal sonography. *AJR.* 1990;155:307–310.
45. Kivikoski AI, Martin CM, Smeltzer JS: Transabdominal and transvaginal ultrasonography in the diagnosis of ectopic pregnancy: A comparative study. *Am J Obstet Gynecol.* 1990;163:123–128.
46. Cacciatore B: Can the status of tubal pregnancy be predicted with transvaginal sonography? A prospective comparison of sonography, surgical and serum hCG findings. *Radiology.* 1990;177:481–484.
47. Schwab RA: Ultrasound versus culdocentesis in the evaluation of early and late ectopic pregnancy. *Ann Emerg Med.* 1988; 17:801–803.
48. Mendelson EB, Bohm-Velez M, Neiman HL, et al: Transvaginal sonography in gynecologic imaging. *Semin Ultrasound CT MR.* 1988;9:102–121.
49. Gussow LM, Alberto G: Performance and interpretation of pelvic ultrasound by emergency physicians in patients with suspected ectopic pregnancy: A prospective study [abstract]. *Ann Emerg Med.* 1990;19:1224.
50. Mateer J, Aiman EJ, Brown M. Ultrasound evaluation of ectopic pregnancy by emergency physicians [abstract]. *Ann Emerg Med.* 1993;22:210.
51. Fleischer AC, Gordon AN, Entman SS: Transabdominal and transvaginal sonography of pelvic masses. *Ultrasound Med Biol.* 1989;15:529–533.
52. Tessler FN, Schiller VL, Perrella RR, et al: Transabdominal versus endovaginal pelvic sonography: Prospective study. *Radiology.* 1989;170:553–556.
53. Gruessner R, Mentges B, Duber C, et al: Sonography versus peritoneal lavage in blunt abdominal trauma. *J Trauma.* 1989;29:242–244.
54. Kimura A, Otsuka T: Emergency center ultrasonography in the evaluation of hemoperitoneum: A prospective study. *J Trauma.* 1991;31:20–23.
55. Bode PJ, Niezen RA, van Vugt AB, et al: Abdominal ultrasound as a reliable indicator for conclusive laparotomy in blunt abdominal trauma. *J Trauma.* 1993;34:27–31.
56. Chambers JA, Pilbrow WJ: Ultrasound in abdominal trauma: An alternative to peritoneal lavage. *Arch Emerg Med.* 1988;5:26–33.
57. Forster R, Pillasch J, Zielke A, et al: Ultrasonography in blunt abdominal trauma: Influence of the investigators' experience. *J Trauma.* 1993;34:264–269.
58. Pearlman MD, Tintinnalli JE, Lorenz RP: Blunt trauma during pregnancy. *N Engl J Med.* 1990;323:1609–1613.
59. Prasadarao PR, Naseen M, Devastahli R: Sonographic diagnosis of fractured kidney. *Ill Med J.* 1986;169:167–168.
60. Froehlich JW, Simeone JF, McKusick KA, et al: Radionuclide imaging and ultrasound in liver/spleen trauma: A prospective comparison. *Radiology.* 1982;145:457–461.
61. Asher WM, Parvin S, Virgillio RW, et al: Echographic evaluation of splenic injury after blunt trauma. *Radiology.* 1976;118:411–415.
62. Rohmer FW, Didier D, Coche G: Ultrasound of the traumatized spleen: Left butterfly sign in lesions masked by echogenic blood clots. *Gastrointest Radiol.* 1988;13:169–172.

63. Bihr FW, Rohmer P, Zeltner F, et al: Ultrasonic study of hepatic and splenic traumatic lesions. *Eur J Radiol.* 1981;1:245–249.
64. Jeffrey RB, Laing FC, Hricak H, et al: Sonography of testicular trauma. *AJR.* 1983;141:993–995.
65. McCort JJ: Caring for the major trauma victim: The role for radiology. *Radiology.* 1987;163:1–9.
66. Flaviis LD, Scaglione P, Del Bo P, et al: Detection of foreign bodies in soft tissues: Experimental comparison of ultrasonography and xerography. *J Trauma.* 1988;28:400–404.
67. Fornage BD, Schernberg FL: Sonographic diagnosis of foreign bodies of the distal extremities. *AJR.* 1986;147:567–569.
68. Schlager D, Sanders AB, Wiggins D, et al: Ultrasound for the detection of foreign bodies. *Ann Emerg Med.* 1991;20:189–191.
69. Shiels WE, Babcock DS, Wilson JL, et al: Localization and guided removal of soft-tissue foreign bodies with sonography. *AJR.* 1990;155:1277–1281.
70. Chance JF, Abbitt PL, Tegtmeyer CJ, et al: Real-time ultrasound for the detection of deep venous thrombosis. *Ann Emerg Med.* 1991;20:494–496.
71. Cronan JJ: Venous thromboembolic disease: The role of US. *Radiology.* 1993;186:619–630.
72. Bond DM, Champion LK: Real-time ultrasound imaging aids jugular venipuncture [letter]. *Anesth Analg.* 1989;68:698–701.
73. Denys BG, Uretsky BF, Reddy PS, et al: An ultrasound method for safe and rapid central venous access. *N Engl J Med.* 1991;324:566–570.
74. Gochman RF, Karasic RB, Heller MB: Use of portable ultrasound to assist urine collection by suprapubic aspiration. *Ann Emerg Med.* 1991;20:631–635.

Chapter

Ventilation/Perfusion Nuclear Lung Scan

Steven J. White

Pulmonary embolism (PE) is a common event with life-threatening potential. Although the mortality of untreated PE has been reported to approach 30%, the mortality of treated PE is only about 8%.[1] Treatment itself is not without risk, however: Heparin therapy represents one of the most common causes of drug-related complications and death in hospitalized patients.[2, 3] Long-term therapy with coumadin carries a similar risk.[4] The mandate for accurate diagnosis is clear. Unfortunately, the diagnosis of PE is neither straightforward nor uniformly approached.

Many clinical features and laboratory data may weigh into the decision to consider and further pursue the ultimate diagnosis of PE. Once that decision has been reached, the next step in diagnostic workup is almost invariably the technetium-99m nuclear lung scan (ventilation/perfusion scan, V/Q scan).

After nuclear lung scans came into widespread clinical use in about 1970, clinicians quickly came to rely heavily on the results of this readily available, noninvasive test as a replacement for the less available and more invasive pulmonary angiogram, the accepted standard. Interpretation initially consisted of negative scans and positive scans, with little consideration of "gray zones." Ventilation scanning was added to perfusion scanning, and interpretation criteria evolved to increase diagnostic accuracy. Controversy over accuracy and interpretation continued until a large, prospective, multicenter study known as PIOPED (Prospective Investigation of Pulmonary Embolism Diagnosis) was carried out to determine the sensitivities and specificities of V/Q lung scans in the diagnosis of PE.[5]

EQUIPMENT AND TECHNIQUE

There is no accepted uniform technique with regard to the relative order of ventilation and perfusion scanning, choice of radiopharmaceutical agent, or patient position.

Ventilation Scanning

Radiopharmaceutical Agent

Xenon-133 gas is the most commonly employed agent. Because this agent has lower energy than the technetium-99m used in perfusion scanning, xenon-133 scanning must be performed before the perfusion study unless computer subtraction is used.

Krypton-81m gas is more expensive, but its higher energy provides for better image resolution. It also enables the ventilation scan to be performed after the perfusion scan, allowing one to forgo the ventilation scan if the perfusion scan is normal.

In contrast to these inert gases, which provide for scanning in only the posterior projection, technetium 99m–labeled monodispersed aerosol (^{99m}Tc MDA) remains in the lungs for up to an hour, allowing for six-projection imaging analogous to the views obtained during perfusion scanning. Perfusion scanning, with ten times the number of particles, must follow ventilation so as not to obscure the ventilation images. Technetium-99m also provides better spatial resolution than xenon-133.

Technique

The patient breathes via a closed breathing circuit. When xenon or krypton is used, radioactive gas (approximately 20 mCi) is injected into the circuit during maximal inspiration (the *wash-in phase*) to image normally ventilated portions of lung. Normal breathing for 3 to 5 minutes enables gas to enter abnormally ventilated lung areas and yields the *equilibration phase* images. An additional 5-minute period of breathing nonradioactive gas allows those areas of air-trapping to be imaged (the *wash-out phase*). When technetium-99m aerosol is used, because the radioactive particles persist in the capillaries, only equilibration phase images are possible. The choice of radionuclide for ventilation scanning does not appear to affect diagnostic accuracy.[6]

Perfusion Scanning

Technique

Following intravenous injection, technetium 99m–labeled albumin macroaggregate (^{99m}Tc-MAA) is carried to the pulmonary capillary bed. The radiolabeled particles, ranging in size from 10 to 60 μm, are trapped in the pulmonary capillaries or prepulmonary arterioles; the distribution of particles parallels regional pulmonary blood flow. With the usual administered dose of 500,000 particles, less than 0.1% of the pulmonary vascular cross-sectional area is occluded. Films are exposed in six projections: posterior, anterior, right and left lateral, and right and left posterior oblique.

INTERPRETATION OF V/Q SCAN

Several sets of interpretation criteria have been employed, in conjunction with the chest radiograph findings, in the interpretation of V/Q scan findings. The criteria introduced by Biello and colleagues[7] in 1979 were long the standard. Criteria developed in the PIOPED study[5] have become more widely employed (Table 66–1). One retrospective study applying both sets of criteria to a pool of angiographically and scintigraphically studied patients found that there was no significant difference in interpretation, although the investigators judged that the PIOPED criteria were better defined and simpler to apply.[8]

TABLE 66–1. BIELLO AND PIOPED CRITERIA FOR INTERPRETATION OF VENTILATION/PERFUSION SCANS

V/Q Scan Interpretation	Biello Criteria[a]	PIOPED Criteria[b]
Normal	No perfusion (Q) defects	No Q defects, Q outlines parallel lung shape on CXR
Very low probability	Not defined	≤3 small (<25% segment) Q defects, normal CXR
Low probability	Small ventilation/perfusion (V/Q) mismatches without corresponding CXR abnormalities	Nonsegmental Q defects (e.g., corresponding to hila, effusion)
	Q defect much < CXR defect	Q defect much < CXR defect
	V/Q match defect (<50% lung or corresponding to pleural effusion)	Single moderate (≥25% and ≤75% segment) V/Q mismatch, normal CXR
		Large (>75% segment) or moderate Q defects involving ≤4 segments in 1 lung and ≤3 segments in 1 lung region with *matching* $\dot{V}$ defects ≥ Q defects *and* CXR normal or defects much < Q defects
Indeterminate/intermediate probability	Diffuse V/Q matching defects (>0% lung field V abnormal)	Not easily into high or low, borderline high, borderline low
	Matched Q and CXR defects	
	Single moderate Q > V mismatch with regional CXR normality	
High probability	Q defect much > than CXR defect	≥2 large segmental Q > V defects, no or smaller CXR defects
	≥1 large or ≥ 2 moderate Q/V mismatched with regionally normal CXR	≥2 moderate segmental Q defects, no matching V defects + 1 large segmental Q > V mismatched defect, no matching CXR defect
		≥4 moderate segmental Q defects, no matching V or CXR defects

[a]Data from Hull RD, Hirsh J, Carter CJ: Diagnostic value of ventilation-perfusion lung scanning in patients with suspected pulmonary embolism. *Chest*. 1985;88:819–828.

[b]Data from Woods ER, Iles S, Jackson S: Comparison of scintigraphic diagnostic criteria in suspected pulmonary embolism. *J Can Assoc Radiol*. 1989;40:194–197.

The unfortunate use of descriptions such as "low probability," "intermediate probability" and "high probability" scan results has implied a mathematic precision that is not inherent in the interpretation of the V/Q scan. Many studies correlating V/Q scans with angiographically proven PE have demonstrated a PE prevalence rate of at least 15 to 20% when the V/Q scan is interpreted as indicating "low probability" by established criteria.[5, 8–10] Although the term "low" is correct in the relative sense compared with the other categories, it is by no means *low* in terms of potential lethality. Similarly, "high probability" should not connote *certainty*. In the PIOPED study, 12% of patients with high-probability V/Q scans did not have PE demonstrated on angiogram.[5] Intermediate-probability scans provide little better than a 50-50 chance of PE.

That clinicians inordinately rely on V/Q scans to make management decisions is well documented. In a large prospective study involving 566 patients referred for V/Q scans for suspected PE, Frankel and associates[11] asked the physicians who were managing care to estimate pretest likelihood of PE as low (<20%), medium (20 to 80%), or high (>80%). Of 495 patients considered eligible for angiography (ie, no other reason to anticoagulate, not too unstable for study), management decisions were recorded as "pulmonary angiography," "anticoagulation," or "no treatment." Regardless of pretest estimate, high-probability V/Q scan results led to anticoagulation in 41 of 47 patients (87%), with the remainder (six) having angiograms. Only eight of 48 (17%) patients with pretest estimation of >80% and low-probability lung scans proceeded to angiography; the remainder were not treated.[11] Lung scan was the most heavily weighted variable in a decision-making study by Wigton and colleagues[12] on how physicians diagnose pulmonary embolism. The study further demonstrated a lack of uniformity in diagnostic workup, which did not improve with increasing clinical experience.

The PIOPED Study

Before the PIOPED study,[5] much of the data regarding the clinical efficacy of lung scans were open to question because of concerns about selection bias or variability in scan interpretation. To address this situation, the National Institutes of Health organized this large, multicenter, prospective, randomized, and standardized study of patients undergoing both V/Q scanning and pulmonary angiography for evaluation of suspected PE. All patients older than 18 years with symptoms suggestive of PE within 24 hours of presentation and without contraindication to angiography were considered eligible for entry in the study. Angiograms were completed in 755 of the 933 randomized patients, and lung scans were interpretable in 931. Telephone follow-up was performed at 1, 3, 6, and 12 months in an effort to determine whether patients ever exhibited clinical evidence of PE.

V/Q scanning was performed following a standardized protocol, and interpretation was carried out according to explicit standard criteria by two specialists who were not affiliated with the treating hospital. Disagreements were adjudicated by a panel of nuclear medicine specialists. Lung scans were categorized as high-probability (13%), intermediate-probability (39%), low-probability (34%), or near-normal/normal (14%). The last category included cases for which scan interpretations by the two readers were discrepant.

Of the 755 patients who underwent angiography, 251 (33%) had PE, and presence of PE in 24 (3%) was uncertain. Interestingly, four cases with negative angiograms had autopsy findings of PE 2 to 6 days following angiogram. V/Q scans had low-probability results in three of these cases and intermediate-probability results in the fourth.

A high-probability scan had a sensitivity of 41% and a specificity of 98%. The positive predictive value in this population was 88%. The rates of PE in the intermediate-probability, low-probability, and near-normal/normal categories were 105/322 (33%), 39/238 (16%), and 5/55 (9%), respectively.

Only 21 of the 931 (2%) patients who underwent lung scanning had normal V/Q scans interpretations from both readers; of these, only three patients underwent angiography, which in all three was normal. The remaining 18 had no clinical evidence of PE at 1-year follow-up.

An additional objective of the study was to correlate pretest probability of PE based on clinical assessment with both scan and angiogram results. Clinicians were asked to assess prescan probability as high (80 to 100%), medium (20 to 79%), or low (0 to 19%). A high pretest probability raised the positive predictive value of a high-probability scan from 88% to 96% and that of an intermediate-probability scan from 66% to 30%. Of the patients with a near-normal/normal scan and low pre-test likelihood of PE, only one of 61 (< 2%) had PE.

The Normal Scan

Clinicians have long relied on the premise that a normal perfusion scan rules out PE. Animal studies demonstrate, however, that although the lung scan detects 97% of emboli > 2 mm in diameter, it may fail to detect smaller or incompletely occlusive emboli.[13] A more carefully worded axiom would be that a normal perfusion scan rules out *clinically significant* PE. The PIOPED study appears to support this supposition, in that none of the patients in whom both readers interpreted the scan as normal had clinical evidence of PE at follow-up. Patients with normal scans, however, constituted only 2% of the study population. Among the other patients in the near-normal/normal category, a worst-case assumption gives a positive predictive value of 4%. The true probability of clinically significant PE in this group of patients is most likely to lie between 0 and 4%.

This assumption is supported by other studies. For example, Hull and colleagues[14] followed 515 patients with normal (Biello criteria)[7] lung scans from 1420 consecutive patients referred to their specialty center. This normal rate of 36% is substantially higher than the rate for the near-normal/normal PIOPED group. Only one of 515 (0.2%) patients had symptomatic pulmonary embolism during 3 months of follow-up. One additional patient with documented proximal vein thrombosis at study entry died within 24 hours; no autopsy was performed, but the death was clinically consistent with massive PE. Therefore, the worst-case scenario in the Hull study would be two of 515 (0.4%) patients who had PE but a normal (Biello criteria) V/Q scan.

Normal scans are obtained, though very rarely, in the presence of extensive embolic disease.[15] Some would argue that the PE-positive rate of 4 to 9% in the PIOPED near-normal/normal group is too high to consider that PE is excluded.

The High-Probability Scan

At the other extreme, physicians have come to rely on the high-probability scan as a means of avoiding pulmonary angiography. As previously mentioned, high-probability scans in patients with a high pretest likelihood of PE were associated with a 96% positive rate, whereas in patients with a low pretest likelihood of disease, the corresponding predictive value was only 56%. It is therefore important to assess one's personal clinical impression as well as the relative risk of anticoagulation compared with the risk of angiography when deciding whether to forgo angiogram and initiate presumptive therapy.

ALTERNATIVES TO V/Q SCANNING

The association of deep vein thrombosis (DVT) of the iliofemoral veins (proximal DVT) with PE is well known. DVT is present in up to 80% of patients with pulmonary embolism.[16] Because a diagnosis of DVT almost invariably leads to the institution of anticoagulant therapy, further evaluation for PE becomes moot. The decision whether to proceed first with invasive or noninvasive evaluation for DVT or with V/Q scan depends on test availability, radiologic technical expertise, resources, and clinical circumstances.

LUNG SCANS IN PREGNANCY

Pregnancy represents a definite risk factor for pulmonary embolism and an increased risk for anticoagulation as well. The teratogenic risk of nuclear lung scan is not defined. As for all such tests, the potential risk of fetal malformation from the test must be weighed against the maternal and fetal risk from the disease. Certainly, fetal risk is greatest in, and perhaps limited to, the first trimester.

Every attempt should be made to reduce the radiation dosage to the fetus during this period. This can be accomplished by decreasing the amount of administered radioisotope and increasing the time of image acquisition. Commonly, half the usual dose is administered, and twice the acquisition time is then utilized for image generation. This approach does not seriously affect scan quality.

The technetium-99m MAA does not pass the placental barrier; technetium-99m aerosol does not cross the alveolar membrane. Finally, the radiation dose during inhalation of inert radioactive krypton-81m, xenon-133, or xenon-127 is low and remains confined primarily to the alveoli. Nevertheless, a prudent approach is to attempt noninvasive, nonradiologic imaging via Doppler ultrasound venography or impedance plethysmography as an initial screen. If such test results are positive, the patient is likely to require anticoagulation regardless of lung scan or angiogram results. Nursing mothers are instructed to discontinue breastfeeding for 5 to 7 days after the study.

RECOMMENDATIONS FOR LUNG SCAN UTILIZATION IN THE EMERGENCY DEPARTMENT

1. Emergency physicians should be familiar with the criteria for the diagnosis of PE by V/Q scan. At many institutions, initial readings may be made by relatively inexperienced radiologists-in-training, especially during night and weekend hours.
2. Emergency physicians should formulate a pretest estimate of the likelihood of PE as well as a presumptive plan of evaluation for each potential category of lung scan interpretation. Even patients in whom angiography will be performed regardless of the scan results may benefit from lung scan, which can identify lung segments for *selective* arteriography.
3. A high-probability scan can permit presumptive anticoagulant therapy when the pretest estimate is also high. In patients who have an increased risk from anticoagulation or in whom confirmation of the diagnosis is important (in terms of insurability or employment), the comparatively low risk of pulmonary arteriography may be warranted.

The overall mortality rate of pulmonary angiography is about 0.3%, and the complication rate is about 4%.[17]

4. An intermediate-probability scan does not permit any diagnostic conclusion to be reached. Evaluation should proceed according to the pretest plan. In the PIOPED study,[5] an intermediate-probability scan in patients with a high pretest likelihood of disease was associated with a positive angiogram 66% of the time; of patients with low pretest likelihood, PE was present in 16%.

5. A low-probability scan is associated with an unacceptably high frequency of PE, especially when the pretest likelihood of PE is high (40%) or intermediate (16%). When the pretest likelihood is low, a low-probability scan makes PE quite unlikely (4%) but does not rule it out.

6. A normal scan makes the diagnosis of clinically significant PE extremely unlikely. Further evaluation should be directed toward establishing an alternative diagnosis.

7. Noninvasive evaluations of the lower extremities (Doppler ultrasound, impedance plethysmography) can improve the diagnostic yield of V/Q scanning, especially in patients with intermediate- or low-probability scans. Noninvasive testing shold be the first evaluation in pregnant women and perhaps in patients with preexisting lung disease, in whom an indeterminate scan is to be expected.[18]

REFERENCES

1. Dalen JE, Alpert JS: Natural history of pulmonary embolism. *Prog Cardiovasc Dis.* 1975;27:259–268.
2. Porter J, Hershel J: Drug-related deaths among hospital inpatients. *JAMA.* 1977;237:879–881.
3. Mant MJ, Thong KL, Kirtwhistle RV, et al: Hemorrhagic complications of heparin therapy. *Lancet.* 1977;1:1133–1135.
4. Levine MN, Raskob G, Hirsh J: Risk of haemorrhage associated with long term anticoagulant therapy. *Drugs.* 1985;30:444–460.
5. PIOPED Investigators: Value of the ventilation/perfusion scan in acute pulmonary embolism. *JAMA.* 1990;263:2753–2759.
6. Biello DR: Radiological (scintigraphic) evaluation of patients with suspected pulmonary thromboembolism. *JAMA.* 1987;257:3257–3259.
7. Biello DR, Mattar AG, McKnight RC, et al: Ventilation-perfusion studies in suspected pulmonary embolism. *AJR.* 1979;133:1033–1037.
8. Woods ER, Iles S, Jackson S: Comparison of scintigraphic diagnostic criteria in suspected pulmonary embolism. *J Can Assoc Radiol.* 1989;40:194–197.
9. Hull RD, Hirsh J, Carter CJ: Diagnostic value of ventilation-perfusion lung scanning in patients with suspected pulmonary embolism. *Chest.* 1985;88:819–828.
10. Catania TA, Caride VJ: Single perfusion defect and pulmonary embolism: Angiographic correlation. *J Nucl Med.* 1990;31:296–301.

11. Frankel N, Coleman RE, Pryor DB, et al: Utilization of lung scans by clinicians. *J Nucl Med.* 1986;27:366–369.
12. Wigton RS, Hoellerich VL, Patil KD: How physicians use clinical information in diagnosing pulmonary embolism: An application of conjoint analysis. *Med Decis Making.* 1986;6:2–11.
13. Alderson PO, Doppman JL, Diamond SS, et al: Ventilation-perfusion lung imaging and selective pulmonary angiography in dogs with experimental pulmonary embolism. *J Nucl Med.* 1978;9:164–171.
14. Hull RD, Raskob GE, Coates G, et al: Clinical validity of a normal perfusion lung scan in patients with suspected pulmonary embolism. *Chest.* 1990;97:23–26.
15. Brandstetter RD, Naccarato E, Sperber RJ: Normal lung perfusion scan with extensive thromboembolic disease. *Chest.* 1987;92:565–567.
16. Hirsh J: Diagnosis of venous thrombosis and pulmonary embolism. *Am J Cardiol.* 1990;65:45.
17. Mills SR, Jackson DC, Older RA, et al: The incidence, etiologies, and avoidance of complications of pulmonary arteriography. *Radiology.* 1980;136:295.
18. Stein PD, Coleman RE, Gottschalk A: Diagnostic utility of ventilation/perfusion lung scans in acute pulmonary embolism is not diminished by preexisting cardiac or pulmonary disease. *Chest.* 1991;100:604–606.

Chapter

Cholescintigraphy

John G. Fata

Historically, the oral cholecystogram and intravenous cholangiogram have served the physician as important tools in the evaluation of suspected biliary tract disease. In the last 15 years, they have largely been supplanted by ultrasonography and hepatic cholescintigraphy. This chapter discusses cholescintigraphy, which has excellent sensitivity in the detection of acute cholecystitis.[1–10]

HEPATOBILIARY IMAGING

The introduction in 1975 of ^{99m}Tc-labeled iminodiacetic acid (IDA) analogs made possible the development of this new imaging modality.[11, 12] When given intravenously, this chemical is rapidly absorbed by hepatocytes, secreted into the biliary system, and concentrated in the gallbladder with bile. With bile secretion, IDA enters the duodenum via the common bile duct. Depending on which IDA analog is utilized, elevated bilirubin levels may displace the chemical from receptors and adversely affect the scan.

After the introduction of dimethyliminodiacetic acid (HIDA) in 1975, several derivatives were subsequently introduced. They are paraisopropyl iminodiacetic acid (PIPIDA), diisopropyl iminodiacetic acid (DISIDA), and 3-bromo-2,4,6-trimethyl iminodiacetic acid (mebrofenin). These newer compounds have the advantage of more effectively competing for bilirubin-binding sites. DISIDA and mebrofenin are currently the widely used. Both allow hepatic uptake and biliary excretion despite bilirubin levels as high as 20 to 30 mg/dL, whereas imaging with HIDA may be ineffective when bilirubin levels are only 5 to 8 mg/dL.

Proper preparation is important and consists basically of ensuring that the patient has fasted for 2 to 4 hours before the study. In the nonfasted state, as many as 64% of normal subjects have an abnormal (false-positive) scintigram.[13] This appears to be at least in part caused by the contracted state of the postprandial gallbladder, with a resultant decreased flow of tracer into it.

Prolonged fasting (>24 hours) can also interfere with gallbladder visualization despite cystic duct patency. Additionally, ICU patients with intercurrent infections, patients on hyperalimentation, and alcoholic patients often have false-positive studies.[14–18]

The technique of hepatobiliary scintigraphy is relatively simple. A ^{99m}Tc-IDA compound (3 to 10 mCi) is administered intravenously. Obtaining sequential 3-second images for 1 minute after bolus injection enables evaluation of gallbladder and liver blood flow.[12] After the flow study, standard images are obtained at 5-minute intervals for the first 30 minutes, followed by 45-, 60-, and 90-minute images. In normal individuals, radioactive tracer can be seen to be taken up by the liver, concentrated in the gallbladder, and excreted into the common bile duct, the cystic duct, and, finally, the small bowel. If the gallbladder and/or duodenum has not been visualized at 90 minutes, further images at 2 and 4 hours and even 24 hours are obtained in some centers. The administration of morphine sulfate (0.04 mg/kg) has been shown to decrease the time needed for a complete examination from 24 hours to 2 hours. Morphine causes contraction of the sphincter of Oddi, thereby elevating proximal biliary tract pressure.[19] Bile is then redirected through a patent cystic duct into the gallbladder. This technique has been demonstrated to improve the sensitivity and specificity of scintigraphy in conditions that commonly manifest as delayed gallbladder filling, such as chronic cholecystitis, prolonged fasting, hyperalimentation, alcoholism, and chronic illness.[19–23] Morphine must not be given prior to the appearance of isotope in the intestine (or for several hours prior to the study), because it can cause a functional obstruction of the distal common bile duct that can be very difficult to differentiate from complete mechanical obstruction.

ACUTE CHOLECYSTITIS

Acute cholecystitis is caused by obstruction of the cystic duct, which may be due to stones, inflammation, or edema. Hepatobiliary imaging provides functional evaluation of cystic duct patency and allows differentiation of acute cholecystitis from other causes of abdominal pain, such as pancreatitis, hepatitis, pyelonephritis, peptic ulcer disease, and appendicitis. A normal hepatobiliary scan (demonstrating visualization of the gallbladder by 1 hour) excludes obstruction of the cystic duct with a very high degree of accuracy. Failure to visualize the gallbladder at 1 hour, with persistent nonfilling at 4 hours, is a sensitive sign of obstruction. Examination time can be reduced from 4 hours to 90 to 120 minutes if morphine augmentation is provided, without decreasing accuracy.[19–21, 24] The sensitivity of hepatobiliary scanning in the detection of acute cholecystitis, employing histologic findings as the standard, has been found to range from 68 to 100%, with most studies reporting 95 to 97%. The reported specificity ranges from 82 to 100%; most studies report 90 to 97%.[1–9, 13, 25–29]

Another useful scintigraphic sign of acute cholecystitis is sometimes observed. This is the "rim sign," representing pericholecystic hepatic uptake in the gallbladder fossa.[30–34] This sign suggests acute gangrenous cholecystitis or perforation, both of which are associated with a much higher mortality.

Some studies report a large number of false-positive scans. These depend on the population studied[14–18] and occur predominantly with the conditions mentioned previously (critical illness, prolonged fasting, hyperalimentation, alcoholism) that predispose patients to delayed gallbladder filling.

A number of prospective studies have shown ultrasonography to be less accurate than cholescintigraphy in demonstrating acute cholecystitis.[7, 27, 35, 36] One problem in the interpretation of these findings, however, is the lack of universally accepted ultrasonographic criteria for acute cholecystitis. Ultrasound has been demonstrated to have sensitivity and specificity both >90% in detecting gallstones.[25, 37–41] The presence of gallstones is an important finding, because more than 90% of cases of acute cholecystitis are associated with cholelithiasis.[6, 36, 42, 43] The prevalence of cholelithiasis in the general population is high (over 10% in adults older than age 55),[44] however, so that the presence of gallstones is a nonspecific indicator for acute cholecystitis. These considerations have led to the development of ultrasonographic criteria for an abnormal gallbladder. Major criteria are the presence of gallstones and nonvisualized gallbladder. Wall thickening (>5 mm), focal tenderness (sonographic Murphy sign), gallbladder distension (>5 cm), and pericholecystic fluid are considered minor criteria.[7–9, 45, 46] With major criteria, most studies have found the sensitivity of ultrasonography to be 81 to 86% and the specificity 94 to 98%. If minor criteria are used as well, the sensitivity is increased to >90%, but specificity falls to ~70%.

Ultrasonography offers another benefit that is not reflected in these figures. Because the examination is not organ-specific, it can demonstrate abnormalities in other areas of the abdomen. Detection of nonbiliary causes of abdominal pain is reported in 24 to 35% of patients who are referred for examination because of abdominal pain and whose gallbladders prove to be normal.[47, 48]

CHRONIC CHOLECYSTITIS

Delayed visualization of the gallbladder (1 to 4 hours) following normal hepatic uptake and bile duct visualization is an abnormal finding that is infrequently observed in acute cholecystitis (2% of cases) but often in chronic cholecystitis (82% of cases).[49] Most affected patients have stones or sludge-filled gallbladders with inflamed and fibrotic walls. Many patients with chronic cholecystitis actually have normal hepatobiliary scans, however.[50]

Because scintigraphy has limited anatomic resolution, it plays a secondary role in the diagnosis of chronic cholecystitis, especially since ultrasound can detect gallstones and gallbladder wall thickening with a high degree of accuracy. Cholescintigraphy does have some value, however, in identifying patients with cholelithiasis who present with right upper quadrant pain and an equivocal clinical picture suggestive of acute cholecystitis. This approach can allow some patients with biliary colic secondary to chronic cholecystitis to avoid hospitalization and emergency surgery.

ACUTE COMMON BILE DUCT OBSTRUCTION

With common bile duct obstruction, the biliary tree fails to be visualized because of back-pressure from the point of obstruction. Thus, there is normal hepatic uptake of tracer, but no visualization of the biliary tree, gallbladder, or intestine. This pattern is typical of extrahepatic duct obstruction, usually from a stone.[49, 51, 52] Scintigraphy thus appears to be a sensitive test in detecting acute common duct obstruction, particularly early.[49] In contrast, ultrasonography detects only the anatomic changes that occur much later than the functional changes detected by scintigraphy.[53–55] The sensitivity of ultrasonography is reported to be <60%. Ultrasound is thus helpful only if it is positive; if it is negative, acute common duct obstruction cannot be ruled out.

ACUTE ACALCULOUS CHOLECYSTITIS

Acalculous cholecystitis, although seen uncommonly in the emergency department, is reported to be responsible for 2 to 15% of all cases of acute cholecystitis.[56–65] It typically occurs following surgery, trauma, or burns or in patients who are receiving hyperalimentation.[56–59] The importance of a timely diagnosis is underscored by a very high incidence of gangrene and perforation, approaching 50% in some studies,[60–62] and a mortality rate for untreated disease that is double that of calculous acute cholecystitis.[58] Obstruction of the cystic duct by edema and inflammation occurs in the majority of patients with acalculous cholecystitis, allowing the diagnosis to be made by scintigraphy with a reported sensitivity of 78 to 93%.[5, 56, 63, 64] Ultrasonography, however, has a very low sensitivity in this group.[65] Scintigraphy is thus the optimal study in patients predisposed to acalculous cholecystitis.

SUMMARY

The major controversy in the evaluation of patients with right upper quadrant pain concerns the proper sequence of diagnostic test selection, cholescintigraphy vs ultrasonography. Both tests have well-documented accuracy in the wide range of hepatobiliary disorders, and many observers contend that the tests are not competitive but complementary.[12] The real issue is which disease process one is trying to document.

In the setting of right upper quadrant pain and signs typical of acute cholecystitis in which one wants to confirm cystic duct obstruction, hepatobiliary scanning consistently demonstrates superior sensitivity and specificity in the evaluation of both acute calculous and acute acalculous cholecystitis. It is available 24 hours a day at most centers. With morphine augmentation, the total time required is no more than 2 hours if positive, and usually less than 1 hour if negative.

If one wishes only to confirm symptomatic gallbladder disease in a patient with recurrent right upper quadrant pain, ultrasound is the procedure of choice. This modality is inferior to scintigraphy in diagnosing cystic duct obstruction and inflammation, but in the proper clinical setting, in which one wishes only to document cholelithiasis or chronic cholecystitis, ultrasound is a very accurate tool.

REFERENCES

1. Fiertas JE, Fink-Bennett DM, Thrall JH, et al. Efficacy of hepatobiliary imaging in acute abdominal pain: Concise communication. *J Nucl Med.* 1980;21:919.
2. Cobellon S Jr, Brown JM, Cavanaugh DG: Accuracy of hepatobiliary scan in acute cholecystitis. *Am J Surg.* 1984;148:607.
3. Weissmann HS, Frank MS, Bernstein LH, Freeman LM: Rapid and accurate diagnosis of acute cholecystitis with 99mTc-HIDA cholescintigraphy. *AJR.* 1979;132:523.
4. Cheng TH, Davis MS, Selzer SE, et al: Evaluation of hepatobiliary imaging by radionuclide scintigraphy, ultrasonography and contrast cholangiography. *Radiology.* 1979;133:761.
5. Freitas JE: Cholescintigraphy in acute and chronic cholecystitis. *Semin Nucl Med.* 1982;12:18.
6. Fink-Bennett D, Freitas JE, Ripley SD, Bree RL: The sensitivity of hepatobiliary imaging and real-time ultrasonography in the detection of acute cholecystitis. *Arch Surg.* 1985;120:904.
7. Zewan RK, Burrell MI, Cahow CE, Caride V: Diagnostic utility of cholescintigraphy and ultrasonography in acute cholecystitis. *Am J Surg.* 1981;141:446.
8. Worthen NJ, Uszler JM, Funamura JL: Cholecystitis: Prospective evaluation of sonography and 99m-Tc-HIDA cholescintigraphy. *AJR.* 1981;137:973.
9. Shuman WP, Mack LA, Rudd TG, et al. Evaluation of acute right upper quadrant pain: Sonography and 99mTc PIPIDA cholescintigraphy. *AJR.* 1982;139:61.
10. Bennett MJ, Sheldon MI, dos Remedios LV, et al. Diagnosis of acute cholecystitis using hepatobiliary scan with technetium-99m PIPIDA. *Am J Surg.* 1981;142:338.
11. Loberg MD, Cooper M, Harvey E, et al: Development of new radiopharmaceutical based on N-substitution of iminodiacetic acid. *J Nucl Med.* 1976;17:633.
12. Grossman SJ, Joyce JM: Hepatobiliary imaging. *Emerg Med Clin North Am.* 1991;9:853.
13. Klingersmith WC, Spitzer VM, Fritzberg AR, Kuni CC: The normal fasting and postprandial Tc-99m-diisopropyl 1-IDA hepatobiliary study. *J Nucl Med.* 1981;22:7.
14. Drane WE, Nelp NB, Rudd TG: The need for routine delayed radionuclide hepatobiliary imaging in patients with intercurrent disease. *Radiology.* 1984;84:763.

15. Garner WL, Marx V, Fabri PJ: Cholescintigraphy in the critically ill. *Am J Surg.* 1988;155:727.
16. Larson MJ, Klingensmith WC III, Kuni CL: Radionuclide hepatobiliary imaging: Nonvisualization of the gallbladder secondary to prolonged fasting. *J Nucl Med.* 1982;23:1003.
17. Shuman WP, Gibbs P, Rudd TG, et al. PIPIDA scintigraphy for cholecystitis: False positives for alcoholism and total parenteral nutrition. *AJR.* 1982;138:1.
18. Warner BW, Hamilton FN, Siberstein EB, et al: The value of hepatobiliary scans in the fasted patients receiving total parenteral nutrition. *Surgery.* 1987;102:595.
19. Choy D, Shifer, McLean RG, et al: Cholescintigraphy in acute cholecystitis: Use of intravenous morphine. *Radiology.* 1984;151:203.
20. Kim EE, Nguyen M, Pjura G, et al: Use of morphine in cholescintigraphy for obstructive cholecystitis [abstract]. *J Nucl Med.* 1985;28:P79.
21. Kim EE, Pjuro G, Lowry PA, et al: Use of morphine in the cholescintigraphic diagnosis of acute acalculous cholecystitis [abstract]. *J Nucl Med.* 1987;28:P596.
22. Fig LM, Wahl RL, Steward RE, et al: Morphine-augmented hepatobiliary scintigraphy in the severely ill: Caution is in order. *Radiology.* 1990;175:467.
23. Flancbaum L, Alder SM, Trososkin SZ: Use of cholescintigraphy with morphine in critically ill patients with suspected cholecystitis. *Surgery.* 1989;106:668.
24. Vasquez TE, Greenspan G, Evans DG: Clinical efficacy of intravenous administration of morphine sulfate in hepatobiliary imaging for acute cholecystitis [abstract]. *J Nucl Med.* 1987;28:P596.
25. Matolo NM, Stadolnik RC, McGahan JP: Comparison of ultrasonographic, computerized tomography, and radionuclide imaging in the diagnosis of acute and chronic cholecystitis. *Am J Surg.* 1982;144:678.
26. Berk RN, Ferruci JR Jr, Fordtron TS, et al: The radiological diagnosis of gallbladder disease: An imaging symposium. *Radiology.* 1981;141:49.
27. Freitas JE, Mirkes SH, Fink-Bennett DM, Bree RL: Suspected acute cholecystitis: Comparison of hepatobiliary scintigraphy versus ultrasonography. *Clin Nucl Med.* 1982;7:364.
28. Nicholson RW, Hastings DL, Testa NJ, Torrance B: HIDA scanning in gallbladder disease. *Br J Radiol.* 1980;53:878.
29. Mound MA, McCartney WH, Melamed JR: Hepatobiliary scanning with 99mTc-PIPIDA in acute cholecystitis. *Radiology.* 1982;142:193.
30. Brachman MB, Tanaseseu DE, Ramana L, et al: Acute gangrenous cholecystitis: Radionuclide diagnosis. *Radiology.* 1984;151:209.
31. Bushnell DL, Perlman SB, Wilson MA, et al: The rim sign: Association with acalculous cholecystitis. *J Nucl Med.* 1986;27:353.
32. Cawthon MA, Brown DM, Hartshorne MF, et al: Biliary scintigraphy. The "hot rim" sign. *Clin Nucl Med.* 1984;9:619.
33. Smith R, Rosen JM, Gallo LN, et al: Pericholecystic hepatic activity in cholescintigraphy. *Radiology.* 1985;156:797.
34. Swayne LC, Ginsberg NN: Diagnosis of acute cholecystitis by scintigraphy: Significance of pericholecystic hepatic uptake. *AJR.* 1989;152:1211.
35. Weissman HS, Rosenblatt R, Sugarman LA, et al: An update in radionuclide imaging in the diagnosis of cholecystitis. *JAMA.* 1981;246:1354.
36. Samuals BL, Frietas JE, Bree RL, et al: Comparison of radionuclide hepato-

biliary imaging and real-time ultrasound for the detection of acute cholecystitis. *Radiology.* 1983;174:207.
37. Berk RN, Ferruci JT, Fordtran JS, et al: The radiologic diagnosis of gallbladder disease: An imaging symposium. *Radiology.* 1981;141:49.
38. Bartrum RJ, Jr, Crow HC, Foote SC: Ultrasonographic and radiolographic cholecystography. *N Engl J Med.* 1977;296:538.
39. Crade M, Taylor RJ, Rosenfield AT, et al: Surgical and pathological correlation of cholecystosonography and cholecystography. *AJR.* 1978;131:227.
40. Cooperberg P, Golding RH: Advances in ultrasonography of the gallbladder and biliary tract. *Radiol Clin North Am.* 1982;20:611.
41. Krook PM, Allen FM, Bush WH Jr, et al: Comparison of real-time ultrasonography and oral cholecystography. *Radiology.* 1980;135:145.
42. Byrne JJ: Acute cholecystitis. *Am J Surg.* 1959;97:156.
43. Munster AM, Brown JR: Acalculous cholecystitis. *Am J Surg.* 1967;113:730.
44. Friedman GD, Kannel WB, Dawber TR: The epidemiology of gallbladder disease: Observations in the Framingham study. *J Chronic Dis.* 1966;19:273.
45. Dillon E, Parkus GJ: The role of upper abdominal ultrasonography in suspected acute cholecystitis. *Clin Radiol.* 1980;31:175.
46. Handler SJ: Ultrasound of gallbladder wall thickening and its relation to cholecystitis. *AJR.* 1979;132:581.
47. Laing FC, Federle MP, Jeffrey RB, Brown TW: Ultrasonic evaluation of patients with acute right upper quadrant pain. *Radiology.* 1981;190:449.
48. Reid MH, Phillips NE: The role of computed tomography and ultrasound imaging in biliary tract disease. *Surg Clin North Am.* 1981;61:787.
49. Weissman HS, Badia J, Sugarman LA, et al: Spectrum of 99m-Tc-IDA cholescintigraphic patterns in acute cholecystitis. *Radiology.* 1981;138:167.
50. Freitas JE, Fink-Bennett DM: Asymptomatic cystic duct obstruction in chronic cholecystitis. *J Nucl Med.* 1980;21:17.
51. Lecklitner ML, Austin AR, Benedetto AR, et al: Positive predictive value of cholescintigraphy in common bile duct obstruction. *J Nucl Med.* 1986; 27:1403.
52. Miller DR, Egbert RM, Braustein P: Comparison of ultrasound and hepatobiliary imaging in the early detection of acute total common bile duct obstruction. *Arch Surg.* 1984;119:1233.
53. Weissman HS, Rosenblatt RR, Sugarman LA, et al: Early diagnosis of acute common bile duct obstruction by Tc-99m-IDA cholescintigraphy. *J Nucl Med.* 1980;21:41.
54. Malini S, Sabel J: Ultrasonography in obstructive jaundice. *Radiology.* 1977;123:429.
55. Laing FC, Jeffrey RB Jr: Choledocholithiasis and cystic obstruction: Difficult ultrasonographic diagnosis. *Radiology.* 1981;140:499.
56. Swayne LC: Acute acalculous cholecystitis: Sensitivity in detection using technetium-99m, iminodiacetic acid (IDA) cholescintigraphy. *Radiology.* 1986;160:33.
57. Munster AM, Brown JR: Acalculous cholecystitis. *Am J Surg.* 1967;113:730.
58. Glenn F: Acute acalculous cholecystitis. *Ann Surg.* 1979;189:458.
59. Jonsson PE, Anderson A: Postoperative acute acalculous cholecystitis. *Arch Surg.* 1976;111:1097.
60. Howard RJ: Acute acalculous cholecystitis. *Am J Surg.* 1981;141:194.

61. Robertson RD: Noncalculous acute cholecystitis following surgery, trauma, and illness. *Am J Surg.* 1970;36:610.
62. DuPriest RW, Khaneja SC, Cowley RA: Acute cholecystitis complicating trauma. *Ann Surg.* 1979;188:84.
63. Anderson A, Bergdahl L, Bodquist L: Acalculous cholecystitis. *Am J Surg.* 1971;122:3.
64. Weissmann HS, Berkowitz D, Fox MS, et al: The role of technetium-99m iminodiacetic acid (IDA) cholescintigraphy in acute acalculous cholecystitis. *Radiology.* 1983;146:177.
65. Shuman WP, Rogers JR, Rudd TG, et al: Low sensitivity of sonography and cholescintigraphy in acalculous cholecystitis. *AJR.* 1984;142:531.

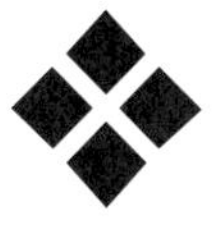

OTHER

Chapter

The 12-Lead Electrocardiogram in Acute Chest Pain

Thomas S. Pannke and Robert Wolford

The 12-lead electrocardiogram (ECG) is usually the first diagnostic test obtained in the ED evaluation of chest pain suggestive of myocardial ischemia.[1] This chapter discusses the ECG as a diagnostic tool, as a guide to immediate intervention, and as a predictor of hospital course.

ECG INTERPRETATION

In order to evaluate the literature concerning the usefulness of the ECG for these purposes, one must first address the reproducibility of the physician's reading of the tracings. Several studies have examined the accuracy of ECG interpretation. One study found that about half of myocardial infarction (MI) patients inappropriately sent home from the ED could have been diagnosed prior to discharge if the initial ECG had been interpreted accurately.[2] Others, comparing the interpretations of house staff and attending physicians, found disagreement about 40% of the time.[3] The opposite conclusion was reached in other studies. One study comparing the ED reading with that of a cardiologist found agreement 81% of the time overall, and 94% of the time in the subgroup of patients with more serious cardiac disease.[4] Another found 90% concordance between an initial reading and the final reading for abnormal ECGs.[5]

The use of computer programs to evaluate ECG findings is routine in many institutions, and readings are often available with the initial ECG. Studies examining these types of computer programs find them to be "almost as accurate" as the best cardiologist,[6] and better than a group of physicians varying from house staff to attending level (correct 86% of the time in diagnosing MI, whereas the physician group was correct in only 64%).[7] A newer technology uses a computer to analyze a 22-lead ECG, consisting of the standard 12 leads and ten other leads, which may improve upon the sensitivity for detection of MI.[18] The availability of computer readings might help the clinician make better diagnostic decisions when using ECGs but is not a substitute for actually reading the ECG and evaluating it in the context of the entire clinical picture.

Any attempt to use the ECG for diagnosis or prognosis must begin with an accurate interpretation of the data presented. The question of emergency department physician accuracy has not been thoroughly investigated.

DIAGNOSTIC ACCURACY OF THE ECG

The initial ECG, used alone, is diagnostic in less than half of patients with acute MI. Conversely, only 38 to 57% of patients with ECGs judged to be abnormal and suggestive of ischemia actually have acute MI.[4, 9–11] Between 3 and 18% of patients with chest pain and "normal" ECGs are eventually diagnosed as having MI.[4, 5, 9–12]

Another way of looking at how often the clinician with few diagnostic tools besides the ECG accurately diagnoses MI is to study all CCU admissions for "rule out MI." The incidence of acute MI among these patients is 18 to 41% in various studies.[4, 5, 9–15] Conversely, among patients with confirmed acute MI, only about half have a correct diagnosis made antemortem.[16–18]

The ECG is generally believed to have a sensitivity of about 50% for the diagnosis of acute MI. In one large study, however, the initial ECG was 81% sensitive in diagnosing MI using the following criteria: (1) new or presumed new ST segment deviation of greater than 0.01 mV in more than two precordial or diaphragmatic leads or in I or aVL; (2) new or presumed new Q waves that are more than 30 ms wide and 0.20 mV deep in the same lead combinations; and (3) left bundle branch block.[19] Nevertheless, the sensitivity of the ECG is clearly not high enough to be relied upon confidently for disposition decisions in the ED. The emergency physician must continue to follow conservative admission policies in order to avoid the discharge of patients with acute MI. Although these admission decisions may become less difficult with the advent of CK-MB screening for early diagnosis, which is more sensitive and specific than the ECG alone,[20, 21] the goal of 100% sensitivity will continue to mandate a conservative approach.

Comparison of the emergent ECG with previous ones, another common practice, is helpful for identifying changes in axis, morphology, bundle branch blocks, and older MIs. It has been shown, however, that in most cases, availability of a prior ECG has no impact on disposition decisions.[22]

Thus, the ECG fails in the majority of patients to be sufficiently sensitive or specific to be relied upon. Comparison with older ECGs also seems to be less helpful than is usually believed. An ECG should be obtained in patients with history of symptoms suggesting cardiac ischemia but should not be relied upon for patient disposition to home if it is not suggestive of acute MI.

THE ECG FOR PROGNOSIS OF HOSPITAL COURSE

If the assumption is made that only the acute MI patient truly deserves to be in a CCU setting, it is obvious that the methods currently used to select CCU admissions are not ideal. If it were possible to initially identify all patients with true MI, the disposition question then might be: Which of these patients actually needs to be in an intensive care setting? Because this identification is not possible at present, perhaps the ECG might help in separating patients admitted with chest pain into two general groups—those with a high risk for sudden death or life-threatening complications and those with much lower risk. Patients in the first group might be presumed to need an intensive care bed, whereas those in the second group might not.

The use of a standard 12-lead ECG for prognosis in acute MI has been examined by various investigators. An interesting retrospective study of patients admitted either to a general unit or to the CCU revealed no difference in overall mortality between the two groups.[25] An older study, done prior to the use of thrombolytics, even suggests that patients managed at home after infarction have the same mortality as those hospitalized.[26] It has been shown that 4 to 8% of patients with acute MIs are inadvertently discharged from the ED.[2, 27]

There is some evidence that a properly read ECG can be helpful in identifying those individuals who are most likely to require admission to an intensive care setting rather than a simple monitored bed. The following sections examine the individual components of the ECG for their potential diagnostic and prognostic value in ED patients.

The Q Wave

The development of a Q wave in an abnormal position (inferior or anterior leads) and of sufficient size to be significant (duration >0.04 sec and/or amplitude >25% of the succeeding R wave) may be associated with acute MI. These findings may be seen, however, in ECGs of normal subjects in leads III, aVr, and V_1.[28] Approximately 60 to 70%

of all MI patients develop true Q waves during their course, at a time that varies from hours to days after the infarct.[28] The Q wave does not accurately distinguish between transmural and nontransmural infarcts, as was once believed.[30–35]

Patients with Q-wave MI have an increased in-hospital mortality, a greater incidence of heart failure, a higher peak CK level, more frequent conduction disturbance, and a greater degree of myocardial tissue damage than those with non–Q-wave MI. The difference in mortality between Q-wave and non–Q-wave MI is small, however, and the occurrence of complications cannot be reliably predicted only on the basis of the presence or absence of the Q wave.

Thus, the Q wave offers only limited prognostic information when considered without other parts of the ECG. Patients with infarctions who develop Q waves are somewhat more likely to die while in the hospital than those with non–Q-wave infarctions. The Q wave alone cannot be utilized in the ED as a predictive tool for decisions regarding which chest pain patient requires a CCU admission or who might have a complicated hospital course.

The ST Segment

ST segment *elevation* of up to 1 mm in the inferior leads and up to 3 mm in precordial leads (especially in V_2 and V_3 in young black males) may be a normal finding. ST elevation can also be seen in patients with left bundle branch block, ventricular hypertrophy, hyperkalemia, myocarditis, and acute cor pulmonale.[36]

ST *depression* is less common in normal individuals but may be as much as 1 mm in inferior leads.[28] ST depression may be seen in nonischemic cardiac conditions such as left ventricular hypertrophy with strain, digitalis therapy, and hypokalemia, and in right or left bundle branch block.[36]

ST segment changes are often among the most dramatic and easily identified changes in acute MI and have an important place in the current criteria for the administration of thrombolytics. In patients admitted for unstable angina, any ST change on the admission ECG correlates with a significantly higher incidence of death, completed MI, and need for emergency revascularization.[58] Although the magnitude and distribution of ST elevation have been linked to infarct size by some investigators, others have not found the ST segment to be a consistently accurate predictor.[41]

ST segment elevation of >5.0 mm above the baseline in anterior leads, or >2.0 mm in inferior leads, has been associated with significantly more episodes of high-grade AV block (21% vs 10%), ventricular tachycardia (VT) (24% vs 14%), cardiac arrest (25% vs 9%), and death (21% vs 8%) during the hospital stay.[42] In one study, patients with ST elevation in more than two leads were more likely to have unfavorable outcomes than those without.[43] This finding would support the belief that the classic ST elevation of acute MI that is seen in some patients is indicative of a larger and more complicated infarction. In another study, false-positive ST elevation was shown to be increased in patients with previous MI.[60]

ST depression in the setting of acute MI was found in one study to increase the likelihood of cardiac arrest (20% vs 8%) and death (15% vs 6%) compared with ST elevation.[29]

ST segment depression during inferior infarctions has also been found to be associated with larger infarcts as well as significantly more frequent heart failure and hypotension compared with no ST segment depression.[56]

The ST segment appears to provide additional prognostic information when it appears in the "reciprocal" position to acute ST elevation in acute MI. These "reciprocal" changes are thought to represent either "mirror" changes of ST elevation in the inferior leads or actual opposite wall ischemia.[45–47] In patients with inferior MI, precordial ST depression (>0.05 mV in V_1 to V_3) correlated significantly with increased mortality. Others have noted significantly more VT and ventricular fibrillation (VF), more common AV block, increased risk of complications, higher peak CK, and worse ejection fractions in patients with reciprocal ST segment changes during inferior MIs.[48–55] Reciprocal ST changes associated with anterior MI have been linked with more extensive coronary artery disease and increased incidence and extent of wall motion abnormalities and in-hospital complications.[57]

Although significant ST changes may be helpful in the diagnosis of acute MI in some patients, relying only on classic ST changes would result in missing many infarcts. Including minor and "nonsignificant" ST changes might increase the sensitivity of the initial ECG for the diagnosis of MI but is likely to decrease its specificity.

In summary, the ST segment provides some indication of whether a patient might be expected to have a complicated in-hospital course. This is particularly true of patients with the most dramatic classic ST changes. Reciprocal ST changes appear to indicate a significantly worse prognosis for patients with acute MI. The clinical use of the ST segment alone, however, is limited. Differences in complications and mortality in MI patients with varying degrees of ST segment changes, although statistically significant, are not large enough to be clinically helpful in making disposition decisions.

The T wave

The earliest ECG findings suggestive of acute MI can often be found in the elevated T wave. The tall, symmetric "hyperacute" T wave is often believed to be diagnostic for acute MI. T-wave elevation alone, however, is not reliable for the diagnosis of infarction, because it is often only a transient early finding that is gone by the time a patient presents to the ED. Tall T waves can be mimicked by hyperkalemia or normal variants, and can be associated with intracranial bleeding.

Another sign of myocardial ischemia and infarction is the T-wave inversion pattern, which can also be misleading. T inversion can be seen as a normal variant as well as with conditions such as posttachycardia, intracranial bleeding, pericarditis, pulmonary embolism, and other myocardial diseases.[28]

The literature does not support sole reliance on the T wave in determining prognosis for patients with presumed MI. Although hyperacute T waves in a patient with a classic history strongly suggest acute MI, peaked T waves in a patient with a less suggestive history should not be given undue weight.

Combination of ECG Findings

Certainly, there is much more information available from an ECG than ST segment, Q waves, and T waves. Additional data include rhythm, rate, axis, and the QRS complex. Several studies have examined the initial emergency department ECG to determine whether a combination of findings can help to distinguish chest pain patients into those who are likely to have in-hospital complications or death and those who are not.

There are several different ways to classify patients and ECGs of patients with complaints of chest pain.[12, 61–65] One method examines several ECG criteria as well as initial clinical information and uses this information to define high- and low-risk groups.[61] Another method of ECG classification is to use the terms ''abnormal,'' ''normal,'' and ''nonspecific'' ST or T changes to describe the findings.[12] A slightly different approach classifies ECGs into two groups. In Group 1, the ECGs either are normal, have nonspecific ST or T changes, or are abnormal but *unchanged* from a prior ECG; in Group 2, the ECGs have either new pathologic Q waves, abnormal significant ST or T changes, junctional or idioventricular rhythm, and bundle branch block, left ventricular hypertrophy, or high-grade AV block.[62]

A landmark study of a combination of findings from the ECG for prognosis in acute MI was published by Brush and colleagues[8] in 1985. These investigators also divided the admission ECG into two groups, which they called positive and negative. Positive ECGs had the following criteria: (1) Q waves; (2) ST segment elevation or depression or T wave inversion consistent with infarction, ischemia, or strain; (3) left ventricular hypertrophy; (4) left bundle branch block; and (5) paced rhythm. Significant differences between the positive and negative groups were noted in several categories. Life-threatening complications were more likely (14% vs 0.6%), as were deaths due to cardiac complications (9.9% vs 0). In the positive group, acute interventions were also much more common, including cardioversion, temporary pacing, and pulmonary artery catherization. These figures are for all admitted patients with possible MI. When Brush and colleagues[8] looked at the data for those in whom MI was ultimately diagnosed, there remained a significant difference in the rate of complications (25% vs 4%).

Others applying the criteria proposed by Brush and colleagues find even more striking differences between the two groups.[4, 9, 10] The positive group of ECGs were associated with significantly more VF (5.2% vs 0), VT (3.1% vs 0), cardiogenic shock (9.4% vs 0), high-grade AV block (3.1% vs 0), and death (8.3% vs 0). Life-threatening complications were seen only in the positive group. A different variation of these groups employed the same criteria but further defined the negative group as normal or abnormal. The normal category allowed only those ECGs with PACs, occasional PVCs, or sinus bradycardia or tachycardia and no other acute changes. The abnormal group contained all the other ECGs that were not positive according to the Brush criteria, and any that were positive but unchanged from a previous ECG. Significant differences were found between the positive group and the normal group. Only interventions (53% vs 31%) and life-threatening complications (35% vs 18%) were found to be significantly different.

The predictive utility of Brush's criteria have not been validated by all investigators, however. In a community hospital, only small differences were found between the two groups for both complications and deaths. This poorer predictive ability may be attributed to the fact that only 25% of these patients developed MI and that many of the sickest patients may have been transferred elsewhere, both of which could significantly bias results.[5]

In summary, it appears that a combination of ECG findings offers the most reliable use of the ECG as a predictive instrument for the suspected MI patient. None of the studies looked at this type of patient population prospectively, nor does any suggest where a patient with a potential myocardial infarction should be admitted if not to a CCU. The criteria proposed by Brush and colleagues[8] and upheld by others probably represent the best currently available utilization of the 12-lead ECG for prognosis in the possible MI patient, as there are significant differences in both complications and deaths between the two groups distinguished by these criteria.

SUMMARY

The ECG has not been shown to be consistently helpful in the diagnosis of acute MI. The information presented here supports the concept that although an initial 12-lead ECG lacks sufficient sensitivity to be consistently useful for diagnosis, it probably has a role in the prediction of hospital course.

Brush and colleagues[8] have shown that simply classifying the ECG as positive or negative can give it a powerful predictive role, although the application of such criteria in rural and community hospital settings may need to be modified. Other studies have shown that the magnitude of the ST elevation or depression, presence of ST depression in "reciprocal" leads in inferior infarctions, and development of new Q waves are prognostic indicators, but none can be used alone to predict hospital course.

Because of various study designs and the retrospective nature of these studies, it is not possible to make general statements about the ECG to "triage" chest pain patients for admission. An important flaw in this type of research is the fact that most studies evaluated all patients admitted to a CCU, of which only up to 41% actually had MIs. When investigators try to apply their criteria to patients who have actually had MIs, the numbers of patients are often too small to reach meaningful conclusions. No study of acute MI patients admitted to "step-down" telemetry units has been done, so that the appropriateness of this approach in such patients can be only indirectly inferred. The literature supports admission of patients with a history suggestive of possible infarction but a benign ECG to a telemetry bed rather than to the CCU. It is still prudent to ensure that all patients with possible MI are admitted to some sort of monitored bed, even if that means transfer to another institution.

REFERENCES

1. American College of Emergency Physicians: *Clinical Policy for Management of Adult Patients Presenting with a Chief Complaint of Chest Pain, with No History of Trauma.* Dallas, ACEP, 1990.
2. Lee TH, Rouan GW, Weisberg MC, et al: Clinical characteristics and natural history of patients with acute myocardial infarction sent home from the emergency room. *Am J Cardiol.* 1987;60:219–224.
3. Gorman PA, Calatayud JB, Abraham S, et al: Observer variation in interpretation of the electrocardiogram. *Med Ann District of Columbia.* 1964;33:97–99.
4. Zalenski RJ, Sloan EP, Chen EH, et al: The emergency department ECG and immediately life-threatening complications in initially uncomplicated suspected myocardial ischemia. *Ann Emerg Med.* 1988;17:221–226.
5. Young MJ, McMahon LF, Stross JK: Prediction rules for patients with suspected myocardial infarction. *Arch Intern Med.* 1987;147:1219–1222.
6. Willems JL, Abreu-Lima C, Arnaud P, et al: The diagnostic performance of

computer programs for the interpretation of electrocardiograms. *N Engl J Med.* 1991;325:1767–1773.
7. Jakobsson A, Ohlin P, Pahlm O: Does a computer-based ECG-recorder interpret electrocardiograms more efficiently than physicians? *Clin Physiol.* 1985;5:417–423.
8. Brush JE, Brand DA, Acampora D, et al: Use of the initial electrocardiogram to predict in-hospital complications of acute myocardial infarction. *N Engl J Med.* 1985;312:1137–1141.
9. Stark ME, Vacek JL: The initial electrocardiogram during admission for myocardial infarction. *Arch Intern Med.* 1987;147:843–846.
10. Fesmire FM, Percy RF, Wears RL, et al: Risk stratification according to the initial electrocardiogram in patients with suspected acute myocardial infarction. *Arch Intern Med.* 1989;149:1294–1297.
11. Slater DK, Hlatky MA, Mark DB, et al: Outcome in suspected acute myocardial infarction with normal or minimally abnormal admission electrocardiographic findings. *Am J Cardiol.* 1987;60:766–770.
12. Tierney WM, Roth BJ, Psaty B, et al: Predictors of myocardial infarction in emergency room patients. *Crit Care Med.* 1985;13:526–531.
13. Lee TH, Cook EF, Weisberg M, et al: Acute chest pain in the emergency room. *Arch Intern Med.* 1985;145:65–69.
14. Gay PC, Nishimura RA, Roth CS, et al: Lipoprotein analysis in the evaluation of chest pain in the emergency department. *Mayo Clin Proc.* 1991;66:885–891.
15. McGuinness JB, Begg TB, Semple T: First electrocardiogram in recent myocardial infarction. *Br Med J.* 1976;2:449–451.
16. McQueen MJ, Holder D, El-Maraghi NRH: Assessment of the accuracy of serial electrocardiograms in the diagnosis of myocardial infarction. *Am Heart J.* 1983;105:258–261.
17. Zarling EJ, Sexton H, Milnor P: Failure to diagnose acute myocardial infarction. *JAMA.* 1983;250:1177–1181.
18. Justis DL, Hession WT: Accuracy of 22-lead ECG analysis for diagnosis of acute myocardial infarction and coronary artery disease in the emergency department: A comparison with 12-lead ECG. *Ann Emerg Med.* 1992;21:1–9.
19. Rude RE, Poole WK, Muller JE, et al: Electrocardiographic and clinical criteria for recognition of acute myocardial infarction based on analysis of 3,697 patients. *Am J Cardiol.* 1983;52:936–942.
20. Gibler WB, Lewis LM, Erb RE, et al: Early detection of acute myocardial infarction in patients with chest pain and nondiagnostic ECGs: Serial CK-MB sampling in the emergency department. *Ann Emerg Med.* 1990;19:1359–1356.
21. Hostetler M, Walling-Braastad L, Wolford R: Serial creatine phosphokinase (CK-MB) and myoglobin assays in the ED evaluation of patients with possible myocardial infarction [abstract]. *Ann Emerg Med.* 1991;20:464.
22. Hoffman JR, Igarashi E: Influence of electrocardiographic findings on admission decisions in patients with acute chest pain. *Am J Med.* 1985;79:699–707.
23. Day HW: An intensive coronary care area. *Dis Chest.* 1963;44:423–427.
24. Lown B, Klein MD, Hershberg PI: Coronary and precoronary care. *Am J Med.* 1969;46:705–724.
25. Hill JD, Holdstock G, Hampton JR: Comparison of mortality of patients

with heart attacks admitted to a coronary care unit and an ordinary medical ward. *Br Med J.* 1977;2:81–83.
26. Mather HG, Morgan DC, Pearson NG: Myocardial infarction: A comparison between home and hospital care for patients. *Br Med J.* 1976;1:925–929.
27. Schor S, Behar S, Modan B, et al: Disposition of presumed coronary patients from an emergency room. *JAMA.* 1976;236:941–943.
28. Chou TC: *Electrocardiography in Clinical Practice.* 2nd ed., Orlando, FL: Grune & Stratton, Inc; 1986:146–156.
29. Willich SN, Stone PH, Muller JE, et al: High-risk subgroups of patients with non–Q wave myocardial infarction based on direction and severity of ST segment deviation. *Am J Heart J.* 1987;114:1110–1118.
30. Nicod P, Gilpin E, Dittrich H: Short- and long-term clinical outcome after Q wave and non–Q wave myocardial infarction in a large patient population. *Circulation.* 1989;79:528–536.
31. Maisel AS, Ahnve S, Gilpin E, et al: Prognosis after extension of myocardial infarct: The role of Q wave or non-Q wave infarction. *Circulation.* 1985;71:211–217.
32. Goldberg RK, Fenster PE: Significance of the Q wave in acute myocardial infarction. *Clin Cardiol.* 1985;8:40–46.
33. Hutter AM, DeSanctis RW, Flynn T, et al: Nontransmural myocardial infarction: A comparison of hospital and late clinical course with that of matched patients with transmural anterior and transmural inferior myocardial infarction. *Am J Cardiol.* 1981;48:595–602.
34. Thanavaro S, Krone RJ, Kleiger RE, et al: In-hospital prognosis with first nontransmural and transmural infarctions. *Circulation.* 1980;61:29–33.
35. Coll S, Castaner A, Sanz G, et al: Prevalence and prognosis after a first nontransmural myocardial infarction. *Am J Cardiol.* 1983;51:1584–1588.
36. Selker HP: Sorting out chest pain. *Emergency Decisions.* 1985;June:8–17.
37. Yusuf S, Lopez R, Maddison A, et al: Value of electrocardiogram in predicting and estimating infarct size in man. *Br Heart J.* 1979;42:286–293.
38. Aldrich HR, Wagner NB, Boswick J: Use of initial ST-segment deviation for prediction of final electrocardiographic size of acute myocardial infarcts. *Am J Cardiol.* 1988;61:749–753.
39. Feiring AJ, Johnson MR, Kioschos JM, et al: The importance of the determination of the myocardial area at risk in the evaluation of the outcome of acute myocardial infarction in patients. *Circulation.* 1987;75:980–987.
40. Lee JT, Idecker RE, Reimer KA, et al: Myocardial infarct size and location in relation to the coronary vascular bed at risk in man. *Circulation.* 1981;64:526–530.
41. Clements IP, Kaufmann UP, Bailey KR, et al: Electrocardiographic prediction of myocardial area at risk. *Mayo Clin Proc.* 1991;66:985–990.
42. Nielsen BL: ST-segment elevation in acyte myocardial infarction. *Circulation.* 1973;48:338–345.
43. Cohen M, Hawkins L, Greenberg S, et al: Usefulness of ST-segment changes in two or more leads on the emergency room electrocardiogram in either unstable angina pectoris or non-Q-wave myocardial infarction in predicting outcome. *Am J Cardiol.* 1991;67:1368–1373.
44. Abbott JA, Scheinman MM: Nondiagnostic electrocardiogram in patients with acute myocardial infarction. *Am J Med.* 1973;55:608–613.

45. Tzivoni D, Chenzbraun A: The significance of ST abnormalities in myocardial infarction. *Cardiol Clin.* 1987;5:419–426.
46. Mirvis DM: Physiologic bases for anterior ST segment depression in patients with acute inferior wall myocardial infarction. *Am Heart J.* 1988;116:1308–1322.
47. Croft CH, Woodward W, Nicod P, et al: Clinical implications of anterior S-T segment depression in patients with acute inferior myocardial infarction. *Am J Cardiol.* 1982;50:428–436.
48. Hlatky MA, Califf RM, Lee KL, et al: Prognostic significance of precordial ST-segment depression during inferior acute myocardial infarction. *Am J Cardiol.* 1985;55:325–329.
49. Bates ER, Clemmensen PM, Califf RM: Precordial ST segment depression predicts a worse prognosis in inferior infarction despite reperfusion therapy. *J Am Coll Cardiol.* 1990;16:1538–1544.
50. Roubin S, Shen WF, Nicholson M, et al: Anterolateral ST segment depression in acute inferior myocardial infarction: Angiographic and clinical implications. *Am Heart J.* 1984;107:1177–1182.
51. Salcedo JR, Baird MG, Chambers RJ, et al: Significance of reciprocal S-T segment depression in anterior precordial leads in acute inferior myocardial infarction: Concomitant left anterior descending coronary artery disease? *Am J Cardiol.* 1981;48:1003–1008.
52. Gelman JS, Saltups A: Precordial ST segment depression in patients with inferior myocardial infarction: Clinical implications. *Br Heart J.* 1982;48:560–565.
53. Lembo NJ, Starling MR, Dell'Italia LJ, et al: Clinical and prognostic importance of persistent precordial (V1–V4) electrocardiographic ST segment depression in patients with inferior transmural infarction. *Circulation.* 1986;74:56–63.
54. Shah PK, Pichler M, Berman DS, et al: Noninvasive identification of a high risk subset of patients with acute inferior myocardial infarction. *Am J Cardiol.* 1980;46:915–921.
55. Gibson RS, Crampton RS, Watson DD, et al: Precordial ST-segment depression during acute inferior myocardial infarction: Clinical, scintigraphic and angiographic correlations. *Circulation.* 1982;66:732–741.
56. Herlitz J, Hjalmarson A: Occurrence of anterior ST depression in inferior myocardial infarction and relation to clinical outcome. *Clin Cardiol.* 1987;10:529–534.
57. Balla S, Shenoy MM, Nejat M, et al: ST segment depression in acute anterior myocardial infarction. *South Med J.* 1985;78:673–676.
58. Langer A, Freeman MR, Armstrong PW: ST segment shift in unstable angina: Pathophysiology and association with coronary anatomy and hospital outcome. *J Am Coll Cardiol.* 1989;13:1495–1502.
59. Short D: The earliest electrocardiographic evidence of myocardial infarction. *Br Heart J.* 1970;32:6–15.
60. Miller DH, Kligfield P, Schreiber TL, et al: Relationship of prior myocardial infarction to false-positive electrocardiographic diagnosis of acute injury in patients with chest pain. *Arch Intern Med.* 1987;147:257–261.
61. Gheorghiade M, Anderson J, Rosman H: Risk identification at the time of admission to coronary care unit in patients with suspected myocardial infarction. *Am Heart J.* 1988;116:1212–1217.

62. Bell MR, Montarello JK, Steele PM: Does the emergency room electrocardiogram identify patients with suspected myocardial infarction who are at low risk of acute complications? *Aust N Z J Med.* 1990;20:564–569.
63. Yusuf S, Pearson M, Sterry H: The entry ECG in the early diagnosis and prognostic stratification of patients with suspected acute myocardial infarction. *Eur Heart J.* 1984;5:690–696.
64. Fuchs R, Scheidt S: Improved criteria for admission to cardiac care units. *JAMA.* 1981;246:2037–2041.
65. Ricou F, Nicod P, Gilpin E, et al: Influence of right bundle branch block on short- and long-term survival after inferior wall Q-wave myocardial infarction. *Am J Cardiol.* 67;1991:1143–1146.
66. Green L, Smith M: Evaluation of two acute cardiac ischemia decision-support tools in a rural family practice. *J Fam Pract.* 1988;26:627–632.

Chapter

Pulse Oximetry

Kevin R. Ward

Perhaps in no other specialty is the rapid assessment of oxygenation as critical as it is in emergency medicine. Yet the traditional clinical findings of hypoxemia (such as cyanosis, tachypnea, altered mental status, and arrhythmias) are not uniformly reliable and may be present only when hypoxia is severe.

The standard for assessing arterial blood oxygenation, ventilation, and acid-base status has been and remains the arterial blood gas (ABG) analysis. Yet ABG has several drawbacks. It provides data at only one point in time, making it difficult to use in following trends in oxygenation or as an early warning system. Using frequent blood gas analysis to detect hypoxia and to titrate oxygen therapy is expensive, invasive, and prone to potential sampling errors. Thus, the availability of simple, accurate, noninvasive, and continuous oxygen monitoring has many advantages.

Pulse oximetry is now in widespread use. This chapter discusses the utilizations and limitations of this relatively new technology as they apply to emergency medicine.

Nevertheless, certain limitations of pulse oximetry must be kept in mind. Because oxygen delivery depends on a number of factors, $Pa{O_2}$ and $Sa{O_2}$ values alone do not indicate tissue oxygenation status.

PRINCIPLES OF OPERATION

The instantaneous in vivo measurement of the percentage of oxygenated hemoglobin (Sao_2) by pulse oximetry is based on the fact that the total absorbance of a system of absorbers is the sum of their independent absorbances. The pulse oximetry apparatus consists of two light-emitting diodes (LEDs) that emit red light (660 nm) and infrared light (940 nm). Differences in light absorption between hemoglobin and reduced hemoglobin are maximal near these wavelengths. When light of these wavelengths is passed through an arterial bed, the percentage of deoxyhemoglobin and oxyhemoglobin in that bed can be determined by measuring the ratio of transmitted red and infrared light.[1] Pulse oximetry measures the amount of oxyhemoglobin as a percentage of the total of deoxygenated and oxygenated hemoglobin.

Skin, bone, and connective tissue absorb the majority of transmitted light from the LEDs, and a smaller amount is absorbed by the static volume of arterial and venous blood between the LEDs and sensor. At the peak of the cardiac cycle, there is a small increase in the amount of arterial capillary blood in the tissue bed. The change in light absorption produced by this small increase in arterial blood with each pulse, coupled with the absorbance data from the trough of the cycle, is used to calculate arterial saturation. Variations in absorption because of skin color or skin thickness have little influence on the accuracy of the reading, because only peak absorptions are considered.[1]

The most common site of pulse oximetry sampling is the finger. Other sites that have proved valuable in low-amplitude flow states are the earlobe and the nasal septum. The earlobe has been found to be the least vasoactive site compared with the nail bed and finger pad. Nitroglycerin applied to the probe area has been reported to overcome some of the problems associated with low flow to the probe site.

ACCURACY

Pulse oximeters are generally accurate to within ±5% of in vitro oximetry when the Sao_2 is in the range of 70 to 100%.[2, 3] This degree of accuracy is acceptable for applications such as the initial assessment of hemoglobin saturation or for monitoring trends in oxygenation, but it is not acceptable for calculating right-to-left shunts or arterial-to-alveolar (A–a) oxygen gradients.

The standard against which pulse oximetry is assessed is the co-oximeter, which employs four-wavelength in vitro oximeters that can distinguish hemoglobin, oxyhemoglobin, carboxyhemoglobin, and methemoglobin. The co-oximeter measures Sao_2 directly, whereas arterial blood gas analyzers measure PaO_2 and then calculate SaO_2 using concomitant pH and temperature data. The ABG is thus less accurate than pulse oximetry in certain situations.

The accuracy of pulse oximetry at levels of saturation below 70% is problematic[4] but probably does not represent much of a disadvantage for emergency physicians, because initial readings in this range prompt physicians to obtain arterial blood gas analysis immediately.

Of more concern are relative inaccuracies of the SaO_2 as an indicator of true PaO_2 at the higher end of the oxyhemoglobin curve (Fig. 69–1). When the PaO_2 is greater than 100, the SaO_2 correlates poorly with it—large changes in PaO_2 may occur while SaO_2 remains unchanged. Likewise, small changes in SaO_2 in the 94 to 96% range can mask potentially important falls in PaO_2. Thus, an SaO_2 value in this range may or may not represent an abnormal PaO_2.

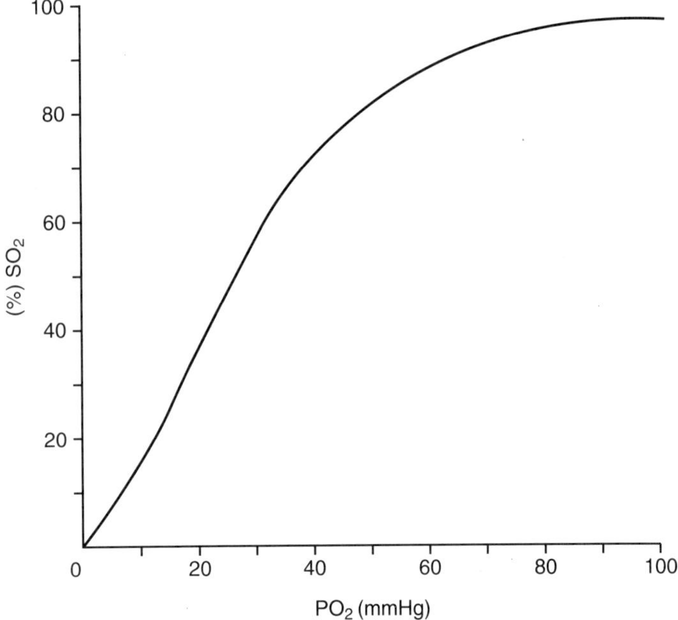

FIGURE 69–1. The oxyhemoglobin dissociation curve (HbO_2 curve). The HbO_2 curve is a graphic representation of the relationship between hemoglobin oxygen saturation and the partial pressure of oxygen in blood. This graph depicts the percentage of available hemoglobin combined with oxygen (percent saturation) and its corresponding relationship to blood PO_2.

Several other limitations of pulse oximetry are of potential concern. Because the oxyhemoglobin dissociation curve is not fixed, changes in pH, temperature, and 2,3-diphosphoglycerate levels can adversely effect tissue oxygenation while SaO_2 stays normal.

Another concern is that because most pulse oximeters display a value after averaging data from the previous 5 to 8 seconds, the time required to respond to a change in saturation can be as much as 25 seconds.[5] Ear probes have been found to respond faster to changes in SaO_2 than finger probes, probably because of shorter circulation times.

Because pulse oximetry uses plethysmography to determine SaO_2, it reports the saturation only if the machine is able to detect an adequate pulse. Unfortunately, some pulse oximeters display SaO_2 values even when an adequate pulse is not detected, such as when there is motion artifact or a low-flow state in which an adequate pulse is only intermittently present. Other devices use advanced signal processing algorithms to distinguish valid pulsatile signals from signals generated by motion or other artifact.

Some pulse oximeters provide only an SaO_2 reading and no other information, such as pulse rate or indication of signal intensity. Others provide signal intensity bars and various beeping tones to indicate the signal strength and simultaneously provide a pulse rate. Thus, if the pulse rate displayed on the pulse oximeter does not match the patient's, the SaO_2 reading is suspect. Nevertheless, it may still be difficult to be sure that SaO_2 readings in low-flow states (in which SaO_2 would be most valuable) are accurate.

The best means to ensure proper tracking and signal verification is with displayed plethysmographic waveforms. Viewing the waveform and pulse rate gives the operator the maximum ability to assess the validity of the SaO_2 and pulse rate displays. This approach may be of particular importance in patients who are critically ill or are being transported.

Another advantage of the displayed waveform is in determining systolic blood pressure. Placing the blood pressure cuff on the same extremity as the pulse oximeter probe enables the appearance and disappearance of the pulse wave to be correlated with sphygmomanometer readings to determine systolic blood pressure.[6] This technique has been found to have an excellent correlation with Doppler readings ranging from 85 to 250 mm Hg and is likely to be most useful when critically ill patients are transported.

A number of factors can affect the accuracy of pulse oximetry. They include low-amplitude states, dyshemoglobinemias, anemia, dyes, ambient light, skin pigment, electrocautery, motion artifact, and nail products.

In conditions in which *pulses are absent* (such as cardiac arrest or tourniquet or blood pressure cuff inflation proximal to the probe) and in conditions of very-low-amplitude pulse waves (such as hypotension, hypovolemia, hypothermia, vasopressor infusions, or nonpulsatile cardiopulmonary bypass), readings may be unobtainable.[7] These conditions unfortunately represent many situations in which rapid noninvasive indicators of oxygenation would be extremely useful. Nevertheless, it has been shown that flow as low as 4 to 8.6% of baseline can trigger a pulse signal.[8]

Because pulse oximetry employs only two wavelengths to estimate Sao_2, the presence of *abnormal hemoglobin species*, such as methemoglobin and carboxyhemoglobin, leads to inaccurate estimates of true Sao_2.[9, 10] Carboxyhemoglobin is misinterpreted as oxygenated hemoglobin, and increasing concentrations of methemoglobin cause saturation readings to move toward a value of 84%.[9] In vitro co-oximeters, which use more than two wavelengths, can quantify other hemoglobin species directly.

Anemia does not appear to significantly affect the accuracy of pulse oximetry until the hematocrit is below 10%.[11, 12] Some *intravenous dyes* can affect the accuracy of pulse oximetry.[13] For example, methylene blue causes spuriously low readings.

There are sporadic reports that different *ambient lighting* sources (ranging from common fluorescent lights to xenon arc surgical lamps) may cause misleadingly high readings. Using Sao_2 probes that are well secured and covering them to exclude extrinsic light should eliminate these problems.

For the most part, *skin pigment* does not affect Sao_2 readings. Pulse oximetry readings cannot be obtained in some patients because of their dark skin pigmentation. In these cases, lightly pigmented areas such as the nail bed should be tried.

Although not as common a problem for emergency physicians as for surgeons and anesthesiologists, *electrocautery* can produce artifactually low Sao_2 readings.

As noted earlier, the accuracy of pulse oximetry readings can be affected by *motion*.

Nail products (both fingernail polish and synthetic nails) have been noted to interfere with pulse oximetry readings. With nail polishes (mainly, certain shades of blue), the effect depends on the absorption characteristics of the specific color as well as the number of coats applied.[14]

PULSE OXIMETRY IN THE EMERGENCY DEPARTMENT AND PREHOSPITAL SETTING

Despite the inability of pulse oximetry to provide all the information needed to assess tissue oxygenation, it has clearly been shown to be of great value in the early identification and semiquantitative assessment of hypoxia.[15–20] In addition to helping guide oxygen therapy, its real-time capabilities make pulse oximetry valuable in monitoring improvement or deterioration in the patient's clinical condition.[21, 22]

Caution should be exercised in the use of pulse oximetry to exclude pulmonary causes of chest pain, such as pulmonary embolus. Although not studied to date, the absence of an A–a oxygen gradient can probably not be ascertained with a great deal of confidence unless the Sao_2 is above 97% and one is reasonably sure that there is no occult hypocapnia. (With combinations of pulse oximetry and capnography, this determination may be possible in the future.) Readings less than 97% would mandate an arterial blood gas analysis, because the Pao_2 can vary over a wide range when the Sao_2 is between 94 and 96%. Of course, in patients who are dyspneic or those in whom there is a strong suspicion of pulmonary embolism, the A–a gradient should be calculated, and for this, an ABG is required.

Pulse oximetry may be useful in detecting occult hypoxemia at the bedside and in the field, because clinical indicators of hypoxia are so insensitive. Obtaining a reading before and after oxygen therapy probably provides the most information. Of course, in patients with obvious dyspnea, chest pain, or other critical conditions, high-flow oxygen should be applied without delay.

An arterial blood gas analysis should be obtained after initial pulse oximetry when (1) hypocarbia or hypercarbia is a real concern, (2) knowledge of blood pH is critical, (3) accuracy of the Sao_2 in predicting the true Pao_2 is in doubt and is clinically important, (4) dyshemoglobinemia is suspected, and (5) Pao_2 is outside the sensitive range of pulse oximetry.

COST

Several cost-benefit studies have been published regarding pulse oximetry. One study from the anesthesia literature found that pulse oximetry is cost-effective if only one in 40,000 intraoperative hypoxic episodes ($Sao_2 < 90\%$) is associated with mortality.[23] On a case-by-case basis, the actual cost of pulse oximetry has been estimated to be from $1.35 to $2.40 per case (probes average about $10 apiece).[24] Another study found that pulse oximetry eliminated the need for diagnostic arterial blood gas analyses in 16% of cases, and in 48% of cases for which ABGs were ordered to assess oxygen therapy.[18] The only study examining cost in the emergency department found that after the introduction of pulse oximetry, the number of arterial blood gas analyses performed actually increased; this may have been because of the more frequent uncovering of occult hypoxia.[19]

REFERENCES

1. Alexander CM, Teller LE, Gross JB: Principles of pulse oximetry: Theoretical and practical considerations. *Anesth Analg.* 1989;68:368–376.
2. Nickerson BG, Sarkisian C, Tremper K: Bias and precision of pulse oximeters and arterial oximeters. *Chest.* 1988;93:515–517.
3. The Technology Assessment Task Force SCCM: A model of technology assessment applied to pulse oximetry. *Crit Care Med.* 1993;21:615–624.
4. Severinghaus JW, Naifeh KH, Khoh SO: Errors in 14 pulse oximeters during profound hypoxia. *J Clin Monit.* 1989;5:72–81.
5. Young D, Jewkes C, Spittal M, et al: Response times of pulse oximeters assessed using acute decompression. *Anesth Analg.* 1992;72:189–195.
6. Talke PO: Measurement of systolic blood pressure using pulse oximetry during helicopter flight. *Crit Care Med.* 1991;19:934–937.
7. Severinghaus JW, Spellman MJ: Pulse oximeter failure thresholds in hypotension and vasoconstriction. *Anesthesiology.* 1990;73:532–537.
8. Lawson D, Norley I, Korbon G, et al: Blood flow limits and pulse oximeter signal detection. *Anesthesiology.* 1987;67:599–603.
9. Tremper KK, Barker SJ: Using pulse oximetry when dyshemoglobin levels are high. *J Crit Illness.* 1988;3:103–107.
10. Barker SJJ, Tremper FF: The effect of carbon monoxide inhalation on pulse oximeter signal detection. *Anesthesiology.* 1987;66:677–679.
11. Lee S, Tremper KK, Barker SJ: Effects of anemia on pulse oximetry and continuous mixed venous hemoglobin saturation monitoring in dogs. *Anesthesiology.* 1991;75:118–122.
12. Severinghaus JW, Koh SO: Effect of anemia on pulse oximeter accuracy at low saturation. *J Clin Monit.* 1990;6:85–88.
13. Scheller MS, Unger RJ, Kelner MJ: Effects of intravenously administered dyes on pulse oximetry readings. *Anesthesiology.* 1986;65:550–552.
14. Cotte CJ, Goldstein EA, Fuchsman WHH, Hoagglin DJ: The effect of nail polish on pulse oximetry. *Anesth Analg.* 1988;67:683–686.
15. Mellon J, Healer M, Chaplain R, et al: Occult hypoxemia during aeromedical transport: Detection by pulse oximetry. *Prehospital and Disaster Medicine.* 1989;4:115–121.
16. Aughey K, Hess D, Eitel D, et al: An evaluation of pulse oximetry in prehospital care. *Ann Emerg Med.* 1991;20:887–891.
17. Dunmire SM, Paris PM, Menegazzi JJ, Tisherman SA: Value of pulse oximetry in prehospital care [abstract]. *Ann Emerg Med.* 1991;20:492.
18. Kellerman AL, Cofer CA, Joseph S, Hackman BB: Impact of portable pulse oximetry on arterial blood gas test ordering in an urban emergency department. *Ann Emerg Med.* 1991;20:130–134.
19. Singer A, Jouriles NJ, Rutherford WF, Panacek EA: Impact of bedside pulse oximetry on the utilization of arterial blood gas measurements in the ED [abstract]. *Ann Emerg Med.* 1991;20:493.

20. Cydulka RK, Shade B, Emmerman CL, et al: Prehospital pulse oximetry: Useful or misused? *Ann Emerg Med.* 1992;21:675–679.
21. McKay WPS, Noable WH: Critical incidents detected by pulse oximetry during anesthesia. *Can J Anaesth.* 1988;35:265–269.
22. Mateer JR, Olson DW, Steven HA, Aufderheide TP: Continuous pulse oximetry during emergency endotracheal intubation. *Ann Emerg Med.* 1993;222:675–679.
23. Raemer DB, Warren DL, Moarris R, et al: Hypoxemia during ambulatory gynecologic surgery as evaluated by the pulse oximeter. *J Clin Monit.* 1987;3:244–248.
24. Emergency Care Research Institute: Pulse oximeter evaluation. *Health Devices.* 1989;18:185–230.

INDEX

Note: Page numbers in *italics* refer to illustrations; page numbers followed by t refer to tables.

A

B

C

E

F

N

O

P

Q

R

S

T